Antimicrobial Therapy in Intensive Care Unit

Antimicrobial Therapy in Intensive Care Unit

Editors

Elizabeth Paramythiotou
Christina Routsi
Antoine Andremont

MDPI • Basel • Beijing • Wuhan • Barcelona • Belgrade • Manchester • Tokyo • Cluj • Tianjin

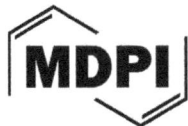

Editors

Elizabeth Paramythiotou
2nd Department of Critical Care
National and Kapodestrian University of Athens
Athens
Greece

Christina Routsi
1st Department of Critical Care
National and Kapodestrian University of Athens
Athens
Greece

Antoine Andremont
Microbiology Department
INSERM U 263
Paris
France

Editorial Office
MDPI
St. Alban-Anlage 66
4052 Basel, Switzerland

This is a reprint of articles from the Special Issue published online in the open access journal *Antibiotics* (ISSN 2079-6382) (available at: www.mdpi.com/journal/antibiotics/special_issues/Antimicrobial_ICU).

For citation purposes, cite each article independently as indicated on the article page online and as indicated below:

LastName, A.A.; LastName, B.B.; LastName, C.C. Article Title. *Journal Name* **Year**, *Volume Number*, Page Range.

ISBN 978-3-0365-6769-3 (Hbk)
ISBN 978-3-0365-6768-6 (PDF)

© 2023 by the authors. Articles in this book are Open Access and distributed under the Creative Commons Attribution (CC BY) license, which allows users to download, copy and build upon published articles, as long as the author and publisher are properly credited, which ensures maximum dissemination and a wider impact of our publications.

The book as a whole is distributed by MDPI under the terms and conditions of the Creative Commons license CC BY-NC-ND.

Contents

About the Editors vii

Preface to "Antimicrobial Therapy in Intensive Care Unit" ix

Elizabeth Paramythiotou and Christina Routsi
Editorial for Special Issue "Antimicrobial Therapy in Intensive Care Unit"
Reprinted from: *Antibiotics* **2023**, *12*, 278, doi:10.3390/antibiotics12020278 1

Konstantinos Mantzarlis, Konstantina Deskata, Dimitra Papaspyrou, Vassiliki Leontopoulou, Vassiliki Tsolaki and Epaminondas Zakynthinos et al.
Incidence and Risk Factors for Blood Stream Infection in Mechanically Ventilated COVID-19 Patients
Reprinted from: *Antibiotics* **2022**, *11*, 1053, doi:10.3390/antibiotics11081053 5

Helen Giamarellou and Ilias Karaiskos
Current and Potential Therapeutic Options for Infections Caused by Difficult-to-Treat and Pandrug Resistant Gram-Negative Bacteria in Critically Ill Patients
Reprinted from: *Antibiotics* **2022**, *11*, 1009, doi:10.3390/antibiotics11081009 15

Nesrine A. Rizk, Nada Zahreddine, Nisrine Haddad, Rihab Ahmadieh, Audra Hannun and Souad Bou Harb et al.
The Impact of Antimicrobial Stewardship and Infection Control Interventions on *Acinetobacter baumannii* Resistance Rates in the ICU of a Tertiary Care Center in Lebanon
Reprinted from: *Antibiotics* **2022**, *11*, 911, doi:10.3390/antibiotics11070911 39

Chee Lan Lau, Petrick Periyasamy, Muhd Nordin Saud, Sarah Anne Robert, Lay Yen Gan and Suet Yin Chin et al.
Plethora of Antibiotics Usage and Evaluation of Carbapenem Prescribing Pattern in Intensive Care Units: A Single-Center Experience of Malaysian Academic Hospital
Reprinted from: *Antibiotics* **2022**, *11*, 1172, doi:10.3390/antibiotics11091172 55

Sofie A. M. Dhaese, Eric A. Hoste and Jan J. De Waele
Why We May Need Higher Doses of Beta-Lactam Antibiotics: Introducing the 'Maximum Tolerable Dose'
Reprinted from: *Antibiotics* **2022**, *11*, 889, doi:10.3390/antibiotics11070889 75

Dalia Adukauskiene, Ausra Ciginskiene, Agne Adukauskaite, Despoina Koulenti and Jordi Rello
Clinical Features and Outcomes of Monobacterial and Polybacterial Episodes of Ventilator-Associated Pneumonia Due to Multidrug-Resistant *Acinetobacter baumannii*
Reprinted from: *Antibiotics* **2022**, *11*, 892, doi:10.3390/antibiotics11070892 85

Christina Routsi, Joseph Meletiadis, Efstratia Charitidou, Aikaterini Gkoufa, Stelios Kokkoris and Stavros Karageorgiou et al.
Epidemiology of Candidemia and Fluconazole Resistance in an ICU before and during the COVID-19 Pandemic Era
Reprinted from: *Antibiotics* **2022**, *11*, 771, doi:10.3390/antibiotics11060771 99

Marios Karvouniaris, Garyphallia Poulakou, Konstantinos Tsiakos, Maria Chatzimichail, Panagiotis Papamichalis and Anna Katsiaflaka et al.
ICU-Associated Gram-Negative Bloodstream Infection: Risk Factors Affecting the Outcome Following the Emergence of Colistin-Resistant Isolates in a Regional Greek Hospital
Reprinted from: *Antibiotics* **2022**, *11*, 405, doi:10.3390/antibiotics11030405 111

Evdoxia Kyriazopoulou and Evangelos J. Giamarellos-Bourboulis
Antimicrobial Stewardship Using Biomarkers: Accumulating Evidence for the Critically Ill
Reprinted from: *Antibiotics* **2022**, *11*, 367, doi:10.3390/antibiotics11030367 . . . . **127**

Khalil Chaïbi, Gauthier Péan de Ponfilly, Laurent Dortet, Jean-Ralph Zahar and Benoît Pilmis
Empiric Treatment in HAP/VAP: "Don't You Want to Take a Leap of Faith?"
Reprinted from: *Antibiotics* **2022**, *11*, 359, doi:10.3390/antibiotics11030359 . . . . **143**

Alexis Tabah, Jeffrey Lipman, François Barbier, Niccolò Buetti, Jean-François Timsit and on behalf of the ESCMID Study Group for Infections in Critically Ill Patients—ESGCIP
Use of Antimicrobials for Bloodstream Infections in the Intensive Care Unit, a Clinically Oriented Review
Reprinted from: *Antibiotics* **2022**, *11*, 362, doi:10.3390/antibiotics11030362 . . . . **161**

Francisco Gomez, Jesyree Veita and Krzysztof Laudanski
Antibiotics and ECMO in the Adult Population—Persistent Challenges and Practical Guides
Reprinted from: *Antibiotics* **2022**, *11*, 338, doi:10.3390/antibiotics11030338 . . . . **181**

Alex R. Schuurman, Robert F. J. Kullberg and Willem Joost Wiersinga
Probiotics in the Intensive Care Unit
Reprinted from: *Antibiotics* **2022**, *11*, 217, doi:10.3390/antibiotics11020217 . . . . **199**

Soo-Min Jang, Alex R. Shaw and Bruce A. Mueller
Size Matters: The Influence of Patient Size on Antibiotics Exposure Profiles in Critically Ill Patients on Continuous Renal Replacement Therapy
Reprinted from: *Antibiotics* **2021**, *10*, 1390, doi:10.3390/antibiotics10111390 . . . . **213**

Stamatis Karakonstantis, Petros Ioannou, George Samonis and Diamantis P. Kofteridis
Systematic Review of Antimicrobial Combination Options for Pandrug-Resistant *Acinetobacter baumannii*
Reprinted from: *Antibiotics* **2021**, *10*, 1344, doi:10.3390/antibiotics10111344 . . . . **225**

About the Editors

Elizabeth Paramythiotou

Dr. Paramythiotou Elisabeth is an NHS director in Second Department of Critical Care, Attikon University Hospital. She is an internist, intensive care, and infectious diseases specialist. Her research interests are in the areas of critical care, and ICU-acquired infections from multiresistant bacteria as well as fungal infections. Dr. Paramythiotou is the author or co-author of numerous publications in well-known journals that have over 900 citations, and she has served as a reviewer in more than 15 International Medical Journals.

Christina Routsi

Christina Routsi is a Professor in Pulmonology and Intensive Care Medicine, National and Kapodistrian University of Athens, Athens, Greece. Her research interests are in Critical Care and Respiratory Medicine, particularly tissue oxygenation, ventilator weaning, and ICU-acquired infections. She is the author or co-author of over 130 peer-review journal papers that have over 5600 citations. Additionally, she has served as a reviewer in more than 20 international Medical Journals.

Antoine Andremont

Professor Antoine Andremont is an emeritus professor of microbiology in Paris, France. During his career, he has published more than 300 articles and his main interests included nosocomial infections and their prevention.

Preface to "Antimicrobial Therapy in Intensive Care Unit"

Dear Reader,

In this reprint, there will be interesting articles about multiresistant bacteria and fungi, and their treatment in the Intensive Care Unit.

Several topics concerning pharmacokinetics, antibiotic stewardship, and probiotics are also included. The reprint is addressed mainly to physicians treating critically ill patients but also to other specialists, such as infectious diseases specialists.

The authors involved are well-known globally due to their important scientific work and their contribution to important scientific fields.

We are very thankful for their valuable contribution.

Elizabeth Paramythiotou, Christina Routsi, and Antoine Andremont
Editors

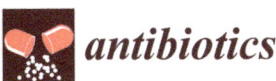

Editorial

Editorial for Special Issue "Antimicrobial Therapy in Intensive Care Unit"

Elizabeth Paramythiotou [1,*] and Christina Routsi [2,*]

1. 2nd Department of Intensive Care, School of Medicine, National and Kapodistrian University of Athens, 'Attikon' Hospital, 12462 Athens, Greece
2. 1st Department of Intensive Care, School of Medicine, National and Kapodistrian University of Athens, ICU "Evangelismos" Hospital, 10676 Athens, Greece
* Correspondence: icuattiko2@med.uoa.gr (E.P.); chroutsi@med.uoa.gr (C.R.)

Life-threatening infections, either as the initial reason for an admission to the intensive care unit (ICU) or acquired in the ICU, are especially common among critically ill patients. As a result, patients hospitalized in the ICU have a great exposure to multiple antimicrobial and antifungal agents. Antimicrobial therapy in the ICU has been challenging due to the emergence and the increasing incidence of difficult-to-treat and multidrug-resistant pathogens. Furthermore, during the ongoing pandemic, the number of patients who are hospitalized in the ICU due to COVID-19 has greatly increased with the concomitant increase in antimicrobial exposure. In addition, organ support techniques, including renal replacement therapy and extracorporeal membrane oxygenation (ECMO), further complicate the appropriate antimicrobial treatment in terms of dosing and the way the drug is administered.

The current special edition of *Antibiotics* entitled "Antimicrobial Therapy in Intensive Care Unit" brings together 15 important articles which are presenting the current evidence on the antimicrobial treatment in the ICU and the associated issues. It includes seven original articles and eight comprehensive reviews dealing with a great diversity of subjects and the factors affecting the outcome of the frail and the often subdued to long treatments in the ICU.

This Special Issue begins with an excellent review article by Tabah et al. [1] on the antimicrobial management of bloodstream infections focusing on the importance of microbiology specimens, the timing and choice of the empirical antimicrobial therapy, the role of spectrum and dose optimization, the importance of source control, and, finally, strategies for stopping antimicrobials.

Next, Karaiskos and Giamarellou [2] place emphasis on the difficult-to-treat and pandrug-resistant Gram-negative bacteria in critically ill patients by reviewing salvage antibiotics treatments, synergistic combinations, as well as an increased exposure regimen adapted to the MIC of the pathogen. Furthermore, this review article contains a report on novel antimicrobial agents, namely the lactam-beta-lactamase inhibitor combinations cefiderocol and eravacycline.

In their systematic review, Karakonstantis and colleagues [3] summarize well the currently available approaches to the management of pandrug-resistant *Acinetobacter baumannii*. The authors propose antimicrobial combinations which have been guided by an in vitro synergy evaluation as the most appropriate treatment option.

Excess antibiotic use is one of the factors contributing to the emergence of bacterial resistance. Therefore, the de-escalation of empirical regimens is a principal component of antimicrobial stewardship programs. Cumulative evidence supporting the use of procalcitonin guidance in promoting antimicrobial stewardship for critically ill patients by the restriction of an injudicious antimicrobial treatment has been presented by Kyriazopoulou

Citation: Paramythiotou, E.; Routsi, C. Editorial for Special Issue "Antimicrobial Therapy in Intensive Care Unit". *Antibiotics* 2023, 12, 278. https://doi.org/10.3390/antibiotics12020278

Received: 17 January 2023
Accepted: 27 January 2023
Published: 31 January 2023

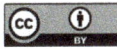

Copyright: © 2023 by the authors. Licensee MDPI, Basel, Switzerland. This article is an open access article distributed under the terms and conditions of the Creative Commons Attribution (CC BY) license (https://creativecommons.org/licenses/by/4.0/).

and Giamarellos-Bourboulis in their review article [4]. The authors conclude that according to the current evidence biomarkers, mainly procalcitonin should be implemented in antimicrobial stewardship programs, including also the COVID-19 pandemic.

In their nice study, Rizk et al. [5] describe the impact of combining antimicrobial stewardship and infection control measures on resistance rates and colonization pressure of carbapenem-resistant *Acinetobacter baummanni* (CRAb) in the ICUs of a tertiary care center in Lebanon before the COVID-19 pandemic. They demonstrate that a multidisciplinary approach and combined interventions between the stewardship and infection control teams can lead to a sustained reduction in resistance rates and the spread of CRAb in ICUs.

The article by Routsi et al. [6] confirms that the incidence of candidemia in the ICU has increased in COVID-19 patients compared to the pre-pandemic era and it highlights the marked increase in the resistance to fluconazole as well as the emergence of *C. auris*.

Lau et al. [7] provides important information regarding the utilization of antibiotics in the South East Asia region. In a retrospective study over the past six years, the authors recorded antibiotics and specifically the consumption of carbapenem in the general and in the COVID-19 ICUs of a Malaysian hospital. They found that the consumption of antibiotics increased markedly in the year 2021 compared to previous years. The excessive consumption of antibiotics was partially attributed to an unwarranted empirical use over a prolonged period and to the infrequent application of antimicrobial de-escalation.

There are two separate papers that examined ICU-acquired blood stream infections. In the first one is by Mantzarlis et al. [8]. The investigators examined secondary infections in patients admitted to the ICU due to COVID-19 over a period of 9 months. They demonstrated a high incidence of 57% of blood stream infections. Multidrug-resistant *Acinetobacter baumannii* and *Klebsiella pneumoniae* were the most common isolated pathogens. However, in the multivariate analysis, the illness severity on ICU admission was the only independent risk factor for mortality. The second paper by Karvouniaris et al. [9] examined retrospectively the impact of ICU-acquired Gram-negative blood stream infections on mortality in a regional Greek hospital. Patients with blood stream infections due to colistin-resistant strains were compared to those with colistin-sensitive strains. The authors demonstrate that the sepsis severity was the independent predictor of mortality regardless of the colistin-resistance phenotype or empirical colistin treatment.

Two studies published in this issue of *Antibiotics* address ventilator-associated pneumonia (VAP). Given the global increase in antibiotic resistance, particularly among Gram-negative bacilli and the difficulty in choosing empiric therapy, Chaibi et al. [10], in their review article, present the difficulties in the management of VAP. The empiric use of newly available antibiotics is discussed along with the presentation of the current epidemiological data in terms of multidrug-resistant pathogens, as well as the clinical and microbiological elements that should be considered when an empirical therapy is started. In the same context, Adukauskiene et al. [11], in their research article, have investigated the clinical features and the 30-day mortality of VAP due to multidrug-resistant *A. baumannii* (MDRAB) in a reference Lithuanian university hospital. Both monobacterial and polybacterial MDRAB VAP episodes during a two-year period were retrospectively studied. It was demonstrated that monobacterial MDRAB VAP had different demographic/clinical characteristics compared to polybacterial and carried worse outcomes.

One of the main problems in treating infections in critically ill patients is the difficulty to achieve the pharmacodynamic targets. This Special Issue offers three articles addressing this topic. Extracorporeal membrane oxygenation (ECMO), a temporary mechanical cardiorespiratory support, is a relatively new development increasingly used in modern ICU as a bridge to recovery in otherwise irrecoverable patients. Both critical illness and ECMO alter the pharmacokinetics (PK) and pharmacodynamics (PD) of administered drugs and challenge appropriate antibiotic regiments. The review by Gomez et al. [12] thoroughly summarizes PK/PD alterations in critically ill patients receiving ECMO, emphasizing the practical application and reviewing patient-, illness-, and ECMO hardware-related factors. Jang and colleagues [13] have provided an interesting analysis to determine whether a patient's weight influences the probability of target attainment (PTA) over 72 h of initial therapy with beta-lactam and carbapenem antibiotics in critical care patients under continuous renal replacement therapy. By using Monte Carlo simulations, it was shown that patients in lower weight quartiles tended to achieve higher antibiotic pharmacodynamic target attainment compared to heavier patients. In addition, in the context of the increasing incidence of multidrug resistance, Dhaese et al. [14] in a great perspective article suggest the new concept of the maximum tolerable dose (MTD. MTD has been defined as the highest dose of an antimicrobial drug deemed safe for the patient. Maximizing the death of bacterial cells and minimizing the risk of antimicrobial resistance and toxicity is the goal in the introduction of this concept. The authors provide a theoretical approach of how increasing uremic toxin concentrations could be used as a quantifiable marker of beta-lactam antibiotic toxicity, thus suggesting directions for future research.

Finally, Schuurman et al. [15], in a thorough review, describe the gut microbiome in health and disease. The authors discuss the concept of a probiotic intervention to positively modulate the gut microbiome. They summarize the evidence from randomized clinical trials and focus on the prevention of ventilator-associated pneumonia.

We wish to thank all the authors for their comprehensive contributions to this Special Issue of *Antibiotics* and hope that the readers will find interest in the content.

Acknowledgments: We would like to express our sincere gratitude to the Editorial Office of the Microorganisms for their assistance in managing and organizing this Special Issue and also to all contributing authors and reviewers for their excellent work.

Conflicts of Interest: The authors declare no conflict of interest.

References

1. Tabah, A.; Lipman, J.; Barbier, F.; Buetti, N.; Timsit, J.-F.; on behalf of the ESCMID Study Group for Infections in Critically Ill Patients. Use of Antimicrobials for Bloodstream Infections in the Intensive Care Unit, a Clinically Oriented Review. *Antibiotics* **2022**, *11*, 362. [CrossRef] [PubMed]
2. Giamarellou, H.; Karaiskos, I. Current and Potential Therapeutic Options for Infections Caused by Difficult-to-Treat and Pandrug Resistant Gram-Negative Bacteria in Critically Ill Patients. *Antibiotics* **2022**, *11*, 1009. [CrossRef] [PubMed]
3. Karakonstantis, S.; Ioannou, P.; Samonis, G.; Kofteridis, D.P. Systematic Review of Antimicrobial Combination Options for Pandrug-Resistant Acinetobacter baumannii. *Antibiotics* **2021**, *10*, 1344. [CrossRef] [PubMed]
4. Kyriazopoulou, E.; Giamarellos-Bourboulis, E.J. Antimicrobial Stewardship Using Biomarkers: Accumulating Evidence for the Critically Ill. *Antibiotics* **2022**, *11*, 367. [CrossRef] [PubMed]
5. Rizk, N.A.; Zahreddine, N.; Haddad, N.; Ahmadieh, R.; Hannun, A.; Bou Harb, S.; Haddad, S.F.; Zeenny, R.M.; Kanj, S.S. The Impact of Antimicrobial Stewardship and Infection Control Interventions on Acinetobacter baumannii Resistance Rates in the ICU of a Tertiary Care Center in Lebanon. *Antibiotics* **2022**, *11*, 911. [CrossRef] [PubMed]
6. Routsi, C.; Meletiadis, J.; Charitidou, E.; Gkoufa, A.; Kokkoris, S.; Karageorgiou, S.; Giannopoulos, C.; Koulenti, D.; Andrikogiannopoulos, P.; Perivolioti, E.; et al. Epidemiology of Candidemia and Fluconazole Resistance in an ICU before and during the COVID-19 Pandemic Era. *Antibiotics* **2022**, *11*, 771. [CrossRef] [PubMed]
7. Lau, C.L.; Periyasamy, P.; Saud, M.N.; Robert, S.A.; Gan, L.Y.; Chin, S.Y.; Pau, K.B.; Kong, S.H.; Tajurudin, F.W.; Yin, M.K.; et al. Plethora of Antibiotics Usage and Evaluation of Carbapenem Prescribing Pattern in Intensive Care Units: A Single-Center Experience of Malaysian Academic Hospital. *Antibiotics* **2022**, *11*, 1172. [CrossRef] [PubMed]
8. Mantzarlis, K.; Deskata, K.; Papaspyrou, D.; Leontopoulou, V.; Tsolaki, V.; Zakynthinos, E.; Makris, D. Incidence and Risk Factors for Blood Stream Infection in Mechanically Ventilated COVID-19 Patients. *Antibiotics* **2022**, *11*, 1053. [CrossRef] [PubMed]
9. Karvouniaris, M.; Poulakou, G.; Tsiakos, K.; Chatzimichail, M.; Papamichalis, P.; Katsiaflaka, A.; Oikonomou, K.; Katsioulis, A.; Palli, E.; Komnos, A. ICU-Associated Gram-Negative Bloodstream Infection: Risk Factors Affecting the Outcome Following the Emergence of Colistin-Resistant Isolates in a Regional Greek Hospital. *Antibiotics* **2022**, *11*, 405. [CrossRef] [PubMed]
10. Chaïbi, K.; Péan de Ponfilly, G.; Dortet, L.; Zahar, J.-R.; Pilmis, B. Empiric Treatment in HAP/VAP: "Don't You Want to Take a Leap of Faith?". *Antibiotics* **2022**, *11*, 359. [CrossRef] [PubMed]
11. Adukauskiene, D.; Ciginskiene, A.; Adukauskaite, A.; Koulenti, D.; Rello, J. Clinical Features and Outcomes of Monobacterial and Polybacterial Episodes of Ventilator-Associated Pneumonia Due to Multidrug-Resistant Acinetobacter baumannii. *Antibiotics* **2022**, *11*, 892. [CrossRef] [PubMed]
12. Gomez, F.; Veita, J.; Laudanski, K. Antibiotics and ECMO in the Adult Population—Persistent Challenges and Practical Guides. *Antibiotics* **2022**, *11*, 338. [CrossRef] [PubMed]
13. Jang, S.-M.; Shaw, A.R.; Mueller, B.A. Size Matters: The Influence of Patient Size on Antibiotics Exposure Profiles in Critically Ill Patients on Continuous Renal Replacement Therapy. *Antibiotics* **2021**, *10*, 1390. [CrossRef] [PubMed]

14. Dhaese, S.A.M.; Hoste, E.A.; De Waele, J.J. Why We May Need Higher Doses of Beta-Lactam Antibiotics: Introducing the 'Maximum Tolerable Dose'. *Antibiotics* **2022**, *11*, 889. [CrossRef] [PubMed]
15. Schuurman, A.R.; Kullberg, R.F.J.; Wiersinga, W.J. Probiotics in the Intensive Care Unit. *Antibiotics* **2022**, *11*, 217. [CrossRef] [PubMed]

Disclaimer/Publisher's Note: The statements, opinions and data contained in all publications are solely those of the individual author(s) and contributor(s) and not of MDPI and/or the editor(s). MDPI and/or the editor(s) disclaim responsibility for any injury to people or property resulting from any ideas, methods, instructions or products referred to in the content.

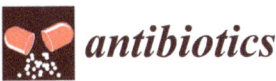

Article

Incidence and Risk Factors for Blood Stream Infection in Mechanically Ventilated COVID-19 Patients

Konstantinos Mantzarlis *, Konstantina Deskata, Dimitra Papaspyrou, Vassiliki Leontopoulou, Vassiliki Tsolaki, Epaminondas Zakynthinos and Demosthenes Makris

Department of Critical Care, University Hospital of Larissa, School of Medicine, University of Thessaly, 41110 Thessaly, Greece; kostadv@gmail.com (K.D.); dimitra.papaspyrou@hotmail.com (D.P.); vasoula_leontop@yahoo.com (V.L.); vasotsolaki@yahoo.com (V.T.); ezakynth@yahoo.com (E.Z.); appollon7@hotmail.com (D.M.)
* Correspondence: mantzk@outlook.com

Abstract: It is widely known that blood stream infections (BSIs) in critically ill patients may affect mortality, length of stay, or the duration of mechanical ventilation. There is scarce data regarding blood stream infections in mechanically ventilated COVID-19 patients. Preliminary studies report that the number of secondary infections in COVID-9 patients may be higher. This retrospective analysis was conducted to determine the incidence of BSI. Furthermore, risk factors, mortality, and other outcomes were analyzed. The setting was an Intensive Care Unit (ICU) at a University Hospital. Patients suffering from SARS-CoV-2 infection and requiring mechanical ventilation (MV) for >48 h were eligible. The characteristics of patients who presented BSI were compared with those of patients who did not present BSI. Eighty-four patients were included. The incidence of BSI was 57%. In most cases, multidrug-resistant pathogens were isolated. Dyslipidemia was more frequent in the BSI group ($p < 0.05$). Moreover, BSI-group patients had a longer ICU stay and a longer duration of both mechanical ventilation and sedation ($p < 0.05$). Deaths were not statistically different between the two groups (73% for BSI and 56% for the non-BSI group, $p > 0.05$). Compared with non-survivors, survivors had lower baseline APACHE II and SOFA scores, lower D-dimers levels, a higher baseline compliance of the respiratory system, and less frequent heart failure. They received anakinra less frequently and appropriate therapy more often ($p < 0.05$). The independent risk factor for mortality was the APACHE II score [1.232 (1.017 to 1.493), $p = 0.033$].

Keywords: SARS-CoV-2 infection; mechanical ventilation; risk factors; blood stream infection; mortality

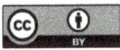

1. Introduction

Severe acute respiratory syndrome coronavirus 2 (SARS-CoV-2) was first identified in Wuhan, China, in December 2019 [1]. Intensive care unit (ICU) admission is required for 20% of patients with coronavirus disease 2019 (COVID-19) due to acute respiratory distress syndrome (ARDS) or other complications [2–4].

The incidence of blood stream infections (BSIs) among non-COVID-19 patients with infection is high [5]. The immune dysregulation induced by severe SARS-CoV-2 infection and the immunosuppressive agents used for treatment can predispose patients to concurrent infections. Studies detected a reduction in both CD4+ T and CD8+ T lymphocyte counts, an increase in neutrophils, a reduction in interferon gamma (IFN-γ) serum concentrations, and a cytokine pattern characterized by excess pro-inflammatory molecules [6–8]. Moreover, the need for vasopressors, renal replacement therapy (RRT), or sometimes extracorporeal membrane oxygenation (ECMO) may increase the risk of developing infectious complications.

There are reports that the incidence of BSIs is higher for COVID-19 patients in comparison with non-COVID-19 patients [9] during the ICU stay. However, there is scarce data regarding secondary infections in patients with severe COVID-19 [10–12], especially for those admitted to the ICU who receive invasive mechanical ventilation. There is also limited evidence on how secondary infections and especially BSIs affect patients' outcomes, such as mortality, duration of mechanical ventilation, or length of stay.

We therefore aimed to assess the incidence rate, identify risk factors for the first episode of BSI, and determine survival and other outcomes in COVID-19, mechanically ventilated patients.

2. Materials and Methods

This is a retrospective analysis of prospectively collected data. The study was conducted from 1 April to 31 December 2020 in an ICU dedicated to patients suffering from SARS-CoV-2 infection and requiring invasive mechanical ventilation in the University Hospital of Larissa, Thessaly, Greece. Inclusion criteria were: (a) ICU admission for SARS-CoV-2 infection, and (b) intubation and mechanical ventilation for >48 h. Exclusion criteria were: (a) age <18 years old, and (b) ICU readmission. The first episode of BSI was reported. Patients were divided in two different groups: the first group consisted of patients that presented BSI, and the second one of patients without BSI.

2.1. Outcome

The primary outcome of this study was the incidence of ICU-acquired BSIs in COVID-19, mechanically ventilated, critically ill patients. The secondary outcome was the identification of risk factors for the first episode of BSI.

2.2. Clinical Assessment

For all study patients, the following characteristics were recorded: age, sex, characteristics of the respiratory system, illness severity based on Acute Physiology and Chronic Health Evaluation Score II (APACHE II), Sequential Organ Failure Assessment (SOFA) score at admission, history of hospitalization during the last 3 months before current admission, history of invasive procedures (gastroscopy, colonoscopy, bronchoscopy, or surgery), medical history, history of antibiotic use, type and duration of antibiotics used, and finally therapies and laboratory findings related to COVID-19 infection. For survivors and non-survivors, several characteristics that might affect mortality were also taken into account.

2.3. Microbiology

Identification and susceptibility testing of the isolated pathogens were performed by the Vitek 2 automated system (bioMerieux, Marcy l' Etoile, France). For the interpretation of the results, EUCAST breakpoints were used.

2.4. Statistical Analysis

The results are presented as the frequency (%) for categorical variables or the median (25th, 75th quartiles) for continuous variables. The normality of data distribution was assessed by a Kolmogorov/Smirnov test. Categorical variables were compared using a chi square test or Fisher's exact test where appropriate; continuous variables were compared by a Mann–Whitney U test. Multivariate analyses were performed to determine variables associated with BSI or mortality. Only variables with a p value <0.05 were used in the stepwise logistic regression models. The analysis was performed between two groups (patients with BSI and patients without BSI). Exposure to potential risk factors was taken into account only before diagnosis of infection. A mortality analysis was performed between two groups (survivors and non survivors). SPSS software (SPSS 17.0, Chicago, IL, USA) was used for the data analysis.

3. Results

A total of 90 cases were studied. One case was a readmission, and data for five cases were incomplete, leaving 84 cases for the analysis. The characteristics of participants are presented in Tables 1–3. The incidence of BSIs was 57%, since 48 patients were infected, and they made up the BSI group, whereas a second group included 36 patients who did not present BSI (non-BSI group). Patients from the first group presented BSI at median day 9 (25th and 75th quartiles were 5 and 11, respectively) after ICU admission. There were 60 pathogens that were isolated; 10 patients presented multi-bacterial bloodstream infection. A total of 77% (46 cases) of the isolates were gram-negative bacteria, and the remaining 23% (14 cases) were gram-positive (Table 4). Seventeen *A. baumannii* and ten *K. pneumoniae* isolates were PDR, and the rest were XDR, susceptible only to colistin, and colistin and aminoglycosides, respectively. The other isolates were MDR. Resistant *A. baumannii* and *K. pneumoniae* strains are endemic in our ICU, as previously described [13,14]. The high prevalence of resistance to antibiotics pathogens and the high antibiotic consumption may explain the abovementioned result. The mechanisms of resistance and transmission between patients were not studied.

Table 1. Baseline characteristics during ICU admission.

	BSI Group (N = 48)	Non-BSI Group (N = 36)	p
Sex (Male)	32 (67)	24 (67)	-
Age (years)	69 (57, 76)	71 (66, 76)	0.274
APACHE II score	13 (10, 19)	16 (12, 22)	0.070
SOFA score	7 (7, 8)	8 (7, 10)	0.204
PaO2/FiO2 ratio	161 (120, 198)	154 (118, 199)	0.953
Crs	36 (30, 44)	34 (22, 45)	0.472
D-dimers	767 (522, 1134)	1042 (566, 2156)	0.093
Lymphocyte Count	640 (400, 847)	600 (413, 790)	0.772
Ferritin	976 (510, 1707)	1488 (861, 2455)	0.068
Hospitalization in the last 3 months	1 (2)	1 (3)	-
Days of hospitalization before ICU admission	1 (1, 4)	2 (1, 7)	0.084
Diabetes Mellitus	18 (38)	10 (28)	0.483
Chronic Lung disease	11 (23)	11 (31)	0.483
Chronic Heart Failure	5 (11)	3 (8)	-
Chronic Renal failure	2 (4)	3 (8)	0.647
Neurological disease	6 (13)	6 (17)	0.754
Arterial Hypertension	26 (54)	26 (72)	0.114
Malignancy	2 (4)	3 (8)	0.647
Dyslipidemia	10 (21)	16 (44)	0.031
Coronary Heart Disease	11	7 (19)	0.792
Autoimmune	2	2 (6)	-

Data is presented as median (25%, 75% quartiles) or n (%); BSI, Blood Stream Infection; ICU, Intensive Care Unit; APACHE, Acute Physiology and Chronic Health Evaluation; SOFA, Sequential Organ Failure Assessment; Crs, Compliance of the respiratory system; p, comparison between the two groups. Results by univariate analysis, chi square test, or Fisher's exact test for categorical variables and by Mann–Whitney U test for continuous variables.

3.1. Risk Factors for BSI

The baseline characteristics between groups are presented in Table 1. In Tables 2 and 3, the characteristics of the patients before BSI or the total length of the ICU stay for the BSI group and non-BSI group are presented, respectively. Patients without dyslipidemia presented BSIs more frequently after univariate analysis ($p < 0.05$, Table 1).

Table 2. Clinical characteristics in the ICU before BSI.

	BSI Group (N = 48)	Non-BSI Group (N = 36)	p
MV duration (days)	8 (4, 11)	7 (4, 12)	0.895
Invasive procedures	2 (4)	2 (6)	-
CVVHDF use	9 (19)	8 (22)	0.786
CVVHDF duration (days)	5 (2, 9)	4 (3, 5)	0.843
Steroids	40 (83)	33 (92)	0.338
Tocilizumab	11 (23)	13 (36)	0.226
Anakinra	7 (15)	12 (33)	0.064
Remdesivir	12 (25)	10 (28)	0.806

Data is presented as median (25%, 75% quartiles) or n (%); BSI, Blood Stream Infection; ICU, Intensive Care Unit; MV, mechanical ventilation; CVVHDF, Continuous veno-venous hemodiafiltration; Invasive procedures, gastroscopy, colonoscopy, or bronchoscopy; p, comparison between the two groups. Results by univariate analysis, chi square test, or Fisher's exact test for categorical variables and by Mann–Whitney U test for continuous variables.

Table 3. Antibiotics administered to participants before BSI.

	BSI Group (N = 48)	Non-BSI Group (N = 36)	p
Antibiotics during the last 3 months	1 (2)	0 (0)	-
Antibiotics during hospitalization prior to infection	48 (100)	36 (100)	-
Use of Carbapenems	22 (45)	19 (53)	0.660
Use of Antipseudomonal Penicillins	13 (27)	9 (25)	0.155
Use of Quinolones	24 (50)	18 (50)	-
Use of Cephalosporins 3d generation	23 (48)	12 (33)	0.263
Use of Ceftarolin	20 (42)	12 (33)	0.500
Use of Colistin	25 (52)	16 (44)	0.516
Use of Tygecycline	21 (44)	19 (52)	0.509
Use of Aminoglycosides	7 (15)	3 (8)	0.504
Gram (+) antibiotics	35 (73)	29 (80)	0.446
TMP/SMX	10 (20)	15 (42)	0.551
Use of CAZ-AVI	9 (19)	2 (6)	0.105

Data is presented as median (25%, 75% quartiles) or n (%); BSI, Blood Stream infection; TMP/SMX, trimethoprim-sulfamethoxazole; CAZ-AVI, ceftazidime-avibactam; Gram (+) antibiotics, teicoplanin, daptomycin, vancomycin, and linezolid; p, comparison between the two groups. Results by univariate analysis, chi square test, or Fisher's exact test for categorical variables and by Mann–Whitney U test for continuous variables.

Table 4. Pathogens detected in blood stream infections.

Pathogen	Number of Cases (N = 60)
Acinetobacter baumannii	20 (33%)
Klebsiella pneumonia	19 (32%)
Stenotrophomonas maltophilia	3 (5%)
Pseudomonas aeruginosa	2 (3%)
Proteus mirabilis	1 (2%)
Serratia marcescens	1 (2%)
Enterococcus spp.	14 (23%)

3.2. Mortality and Morbidity Indices in Patients with BSI

Patients who presented BSI, when compared with patients who did not, had a longer length of ICU stay and a longer duration of mechanical ventilation and sedation ($p < 0.05$, Table 5). In this population, there was a trend towards increased mortality that did not reach statistical significance. Compared with non-survivors, survivors had lower baseline APACHE II and SOFA scores, lower D-dimers levels, and a higher baseline compliance of the respiratory system. They received anakinra less frequently and appropriate therapy more often ($p < 0.05$, Table 6). The multivariate analysis (Table 7) showed that the baseline

APACHE II score [1.232 (1.017 to 1.493), *p* = 0.033] was the only independent risk factor for ICU mortality, while there was an indication towards increased mortality for patients who received anakinra [0.051 (0.003 to 1.026), *p* = 0.051].

Table 5. Outcomes.

	BSI Group (N = 48)	Non-BSI Group (N = 36)	*p*
ICU length of stay (days)	18 (14, 26)	7 (5, 12)	<0.000
Death	35 (73)	20 (56)	0.111
MV duration (days)	14 (18, 23)	7 (4, 12)	<0.000
Duration of Sedation (days)	13 (9, 18)	7 (4, 11)	<0.000

Data is presented as median (25%, 75% quartiles) or n (%); BSI, Blood Stream Infection; ICU, intensive care unit; MV, mechanical ventilation; *p*, comparison between the two groups. Results by univariate analysis, chi square test, or Fisher's exact test for categorical variables and by Mann–Whitney *U* test for continuous variables.

Table 6. Characteristics of survivors and non-survivors in the ICU.

	Survivors (N = 29)	Non-Survivors (N = 55)	*p*
Sex (Male)	18 (62)	38 (69)	0.627
Age (years)	70 (61, 74)	70 (62, 77)	0.296
APACHE II score	12 (11, 15)	17 (12, 22)	0.001
SOFA score	7 (6, 8)	8 (7, 9)	0.009
BSI	13 (45)	35 (64)	0.111
Diabetes Mellitus	6 (20)	22 (40)	0.091
Chronic Lung disease	6 (20)	16 (29)	0.447
Chronic Heart Failure	0 (0)	8 (15)	0.046
Chronic renal disease	1 (3)	4 (7)	0.665
Neurological disease	3 (10)	9 (16)	0.531
Arterial Hypertension	16 (55)	36 (65)	0.479
Malignancy	3 (10)	2 (4)	0.335
Autoimmune disease	1 (3)	3 (5)	-
Dyslipidemia	10 (34)	16 (29)	0.628
Coronary Artery Disease	4 (14)	14 (25)	0.271
Total ICU length of stay (days)	14 (8, 25)	13 (7, 18)	0.349
Total MV duration (days)	11 (6, 19)	7 (4, 12)	0.349
Total duration of sedation (days)	9 (5, 15)	7 (4, 12)	0.193
Appropriate Therapy	9/13 (69)	12/35 (34)	0.049
Steroids	24 (83)	49 (89)	0.501
Tocilizumab	7 (24)	17 (31)	0.615
Anakinra	2 (7)	17 (31)	0.014
Remdesivir	9 (31)	13 (24)	0.602
PaO2/FiO2 ratio	164 (137, 204)	125 (99, 156)	0.078
Crs	40 (30, 47)	34 (27, 42)	0.032
D-dimers	659 (473, 1023)	1180 (1140, 4578)	0.027
Lymphocyte Count	500 (390, 845)	600 (435, 738)	0.556
Ferritin	941 (554, 1997)	1617 (1058, 2795)	0.204

Data is presented as median (25%, 75% quartiles) or n (%); BSI, Blood Stream Infection; ICU, intensive care unit; APACHE, Acute Physiology and Chronic Health Evaluation; SOFA, Sequential Organ Failure Assessment; MV, mechanical ventilation; Crs, compliance of the respiratory system; *p*, comparison between the two groups. Results by univariate analysis, chi square test, or Fisher's exact test for categorical variables and by Mann–Whitney *U* test for continuous variables.

Table 7. Multivariate analysis.

	Odds Ratio	95% CI	*p*
APACHE II Score	1.232	1.017–1.493	0.033
SOFA score	0.460	0.203–1.044	0.063
Dyslipidemia	0.000	0.000	0.999
Appropriate therapy	4.553	0.855–24.257	0.076
Anakinra	0.051	0.003–1.026	0.051
Compliance of respiratory system	0.983	0.917–1.053	0.628
D-Dimers	1.000	1.000–1.001	0.635

4. Discussion

In the present study, we aimed to determine the incidence and to identify risk factors for BSI in critically ill, mechanically ventilated COVID-19 patients. Our results indicate that BSIs are frequent, since more than half of the patients were infected. Dyslipidemia occurs more often in non-infected patients. Furthermore, survivors had a significantly lower APACHE II score, and received anakinra less frequently when compared with non-survivors.

There are several studies on secondary infections in COVID-19 patients. Most of them include several types of infections, such as BSIs or infections of the respiratory tract. The populations included were usually mixed in terms of severity (hospitalizations both in ICUs and medical wards). Even in studies conducted in ICUs, patients may be under invasive mechanical ventilation or other forms of respiratory support, such as high flow oscillatory ventilation (HFOV) or non-invasive mechanical ventilation (NIV) [9,15–18]. To our knowledge, the present study is the first one to be conducted in the ICU, and all patients included were intubated and mechanically ventilated.

The incidence of BSIs in this study is higher when compared with our previously published data where patients did not present SARS-CoV-2 infection [13,14]. The results are also in accordance with other studies that report a higher number of COVID-19 patients with BSIs when compared with non-COVID-19 patients [9,19–21]. The profile of immune dysregulation and the higher percentage of COVID-19 patients that receive immunomodulatory agents may explain the finding.

The only risk factor for BSI that was identified in our study was dyslipidemia; more specifically, patients with dyslipidemia were protected from BSI. Certainly, this association does not imply a causative relationship. The concurrent administration of statins to these patients may play a role [22]. Data on this issue has not been reported previously in the literature; in this respect, this finding needs further investigation in the future with an appropriate methodology.

Despite the fact that the administration of antibiotics is widely known to be a factor responsible for infection, especially by multi-drug-resistant bacteria [13,14], we found no such evidence in this study. The shorter length of the hospital stay and the consequently lower use of antibiotics in comparison with non-COVID-19 patients, as well as the small number of participants in the present study, might be an explanation.

The results for the impact on secondary infections of immunosuppressive agents administered for the treatment of COVID-19 disease are inconclusive. There are studies where these agents are independently associated with increased nosocomial infections [9,17] and others that indicate no correlation [18]. Furthermore, there is no specific data for intubated and mechanically ventilated patients. In our study, the use of steroids, tocilizumab, or anakinra was not associated with BSIs. On the other hand, anakinra was associated with increased mortality. The etiology cannot be specified by the present study. Other factors related to this intervention, such as infections other than BSIs or different actions of anakinra, may be implicated.

BSIs did not affect mortality on a statistically significant level. The same result was identified by other studies [23]. The fact that the clinical outcome in severe COVID-19 patients is multifactorial may be an explanation for this. On the contrary, other indices of disease severity are affected: patients suffering from BSI had prolonged mechanical ventilation and a subsequent need for sedatives, and also a prolonged ICU length of stay, confirming the results from other studies [15,24,25]. Finally, the APACHE II score was higher in non-survivors. The relationship between the severity of illness and mortality is well established in several studies involving COVID-19 patients or non-COVID-19 patients [14,23].

The relationship between respiratory mechanics in patients with ARDS and mortality is not clear. According to the concept of patient self-inflicted lung injury (PSILI), the increased respiratory effort may generate lung injury in spontaneously breathing patients, leading to worse outcomes [26]. Consequently, early intubation and mechanical ventilation may prevent lung damage. Compliance of the respiratory (Crs) can be used as an indicator of the lung injury in ARDS patients. Higher values of Crs indicate less lung injury. In our study, survivors presented higher Crs after intubation and during ICU admission, but Crs was not an independent factor for mortality after the multivariate analysis. The fact that a higher APACHE II score predicted a worse outcome when compared to Crs alone suggests that the overall severity of multi-organ failure is more important than isolated respiratory mechanics.

This study presents limitations. It was performed at a single center, and the results should therefore be interpreted cautiously. The number of participants was relatively small. The fact that most of our pathogens are pan-drug-resistant, as previously described [13,14], may limit the generalizability of the results. However, the findings of this study may form the basis for a further investigation in the future.

5. Conclusions

A considerable percentage of intubated and mechanically ventilated patients with SARS-CoV-2 infection present BSI. Fever or reduced serum concentrations of inflammatory markers may make the diagnosis of BSI difficult if immunomodulatory drugs are used; therefore, close monitoring may improve the outcome. Finally, further studies are required to confirm the aforementioned findings.

6. Definitions

BSI was defined according to Center of Disease Control (CDC) criteria [27]. Previous hospitalization was defined as the admission to hospitals or other healthcare facilities for >48 h during the last three months. Antibiotics against Gram (+) bacteria include teicoplanin, daptomycin, vancomycin, and linezolid. As appropriate therapy was considered to be the administration of in vitro active antibiotics for at least 48 h. EUCAST breakpoints were used for susceptibility testing. SARS-CoV-2 infection was confirmed by reverse transcription polymerase chain reaction (PCR) with nasopharyngeal swabs. No genetic testing was performed. Patients' treatment decision was at the attending physician's discretion, and thus antibiotic combinations were different among patients. Only a single dose of tocilizumab was administered. No antibiotics were given as a prophylaxis in the ICU. Pandrug-resistant (PDR) was defined as a pathogen that was nonsusceptible to all agents in all antimicrobial categories, extensively drug-resistant (XDR) as a pathogen that was susceptible to only one or two antimicrobial categories, and finally multidrug-resistant (MDR) as a pathogen that was resistant to at least one agent in three or more drug classes.

Author Contributions: Data curation, E.Z. and D.M.; Formal analysis, K.M. and D.M.; Investigation, K.M., K.D., D.P., V.L. and V.T.; Methodology, K.M., E.Z. and D.M.; Supervision, E.Z. and D.M.; Writing–original draft, K.M. All authors have read and agreed to the published version of the manuscript.

Funding: This research received no external funding.

Institutional Review Board Statement: The study was approved by the University Hospital of Larissa Institutional Review Board/Research Ethics Committee (approval code 23852).

Informed Consent Statement: Patient consent was waived due to the pandemic.

Acknowledgments: We thank Elena Chatzinikou for her assistance in editing the paper.

Conflicts of Interest: The authors have no conflicts of interest to declare.

References

1. Zhu, N.; Zhang, D.; Wang, W.; Li, X.; Yang, B.; Song, J.; Zhao, X.; Huang, B.; Shi, W.; Lu, R.; et al. A Novel Coronavirus from Patients with Pneumonia in China, 2019. *N. Engl. J. Med.* **2020**, *382*, 727–733. [CrossRef]
2. Wang, Y.; Lu, X.; Li, Y.; Chen, H.; Chen, T.; Su, N.; Huang, F.; Zhou, J.; Zhang, B.; Yan, F.; et al. Clinical Course and Outcomes of 344 Intensive Care Patients with COVID-19. *Am. J. Respir. Crit. Care Med.* **2020**, *201*, 1430–1434. [CrossRef]

3. Zhou, F.; Yu, T.; Du, R.; Fan, G.; Liu, Y.; Liu, Z.; Xiang, J.; Wang, Y.; Song, B.; Gu, X.; et al. Clinical course and risk factors for mortality of adult inpatients with COVID-19 in Wuhan, China: A retrospective cohort study. *Lancet* **2020**, *395*, 1054–1062. [CrossRef]
4. Petrilli, C.M.; Jones, S.A.; Yang, J.; Rajagopalan, H.; O'Donnell, L.; Chernyak, Y.; Tobin, K.A.; Cerfolio, R.J.; Francois, F.; Horwitz, L.I. Factors associated with hospital admis-sion and critical illness among 5279 people with coronavirus disease 2019 in New York City: Prospective cohort study. *BMJ* **2020**, *369*, m1966. [CrossRef]
5. Brown, R.M.; Wang, L.; Coston, T.D.; Krishnan, N.I.; Casey, J.D.; Wanderer, J.P.; Ehrenfeld, J.M.; Byrne, D.W.; Stollings, J.L.; Siew, E.D.; et al. Balanced Crystalloids versus Saline in Sepsis. A Secondary Analysis of the SMART Clinical Trial. *Am. J. Respir. Crit. Care Med.* **2019**, *200*, 1487–1495. [CrossRef] [PubMed]
6. Qin, C.; Zhou, L.; Hu, Z.; Zhang, S.; Yang, S.; Tao, Y.; Xie, C.; Ma, K.; Shang, K.; Wang, W.; et al. Dysregulation of Immune Response in Patients with Coronavirus 2019 (COVID-19) in Wuhan, China. *Clin. Infect. Dis. Off. Publ. Infect. Dis. Soc. Am.* **2020**, *71*, 762–768. [CrossRef] [PubMed]
7. Liu, J.; Liu, Y.; Xiang, P.; Pu, L.; Xiong, H.; Li, C.; Zhang, M.; Tan, J.; Xu, Y.; Song, R.; et al. Neutrophil-to-lymphocyte ratio predicts critical illness patients with 2019 coronavirus disease in the early stage. *J. Transl. Med.* **2020**, *18*, 206. [CrossRef]
8. Mehta, P.; McAuley, D.F.; Brown, M.; Sanchez, E.; Tattersall, R.S.; Manson, J.J. COVID-19: Consider cytokine storm syndromes and immunosuppression. *Lancet* **2020**, *395*, 1033–1034. [CrossRef]
9. Buetti, N.; Ruckly, S.; de Montmollin, E.; Reignier, J.; Terzi, N.; Cohen, Y.; Siami, S.; Dupuis, C.; Timsit, J.F. COVID-19 increased the risk of ICU-acquired bloodstream infections: A case-cohort study from the multicentric OUTCOMEREA network. *Intensive Care Med.* **2021**, *47*, 180–187. [CrossRef] [PubMed]
10. Huang, C.; Wang, Y.; Li, X.; Ren, L.; Zhao, J.; Hu, Y.; Zhang, L.; Fan, G.; Xu, J.; Gu, X.; et al. Clinical features of patients infected with 2019 novel coronavirus in Wuhan, China. *Lancet* **2020**, *395*, 497–506. [CrossRef]
11. Antinori, S.; Galimberti, L.; Milazzo, L.; Ridolfo, A.L. Bacterial and fungal infections among patients with SARS-CoV-2 pneumonia. *Infez. Med.* **2020**, *28* (Suppl. S1), 29–36. [PubMed]
12. Yang, X.; Yu, Y.; Xu, J.; Shu, H.; Xia, J.; Liu, H.; Wu, Y.; Zhang, L.; Yu, Z.; Fang, M.; et al. Clinical course and outcomes of critically ill patients with SARS-CoV-2 pneumonia in Wuhan, China: A single-centered, retrospective, observational study. *Lancet Respir. Med.* **2020**, *8*, 475–481. [CrossRef]
13. Mantzarlis, K.; Makris, D.; Manoulakas, E.; Karvouniaris, M.; Zakynthinos, E. Risk factors for the first episode of Klebsiella pneumoniae resistant to carbapenems infection in critically ill patients: A prospective study. *BioMed Res. Int.* **2013**, *2013*, 850547. [CrossRef]
14. Mantzarlis, K.; Makris, D.; Zakynthinos, E. Risk factors for the first episode of Acinetobacter baumannii resistant to colistin infection and outcome in critically ill patients. *J. Med. Microbiol.* **2020**, *69*, 35–40. [CrossRef] [PubMed]
15. Bhatt, P.J.; Shiau, S.; Brunetti, L.; Xie, Y.; Solanki, K.; Khalid, S.; Mohayya, S.; Au, P.H.; Pham, C.; Uprety, P.; et al. Risk Factors and Outcomes of Hospitalized Patients with Severe Coronavirus Disease 2019 (COVID-19) and Secondary Bloodstream Infections: A Multicenter Case-Control Study. *Clin. Infect. Dis.* **2020**, *72*, e995–e1003. [CrossRef] [PubMed]
16. Ippolito, M.; Simone, B.; Filisina, C.; Catalanotto, F.R.; Catalisano, G.; Marino, C.; Misseri, G.; Giarratano, A.; Cortegiani, A. Bloodstream Infections in Hospital-ized Patients with COVID-19: A Systematic Review and Meta-Analysis. *Microorganisms* **2021**, *9*, 2016. [CrossRef] [PubMed]
17. Giacobbe, D.R.; Battaglini, D.; Ball, L.; Brunetti, I.; Bruzzone, B.; Codda, G.; Crea, F.; De Maria, A.; Dentone, C.; Di Biagio, A.; et al. Bloodstream infections in critically ill pa-tients with COVID-19. *Eur. J. Clin. Investig.* **2020**, *50*, e13319. [CrossRef] [PubMed]
18. Grasselli, G.; Scaravilli, V.; Mangioni, D.; Scudeller, L.; Alagna, L.; Bartoletti, M.; Bellani, G.; Biagioni, E.; Bonfanti, P.; Bottino, N.; et al. Hospital-Acquired Infections in Critically Ill Patients With COVID-19. *Chest* **2021**, *160*, 454–465. [CrossRef] [PubMed]
19. Shafran, N.; Shafran, I.; Ben-Zvi, H.; Sofer, S.; Sheena, L.; Krause, I.; Shlomai, A.; Goldberg, E.; Sklan, E.H. Secondary bacterial infection in COVID-19 patients is a stronger predictor for death compared to influenza patients. *Sci. Rep.* **2021**, *11*, 12703. [CrossRef]
20. Grasselli, G.; Cattaneo, E.; Florio, G. Secondary infections in critically ill patients with COVID-19. *Crit. Care* **2021**, *25*, 317. [CrossRef]
21. Pandey, M.; May, A.; Tan, L.; Hughes, H.; Jones, J.P.; Harrison, W.; Bradburn, S.; Tyrrel, S.; Muthuswamy, B.; Berry, N.; et al. Comparative incidence of early and late bloodstream and respiratory tract co-infection in patients admitted to ICU with COVID-19 pneumonia versus Influenza A or B pneumonia versus no viral pneumonia: Wales multicentre ICU cohort study. *Crit. Care* **2022**, *26*, 158. [CrossRef]
22. Makris, D.; Manoulakas, E.; Komnos, A.; Papakrivou, E.; Tzovaras, N.; Hovas, A.; Zintzaras, E.; Zakynthinos, E. Effect of pravastatin on the frequency of ventilator-associated pneumonia and on intensive care unit mortality: Open-label, randomized study. *Crit. Care Med.* **2011**, *39*, 2440–2446. [CrossRef] [PubMed]
23. Kokkoris, S.; Papachatzakis, I.; Gavrielatou, E.; Ntaidou, T.; Ischaki, E.; Malachias, S.; Vrettou, C.; Nichlos, C.; Kanavou, A.; Zervakis, D.; et al. ICU-acquired bloodstream infections in critically ill patients with COVID-19. *J. Hosp. Infect.* **2021**, *107*, 95–97. [CrossRef] [PubMed]
24. Bardi, T.; Pintado, V.; Gomez-Rojo, M.; Escudero-Sanchez, R.; Azzam Lopez, A.; Diez-Remesal, Y.; Martinez Castro, N.; Ruiz-Garbajosa, P.; Pestaña, D. Nosocomial infections associated to COVID-19 in the intensive care unit: Clinical characteristics and outcome. *Eur. J. Clin. Microbiol. Infect. Dis. Off. Publ. Eur. Soc. Clin. Microbiol.* **2021**, *40*, 495–502. [CrossRef] [PubMed]

25. Bonazzetti, C.; Morena, V.; Giacomelli, A.; Oreni, L.; Casalini, G.; Galimberti, L.R.; Bolis, M.; Rimoldi, M.; Ballone, E.; Colombo, R.; et al. Unexpectedly High Frequency of Enterococcal Bloodstream Infections in Coronavirus Disease 2019 Patients Admitted to an Italian ICU: An Observational Study. *Crit. Care Med.* **2021**, *49*, e31–e40. [CrossRef] [PubMed]
26. Weaver, L.; Das, A.; Saffaran, S.; Yehya, N.; Scott, T.E.; Chikhani, M.; Laffey, J.G.; Hardman, J.G.; Camporota, L.; Bates, D.G.; et al. High risk of patient self-inflicted lung injury in COVID-19 with frequently encountered spontaneous breathing patterns: A computational modelling study. *Ann. Intensive Care* **2021**, *11*, 109. [CrossRef] [PubMed]
27. Horan, T.C.; Andrus, M.; Dudeck, M.A. CDC/NHSN surveillance definition of health care–associated infection and criteria for specific types of infections in the acute care setting. *Am. J. Infect. Control.* **2008**, *36*, 309–332. [CrossRef] [PubMed]

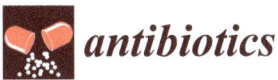

Review

Current and Potential Therapeutic Options for Infections Caused by Difficult-to-Treat and Pandrug Resistant Gram-Negative Bacteria in Critically Ill Patients

Helen Giamarellou and Ilias Karaiskos *

1st Department of Internal Medicine-Infectious Diseases, Hygeia General Hospital, 4, Erythrou Stavrou & Kifisias, Marousi, 15123 Athens, Greece; e.giamarellou@hygeia.gr
* Correspondence: ikaraiskos@hygeia.gr

Abstract: Carbapenem resistance in Gram-negative bacteria has come into sight as a serious global threat. Carbapenem-resistant Gram-negative pathogens and their main representatives *Klebsiella pneumoniae*, *Acinetobacter baumannii*, and *Pseudomonas aeruginosa* are ranked in the highest priority category for new treatments. The worrisome phenomenon of the recent years is the presence of difficult-to-treat resistance (DTR) and pandrug-resistant (PDR) Gram-negative bacteria, characterized as non-susceptible to all conventional antimicrobial agents. DTR and PDR Gram-negative infections are linked with high mortality and associated with nosocomial infections, mainly in critically ill and ICU patients. Therapeutic options for infections caused by DTR and PDR Gram-negative organisms are extremely limited and are based on case reports and series. Herein, the current available knowledge regarding treatment of DTR and PDR infections is discussed. A focal point of the review focuses on salvage treatment, synergistic combinations (double and triple combinations), as well as increased exposure regimen adapted to the MIC of the pathogen. The most available data regarding novel antimicrobials, including novel β-lactam-β-lactamase inhibitor combinations, cefiderocol, and eravacycline as potential agents against DTR and PDR Gram-negative strains in critically ill patients are thoroughly presented.

Keywords: pandrug-resistant; *Klebsiella pneumoniae*; *Acinetobacter baumannii*; *Pseudomonas aeruginosa*; salvage treatment; double carbapenem; newer β-lactam-β-lactamase inhibitors; cefiderocol; eravacycline; antimicrobial combinations

1. Introduction

Antimicrobial resistance poses a major threat to human health all over the world. The global burden associated with bacterial antimicrobial resistance in 2019 was an estimated 4.95 million deaths, of which 1.27 million were directly attributable to drug resistance. There is an emphasis on six common pathogens accountable for nosocomial infections: *Escherichia coli*, *Staphylococcus aureus*, *Klebsiella pneumoniae*, *Streptococcus pneumoniae*, *Acinetobacter baumannii*, and *Pseudomonas aeruginosa*, which were responsible for 73% of deaths attributable to antimicrobial resistance in the same report [1]. Additionally, carbapenem resistance in Gram-negative bacteria has come into sight as a serious global threat [2]. The 2017 World Health Organization (WHO) global priority list of pathogens ranks carbapenem-resistant Enterobacteriaceae (CRE), carbapenem-resistant *Pseudomonas aeruginosa*, and carbapenem-resistant *Acinetobacter baumannii* in the highest priority category [3]. More recent attention has focused on evidence of increased likelihood of morbidity and mortality in patients infected by carbapenem-resistant pathogens in comparison to those infected by susceptible pathogens [4,5]. A new terminology has been proposed for the categorization of resistance in Gram-negative pathogens. Multi-drug resistant (MDR) is defined as the acquired non-susceptibility to at least one agent in three or more categories of antimicrobial agents, and extensively-drug resistant (XDR) is the nonsusceptibility to at least one agent in all but two or fewer categories of antimicrobial agents. Finally, PDR is the nonsusceptibility to all agents in all categories of antimicrobial agents [6]. This statement was proposed by Magiorakos et al. [6] in 2012, when new β-lactam-β-lactamase inhibitors and novel antimicrobial agents were not launched in the market for the treatment of MDR, XDR, and PDR Gram-negative pathogens [7]. Therefore, a new consensus to be established in the era of novel β-lactam-β-lactamase inhibitors is of great matter. However, a new definition of resistance for Gram-negative infections defined as difficult-to-treat resistance (DTR) has recently been proposed as treatment-limiting resistance to all first-line agents, including all β-lactams (carbapenems and β-lactamase inhibitor combinations) and fluoroquinolones [8]. On the other hand, there is a considerable knowledge gap for the treatment of PDR Gram-negative strains, which are linked to extremely high all-cause mortality, ranging from 20 to 71% [9]. Therapeutic options for DTR and PDR *K. pneumoniae*, *A. baumannii*, and *P. aeruginosa* are scarce and based exclusively on few case reports and small case series, initiating salvage treatments counting upon synergistic combinations (in vitro or animal model), increased exposure regimen adapted to the MIC of the pathogen, as well as the introduction of novel antibacterial agents [9].

A narrative review of relevant studies was conducted using the PubMed/MEDLINE, Scopus, and Web of Science databases (from 1970 up to January 2022). The keywords used alone or in combination were pandrug, pandrug-resistant, pan-resistant, epidemiology of PDR, difficult to treat, difficult-to-treat-resistance, salvage treatment, Gram-negative limited options, compassionate use, double carbapenems, ICU patients, critically ill patients, novel β-lactam-β-lactamase inhibitors, cefiderocol, and eravacycline. Information regarding therapy of DTR and PDR Gram-negative infections were included. Full text and abstract screening as well as review articles were searched.

In this review, the latest data regarding the current and potential therapeutic choices for DTR and PDR Gram-negative bacteria are reported and discussed.

2. Carbapenem-Resistant *Klebsiella pneumoniae*

2.1. Epidemiological Issues

In a detailed review of 125 PDR *K. pneumoniae* strains, the geographical distribution was as follows: (i) Europe (71 strains), Greece being the predominant European country (47 strains), accompanied by Italy, France, and the Netherlands; (ii) America (12 strains); (iii) Asia (41 strains), mostly in India (28 strains). Only one strain was observed in Australia and none from Africa [8]. Regarding all-cause mortality, PDR *K. pneumoniae* strains, despite therapeutic manipulations, were reported as lethal in 31% of bloodstream infections (BSI), 50% in respiratory tract infections (RTIs), 29% in complicated urinary tract infections (cUTIs), 100% in CNS and complicated intra-abdominal infections (cIAI), and 67% in osteomyelitis, with a total fatality rate of 47%. The high mortality rates reported are referred to critically ill patients with high severity scores, with almost 37% of the patients hospitalized in the ICU [9].

2.1.1. Salvage Therapies

Salvage treatments for PDR infections caused by Gram-negative pathogens have been analyzed in a retrospective single-center cohort study, including 65 consecutive eligible patients suffering from infections with a PDR profile hospitalized at the University Hospital of Heraklion, Crete, Greece, between January 2010 and June 2018 [10]. Of the 65 PDR isolates, 31 (48%) were *K. pneumoniae*, followed by *A. baumannii* (43%), and *P. aeruginosa* (9%). All strains were resistant to all available antimicrobial agents; however, the mechanism of resistance was not reported. The majority of the patients were hospitalized in the ICU (79%) with multiple comorbidities, whereas severe sepsis and septic shock at the onset of infection was reported in 14% and 22% of cases, respectively. The most common empirical therapy was colistin-based combination, followed by non-colistin, non-tigecycline combination, and carbapenems plus tigecycline. Empiric therapy was defined arbitrarily as "effective empirical therapy" in cases where antimicrobial treatment administered (although in vitro non-susceptible) before the microbiological documentation of the PDR infection resulted in clinical improvement, without the necessity of treatment modification. The empirical therapy was effective in 50%, 37.5%, and 8% of patients receiving colistin combination, carbapenems-tigecycline, and non-colistin, non-tigecycline combination, respectively ($p = 0.003$). The infection-related in-hospital mortality was 32%. Even though the authors do not distinguish empirical therapeutic results regarding *K. pneumoniae*, *P. aeruginosa*, and *A. baumannii*, the obtained cure rates support the use of colistin and/or tigecycline-based combinations as empirical therapy when an infection due to PDR pathogens is suspected [10]. However, the frequent use of the pre-reported older antibiotics has provoked the emergence of strains with high resistance rates, particularly towards colistin; a fact attributed mainly to overconsumption [11]. In another retrospective study from Greece, amongst 412 monomicrobial BSIs due to *K. pneumoniae*, 115 (27.9%) were due to PDR isolates. The majority of infections were primary BSIs (46.1%), followed by catheter-related BSI (30.4%), cIAI (9.6%), and ventilator-associated pneumonia (VAP) (7.0%). bla_{KPC} was the most prevalent carbapenemase gene (85.2%), followed by a co-carriage of bla_{KPC} and bla_{VIM} (6.1%), bla_{VIM} (5.2%), and bla_{NDM} (3.1%). Thirty-day mortality was 39.1%. Among all patients, multivariate analysis identified the development of septic shock, Charlson comorbidity index, and BSI other than primary or catheter-related as independent predictors of mortality, while a combination of at least three antimicrobials was identified as an independent predictor of survival for PDR infections caused by *K.pneumoniae* [12].

2.1.2. Double Carbapenem Combinations (DCC)

The rationale of the application of the so-called DCC, i.e., "Double Carbapenem Combination" in case of PDR or XDR *K. pneumoniae* infections, was based on "ertapenem higher affinity with the carbapenemase enzyme, acting as a suicide inhibitor, thus allowing higher levels of the other carbapenems (meropenem or doripenem) to be active in the vicinity of the pathogen" [13]. The first worldwide report was from Greece in 2013 including 3 ICU patients with complicated UTIs [14], to be followed by another study, comprising 27 Greek patients with untreatable infections suffering from cUTIs with secondary bacteremia (four), primary (six) or catheter related BSI (two), hospital acquired pneumonia (HAP) or ventilator associated pneumonia (VAP) (two), and external ventricular drainage infection (one) [15]. PDR strains were isolated in 14 cases, whereas in the remaining 13 cases an XDR profile was identified. Fifteen patients were hospitalized in the ICU and twelve in the medical ward. The median APACHE score was 17 and the median Charslon index was 3, whereas 41% of the cases presented with severe sepsis or septic shock. Patients were treated exclusively with ertapenem (1 g daily, 1-h infusion, to be administered 1-h prior to meropenem dose) and high-dose prolonged infusion meropenem (2 gr, 3-h infusion, every 8-h). MICs against meropenem ranged between 2 and ≥ 16 mg/L. Clinical and microbiological success was 77.8% and 74.1%, respectively, with an attributable mortality of 11.1%. The results are independent of the height of meropenem MICs. Subsequently, until 2020 ninety patients, after combining ertapenem either with meropenem or doripenem, were published with a successful clinical outcome of 65.5%, and a rather low mortality of 24.2% [15–20]. Although the department of hospitalization was not reported in the majority of cases, all patients were critically ill and at least 53 cases were reported to be hospitalized in the ICU [20]. Despite difficulties in evaluation, the beneficiary addition of another antibiotic (mostly colistin) to which the isolated strains of *K. pneumoniae* were resistant in vitro, should also be mentioned [19,20].

2.1.3. The Novel β-Lactamase Inhibitors

In the chapters to follow, the novel β-lactamase inhibitors combination currently in the market (i.e., ceftazidime/avibactam, meropenem-vaborbactam, imipenem-cilastatin-relebactam) and the forthcoming aztreonam-avibactam are presented and discussed, focusing mainly on clinical issues dealing with DTR pathogens in critically ill patients and ICU patients, illustrated in Table 1. Mechanism of action, spectrum of activity, mechanism of resistance, approved indications, and information on DTR and PDR Gram-negative pathogens are depicted in Table 1 [21–71]. Although in vitro these agents have demonstrated susceptibility against PDR strains [72], clinical experience is limited to case reports, if any applicable. Nonetheless, these newer agents have the potency for treatment of DTR pathogens; however, more clinical studies focusing on PDR *K.pneumoniae* infections are needed.

2.2. Clinical Experience with Diazabicyclooctanes Based β-Lactamase Inhibitors (DBO Inhibitors)

2.2.1. Ceftazidime-Avibactam

Avibactam, a novel non-β-lactam-β-lactamase inhibitor, restores the activity of ceftazidime against the majority of β- lactamases, as outlined in Table 1. In Greece, around 2014–2016, against a collection of 394 KPC (+) *K. pneumoniae* strains, 99.6% were inhibited by ceftazidime-avibactam, whereas only 61.9%, 59.6%, 58.4%, and 51.5% were inhibited by gentamicin, colistin, fosfomycin, and tigecycline, respectively. In addition, 19 (4.8%) of isolates exhibited a PDR phenotype and 124 (31.5%) exhibited an XDR phenotype [73].

The real-world efficacy of ceftazidime-avibactam in the treatment of KPC (+) mostly *K. pneumoniae* strains was shown in clinical post-marketing studies, proving that in general, when compared to the conventionally prescribed antibiotics, not only higher cure rates were observed, but also lower mortality rates [26–32]. A multicenter prospective observational study with 147 patients (140 with KPC-producing K. pneumoniae (KPC-Kp) and seven with OXA-48 K. pneumoniae isolates with a median MIC to ceftazidime-avibactam of 1 mg/L) was conducted between January 2018 and March 2019 in 14 tertiary hospitals located all over Greece. The APACHE II and SOFA scores at the onset of infection were 16.5 ± 7.6 and 6.7 ± 4.2, respectively, whereas 45 (30.6%) patients had an ultimately fatal, 21 (14.3%) patients had a rapidly fatal, and 81 (55.1%) patients had a non-fatal underlying disease. Half of the patients were hospitalized in the ICU (50.3%), 50 (34%) had septic shock and 97 (66%) sepsis (by Sepsis-3), highlighting the severity of infection burden. The outcome and mortality predictors were assessed in a variety of infections including mainly bacteremia (64.6%), cUTI (22.4%), HAP/VAP (25.2%), and cIAI (10.2%). The resistance rates reported were for meropenem, colistin, and tigecycline 99%, 34%, and 44%, accordingly; however, a PDR profile was not subjected in the analysis. Monotherapy was given to 68 (46.3%) patients whereas in 79 (53.7%) patients ceftazidime-avibactam was given in combination with at least another active in vitro antibiotic for a median duration of 13 days. At day 14, in 81% of patients clinical success was observed with microbiological eradication in 50.4% and presumed eradication in 37.4% with emergence of resistance in two patients (1.4%). Mortality rates at 14 and 28 days were 9% and 20%, respectively, the highest percentage observed being in pneumonia patients (38%). The study focused in particular on a subgroup of 71 patients with KPC-Kp BSI treated with ceftazidime-avibactam, which was matched by propensity score with an equal group of bacteremic patients treated with other than ceftazidime-avibactam antibiotics active in vitro. The 28-day mortality in the 71 patients treated with ceftazidime-avibactam versus that in the 71 matched patients given other active in vitro antibacterial was 18.5% vs. 40.8% ($p = 0.005$), respectively. As independent predictors of death, ultimately fatal disease, rapidly fatal disease, and Charlson comorbidity index ≥ 2 were determined, whereas therapy with CAZ-AVI was the only independent predictor of survival [31].

Table 1. Current and potential therapeutic options for DTR and PDR Gram-negative pathogens.

Antibiotic	Mechanism of Action	Spectrum of Activity	Mechanism of Resistance	Clinical Development Program and Approved Indications	Dosage (Normal Renal Function)	Comments on DTR and PDR
Ceftazidime-Avibactam (2.5 g: ceftazidime 2 g, avibactam 500 mg) [7,21]	Avibactam is a non–β-lactam β-lactamase inhibitor that inactivates some β-lactamases and protects ceftazidime from degradation [7,21]	**Activity against**: *K. pneumoniae* and *P. aeruginosa* producing ESBL, KPC, AmpC and some class D enzymes (OXA-10, OXA-48). No active against MBL, *Acinetobacter* spp [7,21]	Amino acid substitutions, insertions or deletions in three loops, the Ω-loop, the Val240 loop and the Lys270 loop and membrane impermeability of porin mutations [22]	**Approval:** FDA in 2015 [23] and EMA in 2016 [24] **Approved indications:** FDA: cIAI and cUTI in adults and pediatric age groups over 3 months of age, HAP and VAP in adults [23] EMA: cIAI and cUTI, HAP and VAP in adults and pediatric age groups over 3 months of age. Treatment of adult patients with bacteremia that occurs in association with, or is suspected to be associated with, any of the infections listed above. Treatment of infections due to aerobic Gram-negative organisms in adults and pediatric patients aged 3 months and older with limited treatment options [24]	2.5 g IV every 8 h, infused over 2–3 h [25]	*K. pneumoniae*: Real life clinical studies on XDR *K. pneumoniae* with favorable clinical outcome around 80%. Superiority of ceftazidime-avibactam against comparators [26–32]. PDR cases limited to case reports [33–38]. *P. aeruginosa*: Real life clinical studies on XDR and DTR *P. aeruginosa* with favorable clinical outcome ranging from 45–100%. Superiority of ceftazidime-avibactam against comparators [29,39–41]. No PDR cases reported.

Table 1. *Cont.*

Antibiotic	Mechanism of Action	Spectrum of Activity	Mechanism of Resistance	Clinical Development Program and Approved Indications	Dosage (Normal Renal Function)	Comments on DTR and PDR
Meropenem-Vaborbactam (2g: meropenem 1g, vaborbactam 1g) [7,21]	Vaborbactam is a non-suicidal, boronic acid β-lactamase inhibitor with no antibacterial activity, preventing β-lactamases, such as KPCs, from hydrolyzing meropenem [7,21]	**Activity against:** *K. pneumoniae* producing ESBL, KPC, AmpC. No active against OXA-48-like, or MBL. As active as meropenem alone against *P. aeruginosa* [7,21]	Porin mutations in OmpK36 and OmpK35 and increased expression rate of the AcrAB-ToeC efflux system [22]	**Approval:** FDA in 2017 [42] and EMA in 2018 [43] **Approved indications:** FDA: cIAI and cUTI in adults [42] EMA: cUTI in adults, HAP and VAP in adults. Treatment of adult patients with bacteremia that occurs in association with, or is suspected to be associated with, any of the infections listed above. Treatment of infections due to aerobic Gram-negative organisms in adults with limited treatment options [43]	4 g IV every 8 h, infused over 3 h [25]	***K. pneumoniae:*** Real life clinical studies on XDR *K. pneumoniae* with favorable clinical outcome around 65–70% [44–46]. No PDR cases reported.
Imipenem-Cilastatin-Relebactam (1.25 g: imipenem 500 mg, cilastatin 500 mg, relebactam 250 mg) [7,21]	Relebactam is a novel β-lactamase inhibitor of class with no intrinsic antibacterial activity, protects imipenem from degradation by some β-lactamases and Pseudomonas-derived cephalosporinase [7,21]	**Activity against:** *K. pneumoniae* and *P. aeruginosa* producing ESBL, KPC, AmpC and porin mutations. Diminished inhibitor activity against OXA-48. No activity against MBL and *A. baumannii* [7,21]	Porin loss of OmpK35 and OmpK36 as well as hyperexpression of *bla*KPC [22]	**Approval:** FDA in 2019 [47] and EMA in 2021 [48] **Approved indications:** FDA: HAP and VAP in adults cUTI and cIAI in adult patients who have limited or no alternative treatment options [47] EMA: HAP and VAP in adults. Treatment of adult patients with bacteremia that occurs in association with, or is suspected to be associated with HAP or VAP in adults. Treatment of infections due to aerobic Gram-negative organisms in adults with limited treatment options [48]	1.25 g IV every 6 h, infused over 30 minutes [25]	***K. pneumoniae:*** Real life clinical studies on XDR *K. pneumoniae* are limited [49] ***P. aeruginosa:*** Real life clinical studies on DTR *P. aeruginosa* with clinical cure of 62% [50] No PDR cases reported.

Table 1. Cont.

Antibiotic	Mechanism of Action	Spectrum of Activity	Mechanism of Resistance	Clinical Development Program and Approved Indications	Dosage (Normal Renal Function)	Comments on DTR and PDR
Ceftolozane-Tazobactam (1 g ceftolozane/0.5 g tazobactam) [51]	Ceftolozane inhibits cell-wall synthesis via binding of PBPs. Tazobactam is a β-lactam sulfone that inhibits most class A β-lactamases and some class C β-lactamases [51]	**Activity against:** K. pneumoniae producing ESBL and AmpC. Activity against P. aeruginosa No activity against carbapenemase producing bacteria [51]	Modification of intrinsic AmpC-related genes and horizontally acquired β-lactamases that hydrolyse ceftolozane and are not inhibited by tazobactam, as well as modification of PBPs [51,52]	**Approval:** FDA in 2014 [53] and EMA in 2015 [54] **Approved indications:** FDA: cUTI, cIAI, HAP and VAP in adults [53] EMA: cUTI, cIAI, HAP and VAP in adults [54]	1.5 g IV every 8 h, infused over 1 h HAP/VAP: 3 g IV every 8 h, infused over 3 h [25]	*K. pneumoniae:* No activity against carbapenemase producing K. pneumoniae [51] *P. aeruginosa:* Real life clinical studies on DTR P. aeruginosa with clinical cure of 62–83% [55–57] No PDR cases reported.
Aztreonam-Avibactam (Administrated currently as a combination of ceftazidime-avibactam and aztreonam until the approval of aztreonam-avibactam) [7,21]	Aztreonam is a monobactam combined with a novel non–β-lactam β-lactamase inhibitor. In contrast to most β-lactams, monobactams are not substrates for MBLs, whereas avibactam reversibly inactivates most Class A and C and some D β-lactamase enzymes [7,21]	**Activity against:** K. pneumoniae producing ESBL, KPC, AmpC, OXA-48 and MBL. As active as aztreonam alone against P. aeruginosa and A. baumannii, including MBL-producing strains [7,21]	The production of β-lactamases (mostly AmpC variants in combination with NDM) and target modifications of PBP-3 [58]	Phase 3	Ceftazidime-avibactam: 2.5 g IV every 8 h, infused over 3 h *plus* Aztreonam: 2 g IV every 8 h, infused over 3 h (infused together) [25]	*K. pneumoniae:* Real life clinical studies on XDR K. pneumoniae (MBL producers) with lower 30-day mortality against in vitro comparator antibiotics and lower clinical failures [59] PDR cases limited to case report [60]

Table 1. *Cont.*

Antibiotic	Mechanism of Action	Spectrum of Activity	Mechanism of Resistance	Clinical Development Program and Approved Indications	Dosage (Normal Renal Function)	Comments on DTR and PDR
Cefiderocol (1 g) [7,61,62]	A new siderophore cephalosporin characterized as the "Trojan horse" because it creates a complex with the extracellular free ferric iron, leading to transportation of the drug through the outer cell membrane as a siderophore into the cell [7,61,62]	Activity against: *K. pneumoniae* producing ESBL, KPC, AmpC, OXA-48 and MBL. Activity against carbapenemase producing *P. aeruginosa* and *A. baumannii* [7,61,62]	The production of β-lactamases (mostly NDM, KPC and AmpC variants), porin mutations, mutations affecting siderophore receptors, efflux pumps and target modifications of PBP-3 [63]	Approval: FDA in 2019 [64] and EMA in 2020 [65] Approved indications: FDA: cUTI, HAP and VAP in adults [64] EMA: Treatment of infections due to aerobic Gram-negative organisms in adults with limited treatment options [65]	2 g IV every 8 h, infused over 3 h [25]	*K. pneumoniae*: No PDR cases reported. *P. aeruginosa*: Real life clinical studies on DTR *P. aeruginosa* with favorable clinical outcome of 70.6% [66] No PDR cases reported. *A. baumannii*: Real life clinical studies on XDR and PDR *A. baumannii* with favorable clinical outcome of 80% [67]
Eravacycline (50 mg) [7,68]	Eravacycline disrupts bacterial protein synthesis by binding to the 30S ribosomal subunit [68]	Activity against: *K. pneumoniae* producing ESBL, KPC, AmpC, OXA-48 and MBL. Activity against carbapenemase producing *A. baumannii*. No activity against *P. aeruginosa* [7,68]	The acquisition of genes encoding efflux pumps and the presence of ribosomal protection proteins, as well as target-site modifications such as the 16S RNA or certain 30S ribosomal proteins [68]	Approval: FDA in 2018 [69] and EMA in 2018 [70] Approved indications: FDA: cIAI in adults [69] EMA: cIAI in adults [70]	1 mg/kg/dose IV every 12 h [25]	*K. pneumoniae*: No PDR cases reported. *A. baumannii*: Clinical studies on DTR *A. baumannii* with similar clinical cure rates compared to best available treatment. Higher mortality in bacteremic patients treated with eravacycline [71]

cIAI, complicated intraabdominal infections; cUTI, complicated urinary tract infections; DTR, difficult to treat resistance; EMA, European Medicines Agency; ESBL, extended-spectrum beta-lactamases; FDA, U.S. Food and Drug Administration; HAP, hospital acquired pneumonia; IV, intravenous; KPC, Klebsiella pneumoniae carbapenemase; MBL, metallo-β-lactamase; NDM, New Delhi metallo-β-lactamase; OXA, oxacillinase; PBP, penicillin-binding proteins; PDR, pandrug-resistant; VAP, ventilator associated pneumonia; XDR, extensively drug-resistant.

The largest study published in 2021 on the evaluation of ceftazidime-avibactam monotherapy was an Italian retrospective observational cohort comprised of 577 patients suffering mainly from bacteremia ($n = 391$, 67.7%), cUTIs ($n = 71$, 12.3%), lower respiratory tract infections (LRTI) ($n = 59$, 10.2%), and cIAI ($n = 35$, 6.1%) [32]. The Charlson comorbidity index ≥ 3 was observed in 85%, 24% were hospitalized in the ICU and 17.3% had septic shock. All were given ceftazidime-avibactam as monotherapy ($n = 165$) or with ≥ 1 other active in vitro antibiotic ($n = 412$), including fosfomycin ($n = 92$), tigecycline ($n = 80$), gentamicin ($n = 68$), meropenem ($n = 69$), colistin ($n = 29$), amikacin ($n = 25$), or other suitable antimicrobials ($n = 18$). All-cause mortality at 30 days post infection onset was 25%, without significant difference between the two groups (26.1% vs. 25.0%, $p = 0.79$). In multivariate analysis, the following factors being present at infection onset were positively connected with mortality: septic shock ($p = 0.002$), neutropenia ($p < 0.001$), INCREMENT score ≥ 8 ($p = 0.01$), lower respiratory tract infection ($p = 0.04$), and dose adjustment of ceftazidime-avibactam in case of renal insufficiency ($p = 0.01$). For the first time reported in the relevant literature, mortality was decreased whenever ceftazidime-avibactam was administered by prolonged infusion (≥ 3 h) in 246 patients ($p = 0.006$) as shown in 34.9% of the non-survivors vs. 45.2% of the survivors [32].

The administration of ceftazidime-avibactam in PDR *K.pneumoniae* infections is limited to case reports. Camargo. et al. [33] reported a case of BSI caused by PDR *K.pneumoniae* in an intestinal transplant patient. After failing multiple antimicrobial regimens (tigecycline, colistin, and meropenem in different combinations), the patient was successfully treated with a combination of ceftazidime-avibactam and ertapenem. In another case report, a combination of pre-adapted bacteriophage therapy with ceftazidime-avibactam was successful for a fracture-related infection due to pandrug-resistant *Klebsiella pneumoniae* [34]. The cure of recurring *K. pneumoniae* carbapenemase-producing PDR *Klebsiella pneumoniae* septic shock episodes due to complicated soft tissue infection using a ceftazidime-avibactam based regimen combined with meropenem, tigecycline, and gentamicin was successful in a case report [35]. Lastly, in a patient with severe pancreatitis, a carbapenem resistant PDR *K. pneumoniae* in the pancreatic tissue was identified and bla_{KPC-2} gene was detected. The patient was treated with a combination of ceftazidime-avibactam, metronidazole, and teicoplanin. The patient demonstrated clinical and microbiological response over the first 3 weeks; however, deteriorated after 6 weeks and died [36]. On the other hand, ceftazidime-avibactam has been administered for PDR *K.pneumoniae* infections (BSI, UTI) in five neonates and children with a favorable outcome in all cases [37,38].

Resistance development to ceftazidime-avibactam is a great matter of concern. The worrisome phenomenon of ceftazidime-avibactam transferable resistance due to a novel VEB β-lactamase variant with a Lys234 Arg substitution in *K. pneumoniae* strains, five out of ten with a pan-drug resistant profile, has been published [74,75]. Epidemiological investigations revealed that the resistance was acquired independently from previous ceftazidime-avibactam exposure. Three patients developed an infection: two catheter-related bloodstream infections and one VAP. The salvage therapeutic regimen chosen was a combination of ceftazidime-avibactam with meropenem or aztreonam plus fosfomycin. The triple combination was successful in two of the cases, while the combination of ceftazidime-avibactam and meropenem was reported as a failure in the remaining one [75].

2.2.2. Aztreonam-Avibactam

In the earliest in vitro evaluation, the new combined molecule was found very active against 114 *K. pneumoniae* MBL producing strains collected between 2016–2017 with an MIC of ≤ 2 mg/L [76]. In a more recent study, aztreonam-avibactam activity was tested against 8787 Enterobacterales collected consecutively in 2019 from 64 countries and 64 medical centers; 99.9% of strains were inhibited at ≤ 8 mg/L with 99.5% at ≤ 1 mg/L [77]. A still ongoing randomized phase 3 clinical trial in the evaluation of the efficacy and tolerability of aztreonam-avibactam in the therapy of serious infections due to MBL-producing Enterobacterales is expected to prove the real efficacy of the combination (clinical trial gov. identifier:

NCT03580044). Currently and while awaiting AZ-AVI to be licensed, the combination of aztreonam and ceftazidime-avibactam has been given with very promising responses in patients with serious infections, in whom MBL producing bacteria were implicated. Dosages are depicted in Table 1. In the largest up-to-date study, which was prospective and observational, 102 cases with MBL bacteremia (82 with NDM and 20 with VIM) were included [59]. Results, when ceftazidime-avibactam plus aztreonam was given, were superior compared to active in vitro comparator antibiotics (mostly combination with colistin, tigecycline, fosfomycin, and aminoglycosides) with a lower 30-day mortality (19% vs. 44%, $p = 0.01$), as well as a lower number of clinical failures at day 14 [59]. In a case report, a PDR *K. pneumoniae* isolate encoding NDM-1, OXA-48, CTX-M-14b, SHV-28, and OXA-1 genes caused an infection of the cardiovascular implantable electronic device and right-sided infective endocarditis, that was treated successfully with the synergistic combinations of aztreonam with ceftazidime-avibactam for 6 weeks [60].

2.2.3. Imipenem-Cilastatin-Relebactam

Against 137 strains of carbapenemase-producing Enterobacterales, relebactam reduced MICs of imipenem to 1 mg/L for 88% of the strains. Similarly, among 199 plasmids encoded KPC carbapenemases producing strains which were at 54% resistant to colistin, relebactam restored imipenem susceptibilities in 96.5% of isolates [78]. Regarding 295 KPC-Kp strains isolated in 2015–2016 from Greek hospitals, relebactam restored susceptibilities to 98% [79]. In the Restore-IMI-1 multicenter, a randomized, double-blind trial compared the safety and efficacy of imipenem-cilastatin-relebactam vs. colistin plus imipenem in 47 patients with imipenem-non-susceptible mostly cUTI and HAP/VAP infection. On day 28, a favorable clinical response was noticed in 71% vs. 40% with a 28-day mortality of 10% vs. 30%, respectively. To be pointed out, nephrotoxicity was observed in 10% vs. 56% ($p = 0.002$) [49]. No PDR infections treated with imipenem-cilastatin-relebactam has been reported to this date.

2.2.4. Meropenem-Vaborbactam

In a phase III clinical trial (TANGO II), the efficacy and safety of meropenem-vaborbactam vs. the best available therapy (BAT) against CRE infections was evaluated in a randomized comparative study in which KPC-Kp represented 63.4% of resistant strains [80]. The cure rates of 65.6% vs. 33.3% ($p = 0.03$), with a 28-day all-cause mortality of 15.6% vs. 33.3% ($p = 0.20$) and microbiological cure reaching 65.6% vs. 40% ($p = 0.09$) were reported, respectively [80]. Accordingly, in two comparative prospective observational studies but with limited number of patients with CRE infections (20 and 40 patients, respectively), clinical success ranged from 65% to 70% with a 30-day mortality of 10% and 7.5% [44,45]. In a real-life based experience retrospective study with 131 patients, 105 were given ceftazidime-avibactam and 26 meropenem-vaborbactam, among whom 40% had bacteremia and the most common pathogen was KPC-Kp, and no significant differences either in clinical success or in mortality rates was reported [46].

3. Pandrug-Resistant *Acinetobacter baumannii*
3.1. Epidemiological Issues

Acinetobacter is an important cause of hospital-acquired infections, occurring mainly in ICU patients and among residents of long-term care facilities [81]. The most common infections encountered in the clinical setting are BSI, including catheter-relating bloodstream infections (CRBSI) and HAP, including VAP [82]. The most worrisome phenomenon of the last couple of years is the rise of PDR strains characterized as non-susceptible to all conventional antimicrobial agents [10]. In a systemic review of the current epidemiology and prognosis of PDR Gram—negative bacteria—a total of 526 PDR isolates were reported with 172 of them being PDR *A. baumannii*. The majority of PDR strains were isolated from ICU units, with a potential to cause hospital outbreaks, dissemination between hospitals and long-term facilities, as well as international transmission to other countries.

PDR infections were associated with excess mortality, mounting up to 71%, and were independently high regardless of the infection source [9]. Notably, in a cohort study of 91 patients infected (n = 62) or colonized (n = 29) with PDR carbapenemase producing *A. baumannii* (CRAB), a three-fold increased hazard of mortality was observed in favor of patients with an infection caused by PDR CRAB [83]. Likewise, the comparison of patients with CRAB infections to patients with infections caused by carbapenem-susceptible *A. baumannii* was linked to increased mortality, prolongation of hospital stay, increased rate of ICU utilization, and hospital charges [5].

3.2. Therapeutic Options

3.2.1. Antibiotics with Activity In Vitro against Carbapenemase Producing *A. baumannii*

The optimal therapeutic strategy for the management of carbapenemase producing *A. baumannii* (CRAB) infections exhibiting extensive drug-resistant phenotypes is very limited [84]. There is no "standard of care" treatment regimen for the therapy of CRAB. Sulbactam, meropenem, tigecycline, as well as polymyxins, the last-resort antibiotics in recent decades, have been used in critically ill patients for the treatment of CRAB infections [85]. Sulbactam, an irreversible β-lactamase inhibitor, has demonstrated activity against *A. baumannii* strains; unfortunately, it is administered in combination with ampicillin (3 gr of ampicillin-sulbactam is comprised of 2 gr of ampicillin and 1 gr of sulbactam) [86]. For the treatment of CRAB infections, a dose of 9 gr ampicillin-sulbactam every 8 h with extended infusion of 4 h (total dose of 27 gr ampicillin-sulbactam in a patient with normal renal function) is suggested [85,87]. Polymyxins and mainly colistin is the most common antibiotic utilized in clinical practice for infections caused by CRAB [88–90]. In a systematic review and meta-analysis of polymyxins-based vs. non-polymyxins-based therapies in infections caused by CRAB, polymyxins-based therapies in terms of clinical efficacy had an advantage over non-polymyxins-based therapies (OR, 1.99; 95% CI, 1.31 to 3.03; p =0.001) [91]. The dosage of polymyxins is illustrated in detail in the International Consensus Guidelines for the Optimal Use of the Polymyxins [92]. Tigecycline, although it demonstrates being in vitro susceptible to *A. baumannii* [93], has been linked with higher mortality and lower microbiological eradication in two meta-analyses [94,95]. Improved clinical rates and lower mortality rates have been demonstrated when administrating a high dose of tigecycline (loading dose of 200 mg followed by 100 mg every 12 h) [96]. Thus, a high dose of tigecycline is recommended for the treatment of CRAB infections. Meropenem as a high-dose extended infusion of 3 gr every 8 h with a 3-h infusion has been utilized in combination therapy for the treatment of CRAB infections [85]. Lastly, in response to the medical need for new treatment options, cefiderocol and eravacycline, two new antimicrobial agents with in vitro susceptibility, have been recently approved [62,68]. The major problem is that the distribution of newly approved antimicrobial agents is suboptimal, with eravacycline being unavailable in Europe [97] and cefiderocol being used in compassionate access [98] or been recently launched in a minority of European markets (i.e., United Kingdom, Germany, and Italy) [99].

A respectable spectrum of antimicrobial combinations has been evaluated in vitro and in animal models, predominately based on polymyxins, rifampicin, fosfomycin, sulbactam, and carbapenems with promising results [100]. On the other hand, a variety of clinical studies evaluating in vitro synergy have failed to demonstrate superiority [101–104]. Indicatively, clinical studies comparing colistin monotherapy to colistin–rifampicin [101], colistin–fosfomycin [102], and colistin–meropenem combinations [103,104] depicted similar mortality rates with no significantly statistical difference in clinical cure. In a multicenter study from Italy, two hundred and ten ICU patients with infections due to XDR *A. baumannii* received either colistin methanesulphate (CMS) as monotherapy at a dose of 2 MU every 8 h intravenously, or CMS plus rifampicin 600 mg every 12 h intravenously. The thirty-day mortality in the combination and in the monotherapy arm was 43.3% and 42.9%, respectively, with no difference observed in terms of infection-related death and length of hospitalization [101]. In another study, ninety-four patients infected with CRAB (mostly HAP or VAP) were randomized to receive a combination of intravenous CMS at a dosage of 5 mg of colistin base activity/kg of body weight daily plus intravenous fosfomycin sodium at a dosage of 4 g every 12 h (47 patients in the combination group) or intravenous CMS (47 patients in the monotherapy group). Favorable clinical outcomes, mortality at the end of study treatment, and mortality at 28 days were not significantly different between groups [102]. The major drawback of both studies was the suboptimal dose of CMS (without a loading dose) utilized [101,102]. It is of great significance to analyze the two clinical trials evaluating the role of colistin monotherapy vs. colistin in combination with meropenem, due to large number of participants and the application of updated dose schemes [103,104]. The effectiveness of colistin monotherapy (9 million unit loading dose, followed by 4.5 million units every 12 h) to colistin–meropenem combination (2 gr prolonged infusion every 8 h) therapy for the treatment of severe infections caused by CRAB was evaluated in a randomized trial (with blinded outcome assessment). The majority of the patients had HAP, VAP, or bacteremia. Clinical failure rates for patients who received monotherapy versus combination therapy were 83% (125/151) vs. 81% (130/161) ($p = 0.64$), whereas mortality at 28 days was 46% (70/151) vs. 52% (84/161) ($p = 0.4$) for patients with *A. baumannii* infections [103]. In the second trial, 214 patients were enrolled in the colistin monotherapy arm and 211 in the meropenem-colistin combination arm. *A. baumannii* was the most common bacteria isolated (77%) and the most prevalent infections were nosocomial pneumonia and BSI. There were no differences between monotherapy and combination therapy in respect to 30-day mortality (43% vs. 37%, $p = 0.21$) and clinical failure rates (45% vs. 38%, $p = 0.18$) [104]. The results of both clinical trials strongly encourage the avoidance of colistin–carbapenem combination therapy for carbapenem-resistant *A. baumannii* infections, regardless of the infection course.

3.2.2. Salvage Treatment

A combination therapy with at least two agents, with in vitro activity whenever applicable, has been proposed by the IDSA guidelines for the treatment of moderate to severe CRAB infections [85]. The major issue, not referred to in the guidelines, is the treatment of PDR CRAB infections. Therapeutic options in these cases are based on in vitro and animal studies [100,105]. Two case series study with triple combination therapy have been reported for the treatment of PDR CRAB and are gradually implemented in clinical practice as salvage treatments due to the lack of other therapeutic choices [106,107], as shown in Table 2. The first study from Greece evaluated the triple combination therapy of intravenous high dose ampicillin-sulbactam (dose of 9 gr every 8 h), high dose of tigecycline (200 mg loading dose followed by 100 mg every 12 h), and intravenous CMS (9 million units loading dose, followed by 4.5 million units every 12 h) in 10 ICU patients with a VAP infection caused by *A. baumannii* with a PDR phenotype. The Charlson comorbidity index was ≥ 3 and the median APACHE score was of 23 ± 3. A successful clinical outcome was observed in 90% (9/10), whereas microbiological eradication was identified in 70% (7/10 patients). The 28-day mortality was of 10%, whereas nephrotoxicity was observed in one patient [106]. In another study, 20 patients with a median APACE score of 19.5 (range, 10–28) with infections caused by colistin-resistant *A. baumannii* were evaluated. The most common infections were VAP and bacteremia in 65% (13/20) and 10% (2/20), respectively. Three patients were characterized as colonization and were not treated, whereas the remaining 17 patients were treated in the majority with various CMS-based combination regimens. The most prevalent combination was a combination of carbapenem, ampicillin-sulbactam and CMS prescribed in seven patients. Mortality was depicted as lower in a statistical matter between triple combination and patients receiving other antimicrobial agents for the treatment of colistin-resistant *A. baumannii* (0% vs. 60%, $p = 0.03$) [108].

3.2.3. New Antimicrobials

Cefiderocol

In the SIDERO-CR-2014-2016 surveillance in vitro study, European clinical isolates comprising MDR non-fermenter *A. baumannii* was tested against cefiderocol and 94.9% had a cefiderocol MIC ≤ 2 mg/L [109]. CREDIBLE-CR was a randomized, open-label, multicenter trial of cefiderocol (n = 101) and the best available treatment (BAT) (n = 49) for the treatment of severe infections (cUTI, nosocomial pneumonia, BSI, or sepsis) caused by carbapenem-resistant Gram-negative pathogens. In 118 patients in the carbapenem-resistant microbiological intent to treat (ITT) population, the most common baseline pathogen was *A. baumannii* in 46% (54/118). Cefiderocol was administrated as monotherapy in 83% (66/80) and combination therapy (mostly colistin-based regimens) was given in 71% (27/38) in the BAT arm. The clinical cure rates in the cefiderocol (22/49) and comparator (13/25) regarding *A. baumannii* were similar (45% vs. 52%). An increase in all-cause mortality was observed in patients treated with cefiderocol as compared to BAT. However, the greatest mortality imbalance disfavoring cefiderocol was noted in the nosocomial pneumonia subgroup, followed by BSI. The difference in 49-day mortality stratified for pathogen was the highest for *Acinetobacter* spp. (50% (21/42) vs. 18% (3/17) in cefiderocol and BAT-treated patients, respectively [110]. Deaths due to treatment failure in the cefiderocol group occurred more often in the patients infected with *Acinetobacter* spp. Of the 16 deaths due to treatment failure, 13 involved *Acinetobacter* spp. [109,110]. In conclusion, treatment failure was linked with infection caused by *Acinetobacter* spp., pulmonary infection at baseline, and by increases in cefiderocol MIC while on therapy [109,110]. An additional phase 3 trial, named APEKS-NP, evaluated hospital-acquired, ventilator-associated, or health-care-associated Gram-negative pneumonia and found cefiderocol was non-inferior to high-dose meropenem in patients. Fourteen-day all-cause mortality, clinical cure, and microbiologic eradication were similar between treatment groups for participants infected with *A. baumannii*; however, this group only comprised 16% of the study population, of which 66% of isolates were carbapenemase-resistant [111]. Cefiderocol has also been administrated as compassionate use in a limited number of case series with infections caused by XDR and PDR *A. baumannii* pathogens, resulting in a clinical success of 80% (20/25) [67,98]. Overall, the necessity of further studies to elucidate the true role of cefiderocol against *A. baumannii* infections in real life patients is needed.

Eravacycline

Eravacycline is a synthetic fluorocycline antibacterial agent that is structurally similar to tigecycline with two modifications at the D-ring of its tetracycline core [68]. In vitro activity of eravacycline against *A. baumannii* isolates (n = 2097) worldwide (from 2013 to 2017) revealed an MIC90s of 1 mg/L, demonstrating improved potency up to 4-fold greater than that of tigecycline [112]. Eravacycline has successfully completed clinical trial phase 3 for the treatment of cIAI; however, *A. baumannii* infections only comprised 3% of the total isolated pathogens [113]. Clinical studies with infections caused by CRAB reporting efficacy of eravacycline are lacking and are limited to one study. In a retrospective report of 93 adults hospitalized for pneumonia with DTR *A. baumannii*, 27 patients received eravacycline and were compared to those receiving the best available therapy. Eravacycline-based combination therapy had similar outcomes to the best available combination therapy. However, when taking under consideration patients with secondary bacteremia and coinfection with severe acute respiratory syndrome coronavirus-2 (SARS-CoV-2), eravacycline was associated with higher 30-day mortality (33% vs. 15%; p = 0.048), lower microbiologic cure (17% vs. 59%; p = 0.004), and longer durations of mechanical ventilation (10.5 vs. 6.5 days; p = 0.016), highlighting the avoidance of use in bacteremic patients [71]. However, eravacycline could be a suitable candidate for the treatment of cIAI caused by XDR, and even PDR pathogens. Therefore, further clinical studies addressing the efficacy of eravacycline in difficult-to-treat infections is required.

New β-Lactamase Inhibitor

Durlobactam, previously known as ETX2514, is a novel diazabicyclooctane class of β-lactamase inhibitor specifically designed to inhibit class D β-lactamases, in addition to class A and C enzymes. Durlobactam is combined with sulbactam, and targets infections caused by *A. baumannii* [21]. It has completed clinical trials in combination with sulbactam for the treatment of hospitalized adults with complicated urinary tract infection (cUTI) (Phase 2, clinicaltrials.gov identifier: NCT03445195) [114] and for the treatment of HAP and VAP caused by *A. baumannii* vs. colistin plus imipenem and the results are pending (Phase 3, clinicaltrials.gov identifier: NCT03894046).

4. *Pseudomonas aeruginosa* with Difficult-to-Treat Resistance
4.1. Epidemiological Issues

Pseudomonas aeruginosa is categorized among the ESKAPE pathogens and is considered one of the major causes of nosocomial infections caused by multi-resistant pathogens worldwide [115]. Resistance to last-resort colistin is still quite low. In vitro activity of colistin against isolates of *P. aeruginosa* collected in Europe as part of the INFORM global surveillance program from 2012 to 2015 revealed resistance to colistin < 0.5% [116]. Higher resistance rates have been observed in Greek isolates and are reported to be around 5–6% [117,118]. From the MagicBullet clinical study (2012–2015), fifty-three *P. aeruginosa* isolates from patients with HAP from 12 hospitals in Spain, Greece, and Italy were recovered. A minority was considered PDR (3.8%), whereas 19 (35.8%) were XDR and most of the isolates reported from Greece were PDR [118]. PDR strains of *P. aeruginosa* are extremely uncommon and are limited to 175 cases reported in a recent review [9]. Geographical distribution of PDR *P. aeruginosa* are mainly from Europe, Asia, and Australia, accumulating for 80, 52, and 34 cases, respectively. Almost one-third of the cases were defined in the ICU setting with a mortality rate ranging from 31–58% [9].

4.2. Therapeutic Options

There is a paucity of new classes of antibiotics active against *P. aeruginosa* resistant to carbapenems. Only four new antibiotics have a promising activity: ceftolozane-tazobactam, ceftazidime-avibactam, imipenem-cilastatin-relebactam, and cefiderocol [119]. However, most of those new antibiotics (excluding cefiderocol) are not active against MBL-producing *P. aeruginosa* isolates [120] and clinical experience with PDR *P. aeruginosa* is lacking. However, they are potent agents for the treatment of DTR *P. aeruginosa*.

4.2.1. Ceftolozane-Tazobactam

MDR *P. aeruginosa* pathogens in the setting of phase 3 trials of ceftolozane-tazobactam treatment were 2.9% of uropathogens at baseline in cUTI, 8.9% in cIAI and in HAP, and VAP made up 25% of the study population [53,54,121]. In a multicenter, retrospective, cohort study at eight U.S. medical centers from 2015 to 2019, efficacy data of ceftolozane-tazobactam based on real-life experience was evaluated for the treatment of MDR and XDR *P. aeruginosa* isolates. Many patients had a high severity of illness at infection onset, with 50.6% residing in the ICU and a median APACHE II score of 21. The most common infection source was the respiratory tract in 62.9%. Clinical failure and 30-day mortality occurred in 85 (37.6%) and 39 (17.3%) patients, respectively [55]. A significant clinical experience of ceftolozane-tazobactam treatment exclusively in 101 various types of *P. aeruginosa* infections was reported from a retrospective study conducted in Italy (2016–2018). At the time of infection, 38.6% presented sepsis or septic shock and 23.8% were admitted to the ICU, with 56.4% classified as life-threating infections. Regarding *P. aeruginosa* strains, 50.5% were XDR and 78.2% were resistant to at least one carbapenem. An overall clinical success of 83.2% was depicted; however, lower rates were observed in patients with sepsis or undergoing continuous renal replacement therapy [56]. In a recent multicenter retrospective cohort of 95 critically ill ICU patients affected by severe infections due to *P. aeruginosa* (mostly nosocomial pneumonia) with different resistance patterns and 83.3% carbapenem-resistant

(XDR 48.4% and MDR 36.8%), a favorable clinical response was observed in 71.6% of patients, with a microbiological eradication rate of 42.1% [57]. Therefore, IDSA guidance on the treatment of *P. aeruginosa* with difficult-to-treat resistance suggests ceftolozane-tazobactam therapy for cystitis, pyelonephritis, or cUTI, as well as for infections outside of the urinary tract [25], and the ESCMID guidelines on Gram-negatives recommend the use of ceftolozane-tazobactam in DTR *P. aeruginosa* infections with the obligation of in vitro susceptibility [122].

4.2.2. Ceftazidime-Avibactam

In clinical trials with hospitalized patients with cUTI, cIAI, and HAP/VAP caused by *P. aeruginosa*, ceftazidime-avibactam was generally effective in terms of clinical cure and favorable microbiological response rates. In a pooled analysis of outcomes for patients with MDR Gram-negative isolates from the adult phase 3 clinical trials, ceftazidime-avibactam demonstrated similar efficacy to comparators against MDR *P. aeruginosa* [39]. The largest real-world study highlighting the clinical effectiveness of ceftazidime-avibactam in infections caused by MDR *Pseudomonas* spp. comprises 63 patients with *Pseudomonas* spp. infection. The most common infection source was the respiratory tract (60.3%). Clinical failure, 30-day mortality, and 30-day recurrence in terms of infections caused by *P. aeruginosa* occurred in 19 (30.2%), 11 (17.5%), and 4 (6.3%) patients, respectively [29]. The effectiveness of ceftazidime-avibactam for the treatment of 61 infections due to MDR/XDR *P. aeruginosa* was evaluated in a retrospective study. The median Charlson comorbidity index was 7, and 9.8% episodes were diagnosed in the ICU. The most common infection was lower respiratory tract infection (34.4%) and almost 15% were BSI and 50.8% presented with sepsis at symptom onset. Global clinical cure was achieved in 56 of 61 episodes (91.8%) and microbiological cure was achieved in 82.5% (33/40) of evaluable episodes, whereas mortality by day 30 was 13.1% [40]. In a systemic literature review with 150 cases of MDR/XDR or DTR *P. aeruginosa* infections treated with ceftazidime-avibactam, a favorable outcome ranging from 45–100% was depicted and superiority in a statistical manner vs. comparators was also illustrated [41]. Recent IDSA treatment guidelines for Gram-negative bacterial antimicrobial-resistant infections suggest ceftazidime-avibactam therapy in the settings of all DTR *P. aeruginosa* infections with limited therapeutic options [25]. However, the true efficacy of ceftazidime-avibactam against PDR *P. aeruginosa* is still lacking, due to deficit of reported cases.

4.2.3. Imipenem-Cilastatin-Relebactam

In RESTORE-IMI 1 a phase 3, multicenter, double-blind trial, *P. aeruginosa* was the most common pathogen and was reported in 77% of cases with the majority of pathogens producing ESBL or *Pseudomonas*-derived cephalosporinases. Favorable overall response in terms of Pseudomonas infections was observed in 81% imipenem-cilastatin-relebactam and 62% colistin and imipenem patients (90% CI for difference, −19.8, 38.2), day 28 favorable clinical response in 71% and 40% (90% CI, 1.3, 51.5), and 28-day mortality in 10% and 30% (90% CI, −46.4, 6.7), respectively [49]. In a real-life retrospective, observational case series of 21 hospitalized patients treated with imipenem-cilastatin-relebactam, was conducted in 2020–2021 in the USA. The median APACHE II score was 21.5 and most patients (76%) were admitted to the ICU. The most common infections were respiratory tract infections, including HAP and VAP (52%), whereas bacteremia occurred in 29% of patients. The most prevalent pathogen was *P. aeruginosa* (16/21, 76%). Clinical cure occurred in 13/21 (62%) of patients treated with imipenem-cilastatin-relebactam, whereas mortality occurred in 33% (7/21) of patients [50]. The IDSA guidance on the treatment of *P. aeruginosa* with difficult-to-treat resistance suggests imipenem-cilastatin-relebactam therapy for cystitis, pyelonephritis, or cUTI, as well as for infections outside of the urinary tract [25]. However, the elucidation of the true clinical efficacy of imipenem-cilastatin-relebactam, as well as ceftazidime-avibactam in the era of PDR profiles is to be clarified in real-life studies.

4.3. Newer Antimicrobials
Cefiderocol

A CREDIBLE-CR study was initiated to evaluate cefiderocol's safety and efficacy in patients with carbapenem resistant Gram-negative infections. Regarding *P. aeruginosa* infections, twelve (15%) were initiated in the cefiderocol arm and 10 (26%) in the BAT arm. All-cause mortality regarding *P. aeruginosa* infections was 35% (6/17) vs. 17% (2/12) in the BAT arm. Data reported also depicted that cefiderocol had a greater all-cause mortality compared with BAT at day 14 (6.6% difference), day 28 (18.4% difference), and day 49 (20.4% difference) of treatment [109]. In another phase III trial, APEKS-NP, when filtering results for *P. aeruginosa* as the cultured organism, a total of 24 (17%) and 24 (16%) were included in the cefiderocol and meropenem arm, respectively. All-cause mortality at 14-day was similar for both groups [8% vs. 13%, −4.7 (−22.4 to 12.9)] and clinical cure was 16/24 (67%) vs. 17/24 (71%) (−4.2, −30.4 to 22.0), respectively [112]. In real life conditions, seventeen patients with MDR *P. aeruginosa* treated with cefiderocol have been reported. The most common infection was associated with VAP infections (41.2%), occurring in COVID-19 patients, with 88.2% of the patients admitted to the ICU. Clinical cure and microbiological cure rates were 70.6% and 76.5%, respectively [66].

4.4. Salvage Therapy

Salvage therapy for the treatment of pandrug *P. aeruginosa* has been proposed with amikacin monotherapy adapted to the MIC of the pathogen. Two patients with severe sepsis (secondary BSI due to IAI and HAP) due to pan-resistant *P. aeruginosa*, were successfully treated with a high daily dose of amikacin, given as monotherapy, and combined with continuous venovenous hemodiafiltration (CVVHDF). Both patients were cured with a high daily dose (25 to 50 mg/kg) of amikacin to obtain a peak/MIC ratio of at least 8 to 10 (MIC of both isolates was 16 mg/L). CVVHDF provided no deterioration in renal function after treatment. High dosage of aminoglycosides combined with CVVHDF may represent a valuable therapeutic option for infection due to PDR *P. aeruginosa*; however, the limited number (only two cases) treated with this unique therapeutic agent [123] should be taken into consideration. Salvage therapeutic options are illustrated in Table 2.

In conclusion, the new β-lactam-β-lactamase inhibitors, i.e., cefepime-taniborbactam and aztreonam-avibactam, seem to be promising agents active in vitro against carbapenem-resistant *P. aeruginosa*, including pathogens producing MBL [124,125]. The combination cefepime–taniborbactam is a potential alternative treatment option for PDR infections, particularly those caused by MBL-producing isolates [124]. However, the combination of aztreonam plus avibactam appears to be an encouraging option against MBL-producing bacteria, especially for Enterobacterales, but much less so for *P. aeruginosa* infections [125].

Table 2. Salvage therapeutic options for DTR and PDR Gram-negative pathogens.

Antibiotic	Spectrum of Activity	Mechanism of Action	Dosage (Normal Renal Function)	Comments on DTR and PDR
Ampicillin-sulbactam *plus* Tigecycline *plus* Colistin [106]	**Activity against:** PDR *A. baumannii* [106]	Based on in vitro synergistic combinations [106]	**Ampicillin-sulbactam:** 9 gr IV every 8 h, infused over 3 h *plus* **Tigecycline:** 100 mg IV every 12 h (Loading dose of 200 mg IV tigecycline) *plus* **CMS (colistin):** 4.5 MU IV every 12 h (Loading dose 9 MU IV CMS) [106]	***A. baumannii:*** Clinical studies on PDR *A. baumannii* (7 cases) with favorable clinical outcome of 100% [106]
Ampicillin-sulbactam *plus* Meropenem *plus* Colistin [107]	**Activity against:** PDR *A. baumannii* [105,107]	Based on in vitro synergistic combinations [100,105]	**Ampicillin-sulbactam:** 9 gr IV every 8 h, infused over 3 h *plus* **Meropenem:** 2 gr IV every 8 h, infused over 3 h *plus* **CMS (colistin):** 4.5 MU IV every 12 h (Loading dose 9 MU IV CMS) [107]	***A. baumannii:*** Clinical studies on PDR *A. baumannii* (10 cases) with favorable clinical outcome of 90% [107]
High daly dose of amikacin in combination with CVVHDF [123]	**Activity against:** PDR *P. aeruginosa* [123]	Increased exposure regimen adapted to MIC of the pathogen [123]	Amikacin: 25 to 50 mg/kg IV (to obtain a peak/MIC of at least 8 to 10) *plus* CVVHDF [123]	***P. aeruginosa:*** Clinical data limited to two cases of PDR *P. aeruginosa* with secondary bacteremia due to cIAI and HAP with favorable clinical outcome [123]
Double carbapenem [13]	**Activity against:** *K. pneumoniae* producing KPC and OXA-48 [13–20]	Ertapenem higher affinity with the carbapenemase enzyme, acting as a suicide inhibitor, thus allowing higher levels of the other carbapenems (meropenem or doripenem) to be active in the vicinity of the pathogen [13]	1 gr IV ertapenem every 24 h, infused over 1 h *plus* 2 gr meropenem every 8 h, infused over 3 h [13–15]	***K. pneumoniae:*** Real life clinical studies on XDR and PDR *K. pneumoniae* with favorable clinical outcome of 65% [13–20]

cIAI, complicated intrabdominal infection; CMS, colistin methanesulfonate; CVVHDF, continuous venovenous hemodiafiltration; DTR, difficult to treat resistance; HAP, hospital acquired pneumonia; IV, intravenous; KPC, *Klebsiella pneumoniae* carbapenemase; MBL, metallo-β-lactamase; MIC, minimum inhibitory concentration; MU, million international units; PDR, pandrug-resistant; XDR, extensively drug-resistant.

5. Conclusions

PDR and DTR Gram-negative infections have increasingly been reported globally in recent years and are linked to high mortality rates. There is "no standard of care" treatment regimen for the therapy of PDR and DTR Gram-negative infections, and therapeutic options are extremely limited. Synergistic combinations (double and triple combinations) seem quite promising; however, data are restricted to case reports and case series. The introduction of novel antimicrobials and mainly β-lactam-β-lactamase inhibitor combinations, as well as cefiderocol and eravacycline, are of great potential. However, the efficacy of novel antimicrobial agents for the treatment of PDR and DTR Gram-negative infections is to be elucidated in real-life studies in the near future.

Author Contributions: H.G. and I.K. have written and revised the manuscript. All authors have read and agreed to the published version of the manuscript.

Funding: This research received no external funding.

Conflicts of Interest: H.G. has received speaker honoraria from Pfizer and MSD. I.K. has received speaker honoraria from Pfizer.

References

1. Murray, C.J.; Ikuta, K.S.; Sharara, F.; Swetschinski, L.; Aguilar, G.R.; Gray, A.; Han, C.; Bisignano, C.; Rao, P.; Wool, E.; et al. Global burden of bacterial antimicrobial resistance in 2019: A systematic analysis. *Lancet* **2022**, *399*, 629–655. [CrossRef]
2. Nordmann, P.; Poirel, L. Epidemiology and diagnostics of carbapenem resistance in Gram-negative Bacteria. *Clin. Infect. Dis.* **2019**, *69* (Suppl. 7), S521–S528. [CrossRef] [PubMed]
3. World Health Organization. Global Priority List of Antibiotic-Resistant Bacteria to Guide Research, Discovery, and Development of New Antibiotics. 2017. Available online: https://www.who.int/news/item/27-02-2017-who-publishes-list-of-bacteria-for-which-new-antibiotics-are-urgently-needed (accessed on 15 July 2022).
4. Tabak, Y.P.; Sung, A.H.; Ye, G.; Vankeepuram, L.; Gupta, V.; McCann, E. Attributable clinical and economic burden of carbapenem-non-susceptible Gram-negative infections in patients hospitalized with complicated urinary tract infections. *J. Hosp. Infect.* **2019**, *102*, 37–44. [PubMed]
5. Pogue, J.M.; Zhou, Y.; Kanakamedala, H.; Cai, B. Burden of illness in carbapenem-resistant *Acinetobacter baumannii* infections in US hospitals between 2014 and 2019. *BMC Infect. Dis.* **2022**, *22*, 36. [CrossRef] [PubMed]
6. Magiorakos, A.P.; Srinivasan, A.; Carey, R.B.; Carmeli, Y.; Falagas, M.E.; Giske, C.G.; Harbarth, S.; Hindler, J.F.; Kahlmeter, G.; Olsson-Liljequist, B.; et al. Multidrug-resistant, extensively drug-resistant and pandrug-resistant bacteria: An international expert proposal for interim standard definitions for acquired resistance. *Clin. Microbiol. Infect.* **2012**, *18*, 268–281. [CrossRef] [PubMed]
7. Karaiskos, I.; Galani, I.; Papoutsaki, V.; Galani, L.; Giamarellou, H. Carbapenemase producing *Klebsiella pneumoniae*: Implication on future therapeutic strategies. *Expert Rev. Anti-Infect. Ther.* **2022**, *20*, 53–69. [CrossRef] [PubMed]
8. Kadri, S.S.; Adjemian, J.; Lai, Y.L.; Spaulding, A.B.; Ricotta, E.; Prevots, D.R.; Palmore, T.N.; Rhee, C.; Klompas, M.; Dekker, J.P.; et al. Difficult-to-treat resistance in Gram-negative bacteremia at 173 US hospitals: Retrospective cohort analysis of prevalence, predictors, and outcome of resistance to all first-line agents. *Clin. Infect. Dis.* **2018**, *67*, 1803–1814. [PubMed]
9. Karakonstantis, S.; Kritsotakis, E.I.; Gikas, A. Pandrug-resistant Gram-negative bacteria: A systematic review of current epidemiology, prognosis and treatment options. *J. Antimicrob. Chemother.* **2020**, *75*, 271–282. [CrossRef]
10. Kofteridis, D.P.; Andrianaki, A.M.; Maraki, S.; Mathioudaki, A.; Plataki, M.; Alexopoulou, C.; Ioannou, P.; Samonis, G.; Valachis, A. Treatment pattern, prognostic factors, and outcome in patients with infection due to pan-drug-resistant gram-negative bacteria. *Eur. J. Clin. Microbiol. Infect. Dis.* **2020**, *39*, 965–970. [CrossRef]
11. Giamarellou, H. Epidemiology of infections caused by polymyxin-resistant pathogens. *Int. J. Antimicrob. Agents* **2016**, *48*, 614–621. [CrossRef]
12. Papadimitriou-Olivgeris, M.; Bartzavali, C.; Georgakopoulou, A.; Kolonitsiou, F.; Papamichail, C.; Spiliopoulou, I.; Christofidou, M.; Fligou, F.; Marangos, M. Mortality of Pandrug-Resistant *Klebsiella pneumoniae* bloodstream infections in critically ill patients: A Retrospective cohort of 115 episodes. *Antibiotics* **2021**, *10*, 76. [CrossRef]
13. Bulik, C.C.; Nicolau, D.P. Double-carbapenem therapy for carbapenemase-producing *Klebsiella pneumoniae*. *Antimicrob. Agents Chemother.* **2011**, *55*, 3002–3004. [CrossRef]
14. Giamarellou, H.; Galani, L.; Baziaka, F.; Karaiskos, I. Effectiveness of a double-carbapenem regimen for infections in humans due to carbapenemase-producing pandrug-resistant *Klebsiella pneumoniae*. *Antimicrob. Agents Chemother.* **2013**, *57*, 2388–2390. [CrossRef] [PubMed]
15. Souli, M.; Karaiskos, I.; Masgala, A.; Galani, L.; Barmpouti, E.; Giamarellou, H. Double-carbapenem combination as salvage therapy for untreatable infections by KPC-2-producing *Klebsiella pneumoniae*. *Eur. J. Clin. Microbiol. Infect. Dis.* **2017**, *36*, 1305–1315. [CrossRef] [PubMed]

16. Tumbarello, M.; Trecarichi, E.M.; De Rosa, F.G.; Giannella, M.; Giacobbe, D.R.; Bassetti, M.; Losito, A.R.; Bartoletti, M.; Del Bono, V.; Corcione, S.; et al. Infections caused by KPC-producing *Klebsiella pneumoniae*: Differences in therapy and mortality in a multicentre study. *J. Antimicrob. Chemother.* **2015**, *70*, 2133–2143. [CrossRef] [PubMed]
17. Oliva, A.; Gizzi, F.; Mascellino, M.T.; Cipolla, A.; D'Abramo, A.; D'Agostino, C.; Trinchieri, V.; Russo, G.; Tierno, F.; Iannetta, M.; et al. Bactericidal and synergistic activity of double-carbapenem regimen for infections caused by carbapenemase-producing *Klebsiella pneumoniae*. *Clin. Microbiol. Infect.* **2016**, *22*, 147–153. [CrossRef] [PubMed]
18. Cprek, J.B.; Gallagher, J.C. Ertapenem-containing double-carbapenem therapy for treatment of infections caused by carbapenem-resistant *Klebsiella pneumoniae*. *Antimicrob. Agents Chemother.* **2015**, *60*, 669–673. [CrossRef] [PubMed]
19. Oliva, A.; Scorzolini, L.; Castaldi, D.; Gizzi, F.; De Angelis, M.; Storto, M.; D'Abramo, A.; Aloj, F.; Mascellino, M.T.; Mastroianni, C.M.; et al. Double-carbapenem regimen, alone or in combination with colistin, in the treatment of infections caused by carbapenem-resistant *Klebsiella pneumoniae* (CR-Kp). *J. Infect.* **2017**, *74*, 103–106. [CrossRef] [PubMed]
20. Li, Y.Y.; Wang, J.; Wang, R.; Cai, Y. Double-carbapenem therapy in the treatment of multidrug resistant Gram-negative bacterial infections: A systematic review and meta-analysis. *BMC Infect. Dis.* **2020**, *20*, 408. [CrossRef] [PubMed]
21. Yahav, D.; Giske, C.G.; Grāmatniece, A.; Abodakpi, H.; Tam, V.H.; Leibovici, L. A new β-lactam-β-lactamase inhibitor combinations. *Clin. Microbiol. Rev.* **2020**, *34*, e00115-20. [CrossRef] [PubMed]
22. Galani, I.; Karaiskos, I.; Giamarellou, H. Multidrug-resistant *Klebsiella pneumoniae*: Mechanisms of resistance including updated data for novel β-lactam-β-lactamase inhibitor combinations. *Expert Rev. Anti Infect. Ther.* **2021**, *19*, 1457–1468. [CrossRef]
23. FDA. AVYCAZ (Ceftazidime and Avibactam) for Injection, for Intravenous Use. 2019. Available online: https://www.accessdata.fda.gov/drugsatfda_docs/label/2019/206494s005,s006lbl.pdf (accessed on 15 July 2022).
24. European Medicines Agency. Zavicefta: Summary of Product Characteristics. 2018. Available online: https://www.ema.europa.eu/en/documents/product-information/zavicefta-epar-product-information_en.pdf (accessed on 15 July 2022).
25. Tamma, P.D.; Aitken, S.L.; Bonomo, R.A.; Mathers, A.J.; van Duin, D.; Clancy, C.J. Infectious Diseases Society of America Guidance on the Treatment of Extended-Spectrum β-lactamase producing Enterobacterales (ESBL-E), Carbapenem-Resistant Enterobacterales (CRE), and *Pseudomonas aeruginosa* with Difficult-to-Treat Resistance (DTR-*P. aeruginosa*). *Clin. Infect. Dis.* **2021**, *72*, e169–e183. [PubMed]
26. Shields, R.K.; Nguyen, M.H.; Chen, L.; Press, E.G.; Potoski, B.A.; Marini, R.V.; Doi, Y.; Kreiswirth, B.N.; Clancy, C.J. Ceftazidime-Avibactam is superior to other treatment regimens against carbapenem-resistant *Klebsiella pneumoniae* bacteremia. *Antimicrob. Agents Chemother.* **2017**, *61*, e00883-17. [CrossRef] [PubMed]
27. Van Duin, D.; Lok, J.J.; Earley, M.; Cober, E.; Richter, S.S.; Pérez, F.; Salata, R.A.; Kalayjian, R.C.; Watkins, R.R.; Doi, Y.; et al. Colistin versus ceftazidime-avibactam in the treatment of infections due to carbapenem-resistant Enterobacteriaceae. *Clin. Infect. Dis.* **2018**, *66*, 163–171. [CrossRef] [PubMed]
28. Castón, J.J.; Cano, A.; Pérez-Camacho, I.; Aguado, J.M.; Carratalá, J.; Ramasco, F.; Soriano, A.; Pintado, V.; Castelo-Corral, L.; Sousa, A.; et al. Impact of ceftazidime/avibactam versus best available therapy on mortality from infections caused by carbapenemase-producing Enterobacterales (CAVICOR study). *J. Antimicrob. Chemother.* **2022**, *77*, 1452–1460. [CrossRef]
29. Jorgensen, S.C.J.; Trinh, T.D.; Zasowski, E.J.; Lagnf, A.M.; Bhatia, S.; Melvin, S.M.; Steed, M.E.; Simon, S.P.; Estrada, S.J.; Morrisette, T.; et al. Real-world experience with ceftazidime-avibactam for multidrug-resistant gram-negative bacterial infections. *Open Forum Infect. Dis.* **2019**, *6*, ofz522. [CrossRef] [PubMed]
30. Tsolaki, V.; Mantzarlis, K.; Mpakalis, A.; Malli, E.; Tsimpoukas, F.; Tsirogianni, A.; Papagiannitsis, C.; Zygoulis, P.; Papadonta, M.E.; Petinaki, E.; et al. Ceftazidime-avibactam to treat life-threatening infections by carbapenem-resistant pathogens in critically ill mechanically ventilated patients. *Antimicrob. Agents Chemother.* **2020**, *64*, e02320-19. [CrossRef] [PubMed]
31. Karaiskos, I.; Daikos, G.L.; Gkoufa, A.; Adamis, G.; Stefos, A.; Symbardi, S.; Chrysos, G.; Filiou, E.; Basoulis, D.; Mouloudi, E.; et al. Ceftazidime/avibactam in the era of carbapenemase-producing *Klebsiella pneumoniae*: Experience from a national registry study. *J. Antimicrob. Chemother.* **2021**, *76*, 775–783. [CrossRef] [PubMed]
32. Tumbarello, M.; Raffaelli, F.; Giannella, M.; Mantengoli, E.; Mularoni, A.; Venditti, M.; De Rosa, F.G.; Sarmati, L.; Bassetti, M.; Brindicci, G.; et al. Ceftazidime-avibactam use for *Klebsiella pneumoniae* carbapenemase-producing *K. pneumoniae* infections: A retrospective observational multicenter study. *Clin. Infect. Dis.* **2021**, *73*, 1664–1676. [CrossRef] [PubMed]
33. Camargo, J.F.; Simkins, J.; Beduschi, T.; Tekin, A.; Aragon, L.; Pérez-Cardona, A.; Prado, C.E.; Morris, M.I.; Abbo, L.M.; Cantón, R. Successful treatment of carbapenemase-producing pandrug-resistant *Klebsiella pneumoniae* bacteremia. *Antimicrob. Agents Chemother.* **2015**, *59*, 5903–5908. [CrossRef] [PubMed]
34. Eskenazi, A.; Lood, C.; Wubbolts, J.; Hites, M.; Balarjishvili, N.; Leshkasheli, L.; Askilashvili, L.; Kvachadze, L.; van Noort, V.; Wagemans, J.; et al. Combination of pre-adapted bacteriophage therapy and antibiotics for treatment of fracture-related infection due to pandrug-resistant *Klebsiella pneumoniae*. *Nat. Commun.* **2022**, *13*, 302. [CrossRef] [PubMed]
35. Parruti, G.; Frattari, A.; Polilli, E.; Savini, V.; Sciacca, A.; Consorte, A.; Cibelli, D.C.; Agostinone, A.; Di Masi, F.; Pieri, A.; et al. Cure of recurring *Klebsiella pneumoniae* carbapenemase-producing *Klebsiella pneumoniae* septic shock episodes due to complicated soft tissue infection using a ceftazidime and avibactam-based regimen: A case report. *J. Med. Case Rep.* **2019**, *13*, 20. [CrossRef] [PubMed]
36. Mandrawa, C.L.; Cronin, K.; Buising, K.L.; Poy Lorenzo, Y.S.; Waters, M.J.; Jeremiah, C.J. Carbapenemase-producing *Klebsiella pneumoniae*: A major clinical challenge. *Med. J. Aust.* **2016**, *204*, 277–278. [CrossRef] [PubMed]

37. Coskun, Y.; Atici, S. Successful treatment of pandrug-resistant *Klebsiella pneumoniae* infection with ceftazidime-avibactam in a preterm infant: A case report. *Pediatr. Infect. Dis. J.* **2020**, *39*, 854–856. [CrossRef] [PubMed]
38. Iosifidis, E.; Chorafa, E.; Agakidou, E.; Kontou, A.; Violaki, A.; Volakli, E.; Christou, E.I.; Zarras, C.; Drossou-Agakidou, V.; Sdougka, M.; et al. Use of Ceftazidime-avibactam for the Treatment of Extensively drug-resistant or Pan drug-resistant *Klebsiella pneumoniae* in Neonates and Children <5 Years of Age. *Pediatr. Infect. Dis. J.* **2019**, *38*, 812–815. [CrossRef] [PubMed]
39. Daikos, G.L.; da Cunha, C.A.; Rossolini, G.M.; Stone, G.G.; Baillon-Plot, N.; Tawadrous, M.; Irani, P. Review of ceftazidime-avibactam for the treatment of infections caused by *Pseudomonas aeruginosa*. *Antibiotics* **2021**, *10*, 1126. [CrossRef] [PubMed]
40. Corbella, L.; Boán, J.; San-Juan, R.; Fernández-Ruiz, M.; Carretero, O.; Lora, D.; Hernández-Jiménez, P.; Ruiz-Ruigómez, M.; Rodríguez-Goncer, I.; Silva, J.T.; et al. Effectiveness of ceftazidime-avibactam for the treatment of infections due to *Pseudomonas aeruginosa*. *Int. J. Antimicrob. Agents* **2022**, *59*, 106517. [CrossRef]
41. Soriano, A.; Carmeli, Y.; Omrani, A.S.; Moore, L.S.P.; Tawadrous, M.; Irani, P. Ceftazidime-Avibactam for the treatment of serious Gram-Negative infections with limited treatment options: A systematic literature review. *Infect. Dis. Ther.* **2021**, *10*, 1989–2034. [CrossRef]
42. Vabomere® (Meropenem/Vaborbactam for Injection) [Prescribing Information]; U.S. Food and Drug Administration (FDA). 2020. Available online: https://www.accessdata.fda.gov/drugsatfda_docs/label/2020/209776s003lbl.pdf (accessed on 15 July 2022).
43. European Medicines Agency (EMA). Vaborem Product Information. 2018. Available online: https://www.ema.europa.eu/en/documents/product-information/vaborem-epar-product-information_en.pdf (accessed on 15 July 2022).
44. Shields, R.K.; McCreary, E.K.; Marini, R.V.; Kline, E.G.; Jones, C.E.; Hao, B.; Chen, L.; Kreiswirth, B.N.; Doi, Y.; Clancy, C.J.; et al. Early experience with meropenem-vaborbactam for treatment of carbapenem-resistant Enterobacteriaceae infections. *Clin. Infect. Dis.* **2020**, *71*, 667–671. [CrossRef] [PubMed]
45. Alosaimy, S.; Jorgensen, S.C.J.; Lagnf, A.M.; Melvin, S.; Mynatt, R.P.; Carlson, T.J.; Garey, K.W.; Allen, D.; Venugopalan, V.; Veve, M.; et al. Real-world multicenter analysis of clinical outcomes and safety of meropenem-vaborbactam in patients treated for serious gram-negative bacterial infections. *Open Forum Infect. Dis.* **2020**, *7*, ofaa051. [CrossRef]
46. Ackley, R.; Roshdy, D.; Meredith, J.; Minor, S.; Anderson, W.E.; Capraro, G.A.; Polk, C. Meropenem-vaborbactam versus ceftazidime-avibactam for treatment of carbapenem-resistant Enterobacteriaceae infections. *Antimicrob. Agents Chemother.* **2020**, *64*, e02313-19. [CrossRef] [PubMed]
47. FDA (RECARBRIO) Imipenem-Cilastatin-Relebactam Injection. 2020. Available online: https://www.accessdata.fda.gov/drugsatfda_docs/label/2020/212819s002lbl.pdf (accessed on 15 July 2022).
48. EMA. Recarbrio (Imipenem-Cilastatin-Relebactam). Summary of Product Characteristics. 2020. Available online: https://www.ema.europa.eu/en/documents/product-information/recarbrio-epar-product-information_en.pdf (accessed on 15 July 2022).
49. Motsch, J.; Murta de Oliveira, C.; Stus, V.; Köksal, I.; Lyulko, O.; Boucher, H.W.; Kaye, K.S.; File, T.M.; Brown, M.L.; Khan, I.; et al. RESTORE-IMI 1: A multicenter, randomized, double-blind trial comparing efficacy and safety of imipenem/relebactam vs colistin plus imipenem in patients with imipenem-nonsusceptible bacterial infections. *Clin. Infect. Dis.* **2020**, *70*, 1799–1808. [CrossRef]
50. Rebold, N.; Morrisette, T.; Lagnf, A.M.; Alosaimy, S.; Holger, D.; Barber, K.; Justo, J.A.; Antosz, K.; Carlson, T.J.; Frens, J.J.; et al. Early multicenter experience with Imipenem-Cilastatin-Relebactam for multidrug-resistant Gram-Negative infections. *Open Forum Infect. Dis.* **2021**, *8*, ofab554. [CrossRef] [PubMed]
51. Giacobbe, D.R.; Bassetti, M.; De Rosa, F.G.; Del Bono, V.; Grossi, P.A.; Menichetti, F.; Pea, F.; Rossolini, G.M.; Tumbarello, M.; Viale, P.; et al. ISGRI-SITA (Italian Study Group on Resistant Infections of the Società Italiana Terapia Antinfettiva). Ceftolozane/tazobactam: Place in therapy. *Expert Rev. Anti Infect. Ther.* **2018**, *16*, 307–320. [CrossRef] [PubMed]
52. Fraile-Ribot, P.A.; Cabot, G.; Mulet, X.; Periañez, L.; Martín-Pena, M.L.; Juan, C.; Pérez, J.L.; Oliver, A. Mechanisms leading to in vivo ceftolozane/tazobactam resistance development during the treatment of infections caused by MDR *Pseudomonas aeruginosa*. *J. Antimicrob. Chemother.* **2018**, *73*, 658–663. [CrossRef] [PubMed]
53. FDA. Drug Approval Package: Zerbaxa (Ceftolozane/Tazobactam). Injection. 2019. Available online: https://www.accessdata.fda.gov/drugsatfda_docs/label/2019/206829s008lbl.pdf (accessed on 15 July 2022).
54. EMA. Drug Approval Package: Zerbaxa (Ceftolozane/Tazobactam). Injection. 2015. Available online: https://www.ema.europa.eu/en/documents/product-information/zerbaxa-epar-product-information_en.pdf (accessed on 15 July 2022).
55. Jorgensen, S.C.J.; Trinh, T.D.; Zasowski, E.J.; Lagnf, A.M.; Simon, S.P.; Bhatia, S.; Melvin, S.M.; Steed, M.E.; Finch, N.A.; Morrisette, T.; et al. Real-world experience with ceftolozane-tazobactam for multidrug-resistant Gram-Negative bacterial infections. *Antimicrob. Agents Chemother.* **2020**, *64*, e02291-19. [CrossRef] [PubMed]
56. Bassetti, M.; Castaldo, N.; Cattelan, A.; Mussini, C.; Righi, E.; Tascini, C.; Menichetti, F.; Mastroianni, C.M.; Tumbarello, M.; Grossi, P.; et al. Ceftolozane/tazobactam for the treatment of serious *Pseudomonas aeruginosa* infections: A multicentre nationwide clinical experience. *Int. J. Antimicrob. Agents* **2019**, *53*, 408–415. [CrossRef]
57. Balandin, B.; Ballesteros, D.; Ruiz de Luna, R.; López-Vergara, L.; Pintado, V.; Sancho-González, M.; Soriano-Cuesta, C.; Pérez-Pedrero, M.J.; Asensio-Martín, M.J.; Fernández-Simón, I.; et al. Multicenter study of ceftolozane/tazobactam for treatment of *Pseudomonas aeruginosa* infections in critically ill patients. *Int. J. Antimicrob. Agents* **2021**, *57*, 106270. [CrossRef]
58. Niu, S.; Wei, J.; Zou, C.; Chavda, K.D.; Lv, J.; Zhang, H.; Du, H.; Tang, Y.W.; Pitout, J.D.D.; Bonomo, R.A.; et al. In vitro selection of aztreonam/avibactam resistance in dual-carbapenemase-producing *Klebsiella pneumoniae*. *J. Antimicrob. Chemother.* **2020**, *75*, 559–565. [CrossRef] [PubMed]

59. Falcone, M.; Daikos, G.L.; Tiseo, G.; Bassoulis, D.; Giordano, C.; Galfo, V.; Leonildi, A.; Tagliaferri, E.; Barnini, S.; Sani, S.; et al. Efficacy of ceftazidime-avibactam plus aztreonam in patients with bloodstream infections caused by metallo-β-lactamase-producing Enterobacterales. *Clin. Infect. Dis.* **2021**, *72*, 1871–1878. [CrossRef]
60. Alghoribi, M.F.; Alqurashi, M.; Okdah, L.; Alalwan, B.; AlHebaishi, Y.S.; Almalki, A.; Alzayer, M.A.; Alswaji, A.A.; Doumith, M.; Barry, M. Successful treatment of infective endocarditis due to pandrug-resistant *Klebsiella pneumoniae* with ceftazidime-avibactam and aztreonam. *Sci. Rep.* **2021**, *11*, 9684. [CrossRef] [PubMed]
61. Sato, T.; Yamawaki, K. Cefiderocol: Discovery, chemistry, and in vivo profiles of a novel siderophore cephalosporin. *Clin. Infect. Dis.* **2019**, *69* (Suppl. 7), S538–S543. [CrossRef] [PubMed]
62. Giacobbe, D.R.; Ciacco, E.; Girmenia, C.; Pea, F.; Rossolini, G.M.; Sotgiu, G.; Tascini, C.; Tumbarello, M.; Viale, P.; Bassetti, M.; et al. Evaluating cefiderocol in the treatment of multidrug-resistant Gram-negative bacilli: A review of the emerging data. *Infect. Drug Resist.* **2020**, *13*, 4697–4711. [CrossRef] [PubMed]
63. Karakonstantis, S.; Rousaki, M.; Kritsotakis, E.I. Cefiderocol: Systematic review of mechanisms of resistance, heteroresistance and in vivo emergence of resistance. *Antibiotics* **2022**, *11*, 723. [CrossRef]
64. FETROJA (Cefiderocol)—U.S. Food and Drug Administration (FDA). 2020. Available online: https://www.accessdata.fda.gov/drugsatfda_docs/label/2020/209445s002lbl.pdf (accessed on 15 July 2022).
65. Fetcroja (Cefiderocol)—European Medicines Agency (EMA). 2020. Available online: https://www.ema.europa.eu/en/documents/product-information/fetcroja-epar-product-information_en.pdf (accessed on 15 July 2022).
66. Meschiari, M.; Volpi, S.; Faltoni, M.; Dolci, G.; Orlando, G.; Franceschini, E.; Menozzi, M.; Sarti, M.; Del Fabro, G.; Fumarola, B.; et al. Real-life experience with compassionate use of cefiderocol for difficult-to-treat resistant *Pseudomonas aeruginosa* (DTR-P) infections. *JAC Antimicrob. Resist.* **2021**, *3*, dlab188. [CrossRef] [PubMed]
67. Babidhan, R.; Lewis, A.; Atkins, C.; Jozefczyk, N.J.; Nemecek, B.D.; Montepara, C.A.; Gionfriddo, M.R.; Zimmerman, D.E.; Covvey, J.R.; Guarascio, A.J. Safety and efficacy of cefiderocol for off-label treatment indications: A systematic review. *Pharmacotherapy* **2022**, *42*, 549–566. [CrossRef]
68. Lee, Y.R.; Burton, C.E. Eravacycline, a newly approved fluorocycline. *Eur. J. Clin. Microbiol. Infect. Dis.* **2019**, *38*, 1787–1794. [CrossRef]
69. XERAVA (Eravacycline) for Injection—FDA. 2018. Available online: https://www.accessdata.fda.gov/drugsatfda_docs/label/2018/211109lbl.pdf (accessed on 15 July 2022).
70. XERAVA (Eravacycline)—EMA. 2018. Available online: https://www.ema.europa.eu/en/documents/product-information/xerava-epar-product-information_en.pdf (accessed on 15 July 2022).
71. Scott, C.J.; Zhu, E.; Jayakumar, R.A.; Shan, G.; Viswesh, V. Efficacy of eravacycline versus best previously available therapy for adults with pneumonia due to difficult-to-treat resistant (DTR) *Acinetobacter baumannii*. *Ann. Pharmacother.* **2022**, 10600280221085551. [CrossRef]
72. Maraki, S.; Mavromanolaki, V.E.; Magkafouraki, E.; Moraitis, P.; Stafylaki, D.; Kasimati, A.; Scoulica, E. Epidemiology and in vitro activity of ceftazidime-avibactam, meropenem-vaborbactam, imipenem-relebactam, eravacycline, plazomicin, and comparators against Greek carbapenemase-producing *Klebsiella pneumoniae* isolates. *Infection* **2022**, *50*, 467–474. [CrossRef]
73. Galani, I.; Karaiskos, I.; Karantani, I.; Papoutsaki, V.; Maraki, S.; Papaioannou, V.; Kazila, P.; Tsorlini, H.; Charalampaki, N.; Toutouza, M.; et al. Epidemiology and resistance phenotypes of carbapenemase-producing *Klebsiella pneumoniae* in Greece, 2014 to 2016. *Eurosurveillance* **2018**, *23*, 1700775. [CrossRef]
74. Voulgari, E.; Kotsakis, S.D.; Giannopoulou, P.; Perivolioti, E.; Tzouvelekis, L.S.; Miriagou, V. Detection in two hospitals of transferable ceftazidime-avibactam resistance in *Klebsiella pneumoniae* due to a novel VEB β-lactamase variant with a Lys234Arg substitution, Greece, 2019. *Eurosurveillance* **2020**, *25*, 1900766. [CrossRef] [PubMed]
75. Galani, I.; Karaiskos, I.; Souli, M.; Papoutsaki, V.; Galani, L.; Gkoufa, A.; Antoniadou, A.; Giamarellou, H. Outbreak of KPC-2-producing *Klebsiella pneumoniae* endowed with ceftazidime-avibactam resistance mediated through a VEB-1-mutant (VEB-25), Greece, September to October 2019. *Eurosurveillance* **2020**, *25*, 2000028. [CrossRef] [PubMed]
76. Esposito, S.; Stone, G.G.; Papaparaskevas, J. in vitro activity of aztreonam/avibactam against a global collection of *Klebsiella pneumoniae* collected from defined culture sources in 2016 and 2017. *J. Glob. Antimicrob. Resist.* **2021**, *24*, 14–22. [CrossRef] [PubMed]
77. Sader, H.S.; Carvalhaes, C.G.; Arends, S.J.R.; Castanheira, M.; Mendes, R.E. Aztreonam/avibactam activity against clinical isolates of Enterobacterales collected in Europe, Asia and Latin America in 2019. *J. Antimicrob. Chemother.* **2021**, *76*, 659–666. [CrossRef] [PubMed]
78. Carpenter, J.; Neidig, N.; Campbell, A.; Thornsberry, T.; Truex, T.; Fortney, T.; Zhang, Y.; Bush, K. Activity of imipenem/relebactam against carbapenemase-producing Enterobacteriaceae with high colistin resistance. *J. Antimicrob. Chemother.* **2019**, *74*, 3260–3263. [CrossRef] [PubMed]
79. Galani, I.; Souli, M.; Nafplioti, K.; Adamou, P.; Karaiskos, I.; Giamarellou, H.; Antoniadou, A.; Study Collaborators. In vitro activity of imipenem-relebactam against non-MBL carbapenemase-producing *Klebsiella pneumoniae* isolated in Greek hospitals in 2015–2016. *Eur. J. Clin. Microbiol. Infect. Dis.* **2019**, *38*, 1143–1150, Correction in *Eur. J. Clin. Microbiol. Infect. Dis.* **2019**, *38*, 1151–1152. [CrossRef]

80. Wunderink, R.G.; Giamarellos-Bourboulis, E.J.; Rahav, G.; Mathers, A.J.; Bassetti, M.; Vazquez, J.; Cornely, O.A.; Solomkin, J.; Bhowmick, T.; Bishara, J.; et al. Effect and safety of meropenem-vaborbactam versus best-available therapy in patients with carbapenem-resistant Enterobacteriaceae infections: The TANGO II randomized clinical trial. *Infect. Dis. Ther.* **2018**, *7*, 439–455. [CrossRef]
81. Nguyen, M.; Joshi, S.G. Carbapenem resistance in *Acinetobacter baumannii*, and their importance in hospital-acquired infections: A scientific review. *Appl. Microbiol.* **2021**, *131*, 2715–2738. [CrossRef]
82. Peleg, A.Y.; Seifert, H.; Paterson, D.L. *Acinetobacter baumannii*: Emergence of a successful pathogen. *Clin. Microbiol. Rev.* **2008**, *21*, 538–582. [CrossRef]
83. Karakonstantis, S.; Gikas, A.; Astrinaki, E.; Kritsotakis, E.I. Excess mortality due to pandrug-resistant *Acinetobacter baumannii* infections in hospitalized patients. *J. Hosp. Infect.* **2020**, *106*, 447–453. [CrossRef]
84. Karaiskos, I.; Lagou, S.; Pontikis, K.; Rapti, V.; Poulakou, G. The "Old" and the "New" antibiotics for MDR Gram-negative pathogens: For whom, when, and how. *Front. Public Health* **2019**, *7*, 151. [CrossRef] [PubMed]
85. Tamma, P.D.; Aitken, S.L.; Bonomo, R.A.; Mathers, A.J.; van Duin, D.; Clancy, C.J. Infectious Diseases Society of America guidance on the treatment of AmpC β-lactamase-producing Enterobacterales, carbapenem-resistant *Acinetobacter baumannii*, and *Stenotrophomonas maltophilia* infections. *Clin. Infect. Dis.* **2022**, *74*, ciab1013. [CrossRef] [PubMed]
86. Abdul-Mutakabbir, J.C.; Griffith, N.C.; Shields, R.K.; Tverdek, F.P.; Escobar, Z.K. Contemporary perspective on the treatment of *Acinetobacter baumannii* infections: Insights from the society of infectious diseases pharmacists. *Infect. Dis. Ther.* **2021**, *10*, 2177–2202. [CrossRef]
87. Betrosian, A.P.; Frantzeskaki, F.; Xanthaki, A.; Georgiadis, G. High-dose ampicillin-sulbactam as an alternative treatment of late-onset VAP from multidrug-resistant *Acinetobacter baumannii*. *Scand. J. Infect. Dis.* **2007**, *39*, 38–43. [CrossRef]
88. Liu, J.; Shu, Y.; Zhu, F.; Feng, B.; Zhang, Z.; Liu, L.; Wang, G. Comparative efficacy and safety of combination therapy with high-dose sulbactam or colistin with additional antibacterial agents for multiple drug-resistant and extensively drug-resistant *Acinetobacter baumannii* infections: A systematic review and network meta-analysis. *J. Glob. Antimicrob. Resist.* **2021**, *24*, 136–147. [PubMed]
89. Giacobbe, D.R.; Karaiskos, I.; Bassetti, M. How do we optimize the prescribing of intravenous polymyxins to increase their longevity and efficacy in critically ill patients? *Expert Opin. Pharmacother.* **2022**, *23*, 5–8. [CrossRef]
90. Karaiskos, I.; Souli, M.; Galani, I.; Giamarellou, H. Colistin: Still a lifesaver for the 21st century? *Expert Opin. Drug Metab. Toxicol.* **2017**, *13*, 59–71. [CrossRef]
91. Lyu, C.; Zhang, Y.; Liu, X.; Wu, J.; Zhang, J. Clinical efficacy and safety of polymyxins based versus non-polymyxins based therapies in the infections caused by carbapenem-resistant *Acinetobacter baumannii*: A systematic review and meta-analysis. *BMC Infect. Dis.* **2020**, *20*, 296. [CrossRef] [PubMed]
92. Tsuji, B.T.; Pogue, J.M.; Zavascki, A.P.; Paul, M.; Daikos, G.L.; Forrest, A.; Giacobbe, D.R.; Viscoli, C.; Giamarellou, H.; Ilias Karaiskos, I.; et al. International Consensus Guidelines for the Optimal Use of the Polymyxins: Endorsed by the American College of Clinical Pharmacy (ACCP), European Society of Clinical Microbiology and Infectious Diseases (ESCMID), Infectious Diseases Society of America (IDSA), International Society for Anti-infective Pharmacology (ISAP), Society of Critical Care Medicine (SCCM), and Society of Infectious Diseases Pharmacists (SIDP). *Pharmacotherapy* **2019**, *39*, 10–39.
93. Pournaras, S.; Koumaki, V.; Gennimata, V.; Kouskouni, E.; Tsakris, A. In Vitro Activity of Tigecycline Against *Acinetobacter baumannii*: Global Epidemiology and Resistance Mechanisms. *Adv. Exp. Med. Biol.* **2016**, *97*, 1–14.
94. Yahav, D.; Lador, A.; Paul, M.; Leibovici, L. Efficacy and safety of tigecycline: A systematic review and meta-analysis. *J. Antimicrob. Chemother.* **2011**, *66*, 1963–1971. [CrossRef] [PubMed]
95. Mei, H.; Yang, T.; Wang, J.; Wang, R.; Cai, Y. Efficacy and safety of tigecycline in treatment of pneumonia caused by MDR *Acinetobacter baumannii*: A systematic review and meta-analysis. *J. Antimicrob. Chemother.* **2019**, *74*, 3423–3431. [CrossRef] [PubMed]
96. Zha, L.; Pan, L.; Guo, J.; French, N.; Villanueva, E.V.; Tefsen, B. Effectiveness and safety of high dose tigecycline for the treatment of severe infections: A systematic review and meta-analysis. *Adv. Ther.* **2020**, *37*, 1049–1064. [CrossRef] [PubMed]
97. Rex, J.H.; Outterson, K. New Antibiotics Are Not Being Registered or Sold in Europe in a Timely Manner. 2020. Available online: https://amr.solutions/2020/09/07/new-antibiotics-are-not-being-registered-or-sold-in-europe-in-a-timely-manner (accessed on 15 July 2022).
98. Oliva, A.; Ceccarelli, G.; De Angelis, M.; Sacco, F.; Miele, M.C.; Mastroianni, C.M.; Venditti, M. Cefiderocol for compassionate use in the treatment of complicated infections caused by extensively and pan-resistant *Acinetobacter baumannii*. *J. Glob. Antimicrob. Resist.* **2020**, *23*, 292–296. [CrossRef] [PubMed]
99. Application for Inclusion of FETCROJA/FETROJA (Cefiderocol) on the WHO Model List of Essential Medicines. 2020. Available online: https://cdn.who.int/media/docs/default-source/essential-medicines/2021-eml-expert-committee/applications-for-addition-of-new-medicines/a.7_cefiderocol.pdf?sfvrsn=db365d99_4 (accessed on 15 July 2022).
100. Karakonstantis, S.; Ioannou, P.; Samonis, G.; Kofteridis, D.P. Systematic review of antimicrobial combination options for pandrug-resistant *Acinetobacter baumannii*. *Antibiotics* **2021**, *10*, 1344. [CrossRef]

101. Durante-Mangoni, E.; Signoriello, G.; Andini, R.; Mattei, A.; De Cristoforo, M.; Murino, P.; Bassetti, M.; Malacarne, P.; Petrosillo, N.; Galdieri, N.; et al. Colistin and rifampicin compared with colistin alone for the treatment of serious infections due to extensively drug-resistant *Acinetobacter baumannii*: A multicenter, randomized clinical trial. *Clin. Infect. Dis.* **2013**, *57*, 349–358. [CrossRef] [PubMed]
102. Sirijatuphat, R.; Thamlikitkul, V. Preliminary study of colistin versus colistin plus fosfomycin for treatment of carbapenem-resistant *Acinetobacter baumannii* infections. *Antimicrob. Agents Chemother.* **2014**, *58*, 5598–5601. [CrossRef]
103. Paul, M.; Daikos, G.L.; Durante-Mangoni, E.; Yahav, D.; Carmeli, Y.; Benattar, Y.D.; Skiada, A.; Andini, R.; Eliakim-Raz, N.; Nutman, A.; et al. Colistin alone versus colistin plus meropenem for treatment of severe infections caused by carbapenem-resistant Gram-negative bacteria: An open-label, randomised controlled trial. *Lancet Infect. Dis.* **2018**, *18*, 391–400. [CrossRef]
104. Kaye, K.; Marchaim, D.; Thamlikitkul, V.; Carmeli, Y.; Chiu, C.H.; Daikos, G.; Dhar, S.; Durante-Mangoni, E.; Gikas, A.; Kotanidou, A.; et al. Results from the OVERCOME Trial: Colistin monotherapy versus combination therapy for the treatment of pneumonia or bloodstream infection due to extensively drug resistant Gram-negative bacilli. In Proceedings of the 31st European Congress of Clinical Microbiology & Infectious Diseases (ECCMID), Vienna, Austria, 9–12 July 2021.
105. Lenhard, J.R.; Smith, N.M.; Bulman, Z.P.; Tao, X.; Thamlikitkul, V.; Shin, B.S.; Nation, R.L.; Li, J.; Bulitta, J.B.; Tsuji, B.T. High-dose ampicillin-sulbactam combinations combat polymyxin-resistant *Acinetobacter baumannii* in a hollow-fiber infection model. *Antimicrob. Agents Chemother.* **2017**, *61*, e01268-16. [CrossRef]
106. Assimakopoulos, S.F.; Karamouzos, V.; Lefkaditi, A.; Sklavou, C.; Kolonitsiou, F.; Christofidou, M.; Fligou, F.; Gogos, C.; Marangos, M. Triple combination therapy with high-dose ampicillin/sulbactam, high-dose tigecycline and colistin in the treatment of ventilator-associated pneumonia caused by pan-drug resistant *Acinetobacter baumannii*: A case series study. *Infez. Med.* **2019**, *27*, 11–16.
107. Qureshi, Z.A.; Hittle, L.E.; O'Hara, J.A.; Rivera, J.I.; Syed, A.; Shields, R.K.; Pasculle, A.W.; Ernst, R.K.; Doi, Y. Colistin-resistant *Acinetobacter baumannii*: Beyond carbapenem resistance. *Clin. Infect. Dis.* **2015**, *60*, 1295–1303. [CrossRef] [PubMed]
108. Longshaw, C.; Manissero, D.; Tsuji, M.; Echols, R.; Yamano, Y. In vitro activity of the siderophore cephalosporin, cefiderocol, against molecularly characterized, carbapenem-non-susceptible Gram-negative bacteria from Europe. *JAC Antimicrob. Resist.* **2020**, *2*, dlaa060. [CrossRef] [PubMed]
109. Bassetti, M.; Echols, R.; Matsunaga, Y.; Ariyasu, M.; Doi, Y.; Ferrer, R.; Lodise, T.P.; Naas, T.; Niki, Y.; Paterson, D.L.; et al. Efficacy and safety of cefiderocol or best available therapy for the treatment of serious infections caused by carbapenem-resistant Gram-negative bacteria (CREDIBLE-CR): A randomised, open-label, multicentre, pathogen-focused, descriptive, phase 3 trial. *Lancet Infect. Dis.* **2021**, *21*, 226–240. [CrossRef]
110. Naseer, S.; Weinstein, E.A.; Rubin, D.B.; Suvarna, K.; Wei, X.; Higgins, K.; Goodwin, A.; Jang, S.H.; Iarikov, D.; Farley, J.; et al. US Food and Drug Administration (FDA): Benefit-risk considerations for cefiderocol (Fetroja®). *Clin. Infect. Dis.* **2021**, *72*, e1103–e1111. [CrossRef] [PubMed]
111. Wunderink, R.G.; Matsunaga, Y.; Ariyasu, M.; Clevenbergh, P.; Echols, R.; Kaye, K.S.; Kollef, M.; Menon, A.; Pogue, J.M.; Shorr, A.F.; et al. Cefiderocol versus high-dose, extended-infusion meropenem for the treatment of Gram-negative nosocomial pneumonia (APEKS-NP): A randomised, double-blind, phase 3, non-inferiority trial. *Lancet Infect. Dis.* **2021**, *21*, 213–225. [CrossRef]
112. Morrissey, I.; Olesky, M.; Hawser, S.; Lob, S.H.; Karlowsky, J.A.; Corey, G.R.; Bassetti, M.; Fyfe, C. In vitro activity of eravacycline against Gram-negative bacilli isolated in clinical laboratories worldwide from 2013 to 2017. *Antimicrob. Agents Chemother.* **2020**, *64*, e01699-19. [CrossRef]
113. Solomkin, J.S.; Gardovskis, J.; Lawrence, K.; Montravers, P.; Sway, A.; Evans, D.; Tsai, L. IGNITE4: Results of a phase 3, randomized, multicenter, prospective trial of eravacycline vs. meropenem in the treatment of complicated intraabdominal infections. *Clin. Infect. Dis.* **2019**, *69*, 921–929. [CrossRef]
114. Sagan, O.; Yakubsevitch, R.; Yanev, K.; Fomkin, R.; Stone, E.; Hines, D.; O'Donnell, J.; Miller, A.; Isaacs, R.; Srinivasan, S. Pharmacokinetics and tolerability of intravenous sulbactam-durlobactam with imipenem-cilastatin in hospitalized adults with complicated urinary tract infections, including acute pyelonephritis. *Antimicrob. Agents Chemother.* **2020**, *64*, e01506-19. [CrossRef] [PubMed]
115. De Oliveira, D.M.P.; Forde, B.M.; Kidd, T.J.; Harris, P.N.A.; Schembri, M.A.; Beatson, S.A.; Paterson, D.L.; Walker, M.J. Antimicrobial resistance in ESKAPE pathogens. *Clin. Microbiol. Rev.* **2020**, *33*, e00181-19. [CrossRef]
116. Kazmierczak, K.M.; de Jonge, B.L.M.; Stone, G.G.; Sahm, D.F. In vitro activity of ceftazidime/avibactam against isolates of *Pseudomonas aeruginosa* collected in European countries: INFORM global surveillance 2012–15. *J. Antimicrob. Chemother.* **2018**, *73*, 2777–2781. [CrossRef] [PubMed]
117. Galani, I.; Papoutsaki, V.; Karantani, I.; Karaiskos, I.; Galani, L.; Adamou, P.; Deliolanis, I.; Kodonaki, A.; Papadogeorgaki, E.; Markopoulou, M.; et al. In vitro activity of ceftolozane/tazobactam alone and in combination with amikacin against MDR/XDR *Pseudomonas aeruginosa* isolates from Greece. *J. Antimicrob. Chemother.* **2020**, *75*, 2164–2172. [CrossRef] [PubMed]
118. Pérez, A.; Gato, E.; Pérez-Llarena, J.; Fernández-Cuenca, F.; Gude, M.J.; Oviaño, M.; Pachón, M.E.; Garnacho, J.; González, V.; Pascual, Á.; et al. High incidence of MDR and XDR *Pseudomonas aeruginosa* isolates obtained from patients with ventilator-associated pneumonia in Greece, Italy and Spain as part of the MagicBullet clinical trial. *J. Antimicrob. Chemother.* **2019**, *74*, 1244–1252. [CrossRef] [PubMed]

119. Nguyen, L.; Garcia, J.; Gruenberg, K.; MacDougall, C.; Gruenberg, K.; MacDougall, C. Multidrug-resistant Pseudomonas infections: Hard to treat, but hope on the horizon? *Curr. Infect. Dis. Rep.* **2018**, *20*, 23. [CrossRef] [PubMed]
120. Bassetti, M.; Vena, A.; Croxatto, A.; Righi, E.; Guery, B. How to manage *Pseudomonas aeruginosa* infections. *Drugs Context.* **2018**, *7*, 212527. [CrossRef]
121. Losito, A.R.; Raffaelli, F.; Del Giacomo, P.; Tumbarello, M. New drugs for the treatment of *Pseudomonas aeruginosa* infections with limited treatment options: A narrative review. *Antibiotics* **2022**, *11*, 579. [CrossRef] [PubMed]
122. Paul, M.; Carrara, E.; Retamar, P.; Tängdén, T.; Bitterman, R.; Bonomo, R.A.; de Waele, J.; Daikos, G.L.; Akova, M.; Harbarth, S.; et al. European Society of Clinical Microbiology and Infectious Diseases (ESCMID) guidelines for the treatment of infections caused by multidrug-resistant Gram-negative bacilli (endorsed by European society of intensive care medicine). *Clin. Microbiol. Infect.* **2022**, *28*, 521–547. [CrossRef]
123. Layeux, B.; Taccone, F.S.; Fagnoul, D.; Vincent, J.L.; Jacobs, F. Amikacin monotherapy for sepsis caused by panresistant *Pseudomonas aeruginosa*. *Antimicrob. Agents Chemother.* **2010**, *54*, 4939–4941. [CrossRef]
124. Meletiadis, J.; Paranos, P.; Georgiou, P.C.; Vourli, S.; Antonopoulou, S.; Michelaki, A.; Vagiakou, E.; Pournaras, S. In vitro comparative activity of the new beta-lactamase inhibitor taniborbactam with cefepime or meropenem against *Klebsiella pneumoniae* and cefepime against *Pseudomonas aeruginosa* metallo-beta-lactamase-producing clinical isolates. *Int. J. Antimicrob. Agents* **2021**, *58*, 106440. [CrossRef]
125. Mauri, C.; Maraolo, A.E.; Di Bella, S.; Luzzaro, F.; Principe, L. The revival of aztreonam in combination with avibactam against metallo-β-lactamase-producing Gram-negatives: A systematic review of in vitro studies and clinical cases. *Antibiotics* **2021**, *10*, 1012. [CrossRef]

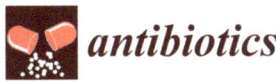

Article

The Impact of Antimicrobial Stewardship and Infection Control Interventions on *Acinetobacter baumannii* Resistance Rates in the ICU of a Tertiary Care Center in Lebanon

Nesrine A. Rizk [1], Nada Zahreddine [2,†], Nisrine Haddad [3,†], Rihab Ahmadieh [2], Audra Hannun [3], Souad Bou Harb [1], Sara F. Haddad [1], Rony M. Zeenny [3] and Souha S. Kanj [1,*]

1. Division of Infectious Diseases, Department of Internal Medicine, American University of Beirut Medical Center, Beirut 1107 2020, Lebanon; nr00@aub.edu.lb (N.A.R.); sb125@aub.edu.lb (S.B.H.); sarahaddad711@gmail.com (S.F.H.)
2. Infection Control and Prevention Program, American University of Beirut Medical Center, Beirut 1107 2020, Lebanon; nk13@aub.edu.lb (N.Z.); ra255@aub.edu.lb (R.A.)
3. Department of Pharmacy, American University of Beirut Medical Center, Beirut 1107 2020, Lebanon; nh126@aub.edu.lb (N.H.); audrahannun@gmail.com (A.H.); rz37@aub.edu.lb (R.M.Z.)
* Correspondence: sk11@aub.edu.lb; Tel.: +961-1-350000; Fax: +961-1-370814
† These authors contributed equally to this work.

Citation: Rizk, N.A.; Zahreddine, N.; Haddad, N.; Ahmadieh, R.; Hannun, A.; Bou Harb, S.; Haddad, S.F.; Zeenny, R.M.; Kanj, S.S. The Impact of Antimicrobial Stewardship and Infection Control Interventions on *Acinetobacter baumannii* Resistance Rates in the ICU of a Tertiary Care Center in Lebanon. *Antibiotics* **2022**, *11*, 911. https://doi.org/10.3390/antibiotics11070911

Academic Editors: Elizabeth Paramythiotou, Christina Routsi and Antoine Andremont

Received: 28 May 2022
Accepted: 5 July 2022
Published: 7 July 2022

Publisher's Note: MDPI stays neutral with regard to jurisdictional claims in published maps and institutional affiliations.

Copyright: © 2022 by the authors. Licensee MDPI, Basel, Switzerland. This article is an open access article distributed under the terms and conditions of the Creative Commons Attribution (CC BY) license (https://creativecommons.org/licenses/by/4.0/).

Abstract: Antimicrobial resistance is a serious threat to global health, causing increased mortality and morbidity especially among critically ill patients. This toll is expected to rise following the COVID-19 pandemic. Carbapenem-resistant *Acinetobacter baumannii* (CRAb) is among the Gram-negative pathogens leading antimicrobial resistance globally; it is listed as a critical priority pathogen by the WHO and is implicated in hospital-acquired infections and outbreaks, particularly in critically ill patients. Recent reports from Lebanon describe increasing rates of infection with CRAb, hence the need to develop concerted interventions to control its spread. We set to describe the impact of combining antimicrobial stewardship and infection control measures on resistance rates and colonization pressure of CRAb in the intensive care units of a tertiary care center in Lebanon before the COVID-19 pandemic. The antimicrobial stewardship program introduced a carbapenem-sparing initiative in April 2019. During the same period, infection control interventions involved focused screening, monitoring, and tracking of CRAb, as well as compliance with specific measures. From January 2018 to January 2020, we report a statistically significant decrease in carbapenem consumption and a decrease in resistance rates of isolated *A. baumannii*. The colonization pressure of CRAb also decreased significantly, reaching record low levels at the end of the intervention period. The results indicate that a multidisciplinary approach and combined interventions between the stewardship and infection control teams can lead to a sustained reduction in resistance rates and CRAb spread in ICUs.

Keywords: *Acinetobacter*; carbapenem-resistant *A. baumannii* (CRAb); infection control; antimicrobial agents; carbapenems; antibiotic resistance; clinical pharmacy services; antimicrobial stewardship; intensive care

1. Introduction

Antimicrobial resistance was recognized as a serious threat to global health several years before the onset of the COVID-19 pandemic [1]. In fact, a report published in 2016 by the World Bank and the World Health Organization (WHO) predicted that antimicrobial resistance could lead to 10 million deaths each year by 2050 [2,3] while a more recent study estimated that, globally, 4.95 million deaths were associated with resistant bacteria in 2019 [4]. In addition to the resulting mortality, the increase in morbidity, disability and hospital length of stay lead to increased costs with direct negative consequences on the global economy [5,6]. Antimicrobial resistance is a major concern for the developing world, with economic- and public health-related repercussions especially due to the spread of resistant Gram-negative pathogens [7,8] that are leading multidrug resistance around the world. Those organisms feature on the critical priority pathogens list of the WHO [9–11]. They are associated with nosocomial infections, specifically in acute care settings and intensive care units (ICUs) [12]. A recent report from the WHO Eastern Mediterranean region revealed alarming rates of multidrug-resistant pathogens including carbapenem-resistant *Acinetobacter baumannii* (CRAb) which is the most common pathogen in Gram-negative bacteremia [13]. As a response to the antimicrobial resistance threat, the WHO launched in 2015 a Global Action Plan against antimicrobial resistance comprising multiple interventions based on five objectives [14]. Among those, Antimicrobial Stewardship and Infection Control are important strategies that aim to guide the judicious use of antimicrobials and control the spread of resistant microorganisms within healthcare institutions [15].

Even prior to the COVID-19 pandemic, antimicrobial misuse and overuse in critical care settings was very common with the frequent utilization of multiple broad-spectrum antibiotics for long courses of therapy [12]. Several risk factors put critically ill patients at higher risk of colonization and infection with multidrug-resistant organisms including treatment with immunosuppressive drugs, use of invasive devices, exposure to a wide range of antibiotics, and prolonged hospitalizations [16]. Following the COVID-19 pandemic, resistance rates are expected to increase [17,18] as COVID-19 has led to an influx of critically ill patients who often receive unnecessary antibiotic therapy [19,20]. A report by the Center for Disease Control published in February 2021 described outbreaks of antimicrobial resistant infections in COVID-19 units such as CRAb and *Candida auris* (*C. auris*) [19] with a noticeable increase in the overall hospital-acquired infections, most of which are caused by multidrug-resistant organisms [21]. On the other hand, the pandemic may have a positive impact on antimicrobial resistance as there may be a possible decrease in the transmission of resistant organisms, as a direct consequence of global travel restrictions, more frequent hand hygiene, social distancing, as well as enhanced infection control practices globally [22].

CRAb is among the most resistant organisms of the *Acinetobacter* species. It is ubiquitous in nature and in addition to its resistance to carbapenems, it is intrinsically resistant to a large number of antimicrobial agents and has the potential to develop additional resistance and cause infections in humans [23]. *A. baumannii* is unique in that it possesses an excellent genome plasticity; it has the ability to take any gene from its surroundings. This feature might have played a crucial role in the evolution of this human opportunistic pathogen towards clinical success and being a multidrug-resistant pathogen [24]. It has an island of drug-resistant genes in its genome that makes it different from other superbugs [25]. *A. baumannii* is the most prevalent carbapenem-resistant organism worldwide [26] and is associated with hospital-acquired infections causing a significant increase in morbidity and mortality [27] especially in patients admitted to ICUs [23,28]. In the East Mediterranean region, CRAb is notoriously implicated in major outbreaks in healthcare settings [29]. During the last decade, wars and violent conflicts have contributed to the spread of this organism from combat areas to hospitals treating the war-injured and refugees [30,31]. The detrimental impact of antimicrobial resistance and CRAb on public health was recognized in this region, prompting governments and experts to collaborate under the WHO umbrella to tackle antimicrobial resistance [32] and develop recommendations for the treatment of CRAb and other multidrug resistant organisms [33].

CRAb is responsible for most of the severe infections in ICUs worldwide [34] in patients colonized or infected with it. CRAb is defined as any *A. baumannii* isolate that is resistant to carbapenems. These isolates are usually also resistant to most antibiotics excluding polymyxin E (colistin) and tigecycline. As early as 1980, and following armed clashes during the Lebanese civil war, an increase in CRAb was reported from our hospital [35]. A recent review on carbapenem resistance among *A. baumannii* isolates revealed increasing resistance rates in Lebanon [36]. In fact, *A. baumannii* comprised 82% of isolates collected from 16 Lebanese hospitals in the years 2011–2013 [37] and 87% among samples from 13 Lebanese hospitals [38] in the years 2015–2016. Other reports from major Lebanese hospitals reveal the burden of CRAb on ICUs, with increased mortality and morbidity and poor patient outcomes [39–42]. Interventions to control CRAb in those hospitals included either infection control measures to break transmission—such as terminal cleaning of an ICU [43]—or antimicrobial stewardship efforts to decrease resistance rates [44,45]. *Acinetobacter baumannii* constitute the large majority of the *Acinetobacter* organisms tested in our microbiology diagnostic laboratory. For the purpose of this study, all *Acinetobacter* species will be referred to as *Acinetobacter baumannii* [46,47].

Similar to the other medical centers in the region, we struggle with high rates of resistance among Gram-negative bacteria, mainly the extended spectrum beta-lactamase-producing (ESBL) Enterobacterales. Therefore, carbapenem use is widespread [29]. Carbapenem consumption has been found to be associated with increasing rates of CRAb [48]. CRAb is a pathogen of concern in our hospital, where according to targeted surveillance efforts, the rates of CRAb sharply increased from 52% in 2010 to peak at 92% in 2012 [49]. A prospective study conducted at our center between 2007 and 2014 showed that the most common site for isolating CRAb was the respiratory tract, notably in patients with ventilator-associated pneumonia (VAP) [39]. CRAb was also the predominant pathogen, both in early- and late-onset VAP, in a retrospective review on VAP published in 2019 [50]. The pattern of resistance of CRAb at AUBMC is quite similar to those reported from neighboring Arab countries, with the predominance of the blaOXA-23 gene. *A. baumannii* isolated from our hospital tend to be multidrug resistant (to trimethoprim–sulfamethoxazole, quinolones, aminoglycosides, and beta-lactam antibiotics) [46].

Accordingly, we find it essential to develop concerted interventions to control the spread of CRAb. In our study, we describe the impact of combined antimicrobial stewardship and infection control interventions on resistance rates of *Acinetobacter baumannii* and colonization pressure of CRAb in our ICU prior to the onset of COVID-19 pandemic.

2. Materials and Methods

2.1. Hospital Setting

The American University of Beirut Medical Center (AUBMC) is a leading tertiary care medical center (364 beds) serving patients from Lebanon and neighboring countries. Its medical and surgical services are the busiest in the nation with a medical and surgical ICU comprising 30 single-bed rooms. The adult ICU population at the AUBMC consists of high-risk patients with multiple comorbidities, immunocompromised patients, trauma patients, as well as patients following major surgical procedures. AUBMC ICU also receives referred patients from other facilities in the country as well as from Syria and Iraq, countries inflicted by war. In November 2018, the AUBMC acquired the EPIC electronic medical record software [51]. EPIC is a cloud-based electronic health record software built for hospitals. The transition to a fully automated health medical record allowed for additional opportunities for antimicrobial monitoring and targeted infection control interventions.

2.2. Antimicrobial Stewardship

Actions led by antimicrobial stewardship programs are essential to control the misuse and abuse of antimicrobials and decrease healthcare costs and antimicrobial resistance [52–54]. Antimicrobial stewardship efforts started at AUBMC in 2007. However, the antimicrobial stewardship program was formally launched in June 2018, with a dedicated team composed of an Infectious Disease physician and a pharmacist [55]. The objectives of the antimicrobial stewardship program are to optimize patient safety, reduce the emergence of antimicrobial resistance and decrease hospitalization costs [54,56,57]. The stewardship team reviews patients' antimicrobial therapies daily and provides prospective audits and feedback on the use of broad-spectrum antibiotics in addition to calculating and reporting overall antimicrobial consumption, developing and implementing guidelines to standardize and optimize antimicrobial use at the institution, and finally offering ongoing educational activities to healthcare providers.

2.2.1. Antimicrobial Stewardship Interventions

Due to the emergence of carbapenem resistance, namely among *Acinetobacter baumannii*, the antimicrobial stewardship team introduced, in April 2019, an initiative for carbapenem sparing with the aim of reducing carbapenem consumption and assessing the impact on *Acinetobacter baumannii* carbapenem resistance rates. Even with carbapenems being the mainstay of therapy for ESBL-producing organisms, recent data and guidance suggest using alternatives to carbapenems in several scenarios (intra-abdominal infections, complicated urinary tract infections and pyelonephritis, oral step-down therapy, and surgical prophylaxis) to try to limit carbapenem use. We implemented a carbapenem-sparing approach focused on the intensive care units during this month [55]. As such, the stewardship team conducted daily stewardship handshake rounds and reviewed the charts of all ICU patients receiving carbapenems. The stewardship team assessed the appropriateness of carbapenem use (appropriate/not appropriate) (opinion of the infectious diseases specialist and pharmacist after chart review). The non-appropriate prescriptions of carbapenems were categorized as follows: duration of therapy, dose adjustment, de-escalation, duplicate coverage, drug–bug mismatch, IV to oral switch. The stewardship team proposed alternatives to the inappropriate carbapenem prescriptions when applicable; those were labeled as "interventions". At the end of this month, we calculated the rate of acceptance of those interventions (accepted/not accepted) and compared the acceptance rates at the beginning versus acceptance rates at the end of the intervention month. Stewardship rounds were coupled with didactic lectures on principles and applications of antimicrobial stewardship to medical interns, residents, infectious diseases fellows, and pharmacists. At the end of this project, the stewardship team resumed their daily operations as described above.

2.2.2. Antimicrobial Stewardship Measures

To assess the impact of the carbapenem-sparing strategy, we adopted the following quantitative metrics to measure carbapenem antibiotic consumption: defined daily dose (DDD) and days of therapy (DOT). Quantitative metrics were calculated at baseline, before the initiative implementation and, subsequently on a monthly and quarterly basis, after implementation [58]. Table 1 illustrates the formulas used to calculate DDD and DOT [58–60] on a quarterly and monthly basis respectively.

Table 1. Equations for Antibiotic Consumption Metrics and colonization pressure DDD, defined daily dose; DOT, days of therapy; CP, colonization pressure.

Metrics	Equations
DDD per 1000 patient days	$\frac{\sum dispensed\ doses\ of\ meropenem,\ ertapenem,\ imipenem}{1000 \times patient\ days\ in\ a\ quarter}$
DOT per 1000 patient days	$\frac{\sum days\ that\ inpatients\ received \geq 1\ dose\ of\ meropenem,\ ertapenem,\ and\ imipenem}{1000 \times patient\ days\ in\ a\ month}$ Days on which patients received more than one carbapenem are counted only once
CP	$\frac{\sum MDR - Ab\ patient\ days\ in\ a\ given\ unit\ in\ a\ month}{1000 \times patient\ days\ in\ a\ month\ in\ same\ unit}$

2.3. Infection Control

The Infection Control and Prevention Program was established at AUBMC in 1980. Infection control strategies have included surveillance, prevention and management of outbreaks, environmental hygiene, and optimization of employee health and education [56]. The Infection Control team at the AUBMC tracks multidrug-resistant organisms in the hospital. Reports for Methicillin-resistant *Staphylococcus aureus* (MRSA), Vancomycin-resistant enterococci (VRE), Carbapenem-resistant Enterobacterales (CRE), multidrug-resistant *A. baumannii*, difficult to treat *Pseudomonas aeruginosa*, and, more recently, *Candida auris* are generated on daily basis. Clusters and outbreaks are closely monitored and investigated especially in critical care units. During the last decade, several CRAb clusters and outbreaks were identified in our ICUs [33]. The infection control team recognized this threat and implemented an active surveillance for CRAb for all ICU admissions to detect colonization or infections: ICU patients are screened for CRAb upon admission and placed on contact isolation pending the culture results. Moreover, the results of the clinical cultures obtained during the patient's stay in ICU are analyzed to differentiate hospital-acquired transmissions from community-acquired infections or colonization with CRAb.

Multiple interventions were introduced by the infection control team throughout the years as part of an intensified effort to curb the spread of CRAb. Screening all ICU admissions was one of the major interventions to detect the carriage of CRAb and other carbapenem-resistant organisms. A screening method was adopted for CRAb and CRE, to collect swabs from the oropharynx, bilateral axilla, umbilical and perianal areas as well as from the rectum. Moreover, all patients admitted to ICU were bathed using Chlorhexidine 4% solutions to decrease the bacterial load on their skin and reduce bacterial transmissions [61]. Furthermore, infection control prevention bundles (ventilator bundle, urinary catheter bundle, and central line bundle) were adopted to improve the processes for care of patients. Certifications for the insertion and care of central lines became mandatory for the medical and nursing teams, and are granted after taking an online course. Several practices were also introduced to reduce environmental contamination outside of the ICU. Practices such as restricting the transport of patients unless urgently needed, cleaning and disinfection of the elevators used and CT premises after imaging, or any other visited area, are used.

Staff education and training on hand hygiene and principles of nosocomial transmission of multidrug-resistant organisms were conducted monthly. Each session included all infection control breaches and observations to improve staff practices in ICU. During these sessions, feedback reports and identified breaches were presented, and opportunities for improvement were discussed. Training on hand hygiene included all five-evidence based key moments as per the WHO recommendations [62]. Alcohol hand rubs, at a concentration of 70% ethanol or propanol, were installed at the door of each patient's room. Compliance was closely monitored with the assistance of anonymous auditors, and feedback reports were regularly communicated to managers and hospital leadership. Closed-circuit television (CCTV) surveillance cameras were installed in three critical care units in 2015. All noted breaches from live and retrospective reviews are promptly reported to nurse managers of the unit for appropriate action. The infection control team conducted intensified rounds to observe practices, raise awareness and improve compliance of the ICU staff with all needed measures. Tiered hand hygiene accountability interventions were adopted based upon a validated model [63] and this was reflected in the hospital hand hygiene policy. Interventions started with direct feedback followed by the awareness intervention, then the authority intervention and ending with the disciplinary intervention. Hand hygiene compliance rates started to improve for the physician group as a result. Hand hygiene compliance rates were sustained and improved further at the start of the COVID-19 pandemic. In addition, visitors were restricted to decrease environmental contamination as per a new visitation policy. An important measure was also added, where nurses were assigned to monitor healthcare workers and visitors during the day shifts; their role was to promptly intervene whenever infection control breaches were observed [50].

The direct patient environment plays a major role in transmitting multidrug-resistant pathogens among patients. Contaminated surfaces contribute to CRAb transmission to vulnerable patients. Routine environmental cultures to identify sources of environmental contamination with CRAb (mattresses, pillows, keyboards) were introduced. After each patient discharge, manual cleaning/disinfection was conducted followed by air decontamination using hydrogen peroxide (H_2O_2) at a concentration of 1% (generating 4.7% boosted H_2O_2). Environmental cultures that were taken initially were discontinued following sustained negative culture results of the patient environment. Obtaining new cleaning and disinfection solutions and changes in housekeeping processes were also instrumental in improving the patient care environment. All the changes were reflected in updated policies and were reinforced through structural staff training.

The carriage on admission and acquisition during ICU stay of CRAb was calculated using the CRAb colonization pressure (Table 1). Colonization pressure is defined as the proportion of patients colonized with CRAb in an ICU during a specific period. It reflects the burden of CRAb in an ICU and can estimate the probability of CRAb transmission in this setting. Thus, any new transmission (colonization or infection) of CRAb is strongly correlated to colonization pressure.

Resistance to carbapenems among *Acinetobacter baumannii* at our hospital was the main outcome of this study. Carbapenem resistance among *Acinetobacter baumannii* is routinely reported by our microbiology laboratory. *Acinetobacter* isolates were identified using the Matrix-Assisted Laser Desorption Ionization (MALDI-TOF) Time-of-Flight Mass Spectrometry (MALDI-TOF) platform, and all isolates were tested using the disk diffusion method based on the Clinical and Laboratory Standards Institute (CLSI) breakpoints. We relied on resistance rates reported by the laboratory to follow the outcome of our interventions on resistance rates.

3. Results

3.1. Antimicrobial Stewardship Results

The antimicrobial stewardship team launched its daily operations in January 2019 and collected data on the appropriateness of broad-spectrum antibiotic use across the hospital. Those recommendations were labeled as "stewardship interventions". Our focused intervention in the ICU (the carbapenem sparing strategy) started in April 2019 and yielded the following results over a one-month period: among patients who were prescribed broad-spectrum antibiotics, 188 patients (or 14.6% of the ICU patients during this month) were receiving carbapenem therapy. A total of 81 interventions were recorded during this month in adult patients and included the de-escalation of therapy (23%), dose change (28%) and limiting the duration of therapy (23%). Therefore, combined recommendations to discontinue carbapenem therapy (de-escalation or stop) comprised 46% of all interventions as shown in Figure 1. The overall acceptance rate of recommendations during this intervention period (April 2019) was 73%. As a result of all antimicrobial stewardship efforts, for 2019, there was an increase in stewardship interventions' acceptance rate from 16.66 to 55.95% when comparing January 2019 to January 2020 ($p = 0.03$). Even though the antimicrobial stewardship team was active, the efforts were less focused and spanned over the whole hospital (vs. April 2019, when the efforts were focused on the ICUs).

In analyzing the indication for use of carbapenems by the antimicrobial stewardship team, we defined an appropriate empiric therapy with carbapenem as follows: patient is a candidate for broad antibiotic therapy and warrants carbapenem usage such as recent culture with ESBL Enterobacterales or other multidrug-resistant organisms, sepsis, or febrile neutropenia. Therefore, 88% of empiric carbapenem prescriptions were deemed appropriate initially and may have required subsequent adjustment based on culture results. As such, the antimicrobial stewardship team found that indication for use, dosing, and duration were appropriate in 88, 80, and 89% of the cases, respectively (Figure 2). As part of our analysis of those results, when comparing the months of January 2019 and January 2020 pre- and post-intervention period, the indication for use in empirical therapy before 48 h changed from 86.4 to 92.9%. Similarly, indication for use in empirical therapy after 48 h from culture results, and indication for targeted therapy was appropriate in 67.1% (January 2019) and 78.9% (January 2020) of cases, and 88.9% (January 2019) and 91.4% (January 2020) of cases, respectively. Duration and dosing regimens were appropriate in 64.3 and 75.8% of cases in January 2019, respectively, as opposed to appropriateness rates of 72.1 and 68.7% in January 2020.

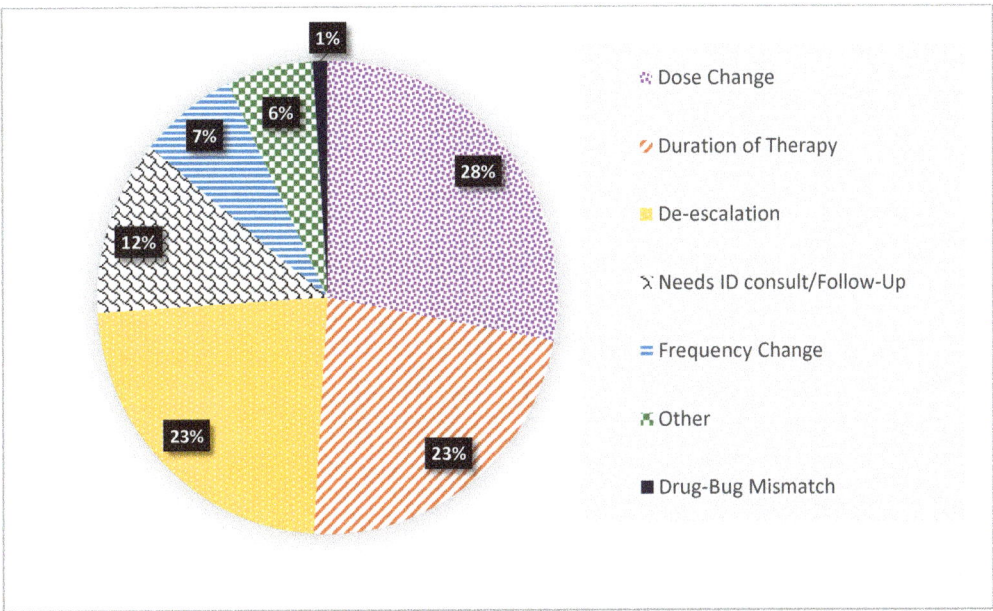

Figure 1. Distribution of antimicrobial stewardship interventions (n = 81) for patients receiving carbapenems during April 2019. ID, Infectious Disease.

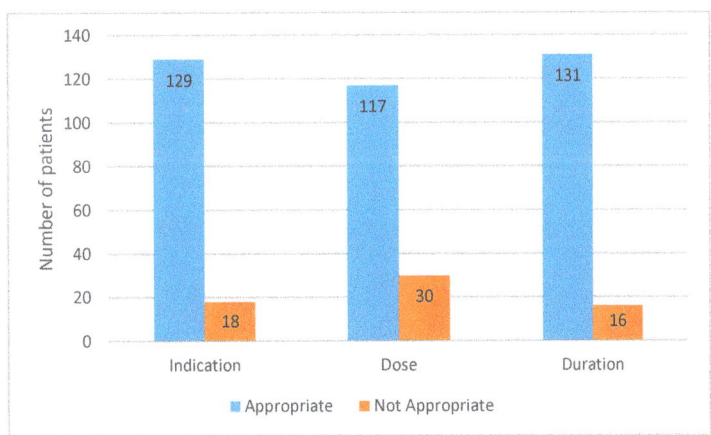

Figure 2. Appropriateness of carbapenem therapy per antimicrobial stewardship team during the implementation of carbapenem sparing strategies (April 2019).

Additional measures such as infection with *Clostridium difficile* rates, hospitalization costs, and the impact of our interventions and recommendations on patient outcomes were not studied during this time.

The overall carbapenem consumption across the hospital was reflected by carbapenem DOT and DDD, with the greatest volume of consumption occurring in the critical care units. Figure 3 demonstrates the decrease in carbapenem DDD since 2018 and until December 2020. Both DOT (shown later in the text) and DDD trends show a decrease in the consumption that is better seen starting in the second quarter (Q2) of 2019 with the intensification of the carbapenem-sparing efforts. This decrease was maintained in 2019, however, there is a noticeable increase in both DDD and DOT in 2020 compared to 2019, albeit the carbapenem consumption was still lower than 2018.

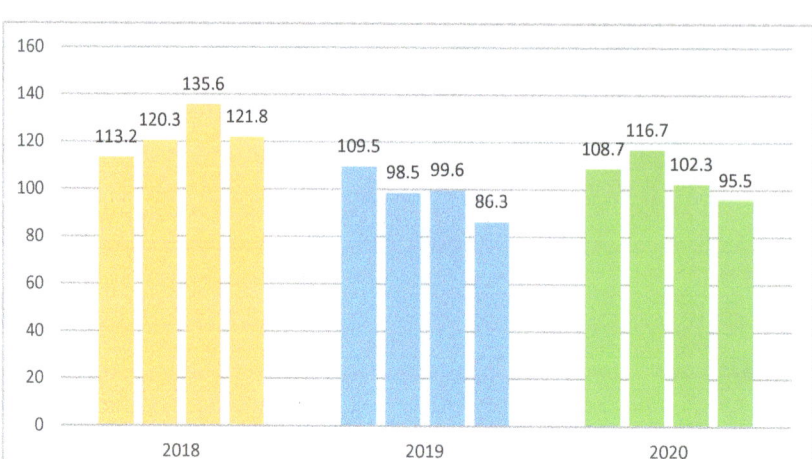

Figure 3. Carbapenems Defined Daily Dose per 1000 Patient Days per quarter and year.

3.2. Infection Control Results

Following the implementation of the intensive infection control measures listed above there was a noticeable improvement in compliance with measures (such as hand hygiene) and reduced colonization pressure of CRAb.

Compliance with hand hygiene is associated with positive patient outcomes. The prevalence of hospital acquired infections was reduced by more than 40% at Geneva University Hospital when compliance rate increased from 48 to 66% over a 5-year period [62]. Figure 4 shows results at our center with improved compliance from 74% to more than 95%.

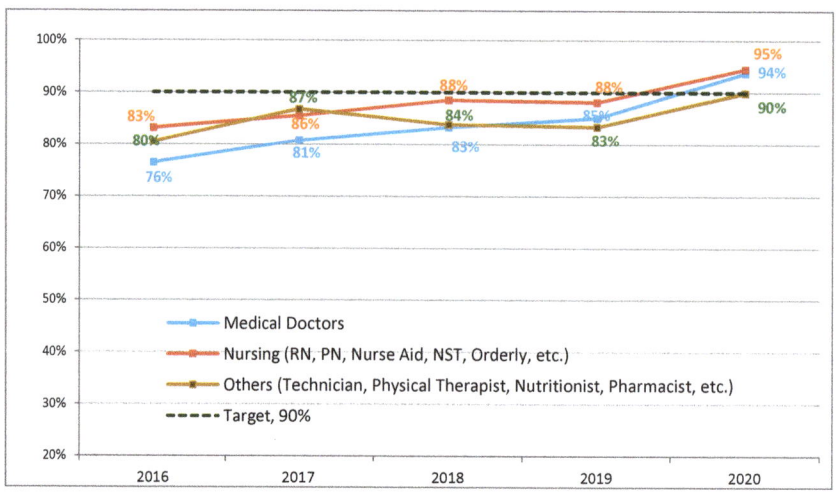

Figure 4. Hand hygiene compliance rates 2016–2020 based on anonymous audits. RN, registered nurse; PN, practical nurse; NST, nurse technician.

A sustained improvement of infection control practices was noticed across the hospital and especially in the ICU. This was reflected in the persistent decrease in the CRAb colonization pressure over the years as shown in Figure 5. CRAb transmission rates in ICU decreased steadily: *A. baumannii* colonization pressure was 340 per 1000 patient days in 2015, 221 per 1000 in 2016, 218 per 1000 in 2017 and 112.7 per 1000 in 2018. The colonization pressure decrease in 2019 became evident and reached 18.4 per 1000 during the second quarter of 2019.

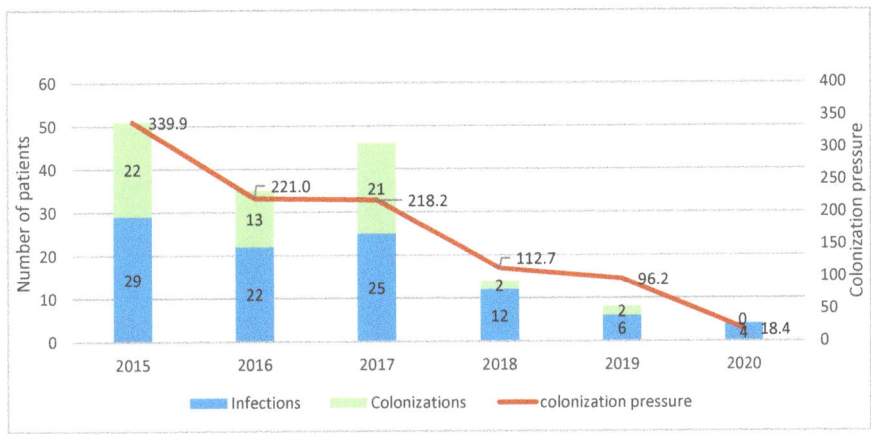

Figure 5. CRAb colonization pressure in ICU over a 7-year period by year.

The carbapenem-sparing strategy, combined with the infection control interventions, led to a significant decrease in CRAb colonization pressure rates among ICU patients. Figure 6 shows the colonization pressure per quarter in relation to carbapenem consumption reflected by the carbapenem DOT for 2018 to 2020. The sustained decrease in CRAb transmissions (infections and colonization) is more clearly seen in Figure 6 where the colonization pressure for CRAb is correlated with DOT per quarter from 2018 to 2020, following the beginning of stewardship efforts in 2019 and the launch of the carbapenem-sparing strategy in April 2019. Colonization pressure rates decreased steadily from 210.4 per 1000 patient days in Q4-2018 to 0 per 1000 patient days in Q1-2020.

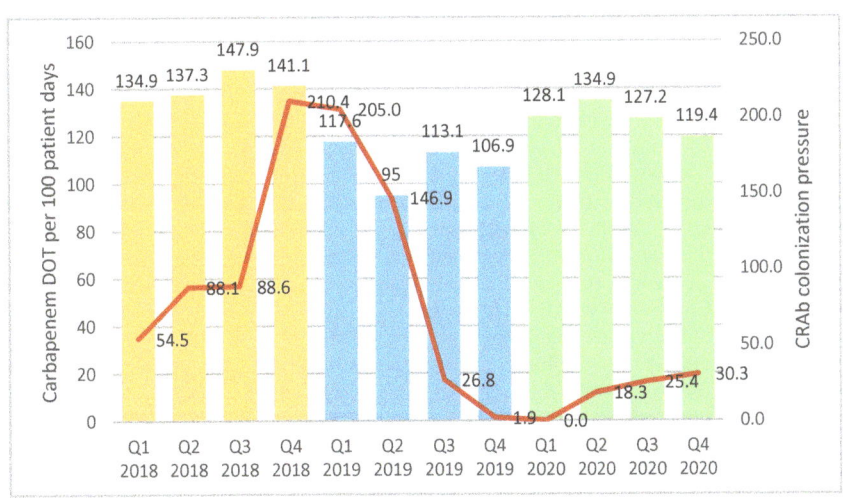

Figure 6. Carbapenem-resistant *Acinetobacter baumannii* colonizing pressure and carbapenem consumption by quarter from 2018 until 2020. DOT, Days of therapy; Q, quarter.

The major finding in our study was the impact on carbapenem resistance rates among *Acinetobacter baumannii* in our institution (Figure 7). The continuous monitoring of resistance rates allows the antimicrobial stewardship and infection control teams to measure the ongoing and long-term effects of their interventions. Figure 7 shows the rates of resistance to carbapenems among the *Acinetobacter baumannii* at the AUBMC over a decade and highlights the continuous but slow decline in resistance rates since 2014, followed by a sharp drop in 2020. The rates of carbapenem resistance among collected CRAb at the AUBMC peaked at 92% in 2012 and were slowly declining with the intensification of infection control measures and some antimicrobial stewardship efforts. However, only following the implementation of the antimicrobial stewardship program at the end of 2018 did the resistance rates among CRAb decreased in 2020 to 63%.

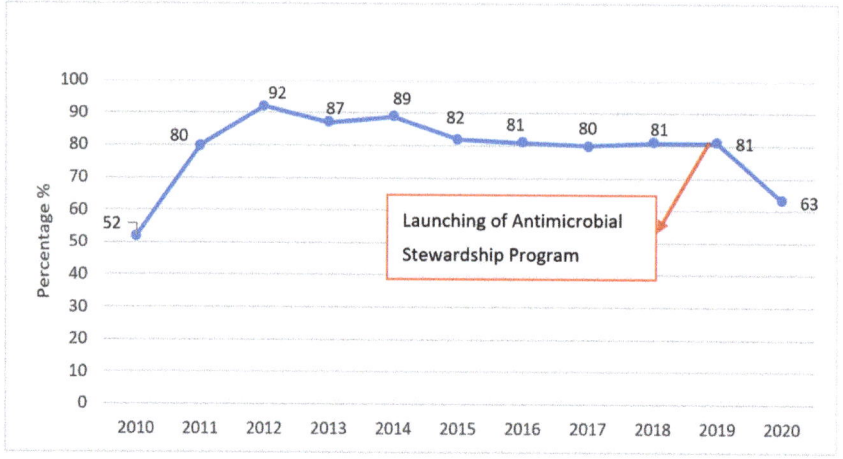

Figure 7. Rates of carbapenem-resistant *Acinetobacter baumannii* over years.

4. Discussion

The containment of CRAb is difficult to achieve in acute care settings; however it is expected to result in a significant reduction of mortality and morbidity especially among critically ill patients [64]. Carbapenem consumption is linked to increasing *Acinetobacter baumannii* resistance rates while nosocomial transmission is linked to environmental contamination, invasive procedures, and patient vulnerabilities [64,65].

Mathematical models have described the potential impact of reducing carbapenem consumption on resistance acquisition among bacteria, including CRAb [66], and antimicrobial stewardship to restrict carbapenem usage has been suggested for controlling outbreaks caused by CRAb in critical care settings [67–69]. There is an abundance of reports and studies on the effectiveness of infection control measures in limiting the transmission of CRAb in hospital ICUs. Environmental cleaning appears to be particularly important [70,71] as well as enforcing strict hand hygiene compliance policies among healthcare workers [72]. Compliance with hand hygiene is associated with positive patient outcomes; the prevalence of hospital acquired infections was reduced by more than 40% at Geneva University Hospital when compliance rate increased from 48 to 66% over a 5-year period [62]. Very few reports describe the impact of combined infection control and antimicrobial stewardship interventions on colonization pressure and resistance rates among CRAb isolates [73,74]. Our results indicate that a multidisciplinary approach and conjoined efforts of antimicrobial stewardship and infection control teams can lead to a sustained reduction in CRAb spread in the ICU.

One main finding of our study relates to the decrease in resistance rates among *Acinetobacter baumannii* to imipenem from 81% in 2018 to 63% in 2020. *A. baumannii* accounts for 99% of *Acinetobacter baumannii* in our hospital. Therefore, this reduction is significant, and reflective of the effectiveness of a carbapenem-sparing strategy at the level of the hospital with an intensification of daily stewardship interventions especially in the ICU and continued educational efforts. A significant reduction in CRAb colonization pressure was demonstrated as a 200-fold decrease during the two-year study period. The decrease in CRAb colonization pressure over the years was mainly the result of ongoing infection control interventions following the identification of each cluster or outbreak of CRAb. The launching of the carbapenem-sparing strategy by the antimicrobial stewardship team during the second quarter of 2019 led to a sustained decrease in colonization pressure over subsequent quarters as shown in Figure 6. Strict antimicrobial stewardship combined with comprehensive infection control measures resulted in successfully controlling the spread of CRAb in our ICU. This effect was maintained even during the first year of the COVID-19 pandemic and until Q4, 2020 after the Beirut blast, despite tremendous strain on our healthcare system [75–78]. The devastating explosion of August 2020 in Beirut caused an influx of trauma patients and was followed by a COVID-19 surge in the last quarter of 2020 leading to an increase in critically ill patients and antibiotic overuse [79].

Our results are particularly encouraging as reports are emerging regarding the potential worsening of antimicrobial resistance following the COVID-19 pandemic [17]. The impact of antimicrobial resistance in the countries of the East Mediterranean region is expected to worsen as well following the COVID-19 pandemic [80]. In addition, our hospital witnessed for the first time an outbreak of *C. auris* during the COVID-19 surge [81]. The lessons learnt during the multiple clusters and outbreaks of CRAb proved successful in controlling the spread of this new pathogen. In addition, the antimicrobial stewardship team adopted elements of antifungal stewardship in an effort to control the *C. auris* outbreaks.

Our study has limitations. First, we did not design our protocol to account for the impact of individual interventions on the outcomes. Thus, our approach was to maintain the infection control interventions and in parallel deploy the antimicrobial stewardship-targeted strategies as an additional combined intervention; ongoing infection control measures had not been fully effective in significantly reducing the colonization pressure of CRAb previously and we assumed that the intensification of the antimicrobial stewardship interventions resulted in the achieved reduction of CRAb rates and colonization pressure. Second, we did not collect data to study the impact of our results on patient outcomes such as cost, *C. difficile* infection, length of stay, and mortality.

5. Conclusions

In conclusion, we have shown a drastic reduction in CRAb colonization in our ICU and decreased resistance rates among *Acinetobacter baumannii* following a combination approach that relied on rigorous infection control practices and antimicrobial stewardship interventions. In our setting, the results are encouraging and could be replicated in hospitals and ICUs suffering from high burdens of CRAb transmission.

It is imperative to build on local experiences in comparable settings to develop successful protocols and implement adapted policies.

Author Contributions: Conceptualization, S.S.K., N.A.R. and R.M.Z.; methodology, S.S.K., N.A.R., N.Z., N.H. and R.M.Z.; software, N.H. and R.M.Z.; formal analysis, N.Z., N.H. and R.M.Z.; investigation, A.H. N.H. and R.A.; resources, S.S.K., N.Z. and R.M.Z.; data curation, N.Z., N.H., R.A. and A.H.; writing—original draft preparation, N.A.R., N.Z., N.H., R.A., A.H. and S.B.H.; writing—review and editing, N.A.R., S.S.K., S.B.H., S.F.H. and R.M.Z.; visualization, N.Z., N.H. and N.A.R. All authors have read and agreed to the published version of the manuscript.

Funding: This research received no external funding.

Institutional Review Board Statement: Not applicable.

Informed Consent Statement: Not applicable.

Data Availability Statement: The data presented in this study are available on request from the corresponding author.

Conflicts of Interest: The authors declare no conflict of interest.

References

1. At UN, Global Leaders Commit to Act on Antimicrobial Resistance. 2016. Available online: https://www.who.int/news/item/21-09-2016-at-un-global-leaders-commit-to-act-on-antimicrobial-resistance (accessed on 17 March 2022).
2. WHO. *Antimicrobial Resistance: Global Report on Surveillance*; WHO: Geneva, Switzerland, 2014.
3. By 2050, Drug-Resistant Infections Could Cause Global Economic Damage on par with 2008 Financial Crisis. 2016. Available online: https://www.worldbank.org/en/news/press-release/2016/09/18/by-2050-drug-resistant-infections-could-cause-global-economic-damage-on-par-with-2008-financial-crisis (accessed on 5 May 2022).
4. Murray, C.J.; Ikuta, K.S.; Sharara, F.; Swetschinski, L.; Aguilar, G.R.; Gray, A.; Han, C.; Bisignano, C.; Rao, P.; Wool, E.; et al. Global burden of bacterial antimicrobial resistance in 2019: A systematic analysis. *Lancet* **2022**, *399*, 629–655. [CrossRef]
5. Maragakis, L.L.; Perencevich, E.N.; Cosgrove, S.E. Clinical and economic burden of antimicrobial resistance. *Expert Rev. Anti-Infect. Ther.* **2008**, *6*, 751–763. [CrossRef] [PubMed]
6. O'Neill, J. *Antimicrobial Resistance: Tackling a Crisis for the Health and Wealth of Nations*; Review on Antimicrobial Resistance: London, UK, 2014.
7. Founou, R.C.; Founou, L.L.; Essack, S.Y. Clinical and economic impact of antibiotic resistance in developing countries: A systematic review and meta-analysis. *PLoS ONE* **2017**, *12*, e0189621. [CrossRef] [PubMed]
8. Dandachi, I.; Chaddad, A.; Hanna, J.; Matta, J.; Daoud, Z. Understanding the Epidemiology of Multi-Drug Resistant Gram-Negative Bacilli in the Middle East Using a One Health Approach. *Front. Microbiol.* **2019**, *10*, 1941. [CrossRef] [PubMed]
9. Boucher, H.W. Bad bugs, no drugs 2002–2020: Progress, challenges, and call to action. *Trans. Am. Clin. Climatol. Assoc.* **2020**, *131*, 65–71. [PubMed]
10. Rice, L.B. Federal Funding for the Study of Antimicrobial Resistance in Nosocomial Pathogens: No ESKAPE. *J. Infect. Dis.* **2008**, *197*, 1079–1081. [CrossRef]
11. Mulani, M.S.; Kamble, E.; Kumkar, S.N.; Tawre, M.S.; Pardesi, K.R. Emerging Strategies to Combat ESKAPE Pathogens in the Era of Antimicrobial Resistance: A Review. *Front. Microbiol.* **2019**, *10*, 539. [CrossRef]
12. Vincent, J.-L.; Rello, J.; Marshall, J.K.; Silva, E.; Anzueto, A.; Martin, C.D.; Moreno, R.; Lipman, J.; Gomersall, C.; Sakr, Y.; et al. International Study of the Prevalence and Outcomes of Infection in Intensive Care Units. *JAMA* **2009**, *302*, 2323–2329. [CrossRef]
13. Talaat, M.; Zayed, B.; Tolba, S.; Abdou, E.; Gomaa, M.; Itani, D.; Hutin, Y.; Hajjeh, R. Increasing Antimicrobial Resistance in World Health Organization Eastern Mediterranean Region, 2017–2019. *Emerg. Infect. Dis.* **2022**, *28*, 717–724. [CrossRef]
14. WHO. *Global Action Plan on Antimicrobial Resistance*; WHO: Geneva, Switzerland, 2016.
15. Teerawattanapong, N.; Kengkla, K.; Dilokthornsakul, P.; Saokaew, S.; Apisarnthanarak, A.; Chaiyakunapruk, N. Prevention and Control of Multidrug-Resistant Gram-Negative Bacteria in Adult Intensive Care Units: A Systematic Review and Network Meta-analysis. *Clin. Infect. Dis.* **2017**, *64*, S51–S60. [CrossRef]
16. Vincent, J.-L.; Sakr, Y.; Singer, M.; Martin-Loeches, I.; Machado, F.R.; Marshall, J.C.; Finfer, S.; Pelosi, P.; Brazzi, L.; Aditianingsih, D.; et al. Prevalence and Outcomes of Infection Among Patients in Intensive Care Units in 2017. *JAMA* **2020**, *323*, 1478–1487. [CrossRef] [PubMed]
17. Ansari, S.; Hays, J.P.; Kemp, A.; Okechukwu, R.; Murugaiyan, J.; Ekwanzala, M.D.; Alvarez, M.J.R.; Paul-Satyaseela, M.; Iwu, C.D.; Balleste-Delpierre, C.; et al. The potential impact of the COVID-19 pandemic on global antimicrobial and biocide resistance: An AMR Insights global perspective. *JAC-Antimicrob. Resist.* **2021**, *3*, dlab038. [CrossRef] [PubMed]
18. Tomczyk, S.; Taylor, A.; Brown, A.; de Kraker, M.E.A.; El-Saed, A.; Alshamrani, M.; Hendriksen, R.S.; Jacob, M.; Löfmark, S.; Perovic, O.; et al. Impact of the COVID-19 pandemic on the surveillance, prevention and control of antimicrobial resistance: A global survey. *J. Antimicrob. Chemother.* **2021**, *76*, 3045–3058. [CrossRef] [PubMed]
19. CDC. COVID-19 & Antibiotic Resistance. 2022. Available online: https://www.cdc.gov/drugresistance/covid19.html (accessed on 27 May 2022).
20. Garcia-Vidal, C.; Sanjuan, G.; Moreno-García, E.; Puerta-Alcalde, P.; Garcia-Pouton, N.; Chumbita, M.; Fernandez-Pittol, M.; Pitart, C.; Inciarte, A.; Bodro, M.; et al. Incidence of co-infections and superinfections in hospitalized patients with COVID-19: A retrospective cohort study. *Clin. Microbiol. Infect.* **2020**, *27*, 83–88. [CrossRef]
21. Weiner-Lastinger, L.M.; Pattabiraman, V.; Konnor, R.Y.; Patel, P.R.; Wong, E.; Xu, S.Y.; Smith, B.; Edwards, J.R.; Dudeck, M.A. The impact of coronavirus disease 2019 (COVID-19) on healthcare-associated infections in 2020: A summary of data reported to the National Healthcare Safety Network. *Infect. Control Hosp. Epidemiol.* **2021**, *43*, 12–25. [CrossRef]
22. Knight, G.M.; E Glover, R.; McQuaid, C.F.; Olaru, I.D.; Gallandat, K.; Leclerc, Q.J.; Fuller, N.M.; Willcocks, S.J.; Hasan, R.; van Kleef, E.; et al. Antimicrobial resistance and COVID-19: Intersections and implications. *eLife* **2021**, *10*, e64139. [CrossRef]
23. Dijkshoorn, L.; Nemec, A.; Seifert, H. An increasing threat in hospitals: Multidrug-resistant *Acinetobacter baumannii*. *Nat. Rev. Genet.* **2007**, *5*, 939–951. [CrossRef]
24. Ayoub Moubareck, C.; Hammoudi Halat, D. Insights into *Acinetobacter baumannii*: A Review of Microbiological, Virulence, and Resistance Traits in a Threatening Nosocomial Pathogen. *Antibiotics* **2020**, *9*, 119. [CrossRef]

25. Howard, A.; O'Donoghue, M.; Feeney, A.; Sleator, R.D. *Acinetobacter baumannii*: An emerging opportunistic pathogen. *Virulence* **2012**, *3*, 243–250. [CrossRef]
26. WHO. *Prioritization of Pathogens to Guide Discovery, Research and Development of New Antibiotics for Drug Resistant Bacterial Infections, Including Tuberculosis*; WHO: Geneva, Switzerland, 2017.
27. Theuretzbacher, U. Global antimicrobial resistance in Gram-negative pathogens and clinical need. *Curr. Opin. Microbiol.* **2017**, *39*, 106–112. [CrossRef]
28. Clark, N.M.; Zhanel, G.G.; Lynch, J.P.I. Emergence of antimicrobial resistance among *Acinetobacter* species: A global threat. *Curr. Opin. Crit. Care* **2016**, *22*, 491–499. [CrossRef] [PubMed]
29. Moghnieh, R.A.; Kanafani, Z.A.; Tabaja, H.Z.; Sharara, S.L.; Awad, L.S.; Kanj, S.S. Epidemiology of common resistant bacterial pathogens in the countries of the Arab League. *Lancet Infect. Dis.* **2018**, *18*, e379–e394. [CrossRef]
30. Dandachi, I.; Azar, E.; Hamouch, R.; Maliha, P.; Abdallah, S.; Kanaan, E.; Badawi, R.; Khairallah, T.; Matar, G.M.; Daoud, Z. *Acinetobacter* spp. in a Third World Country with Socio-economic and Immigrants Challenges. *J. Infect. Dev. Ctries.* **2019**, *13*, 948–955. [CrossRef] [PubMed]
31. Abbara, A.; Rawson, T.M.; Karah, N.; El-Amin, W.; Hatcher, J.; Tajaldin, B.; Dar, O.; Dewachi, O.; Abu Sitta, G.; Uhlin, B.E.; et al. Antimicrobial resistance in the context of the Syrian conflict: Drivers before and after the onset of conflict and key recommendations. *Int. J. Infect. Dis.* **2018**, *73*, 1–6. [CrossRef]
32. WHO. Regional Operational Framework for Implementation of the Global Action Plan on Antimicrobial Resistance. 2016. Available online: https://applications.emro.who.int/docs/Fact_Sheet_2016_EN_19200.pdf?ua=1URL (accessed on 23 March 2022).
33. Al Salman, J.; Al Dabal, L.; Bassetti, M.; Alfouzan, W.A.; Al Maslamani, M.; Alraddadi, B.; Elhoufi, A.; Enani, M.; Khamis, F.A.; Mokkadas, E.; et al. Management of infections caused by WHO critical priority Gram-negative pathogens in Arab countries of the Middle East: A consensus paper. *Int. J. Antimicrob. Agents* **2020**, *56*, 106104. [CrossRef]
34. Henig, O.; Weber, G.; Hoshen, M.B.; Paul, M.; German, L.; Neuberger, A.; Gluzman, I.; Berlin, A.; Shapira, C.; Balicer, R.D. Risk factors for and impact of carbapenem-resistant *Acinetobacter baumannii* colonization and infection: Matched case–control study. *Eur. J. Clin. Microbiol.* **2015**, *34*, 2063–2068. [CrossRef]
35. Matar, G.M.; Gay, E.; Cooksey, R.C.; Elliott, J.A.; Heneine, W.M.; Uwaydah, M.M.; Matossian, R.M.; Tenover, F.C. Identification of an epidemic strain of *Acinetobacter baumannii* using electrophoretic typing methods. *Eur. J. Epidemiol.* **1992**, *8*, 9–14. [CrossRef]
36. Sleiman, A.; Fayad, A.G.A.; Banna, H.; Matar, G.M. Prevalence and molecular epidemiology of carbapenem-resistant Gram-negative bacilli and their resistance determinants in the Eastern Mediterranean Region over the last decade. *J. Glob. Antimicrob. Resist.* **2021**, *25*, 209–221. [CrossRef]
37. Chamoun, K.; Farah, M.; Araj, G.; Daoud, Z.; Moghnieh, R.; Salameh, P.; Saade, D.; Mokhbat, J.; Abboud, E.; Hamze, M.; et al. Surveillance of antimicrobial resistance in Lebanese hospitals: Retrospective nationwide compiled data. *Int. J. Infect. Dis.* **2016**, *46*, 64–70. [CrossRef]
38. Moghnieh, R.; Araj, G.F.; Awad, L.; Daoud, Z.; Mokhbat, J.E.; Jisr, T.; Abdallah, D.; Azar, N.; Irani-Hakimeh, N.; Balkis, M.M.; et al. A compilation of antimicrobial susceptibility data from a network of 13 Lebanese hospitals reflecting the national situation during 2015–2016. *Antimicrob. Resist. Infect. Control* **2019**, *8*, 41. [CrossRef]
39. Kanafani, Z.A.; Zahreddine, N.; Tayyar, R.; Sfeir, J.; Araj, G.F.; Matar, G.M.; Kanj, S.S. Multi-drug resistant Acinetobacter species: A seven-year experience from a tertiary care center in Lebanon. *Antimicrob. Resist. Infect. Control* **2018**, *7*, 9. [CrossRef] [PubMed]
40. Al Atrouni, A.; Hamze, M.; Jisr, T.; Lemarié, C.; Eveillard, M.; Joly-Guillou, M.-L.; Kempf, M. Wide spread of OXA-23-producing carbapenem-resistant *Acinetobacter baumannii* belonging to clonal complex II in different hospitals in Lebanon. *Int. J. Infect. Dis.* **2016**, *52*, 29–36. [CrossRef] [PubMed]
41. Moghnieh, R.; Siblani, L.; Ghadban, D.; El Mchad, H.; Zeineddine, R.; Abdallah, D.; Ziade, F.; Sinno, L.; Kiwan, O.; Kerbaj, F.; et al. Extensively drug-resistant *Acinetobacter baumannii* in a Lebanese intensive care unit: Risk factors for acquisition and determination of a colonization score. *J. Hosp. Infect.* **2015**, *92*, 47–53. [CrossRef] [PubMed]
42. Makke, G.; Bitar, I.; Salloum, T.; Panossian, B.; Alousi, S.; Arabaghian, H.; Medvecky, M.; Hrabak, J.; Merheb-Ghoussoub, S.; Tokajian, S. Whole-Genome-Sequence-Based Characterization of Extensively Drug-Resistant *Acinetobacter baumannii* Hospital Outbreak. *mSphere* **2020**, *5*, e00934-19. [CrossRef]
43. Moghnieh, R.; Tamim, H.; Jadayel, M.; Abdallah, D.; Al-Kassem, R.; Kadiri, H.; Hafez, H.; Al-Hassan, S.; Ajjour, L.; Lakkis, R.; et al. The effect of temporary closure and enhanced terminal disinfection using aerosolized hydrogen peroxide of an open-bay intensive care unit on the acquisition of extensively drug-resistant *Acinetobacter baumannii*. *Antimicrob. Resist. Infect. Control* **2020**, *9*, 108. [CrossRef]
44. Chamieh, A.; Nawfal, T.D.; Ballouz, T.; Afif, C.; Juvelekian, G.; Hlais, S.; Rolain, J.M.; Azar, E. Control and Elimination of Extensively Drug-Resistant *Acinetobacter baumanii* in an Intensive Care Unit. *Emerg. Infect. Dis.* **2019**, *25*, 1928–1931. [CrossRef]
45. Moghnieh, R.; Awad, L.; Abdallah, D.; Jadayel, M.; Sinno, L.; Tamim, H.; Jisr, T.; El-Hassan, S.; Lakkis, R.; Dabbagh, R.; et al. Effect of a "handshake" stewardship program versus a formulary restriction policy on High-End antibiotic use, expenditure, antibiotic resistance, and patient outcome. *J. Chemother.* **2020**, *32*, 368–384. [CrossRef]
46. Kanj, S.S.; Tayyar, R.; Shehab, M.; El-Hafi, B.; Rasheed, S.S.; Kissoyan, K.A.B.; A Kanafani, Z.; Wakim, R.H.; Zahreddine, N.K.; Araj, G.F.; et al. Increased blaOXA-23-like prevalence in *Acinetobacter baumannii* at a tertiary care center in Lebanon (2007–2013). *J. Infect. Dev. Ctries.* **2018**, *12*, 228–234. [CrossRef]

47. Araj, G. Antimicrobial Susceptibility Profiles of Bacterial Isolates at the American University of Beirut Medical Center. 2021. Available online: https://www.aub.edu.lb/fm/PLM/PublishingImages/Pages/AntimicrobialSusceptibilityProfiles/2017-AMR%20-%20AUBMC%20brochure.pdf (accessed on 17 March 2022).
48. Brink, A.J. Epidemiology of carbapenem-resistant Gram-negative infections globally. *Curr. Opin. Infect. Dis.* **2019**, *32*, 609–616. [CrossRef]
49. Moussally, M.; Zahreddine, N.; Kazma, J.; Ahmadieh, R.; Kan, S.S.; Kanafan, Z.A. Prevalence of antibiotic-resistant organisms among hospitalized patients at a tertiary care center in Lebanon, 2010–2018. *J. Infect. Public Health* **2020**, *14*, 12–16. [CrossRef]
50. Kanafani, Z.A.; El Zakhem, A.; Zahreddine, N.; Ahmadieh, R.; Kanj, S.S. Ten-year surveillance study of ventilator-associated pneumonia at a tertiary care center in Lebanon. *J. Infect. Public Health* **2019**, *12*, 492–495. [CrossRef] [PubMed]
51. Lebanon Goes Live with Epic. 2019. Available online: http://www.aubmc.org/Pages/AUBMC-launches-AUBHealth-a-new-comprehensive-health-record-system.aspx#sthash.uulttxN6.b3aSfvPw.dpbs (accessed on 17 March 2022).
52. Karanika, S.; Paudel, S.; Grigoras, C.; Kalbasi, A.; Mylonakis, E. Systematic Review and Meta-analysis of Clinical and Economic Outcomes from the Implementation of Hospital-Based Antimicrobial Stewardship Programs. *Antimicrob. Agents Chemother.* **2016**, *60*, 4840–4852. [CrossRef] [PubMed]
53. Bogan, C.; Marchaim, D. The role of antimicrobial stewardship in curbing carbapenem resistance. *Future Microbiol.* **2013**, *8*, 979–991. [CrossRef] [PubMed]
54. CDC. *Core Elements of Hospital Antibiotic Stewardship Programs/Antibiotic Use*; US Department of Health and Human Services: Atlanta, GA, USA, 2019. Available online: https://www.cdc.gov/antibiotic-use/healthcare/pdfs/hospital-core-elements-H.pdf (accessed on 17 March 2022).
55. El Masri, M.; Haddad, N.; Saad, T.; Rizk, N.A.; Zakhour, R.; Kanj, S.S.; Zeenny, R.M. Evaluation of Carbapenem Use Before and After Implementation of an Antimicrobial Stewardship-Led Carbapenem-Sparing Strategy in a Lebanese Tertiary Hospital: A Retrospective Study. *Front. Cell. Infect. Microbiol.* **2022**, *12*, 729491. [CrossRef]
56. Barlam, T.F.; Cosgrove, S.E.; Abbo, L.M.; MacDougall, C.; Schuetz, A.N.; Septimus, E.J.; Srinivasan, A.; Dellit, T.H.; Falck-Ytter, Y.T.; Fishman, N.O.; et al. Implementing an Antibiotic Stewardship Program: Guidelines by the Infectious Diseases Society of America and the Society for Healthcare Epidemiology of America. *Clin. Infect. Dis.* **2016**, *62*, e51–e77. [CrossRef]
57. The Joint Commission Antimicrobial Stewardship Resources Related to Antimicrobial Stewardship for Health Care Settings. Available online: https://www.jointcommission.org/resources/patient-safety-topics/infection-prevention-and-control/antimicrobial-stewardship/ (accessed on 17 March 2022).
58. Morris, A.M. Antimicrobial Stewardship Programs: Appropriate Measures and Metrics to Study their Impact. *Curr. Treat. Options Infect. Dis.* **2014**, *6*, 101–112. [CrossRef]
59. WHO. *WHO Collaborating Centre for Drug Statistics Methodology: ATC Classification Index with DDDs and Guidelines for ATC Classification and DDD Assignment*; Norwegian Institute of Public Health: Oslo, Norway, 2006.
60. Wieczorkiewicz, S.M.; Sincak, C. *The Pharmacist's Guide to Antimicrobial Therapy and Stewardship*; American Society of Health-System Pharmacists: Bethesda, MD, USA, 2015.
61. Frost, S.A.; Alogso, M.-C.; Metcalfe, L.; Lynch, J.M.; Hunt, L.; Sanghavi, R.; Alexandrou, E.; Hillman, K.M. Chlorhexidine bathing and health care-associated infections among adult intensive care patients: A systematic review and meta-analysis. *Crit. Care* **2016**, *20*, 379. [CrossRef]
62. Pittet, D.; Hugonnet, S.; Harbarth, S.; Mourouga, P.; Sauvan, V.; Touveneau, S.; Perneger, T.V. Effectiveness of a hospital-wide programme to improve compliance with hand hygiene. *Lancet* **2000**, *356*, 1307–1312. [CrossRef]
63. Talbot, T.R.; Johnson, J.G.; Fergus, C.; Domenico, J.H.; Schaffner, W.; Daniels, T.L.; Wilson, G.; Slayton, J.; Feistritzer, N.; Hickson, G.B. Sustained Improvement in Hand Hygiene Adherence: Utilizing Shared Accountability and Financial Incentives. *Infect. Control Hosp. Epidemiol.* **2013**, *34*, 1129–1136. [CrossRef]
64. Karageorgopoulos, D.E.; Falagas, M.E. Current control and treatment of multidrug-resistant *Acinetobacter baumannii* infections. *Lancet Infect. Dis.* **2008**, *8*, 751–762. [CrossRef]
65. Gonzalez-Villoria, A.M.; Valverde-Garduno, V. Antibiotic-Resistant *Acinetobacter baumannii* Increasing Success Remains a Challenge as a Nosocomial Pathogen. *J. Pathog.* **2016**, *2016*, 7318075. [CrossRef] [PubMed]
66. López-Lozano, J.-M.; THRESHOLDS study group; Lawes, T.; Nebot, C.; Beyaert, A.; Bertrand, X.; Hocquet, D.; Aldeyab, M.; Scott, M.; Conlon-Bingham, G.; et al. A nonlinear time-series analysis approach to identify thresholds in associations between population antibiotic use and rates of resistance. *Nat. Microbiol.* **2019**, *4*, 1160–1172. [CrossRef]
67. Lvarez-Marín, R.; López-Cerero, L.; Guerrero-Sánchez, F.; Palop-Borras, B.; Rojo-Martín, M.D.; Ruiz-Sancho, A.; Herrero-Rodríguez, C.; García, M.V.; Lazo-Torres, A.M.; López, I.; et al. Do specific antimicrobial stewardship interventions have an impact on carbapenem resistance in Gram-negative bacilli? A multicentre quasi-experimental ecological study: Time-trend analysis and characterization of carbapenemases. *J. Antimicrob. Chemother.* **2021**, *76*, 1928–1936. [CrossRef] [PubMed]
68. Yusef, D.; A Hayajneh, W.; Issa, A.B.; Haddad, R.; Al-Azzam, S.; A Lattyak, E.; Lattyak, W.J.; Gould, I.; Conway, B.R.; Bond, S.; et al. Impact of an antimicrobial stewardship programme on reducing broad-spectrum antibiotic use and its effect on carbapenem-resistant *Acinetobacter baumannii* (CRAb) in hospitals in Jordan. *J. Antimicrob. Chemother.* **2020**, *76*, 516–523. [CrossRef] [PubMed]
69. Ogutlu, A.; Guclu, E.; Karabay, O.; Utku, A.C.; Tuna, N.; Yahyaoglu, M. Effects of Carbapenem consumption on the prevalence of Acinetobacter infection in intensive care unit patients. *Ann. Clin. Microbiol. Antimicrob.* **2014**, *13*, 7. [CrossRef] [PubMed]

70. Chen, C.-H.; Lin, L.-C.; Chang, Y.-J.; Chen, Y.-M.; Chang, C.-Y.; Huang, C.-C. Infection Control Programs and Antibiotic Control Programs to Limit Transmission of Multi-Drug Resistant *Acinetobacter baumannii* Infections: Evolution of Old Problems and New Challenges for Institutes. *Int. J. Environ. Res. Public Health* **2015**, *12*, 8871–8882. [CrossRef]
71. Wilks, M.; Wilson, A.; Warwick, S.; Price, E.; Kennedy, D.; Ely, A.; Millar, M.R. Control of an Outbreak of Multidrug-Resistant *Acinetobacter baumannii-calcoaceticus* Colonization and Infection in an Intensive Care Unit (ICU) Without Closing the ICU or Placing Patients in Isolation. *Infect. Control Hosp. Epidemiol.* **2006**, *27*, 654–658. [CrossRef]
72. Rodríguez-Baño, J.; García, L.; Ramírez, E.; Martínez-Martínez, L.; Muniain, M.A.; Fernández-Cuenca, F. Long-term control of hospital-wide, endemic multidrug-resistant *Acinetobacter baumannii* through a comprehensive "bundle" approach. *Am. J. Infect. Control.* **2009**, *37*, 715–722. [CrossRef]
73. Cheon, S.; Kim, M.-J.; Yun, S.-J.; Moon, J.Y.; Kim, Y.-S. Controlling endemic multidrug-resistant *Acinetobacter baumannii* in Intensive Care Units using antimicrobial stewardship and infection control. *Korean J. Intern. Med.* **2016**, *31*, 367–374. [CrossRef]
74. Valencia-Martín, R.; Gonzalez-Galan, V.; Alvarez-Marín, R.; Cazalla-Foncueva, A.M.; Aldabó, T.; Gil-Navarro, M.V.; Alonso-Araujo, I.; Martin, C.; Gordon, R.; García-Nuñez, E.J.; et al. A multimodal intervention program to control a long-term *Acinetobacter baumannii* endemic in a tertiary care hospital. *Antimicrob. Resist. Infect. Control* **2019**, *8*, 199. [CrossRef]
75. Abouzeid, M.; Habib, R.R.; Jabbour, S.; Mokdad, A.H.; Nuwayhid, I. Lebanon's humanitarian crisis escalates after the Beirut blast. *Lancet* **2020**, *396*, 1380–1382. [CrossRef]
76. Jabbour, R.; Harakeh, M.; Sailan, S.D.; Nassar, V.; Tashjian, H.; Massouh, J.; Massouh, A.; Puzantian, H.; Darwish, H. Nurses' stories from Beirut: The 2020 explosive disaster on top of a pandemic and economic crises. *Int. Nurs. Rev.* **2021**, *68*, 1–8. [CrossRef]
77. Gebran, A.; Abou Khalil, E.; El Moheb, M.; Albaini, O.; El Warea, M.; Ibrahim, R.; Karam, K.; El Helou, M.O.; Ramly, E.P.; El Hechi, M.; et al. The Beirut Port Explosion Injuries and Lessons Learned: Results of the Beirut Blast Assessment for Surgical Services (BASS) Multicenter Study. *Ann. Surg.* **2022**, *275*, 398–405. [CrossRef] [PubMed]
78. Bizri, A.R.; Khalil, P.B. A Lebanese physician's dilemma: Not how, but with what? *Lancet* **2021**, *398*, 841. [CrossRef]
79. Zahreddine, N.K.; Haddad, S.F.; Kerbage, A.; Kanj, S.S. Challenges of coronavirus disease 2019 (COVID-19) in Lebanon in the midst of the economic collapse. *Antimicrob. Steward. Healthc. Epidemiol.* **2022**, *2*, E67. [CrossRef]
80. Rizk, N.A.; Moghnieh, R.; Haddad, N.; Rebeiz, M.-C.; Zeenny, R.M.; Hindy, J.-R.; Orlando, G.; Kanj, S.S. Challenges to Antimicrobial Stewardship in the Countries of the Arab League: Concerns of Worsening Resistance during the COVID-19 Pandemic and Proposed Solutions. *Antibiotics* **2021**, *10*, 1320. [CrossRef] [PubMed]
81. Allaw, F.; Zahreddine, N.K.; Ibrahim, A.; Tannous, J.; Taleb, H.; Bizri, A.; Dbaibo, G.; Kanj, S. First *Candida auris* Outbreak during a COVID-19 Pandemic in a Tertiary-Care Center in Lebanon. *Pathogens* **2021**, *10*, 157. [CrossRef]

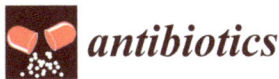

Article

Plethora of Antibiotics Usage and Evaluation of Carbapenem Prescribing Pattern in Intensive Care Units: A Single-Center Experience of Malaysian Academic Hospital

Chee Lan Lau [1,2], Petrick Periyasamy [3], Muhd Nordin Saud [2], Sarah Anne Robert [2], Lay Yen Gan [2], Suet Yin Chin [2], Kiew Bing Pau [2], Shue Hong Kong [2], Farah Waheeda Tajurudin [2], Mei Kuen Yin [2], Sheah Lin Ghan [2], Nur Jannah Azman [2], Xin Yun Chua [2], Poy Kei Lye [2], Stephanie Wai Yee Tan [2], Dexter Van Dort [2], Ramliza Ramli [4], Toh Leong Tan [5], Aliza Mohamad Yusof [6], Saw Kian Cheah [6], Wan Rahiza Wan Mat [6] and Isa Naina-Mohamed [1,*]

1. Pharmacoepidemiology and Drug Safety Unit, Department of Pharmacology, Faculty of Medicine, Universiti Kebangsaan Malaysia, Cheras, Kuala Lumpur 56000, Malaysia
2. Pharmacy Department, Hospital Canselor Tuanku Muhriz, Cheras, Kuala Lumpur 56000, Malaysia
3. Medical Department, Faculty of Medicine, Universiti Kebangsaan Malaysia, Cheras, Kuala Lumpur 56000, Malaysia
4. Department of Medical Microbiology and Immunology, Faculty of Medicine, Universiti Kebangsaan Malaysia, Cheras, Kuala Lumpur 56000, Malaysia
5. Department of Emergency Medicine, Faculty of Medicine, Universiti Kebangsaan Malaysia, Cheras, Kuala Lumpur 56000, Malaysia
6. Department of Anesthesiology & Intensive Care, Faculty of Medicine, Universiti Kebangsaan Malaysia, Cheras, Kuala Lumpur 56000, Malaysia
* Correspondence: isanaina@ppukm.ukm.edu.my

Abstract: Excessive antibiotic consumption is still common among critically ill patients admitted to intensive care units (ICU), especially during the coronavirus disease 2019 (COVID-19) period. Moreover, information regarding antimicrobial consumption among ICUs in South-East Asia remains scarce and limited. This study aims to determine antibiotics utilization in ICUs by measuring antibiotics consumption over the past six years (2016–2021) and specifically evaluating carbapenems prescribed in a COVID-19 ICU and a general intensive care unit (GICU) during the second year of the COVID-19 pandemic. (2) Methods: This is a retrospective cross-sectional observational analysis of antibiotics consumption and carbapenems prescriptions. Antibiotic utilization data were estimated using the WHO Defined Daily Doses (DDD). Carbapenems prescription information was extracted from the audits conducted by ward pharmacists. Patients who were prescribed carbapenems during their admission to COVID-19 ICU and GICU were included. Patients who passed away before being reviewed by the pharmacists were excluded. (3) Results: In general, antibiotics consumption increased markedly in the year 2021 when compared to previous years. Majority of carbapenems were prescribed empirically (86.8%). Comparing COVID-19 ICU and GICU, the reasons for empirical carbapenems therapy in COVID-19 ICU was predominantly for therapy escalation (64.7% COVID-19 ICU vs. 34% GICU, $p < 0.001$), whereas empirical prescription in GICU was for coverage of extended-spectrum beta-lactamases (ESBL) gram-negative bacteria (GNB) (45.3% GICU vs. 22.4% COVID-19 ICU, $p = 0.005$). Despite microbiological evidence, the empirical carbapenems were continued for a median (interquartile range (IQR)) of seven (5–8) days. This implies the need for a rapid diagnostic assay on direct specimens, together with comprehensive antimicrobial stewardship (AMS) discourse with intensivists to address this issue.

Keywords: carbapenems; defined daily dose; antibiotics utilization; intensive care; empiric

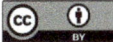

1. Introduction

Antibiotics have been prescribed in 70% of ICU patients due to the high prevalence of suspected or proven infection [1]. Since the outbreak of COVID-19, the hospitalization rate has increased along with an increased tendency of antibiotics prescription. A retrospective study in Malaysia during the early phase of the pandemic found a lower antibiotic usage at a prevalence of only 17.1%, in contrast to findings by two systematic reviews [2,3], though it was observed that ICU/HDU admissions were 2.73 times more likely to be prescribed antibiotics [4]. However, no details on antibiotic dosage and duration were analyzed.

A systematic review of 38 studies consisting of 2715 ICU admissions found a similar frequency of antibiotics prescription at 71%. Yet, incidences of bacterial infections were reported in only 30.8% of the studies reviewed. Furthermore, 69.2% of the antibiotics prescribed were empirical without strong evidence of bacterial infection [5]. In a review by Pasero et al. [6], hospital-acquired infection among COVID-19 patients developed 10–15 days after ICU admissions. However, extensive empirical antibiotics were prescribed, along with prolonged ICU stay leading to the surge of multidrug resistance (MDR) microorganisms, with incidence ranging from 32% to 50%. These data only reflected the use of antibiotics during the first year of the pandemic, and studies on the prescription pattern among critically ill patients in developing countries and the South-East Asia region are scarce. In addition, little is known about the duration of exposure to the prescribed antibiotic(s), which is crucial for antibiotic resistance development [7].

Antimicrobial resistance (AMR) has been a global health threat declared by World Health Organization (WHO) since 2015 [8]. With the high prevalence of antibiotic prescription and infection rates, ICU may potentially be the driver of resistance in hospitals [9]. Furthermore, an increase in antimicrobials resistance (AMR) in ICUs was observed since the COVID-19 pandemic, owing to the compromise in infection control and excessive antimicrobials use [10]. Carbapenems consumption has a positive correlation with increased resistance to carbapenems among gram-negative organisms such as *Acinetobacter baumannii*, *Pseudomonas aeruginosa*, and *Enterobacterales* [11–13]. Till the year 2020, surveillance in local hospitals of Malaysia reported that resistance to meropenem was lower than 10% for most gram-negative organisms, except *Acinetobacter baumannii* (58.5%) [14]. However, it is just a matter of time before carbapenems resistance rate increases beyond 20% as seen with resistance to third-generation cephalosporins in *Klebsiella pneumoniae* [14]. Hence, local antibiotics consumption should be monitored and the reasons for empirical usage of broad-spectrum antibiotics like carbapenems should be explored. This present study attempts to determine antibiotic utilization in ICUs over the past six years and analyze the prescription of carbapenems in COVID-19 ICU and GICU during the second year of the COVID-19 pandemic.

2. Results

The usage of antibiotics was stable from 2016 through 2019. Comparing the year 2019 and year 2021, the total consumption of selected antibiotics (Figure 1) in both ICUs had increased from 823.9 DDD per 1000 patient days to 1307.6 DDD per 1000 patient days (Supplementary File S1). In contrast to the increase in ceftriaxone from 117.4 to 146.9 DDD per 1000 days, amoxicillin/clavulanic acid was raised more than two-fold from 47.9 to 112.7 DDD per 1000 patient days, while ampicillin/sulbactam was raised from 140.5 to 240.3 DDD per 1000 patient days. Notably, the utilization of colistin surged and was almost 10 times higher; it increased from 2.95 to 32.04 DDD per 1000 patient days while that of polymyxin B dropped 15% from 52.6 to 44.5 DDD per patient days. Piperacillin/tazobactam consumption increased from 187.4 to 246.7 DDD per 1000 patient days, but cefepime usage increased and was more than three times higher; it went from from 46 to 134.8 DDD per 1000 patient days. Meanwhile, vancomycin utilization was also raised by 81.7%, from 52 to 94.5 DDD per 1000 patient days.

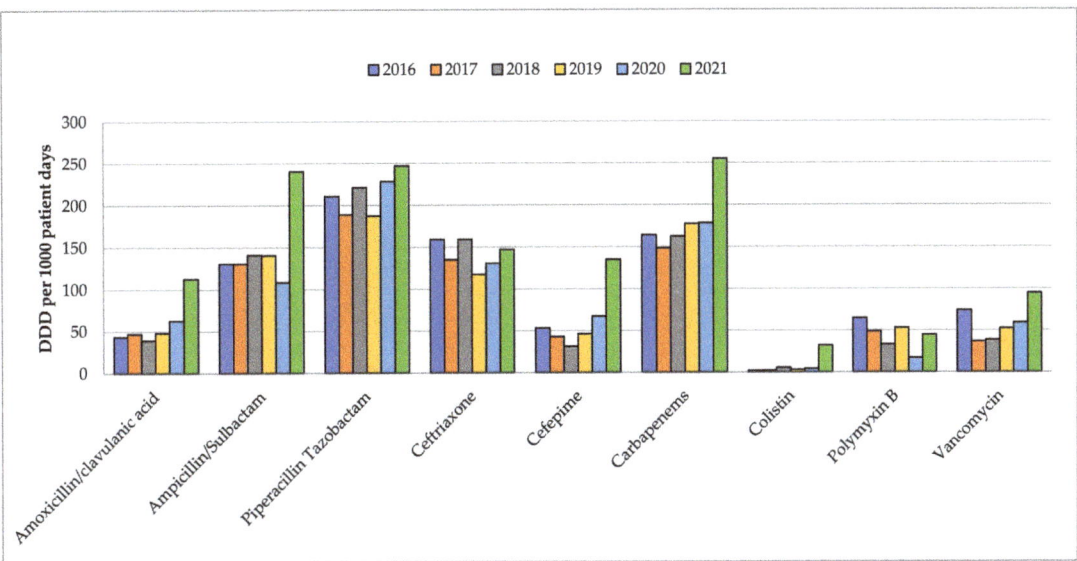

Figure 1. Annual Antibiotic Utilization in COVID-19 ICU and GICU from the year 2016 to the year 2021.

2.1. Carbapenems Consumption

Considering the past six years, the total admissions had dropped since 2020 and were the lowest in 2021. However, the average length of stay per patient and total patient days in both ICUs were the longest in 2021 at 8.02 days and 6229 days, respectively (Table 1). The average consumption of type-2 carbapenems in 2016 to 2019 was maintained at a median (IQR) of 153.3 (140.6–161.0) DDD per 1000 patient days. Subsequently, the usage increased by 53.6% in 2021 compared to 2019.

Table 1. Annual consumption of carbapenems in COVID-19 ICU and GICU.

	2016	2017	2018	2019	2020	2021	
Annual Census							
Number of Admissions, no	849	865	842	794	690	567	
Patient days, day	4636	5422	5504	5605	4228	6229	
Average length of stay, day	5.62	6.33	6.65	7.08	6.15	8.02	
Carbapenems	Consumption (DDD per 1000 patient days)						Increment in 2021 versus 2019 usage (%)
Ertapenem	12.66	−65.5	7.09	14.27	15.37	4.93	−65.5
Imipenem	43.67		15.99	27.25	12.89	23.16	
Meropenem	107.63		139.29	135.65	150.03	227.04	
Group-2 Carbapenems	151.30	53.6	155.28	162.90	162.92	250.20	53.6

2.2. Carbapenems Prescribing in COVID-19 ICU & GICU

2.2.1. Carbapenems Prescriptions

In 2021, a total of 605 carbapenems prescription requests were retrieved from the preauthorization forms, of which 159 prescriptions for 149 patients in the GICU and the COVID-19 ICU were eligible to be included (Figure 2). Meanwhile, a total of five prescriptions were excluded because they were missed, or patients passed away before being reviewed by pharmacists.

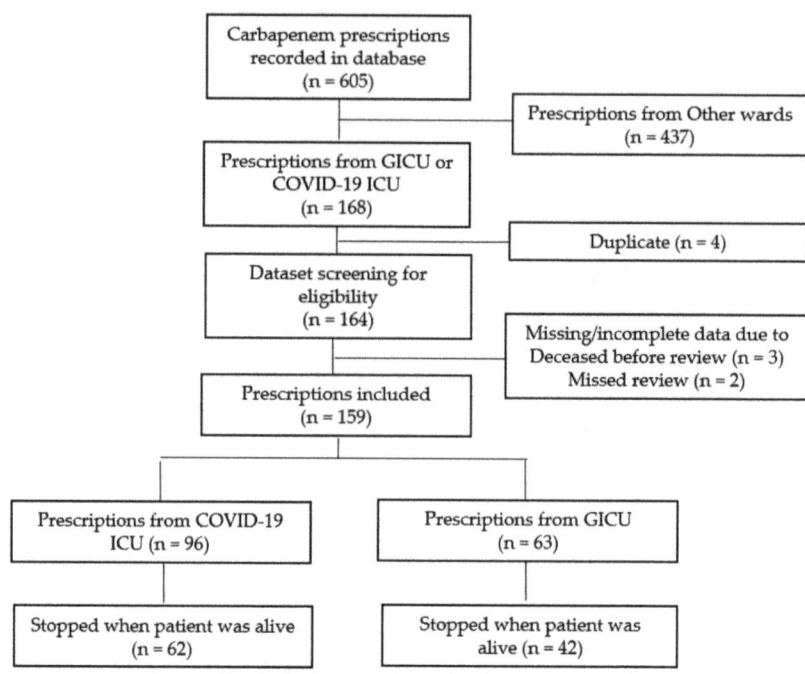

Figure 2. The selection process for eligible carbapenems prescriptions.

2.2.2. Patients' Demographics & Infection Control Surveillance

In 2021, there were 336 admissions to COVID-19 ICU and 231 admissions to GICU. The all-cause in-ICU mortality was higher (127, 37.8% vs. 40, 17.3%, $p < 0.0001$) and the median (IQR) length of ICU stay was longer (9 (5–15) days vs. 5 (3–10) days, $p < 0.0001$) in the COVID-19 ICU compared to the GICU.

Among patients who were prescribed carbapenems, the majority were male patients (94/149, 63.1%) with a median (IQR) age of 61 (44–69) years old. The male proportion (56/91 vs. 40/58, $p = 0.297$) and patients' age (median (IQR): 61 (46–68) years old vs. 60 (37–71) years old, $p = 0.806$) were comparable between COVID-19 ICU and GICU. Notably, GICU had significantly more patients colonized with resistant organisms who were prescribed carbapenems ($p = 0.003$) (Table 2).

Table 2. Rectal colonization among patients who were prescribed carbapenems.

Rectal Colonization by ESBL/MDR	Overall, n = 149	COVID-19 ICU, n = 91	GICU, n = 58	p
n (%)				0.003 [a,*]
Yes [^]	50 (35.7)	22 (25.9)	28 (50.9)	
No	90 (64.3)	63 (74.1)	27 (49.1)	
Unknown [#]	9	6	3	

[#] This group is not included in the analysis as rectal swab is not done; [^] 1 is *Citrobacter* spp.; [a] Pearson Chi-square. MDR, Multidrug-resistant. * $p < 0.05$ indicates statistically significant.

2.2.3. Characteristics of Carbapenems Prescriptions

At the time of prescription, most of the carbapenems were intended for nosocomial infection (type-3) (79.9%), followed by healthcare-associated infection (type-2), and six prescriptions were for community-acquired infection (type-1). Most prescriptions were for nosocomial infections in COVID-19 ICU (83/96 vs. 44/63, $p = 0.011$). In the GICU, the majority were for healthcare-associated infections in the GICU (11/96 vs. 15/63, $p = 0.039$)

(see Table 3). Meropenem accounted for most of the carbapenems prescribed across both ICUs. Overall, only 21 (13.2%) of carbapenems prescriptions were for definitive therapy according to the microbiological reports, and 86.8% were for empirical therapy.

Table 3. Characteristics of all carbapenem prescriptions.

	Overall, n = 159	COVID-19 ICU, n = 96	GICU, n = 63	p
Patient types at the time of prescription, no (%)				0.033 [a]
Type-1 (CA)	6 (3.8)	2 (2.1)	4 (6.3)	0.215 [b,^]
Type-2 (HA)	26 (16.4)	11 (11.3)	15 (23.8)	0.039 [a,*,^]
Type-3 (NI)	127 (79.9)	83 (86.5)	44 (69.8)	0.011 [a,*,^]
Carbapenem, no (%)				<0.001 [b,*]
Meropenem	148 (93.1)	95 (98.9)	53 (84.1)	
Imipenem	8 (5.0)	0 (0.0)	8 (12.7)	
Ertapenem	3 (1.9)	1 (1.0)	2 (3.2)	
Indication, no (%)				0.310 [a]
Definitive	21 (13.2)	11 (11.5)	10 (15.9)	
Empirical	138 (86.8)	85 (88.5)	53 (84.1)	

CA, Community-Acquired infection; HA, Healthcare-associated Infection; NI, Nosocomial Infection; [a] Pearson Chi-square, [b] Fisher Exact test. ^ based on individual groups. * $p < 0.05$ indicates statistically significant.

2.2.4. Empirical Carbapenems Therapy

More than half of the carbapenems were prescribed for escalation therapy, followed by the consideration of ESBL GNB risk (Table 4). Conversely, only 10 (7.2%) prescriptions were initiated after infectious disease (ID) consultation. Type-2 patients were more often prescribed for consideration of ESBL GNB risk (15/24, 62.5%, $p < 0.001$). Empirical escalation to carbapenems was often prescribed for type-3 patients (65/108, $p = 0.001$), and predominantly observed in COVID-19 ICU (55/85 vs. 18/53, $p < 0.001$). The initiation of empirical therapy considering ESBL GNB risk was more frequent (19/85 vs. 24/53, $p = 0.005$) in GICU. No association was found between reasons for empirical therapy with sites of infection. However, empirical therapy was more often intended for respiratory infections in the COVID-19 ICU ($p = 0.017$).

Table 4. Characteristics of empirical carbapenem prescriptions.

Reason for Empirical Therapy, no (%)	Overall, n = 138	COVID-19 ICU, n = 85	GICU, n = 53	p
Therapy escalation/switch	73 (52.9)	55 (64.7)	18 (34.0)	<0.001 [a,*]
Considering ESBL GNB risk	43 (31.2)	19 (22.4)	24 (45.3)	0.005 [a,*]
With ID consultation	10 (7.2)	7 (8.2)	3 (5.7)	0.741 [b]
Others	12 (8.7)	4 (4.7)	8 (15.1)	0.059 [b]
Suspected site of infection, no (%)				
Blood	45 (32.6)	31 (36.5)	14 (26.4)	0.220 [a]
Central nervous system	6 (4.3)	3 (3.5)	3 (5.7)	0.675 [b]
Intra-abdominal	20 (14.5)	4 (4.7)	16 (30.2)	<0.001 [a,*]
Respiratory	62 (44.6)	45 (52.9)	17 (32.1)	0.017 [a,*]
Skin and soft tissue	1 (0.7)	0 (0.0)	1 (1.9)	0.384 [b]
Urinary tract	2 (1.4)	2 (2.3)	0 (0.0)	0.523 [b]
Unknown	2 (1.4)	0 (0.0)	2 (3.8)	0.146 [b]

[a] Pearson Chi-square, [b] Fisher Exact test. * $p < 0.05$ indicates statistically significant.

2.2.5. Microbiological Growth & Organisms

Overall, out of 159 prescriptions, 101 (63.5%) had positive growth from cultures and 66 (41.5%) from blood cultures. The remaining 58 (36.5%) prescriptions had no growth, mixed growth, or candida species from respiratory samples or urine samples.

Among definitive therapies, *Klebsiella pneumoniae* and *Klebsiella* spp. (14/23, 60.9%) were frequently isolated, and the majority were ESBL producers. Two *Klebsiella* isolates were carbapenemases producers (Table 5). This was followed by ESBL-producing *Escherichia coli* (5/23, 21.7%). All isolates were from type-2 and type-3 patients. Among 50 patients with rectal colonization, only eight patients (16.0%) had ESBL GNB bacteremia, compared to eight (8.9%) among 90 patients without colonization ($p = 0.268$). For the empirical prescriptions, the isolated organisms are listed in Table 5. MDR *Acinetobacter* spp. were frequently isolated, especially from COVID-19 ICU ($p = 0.143$), whereas *Enterobacterales* and *Pseudomonas aeruginosa* were isolated more often from GICU.

Table 5. Microbiological profiles and organisms isolated prior to carbapenems therapy.

	Overall, n = 159	COVID-19 ICU, n = 96	GICU, n = 63	p
Growth from cultures [1]				0.952 [a]
Negative	10 (6.3)	6 (6.3)	4 (6.3)	
Mixed growth/*Candida* spp. [2]	48 (30.2)	30 (31.3)	18 (28.5)	
Positive culture	101 (63.5)	60 (62.5)	41 (65.1)	
Site of positive cultures (n = 101)				0.736 [a]
Positive blood cultures	66 (41.5)	40 (41.7)	26 (41.3)	
Other sites	35 (22.0)	20 (20.8)	15 (23.8)	
Organisms isolated from blood cultures				
Definitive therapy:				
Escherichia coli ESBL	4 (4.8)	1 (2.0)	3 (9.4)	
Klebsiella pneumoniae/spp. ESBL	9 (10.8)	5 (9.8)	4 (12.5)	
Klebsiella pneumoniae [#] CRE	1 (1.2)	1 (2.0)	0 (0.0)	
Pseudomonas aeruginosa **	1 (1.2)	1 (2.0)	0 (0.0)	
Achromobacter Xylosoxidans	1 (1.2)	0 (0.0)	1 (3.1)	
Empirical therapy:				
Escherichia coli	4 (4.8)	0 (0.0)	4 (12.5)	
Klebsiella pneumoniae/spp.	7 (8.4)	2 (3.9)	5 (15.6)	
Enterobacter aerogenes/spp.	1 (1.2)	0 (0.0)	1 (3.1)	
Acinetobacter baumannii/spp.	1 (1.2)	0 (0.0)	1 (3.1)	
Acinetobacter baumannii/spp. MDR	9 (10.8)	8 (15.7)	1 (3.1)	
Burkholderia cepacia	1 (1.2)	1 (2.0)	0 (0.0)	
Pseudomonas aeruginosa ***	5 (6.0)	3 (5.9)	2 (6.3)	
Stenotrophomonas maltophilia	3 (3.6)	3 (5.9)	0 (0.0)	
Enterococcus faecium/faecalis/spp.	5 (6.0)	3 (5.9)	2 (6.3)	
Streptococcus spp.	3 (3.6)	1 (2.0)	2 (6.3)	
CoNS	13 (15.7)	10 (19.6)	3 (9.4)	
Candida spp.	5 (6.0)	4 (7.8)	1 (3.1)	
Others	10 (12.0)	8 (15.7)	2 (6.3)	
Organisms isolated from respiratory/tissue/pus/urine cultures				
Definitive therapy:				
Escherichia coli ESBL	1 (2.0)	1 (3.6)	0 (0.0)	
Klebsiella pneumoniae/spp. ESBL	3 (6.0)	2 (7.1)	1 (4.5)	
Klebsiella pneumoniae [#] CRE	1 (2.0)	0 (0.0)	1 (4.5)	
Enterococcus spp.	1 (2.0)	1 (3.6)	0 (0.0)	
CoNS	1 (2.0)	1 (3.6)	0 (0.0)	

Table 5. *Cont.*

	Overall, n = 159	COVID-19 ICU, n = 96	GICU, n = 63	p
Empirical therapy:				
Escherichia coli	2 (4.0)	1 (3.6)	1 (4.5)	
Klebsiella pneumoniae/spp.	5 (10.0)	1 (3.6)	4 (18.2)	
Klebsiella pneumoniae ## CRE	1 (2.0)	1 (3.6)	0 (0.0)	
Enterobacter aerogenes/spp.	2 (4.0)	1 (3.6)	1 (4.5)	
Acinetobacter baumannii/spp. MDR	14 (28)	10 (35.7)	4 (18.2)	
Pseudomonas aeruginosa ***	10 (20.0)	5 (17.9)	5 (22.7)	
Stenotrophomonas maltophilia	2 (4.0)	1 (3.6)	1 (4.5)	
Enterococcus faecium/faecalis/spp.	2 (4.0)	2 (7.1)	0 (0.0)	
Staphylococcus aureus	2 (4.0)	0 (0.0)	2 (9.1)	
MRSA	1 (2.0)	0 (0.0)	1 (4.5)	
Mycobacterium tuberculosis	2 (4.0)	1 (3.6)	1 (4.5)	

[a] Pearson Chi-square; CoNS: coagulase-negative *Staphylococci*; CRE, carbapenem-resistant *Enterobacterales*; ESBL, extended-spectrum beta-lactamase; MIC, minimum inhibitory concentration; MDR, multidrug-resistant; MRSA, methicillin-resistant *Staphylococcus aureus*. # MIC = 4; ## MIC more than 24 for all carbapenems tested; ** Resistant to ceftazidime, cefepime, and piperacillin/tazobactam; *** Sensitive to ceftazidime. [1] Based on cultures reports prior to carbapenems therapy. [2] From tracheal aspirates/sputum/urine/pus.

2.2.6. Duration of Carbapenems Therapy

During the carbapenems therapy, 55 patients passed away before completing the treatment. Overall, the median (IQR) duration of carbapenems prescriptions was seven (5–8) days. The duration of definitive therapy was significantly longer than that of empirical therapy by one day ($p = 0.015$). Compared to GICU, a shorter duration of definitive therapy ($p = 0.463$), but a longer duration of empirical therapy ($p = 0.654$) was observed in COVID-19 ICU (Table 6). In addition, among empirical prescriptions, only seven (13.0%) in COVID-19 ICU and seven (20.0%) in GICU were discontinued within three days ($p = 0.624$).

Table 6. Duration of carbapenems prescriptions.

Duration of Therapy	Overall, n = 104	COVID-19 ICU, n = 62	GICU, n = 42	p
Overall median, days (IQR)	7 (5–8)	7 (5–8)	7 (4–9)	0.963 [a]
Definitive therapy, median, days (IQR)	(n = 15) 8 (7–11) *	(n = 8) 8 (7–8)	(n = 7) 9 (7–14)	0.463 [a]
Empirical therapy, median, days (IQR)	(n = 89) 7 (4–8)	(n = 54) 7 (5–8)	(n = 35) 6 (4–8)	0.654 [a]

[a] Mann Whitney; * $p = 0.010$; IQR, interquartile range.

3. Discussion

The high prevalence of antibiotics prescription for critically ill patients admitted to ICU is common [1,15]. Interestingly, the same proportion at 70% was found during the pandemic period [5]. However, the issue of increased antibiotic consumption during the pandemic period is mostly reflected in the proportion of patients being prescribed antibiotics [2,5], where few reported the magnitude of antibiotic utilization in ICU with the measure of DDD [3], which is also an important indicator for usage trend monitoring, the impact of intervention, global comparison [16], as well as correlation with resistance trends [12,17,18]. The decrease in total ICU admissions was attributed to the opening of the COVID-19 ICU with redistribution of manpower and the closure of the operating theatre elective list during the COVID-19 pandemic. However, this was followed by longer ICU stays and higher antibiotics consumption. Notably, during the pre-pandemic period, 2016–2019, the utilization of carbapenems, vancomycin, and polymyxins consumption was found to be lower than that in surgical ICUs in Serbia (135–340, 83–64, 73–66 DDD per 1000 patient days) [17] and medical-surgical ICUs in Saudi Arabia (345.9, 180.0 and 157.1 DDD per 1000 patient days) [19], in both of which AMS interventions were absent. On the other hand, despite the different measures and denominators used, which made it difficult to perform a direct comparison, this study found an increase in annual consumption of most antibiotics during the pandemic year, similar to a Brazilian ICUs [20], yet contrary to the findings in Spanish ICUs that observed a decrease in meropenem and piperacillin/tazobactam [21]. The relatively lower prevalence of antibiotic prescription found by the study in Malaysia [4] could have been masked by various populations across disciplines. Nevertheless, the trajectory increases in antibiotic usage demanded the need to probe into the prescription rationale and the difference between the COVID-19 ICU and the GICU.

Following the CLSI revision in 2020 on the breakpoint and questioning the clinical value of polymyxin(s) [22,23], empirical use of polymyxins was discouraged and the restriction on polymyxins was further enhanced to definitive therapy only with microbiological evidence, in addition to consent by an ID consultant. Therefore, the consumption in 2021 likely reflected the definite use of polymyxins according to culture reports. In this hospital, intravenous polymyxin B was the primary polymyxin of choice for infection due to carbapenem-resistant gram-negative organisms (CRGNB) [24], whereas colistin was preferred and used intravenously for urinary tract infection [24] or as an inhalation therapy for pneumonia [25]. The sharp increase in colistin implied the higher tendency to treat carbapenem-resistant organisms such as *Acinetobacter baumannii* (CRAb) isolated from respiratory cultures, although the clinical significance is debatable, especially in COVID-19 infected critically ill patients [26]. In contrast, the use of polymyxin B did not increase but was similar to the previous years; it was persistent for carbapenem-resistant gram-negative organisms isolated from blood cultures.

Carbapenems are broad-spectrum antibiotics belonging to the WATCH group under the WHO AWaRe classification, which should be the focus of stewardship [27]. Furthermore, the resistance rate among gram-negative organisms towards carbapenems is on the rise globally, which is attributed to carbapenems use [28,29]. In the setting of limited human resources in our hospital, efforts were, therefore, mainly focused on carbapenems instead of targeting all antibiotics. Following the introduction of local ICU antibiotic treatment protocol (Supplementary File S2) and a weekly visit of ID consultants to ICUs since 2016, the consumption of carbapenems in the ICU was maintained at lower than 200 DDD per 1000 patient days. However, the weekly ID rounds were halted in 2020 due to the pandemic and antibiotics usage has increased since then.

To our knowledge, this was the first study to compare the carbapenems prescription pattern between the COVID-19 ICU and the GICU. Meropenem was the preferred agent used, as it had better activities on gram-negative bacteria and central nervous system penetration [30]. This is consistent with the observations in the recent systematic reviews [3,5]. Good compliance to local treatment protocol (Supplementary File S2) was observed as carbapenems were prescribed mainly for type-3 patients who were at risk of infection by multi-drug resistant organisms [25]. Broad spectrum antibiotics were recommended by the last surviving sepsis guideline for the critically ill, as failure to cover possible pathogens in sepsis will lead to higher mortality [31,32]. Patient types were determined at the point of carbapenems prescription; hence, a higher proportion of type-3 patients in the COVID-19 ICU was likely a result of longer ICU stay. Predictably, carbapenems were prescribed empirically in most cases. The fraction of empirical carbapenems prescriptions from the GICU alone was still higher than the reported 66.1% in French ICUs [33], though the latter was studied during the pre-COVID-19 pandemic period. A similar proportion in either ICU indicated that clinicians were practicing high rates of empirical carbapenems, despite the negative culture or growth of the organism(s) susceptible to narrower spectrum beta-lactam antibiotics or alternatives. Although carbapenems were the recommended empirical choice for ICU patients with severe sepsis [13], only a small percentage of prescriptions had positive growth of ESBL-producing *Enterobacterales*, which were predominantly *Klebsiella* spp., similar to another tertiary hospital in the same region in Malaysia [18].

The reasons for empirical prescription differed between the COVID-19 ICU and the GICU, associated with the distribution of the patient types. Rectal colonization with ESBL/MDR GNB was listed as a risk factor for infection [34–36]. Therefore, this drove the carbapenems prescription [36], as seen with the GICU. However, the clinical value is debatable as the positive predictive value is up to 50%, and the screening is unreliable for ICU patients [37]. The current risk stratification for predicting ESBL GNB infection was derived from criteria commonly listed in other predicting models with the same flaw of lacking external validity [38]. To have a better balance between the consequence of carbapenems exposure and management of infection, a validated scoring system is urgently needed to allow more objective judgment.

Empirical carbapenems prescription was seen to be mainly driven by the intention to escalate therapy in the COVID-19 ICU and expectably more for respiratory infection. Diagnosing hospital or ventilator-acquired pneumonia was challenging in which overdiagnosis and overtreatment were commonly practiced [39]. Respiratory sampling was less preferable in ventilated COVID-19 patients due to the concern of aerosolized transmission from the ventilator circuit, leading to a reduction in frequency and quality of microbiological investigation [40]. This further increased the uncertainty in infection diagnosis as well as lessened the reliance on microbiological results [41]. An international survey by Beovic et al. [42] reported that the preference for broad-spectrum antibiotics in COVID-19 patients and the decision on antibiotic prescription are mainly based on clinical presentation. However, it is challenging to differentiate bacterial etiology from COVID-19 pneumonia. Clinicians would proceed to escalate therapy when the patient's progress was not satisfactory [43]. Moreover, broadening the antibiotic spectrum in managing infection of the critically ill could be a reaction to the fear of missing diagnosis, which needs to be addressed [39,44]. To date, there is no standard recommendation to guide escalation therapy. The current guidelines often recommend the initial choice but lack the guidance on next option when the patient worsens or is not progressing well. The usual practice is mainly broadening the spectrum of the antibiotic while pending microbiological reports [45]. Teitelbaum et al. [46] suggested employing antibiogram to guide the next empirical agents [46]. The study found that the escalation antibiogram did not support the usual exercise of switching from ceftriaxone to ceftazidime or piperacillin/tazobactam among ceftriaxone resistant GNR, but meropenem or amikacin instead. Predictably, this appears to encourage carbapenems prescription when ceftriaxone therapy fails. However, this approach should be applied on the caveat that antibiogram was derived from positive cultures and might not apply to all infections.

During the pandemic period, both the COVID-19 ICU and the GICU experienced a shortage in staffing as they were managed by the same clinician teams. Apart from the uncertainty in COVID-19 management, overwhelming workload and exhaustion could cause clinicians to rely on broad-spectrum antibiotics in the dread of missing possible infecting microbes [44]. However, this appeared to be true in only a small proportion of prescriptions evaluated as definitive therapy for ESBL organisms. When pathogens such as MDR *Acinetobacter* spp. and *Stenotrophomonas maltophilia* are isolated, carbapenems might be inadequate. Carbapenem-resistant *Acinetobacter baumannii* (CRAb) was isolated in substantial proportion among positive cultures from the COVID-19 ICU, compared to the GICU. This was consistent with studies by Rangel et al. [47] and Russo et al. [48], which noted that the incidence of CRAb was heightened among COVID-19 patients. According to the recent treatment guideline by IDSA, high dose ampicillin-sulbactam could be considered, but in reality, there is no antibiotic proven to be effective [49]. A cohort study among ICU patients found that mortality risk was further increased to twice as high for bloodstream infection without adequate therapy within the first 24 h [50]. Although carbapenems might have a role when used as a third agent in combination with ampicillin-sulbactam and polymyxin, this suggestion is based on in vitro studies and remains to be proven by robust clinical studies. The present results indicated that carbapenems were continued as empirical therapy when CRAb was isolated, for which a combination of high dose ampicillin-sulbactam at 9 g every 8 h with polymyxin is the recommended therapy by the current local ICU guideline [51]. Referring to the pathogens isolated from the blood cultures, carbapenems were overly broad for more than three-quarters of empirical prescriptions. Both inadequate and overbroad antibiotic spectrum could lead to poorer survival rates in patients at the odds of a 20% increase in mortality, as revealed in a large cohort study among US hospitals by Rhee et al. [52]. It was beyond the scope of the current study to correlate the association with mortality. However, this highlighted the need for enhancing antimicrobial stewardship and rapid diagnostic tools so that appropriate therapy could be optimized or deescalated promptly.

When ESBL-producing organism(s) is isolated, carbapenem is the preferred choice as there is yet an alternative agent proven non-inferiority as in the case of piperacillin/tazobactam in bacteremia [53]. While the empirical initiation of carbapenem might be rational considering the ESBL acquisition risk and unsatisfactory response requiring escalation, the duration was questionable. This study revealed that the carbapenems were empirically continued for about one week and the COVID-19 ICU had a longer course duration than the GICU. This was shorter than the median eight days in five French ICUs [32]. A recent position statement from European Societies of Intensive Care Medicine (ESICM), Clinical Microbiology and Infectious Diseases (ESCMID) advocates that daily review of antibiotics and de-escalation to narrower spectrum antibiotics should be performed for the critically ill according to microbiological results. Several studies supported that de-escalation is safe and associated with lower mortality [54]. When no growth is detected, the non-infectious cause should be investigated and antibiotics may be stopped [45,54]. The initiation and continuity of broad-spectrum carbapenems despite microbiological reports suggesting viable alternatives are concerning, as the risk of developing resistance increases endlessly by 2% for each day of meropenem exposure [7,55]. One of the possible explanations could be the time lapse required for the microbiological reports. In general, it took about two to four days to have organism identification and susceptibility reports from cultures [56]. Molecular methods such as multiplex polymerase chain reaction (PCR) and microarray or matrix-assisted laser desorption/ionization-time of flight mass spectrometry (MALDI-TOF MS) allow for rapid identification of organisms and resistance determination within hours, which would potentially enable clinicians to optimize antibiotic earlier [57]. Several studies showed that rapid testing, together with AMS, improves the time to appropriate antibiotics [58,59] and can potentially lead to better patient outcomes [60].

Negative cultures are also common among the critically ill. It usually takes five days of blood culture incubation before confirming negative growth [61], during which clinicians might choose to continue antibiotics before the report is finalized. A shorter incubation time might allow earlier decision-making on antibiotic prescription. An incubation period of up to four days [61] or even one day [62] might be possible with certain modern blood culture systems [61,62], which are often unavailable in resource-limited settings. Biomarkers including procalcitonin (PCT) could be used to guide the duration of therapy; however, a rise in PCT in the absence of microbiological evidence might compel the escalation or initiation of antibiotics [63,64] due to the knowledge gap and skepticism on PCT over clinical judgment [65,66], especially among COVID-19 patients who are critically ill and given concurrent steroid and tocilizumab [67].

Antibiotic prescription is often executed by focusing on the immediate benefit instead of the potential detrimental effect in the distant future, which was described by Langford et al. [68] as cognitive bias. Clinicians might prefer maintaining broad-spectrum antibiotics as a "safe option" despite the microbiological reports [43,69]. The perception and attitude could be a consequence of a deficiency in education and training during medical residency and undergraduate years [70]. Education is one of the objectives of the WHO global action plan for AMR [8]. Therefore, AMR and AMS modules should be part of training in critical care practitioners [71] who could act as synergistic AMS champions in ICU management. These would cultivate confident and judicious antibiotic prescribers [72] who are the key to combat against AMR, which is aggravated by antibiotics exposure [10].

The findings add to the existing paucity of information on exposure to broad-spectrum antibiotics in critical care areas in the South-East Asia region. We have demonstrated that the excessive antibiotic consumption is likely a result of unwarranted empirical use over a prolonged period and de-escalation is not performed promptly. Furthermore, we report the duration of therapy adjusted to indication, which provides more meaningful feedback to critical care clinicians for engagement in AMS initiatives. The same measurement can be adopted as a benchmarking across institutions and to design a standard tool of appropriateness assessment, which is currently lacking for critical care areas [71,73]. MDR organisms rate and prescription appropriateness in ICUs should be listed in the critical care units benchmarking worldwide [74] and be added as one of the foci of the global surveillance on antimicrobial resistance initiatives [75,76].

There were many limitations due to the nature of the retrospective observational study based on a single center. Furthermore, the data were retrieved from datasets focusing on carbapenems prescriptions and might not provide the whole picture of antibiotic prescription practice. There could also be missing data that were likely lost due to limited physical access to the COVID-19 ICU. The indication and prescription duration for COVID-19 ICU was extracted during table round discussion and, therefore, subjected to recall bias though data availability and accuracy became better when documents were made available electronically. This study reflected the practice during the COVID-19 pandemic year, which might be different from the usual practice before that. In addition, therapy was evaluated according to the microbiological reports and did not assess the correlation with infection severity [77]. However, this study appraised the reason for carbapenems prescription, which was closer to identifying that prescriber intention as a clinical judgment of severity could be subjective [39].

This current study provides a snapshot of the difference in the prescription practice and the microbiological profile among patients prescribed carbapenems between the COVID-19 ICU and the GICU. This is important as AMS strategies should cater to the circumstances under which broad-spectrum antibiotics are used [78]. ICU could be the epicenter for the spread of MDR organisms that are associated with higher patient mortality and the situation worsens with the pandemic. The AMS efforts should couple with infection control measures such as hand hygiene, resistance tracking, and transmission prevention to work synergistically in improving infection prevention and antibiotic use [79,80], to be better prepared for the ongoing and future pandemic wave(s). Further study should be done to identify risk factors and determine the consequence of carbapenem use on resistance trends and patient outcomes. The current data should alert the government and healthcare institutions to prioritize the effort in optimizing antibiotics use in ICUs. There is an urgent need to improve the epidemiological reporting and infrastructure for rapid microbiological diagnostics and reliable biomarkers, in addition to effective communication and knowledge dissemination to guide antibiotic prescription and exercise de-escalation early.

4. Materials and Methods

4.1. Study Design and Settings

This was a cross-sectional retrospective observational study conducted at the Hospital Canselor Tuanku Muhriz (HCTM), a 1054 bedded tertiary care university hospital located in Kuala Lumpur, Malaysia. This study included antibiotic prescriptions dispensed to ICU(s) during the period from 2016 to 2021. The unit used to be a 17-bedded medical/surgical ICU. In 2020, another ward was repurposed as COVID-19 ICU with only 3 beds initially. Following the worsening of the COVID-19 pandemic, the total ICUs' capacity was configured as the COVID-19 ICU operated fully and expanded to be 22-bedded, while the GICU was 8-bedded since December 2020.

The GICU was a mixed medical and surgical-based intensive care unit and the COVID-19 ICU was designed specifically for patients with confirmed COVID-19 infection. The triaging for admission was based on the admission and discharge protocol of the local institution, which was adapted from Malaysia National Protocol [81] and criteria proposed by Malaysia Society of Intensive Care (MSIC) [82–85]. The severity of patients infected by the COVID-19 virus was categorized into 5 clinical stages from asymptomatic to severely ill based on syndromes [81]. Those who were admitted to COVID-19 ICU were stage 4 (symptomatic with pneumonia requiring supplemental oxygen) or stage 5 (critically ill with multi-organ derangement) or those with medical and surgical conditions that required ICU care with concomitant COVID-19 infection. The severity of illness was assessed using APACHE II score [86] upon admission to GICU only.

The GICU and COVID-19 ICU were primarily managed by clinicians of specialty in anesthesiology and intensive care. One ICU pharmacist was assigned to deliver pharmaceutical care service by participating in the daily handover rounds/discussions with a team remotely for COVID-19 ICU and performing bedside reviews for GICU. Medications were prescribed by medical officers on duty in both ICUs.

The ICUs practiced a routine infection control measure of collecting nasal and rectal swabs from newly admitted patients. All microbiological investigations were done by an in-house microbiological diagnostic laboratory service. Organisms were identified by automated VITEK® 2 system (bioMérieux, Marcy-l'Etoile, France). Antibiotic susceptibility testings (AST) were performed using the Kirby–Bauer disk diffusion method and results were interpreted according to Clinical and Laboratory Standard Institute (CLSI) guidelines [87].

Antibiotics were electronically prescribed using the hospital electronic prescription system Medipro® to initiate the dispensing process based on the unit of use system by the pharmacy. Meanwhile, the administration of antibiotic(s) was manually documented using a paper-based prescription with columns for prescribers to note the indication of the antibiotic as empirical, definitive, or prophylaxis, and columns for administration by nurses for up to 7 days. Both electronic and manual prescriptions were renewed if the duration of antibiotic was beyond 7 days. Antibiotics prescriptions were guided by the national ICU antimicrobial prescribing guide [51] and local hospital ICU-specific antibiotic treatment protocol, which was based on a local antibiogram introduced in 2016. The dosage regimes in the GICU and the COVID-19 ICU were based on the same principle, including prolonged infusion and renal adjustment [51], as COVID-19 infection is not known to affect antibiotic pharmacokinetics [88]. Antibiotics including broad-spectrum beta-lactams such as piperacillin/tazobactam, cefepime, meropenem, and polymyxins were readily available as limited floor stock to administer the first dose. However, the subsequent continuation of carbapenems or piperacillin/tazobactam required specialists' consent and authorization, whereas initiation of polypeptides required consent from the infectious disease consultant on duty. Hence, the consent was obtained using a paper-based pre-authorization form stating the indication and duration completed with signatures by relevant specialists to be submitted to the pharmacy department for screening and dispensing. Beginning from 2021, during daily work routine, for each carbapenem prescription, the ward pharmacist would document further details, which include the type of patients/infections, prescription indication (definitive/empirical/prophylaxis or from infectious disease consultation), the reason for empirical initiation, suspected site of infection, date of initiation and completion, and mortality during therapy. The dataset of the antibiotics, pre-authorized forms, and carbapenems monitoring details were kept in the pharmacy department.

4.2. Data Collection

Data on antibiotics consumption were extracted from the manually recorded dispensing documents from the pharmacy department. The cumulative admissions and patient days data were acquired from the hospital department of health information. Prescriptions of carbapenems were extracted from antibiotics preauthorization forms and carbapenems monitoring datasets in the pharmacy department. Microbiological reports were accessed using the hospital's online microbiological reports system (OMS). The duration of carbapenems therapy was calculated by subtracting the date of initiation from the date of completion and adjusted by adding one day. All carbapenems prescriptions for patients admitted to COVID-19 ICU and GICU wards during 2021 were included. Carbapenems prescriptions of patient(s) who died or were transferred out before pharmacist review were excluded due to incomplete data. Carbapenems courses during which the patient(s) died before doctors' order to stop/complete therapy were excluded from the evaluation of therapy duration.

4.3. Antibiotic Utilization

With reference to WHO methodology [14], the DDD used to estimate the parenteral antibiotic utilization was standardized according to the latest updated value. Therefore, the DDD for the commonly used antibiotics are amoxicillin/clavulanic acid: 3 g; ampicillin/sulbactam: 6 g; ceftriaxone: 2 g; cefepime: 4 g; piperacillin/tazobactam: 14 g; imipenem: 2 g; meropenem: 3 g; vancomycin: 2 g; polymyxin B: 0.15 g; colistin: 9 g. The utilization is estimated by the cumulative data based on the number of vials dispensed as follows:

$$\text{Number of DDD for the year} = \frac{\text{Total number of dispensed vials} \times \text{strength of vial in a year (g)}}{\text{DDD (from WHO)}}$$

$$\text{Number of DDD per 1000 patient days} = \frac{\text{Total number of DDD for the year}}{\text{Total patient days for the year}} \times 1000$$

Antibiotic usage before the pandemic was estimated for the year 2016 to 2019. The antibiotic usage during the pandemic was estimated for 2021. The utilization during 2020 did not belong to either group due to the transitional operation of the COVID-19 ICU.

4.4. Definition

4.4.1. Definitive/Empirical Prescribing

Carbapenems prescriptions were considered definitive when it was initiated or continued following the availability of microbiological results, with pathogen or susceptibility requiring coverage with carbapenems' spectrum, from cultures of relevant sites except those from nasal swab and/or rectal swab for infection control surveillance purposes. If carbapenem-resistant *Enterobacterales* were isolated, carbapenem was considered indicated when MIC was less than 8 [89]. Conversely, empirical therapy was considered when carbapenems were initiated for presumed infection, continued, or completed without microbiological evidence [90] or the isolate(s) were susceptible to other beta-lactam antibiotics of a narrower spectrum, such as penicillins, second/third/fourth generation cephalosporins and/or penicillin/inhibitors; or the isolate(s) was resistant where carbapenems were deemed unsuitable. Empirical escalation was considered when carbapenems were switched from ongoing narrower spectrum beta-lactam therapy or added to ongoing antibiotic(s) therapy due to unsatisfactory response.

4.4.2. Classification of Patient Types

Patient types were classified according to the risk factors of infection by resistant organisms. Type-1 or community-acquired infection referred to young patients with no or few comorbid conditions who had no contact with the health care system and no prior antibiotic treatment in the last 90 days; Type-2 or healthcare-associated infection referred to patients who had contact with the healthcare system in the past 3 months or less than 1 week in the hospital or less than 48 h in the ICU (e.g., admission into hospital or nursing home), had an invasive procedure or recent antibiotic therapy in the last 3 months or were more than 65 years old with few comorbidities [91,92]; Type-3 or nosocomial infections referred to patients who had hospitalization more than 5 to 7 days with or without infections following major invasive procedures or had recent and multiple antibiotic therapies or were more than 65 years old with multiple comorbidities (e.g., structural lung disease, immunodeficiency) [93].

4.4.3. ESBL GNB Risk

The risk of infection with ESBL GNB was considered when a patient had received antibiotics in the past 90 days, especially second and third generation cephalosporins; hospitalization for more than 2 days in the past 90 days; was a resident in a nursing home; had chronic dialysis in the past 1 month; had home wound care, immunosuppressive disease, and/or therapy, catheter colonized by ESBL GNB and rectal swab with ESBL GNB. This was adapted from local guidelines [94,95].

4.5. Statistical Analysis

Antibiotic utilization was measured in units of DDD per 1000 patient days in aggregate annual data. All analyses were carried out using Statistical Package for the Social Sciences (SPSS), version 27.0 (IBM Corp, Armonk, NY, USA for descriptive analysis (percentage and frequency), categorical, and continuous data variables. Univariable analyses were performed with Chi-Squared test or Fisher Exact test to compare categorical variables where appropriate. The median of continuous variables was compared using the Mann–Whitney test. A p-value of <0.05 was used as the level of significance.

5. Conclusions

Antibiotics' consumption in ICU increased markedly during the pandemic year, with near to two-fold increments in carbapenems utilization. Most carbapenem therapies were empirical and the reasons for prescribing differed between the two ICUs. Carbapenems were frequently prescribed to escalate therapy in the COVID-19 ICU, while in the GICU, it was for concern of ESBL GNB risk. Both ICUs had a similar duration of empirical carbapenems' usage.

Supplementary Materials: The following are available online at https://www.mdpi.com/article/10.3390/antibiotics11091172/s1, Supplementary File S1: ICUs antibiotic consumption 2016–2021; Supplementary File S2: Local hospital ICU treatment protocol.

Author Contributions: Conceptualization, C.L.L. and I.N.-M.; methodology, C.L.L., M.N.S., S.A.R., S.Y.C., L.Y.G., K.B.P., S.H.K., F.W.T., M.K.Y., S.L.G., N.J.A., X.Y.C., P.K.L., S.W.Y.T., P.P., R.R. and T.L.T.; formal analysis, C.L.L., M.K.Y. and I.N.-M.; investigation, C.L.L., M.N.S., S.A.R., S.Y.C., L.Y.G., K.B.P., S.H.K., F.W.T., M.K.Y., S.L.G., N.J.A., X.Y.C., P.K.L. and S.W.Y.T.; resources, C.L.L., M.N.S., S.A.R., S.Y.C., L.Y.G., K.B.P., S.H.K., F.W.T., M.K.Y., S.L.G., N.J.A., X.Y.C., P.K.L., S.W.Y.T., D.V.D., A.M.Y. and S.K.C.; data curation C.L.L., M.N.S., S.A.R., S.Y.C., L.Y.G., K.B.P., S.H.K., F.W.T., M.K.Y., S.L.G., N.J.A., X.Y.C., P.K.L. and S.W.Y.T.; writing—original draft preparation, C.L.L.; writing—review and editing, C.L.L., I.N.-M., P.P., R.R., T.L.T., A.M.Y. and W.R.W.M.; supervision, I.N.-M., P.P., R.R. and T.L.T.; project administration, I.N.-M., C.L.L., S.A.R., P.P., R.R. and T.L.T. All authors have read and agreed to the published version of the manuscript.

Funding: This research received no external funding.

Institutional Review Board Statement: The study was approved by the Research Ethics Committee, University Kebangsaan Malaysia (JEP-2019-245) on 11 April 2019. The study was also conducted according to the guidelines of the Declaration of Helsinki.

Informed Consent Statement: Patient consent was waived due to the retrospective nature of the study and analysis of anonymous clinical data.

Data Availability Statement: All data generated and analyzed during this study are included in this article.

Acknowledgments: The study would not have been possible without the contribution and involvement of all staff from the Department of Pharmacy and Department of Anesthesiology and Intensive Care of HCTM and statistical advice from Tg Mohd Ikhwan Bin Tg Abu Bakar Sidik.

Conflicts of Interest: The authors declare no conflict of interest.

References

1. Vincent, J.-L.; Sakr, Y.; Singer, M.; Martin-Loeches, I.; Machado, F.R.; Marshall, J.C.; Finfer, S.; Pelosi, P.; Brazzi, L.; Aditianingsih, D.; et al. Prevalence and Outcomes of Infection Among Patients in Intensive Care Units in 2017. *JAMA* **2020**, *323*, 1478–1487. [CrossRef] [PubMed]
2. Langford, B.J.; So, M.; Raybardhan, S.; Leung, V.; Soucy, J.-P.R.; Westwood, D.; Daneman, N.; MacFadden, D.R. Antibiotic prescribing in patients with COVID-19: Rapid review and meta-analysis. *Clin. Microbiol. Infect.* **2021**, *27*, 520–531. [CrossRef] [PubMed]

3. Khan, S.; Hasan, S.S.; Bond, S.E.; Conway, B.R.; Aldeyab, M.A. Antimicrobial consumption in patients with COVID-19: A systematic review and meta-analysis. *Expert Rev. Anti-Infect. Ther.* **2021**, *20*, 749–772. [CrossRef] [PubMed]
4. Mohamad, I.-N.; Wong, C.K.-W.; Chew, C.-C.; Leong, E.L.; Lee, B.-H.; Moh, C.-K.; Chenasammy, K.; Lim, S.C.-L.; Ker, H.-B. The landscape of antibiotic usage among COVID-19 patients in the early phase of pandemic: A Malaysian national perspective. *J. Pharm. Policy Pract.* **2022**, *15*, 4. [CrossRef] [PubMed]
5. Abu-Rub, L.I.; Abdelrahman, H.A.; Johar, A.-R.A.; Alhussain, H.A.; Hadi, H.A.; Eltai, N.O. Antibiotics Prescribing in Intensive Care Settings during the COVID-19 Era: A Systematic Review. *Antibiotics* **2021**, *10*, 935. [CrossRef] [PubMed]
6. Pasero, D.; Cossu, A.P.; Terragni, P. Multi-Drug Resistance Bacterial Infections in Critically Ill Patients Admitted with COVID-19. *Microorganisms* **2021**, *9*, 1773. [CrossRef] [PubMed]
7. Teshome, B.F.; Vouri, S.M.; Hampton, N.; Kollef, M.H.; Micek, S.T. Duration of Exposure to Antipseudomonal β-Lactam Antibiotics in the Critically Ill and Development of New Resistance. *Pharmacotherapy* **2019**, *39*, 261–270. [CrossRef]
8. World Health Organization (WHO). Global Action Plan on Antimicrobial Resistance. Available online: https://www.who.int/publications/i/item/9789241509763 (accessed on 14 October 2021).
9. Dondorp, A.M.; Limmathurotsakul, D.; Ashley, E.A. What's wrong in the control of antimicrobial resistance in critically ill patients from low- and middle-income countries? *Intensive Care Med.* **2018**, *44*, 79–82. [CrossRef]
10. Segala, F.V.; Bavaro, D.F.; Di Gennaro, F.; Salvati, F.; Marotta, C.; Saracino, A.; Murri, R.; Fantoni, M. Impact of SARS-CoV-2 Epidemic on Antimicrobial Resistance: A Literature Review. *Viruses* **2021**, *13*, 2110. [CrossRef]
11. Liang, C.; Zhang, X.; Zhou, L.; Meng, G.; Zhong, L.; Peng, P. Trends and correlation between antibacterial consumption and carbapenem resistance in gram-negative bacteria in a tertiary hospital in China from 2012 to 2019. *BMC Infect. Dis.* **2021**, *21*, 444. [CrossRef]
12. Paiboonvong, T.; Tedtaisong, P.; Montakantikul, P.; Gorsanan, S.; Tantisiriwat, W. Correlation between Carbapenem Consumption and Carbapenems Susceptibility Profiles of Acinetobacter baumannii and Pseudomonas aeruginosa in an Academic Medical Center in Thailand. *Antibiotics* **2022**, *11*, 143. [CrossRef]
13. Patrier, J.; Timsit, J.-F. Carbapenem use in critically ill patients. *Curr. Opin. Infect. Dis.* **2020**, *33*, 86–91. [CrossRef]
14. Institute of Medical Research (IMR). *National Surveillance of Antimicrobial Resistance, Malaysia*; Ministry of Health (MOH): Kuala Lumpur, Malaysia, 2020. Available online: https://www.imr.gov.my/MyOHAR/index.php/site/archive_rpt. (accessed on 15 August 2020).
15. Bitterman, R.; Hussein, K.; Leibovici, L.; Carmeli, Y.; Paul, M. Systematic review of antibiotic consumption in acute care hospitals. *Clin. Microbiol. Infect.* **2016**, *22*, 561.e7–561.e19. [CrossRef]
16. WHO. WHO Collaborating Centre for Drug Statistics Methodology: ATC/DDD Index. Available online: https://www.whocc.no/atc_ddd_index/?code=J&showdescription=no (accessed on 18 May 2022).
17. Popović, R.; Tomić, Z.; Tomas, A.; Anđelić, N.; Vicković, S.; Jovanović, G.; Bukumirić, D.; Horvat, O.; Sabo, A. Five-year surveillance and correlation of antibiotic consumption and resistance of Gram-negative bacteria at an intensive care unit in Serbia. *J. Chemother.* **2020**, *32*, 294–303. [CrossRef]
18. Tan, S.Y.; Khan, R.A.; Khalid, K.E.; Chong, C.W.; Bakhtiar, A. Correlation between antibiotic consumption and the occurrence of multidrug-resistant organisms in a Malaysian tertiary hospital: A 3-year observational study. *Sci. Rep.* **2022**, *12*, 3106. [CrossRef]
19. Balkhy, H.H.; El-Saed, A.; El-Metwally, A.; Arabi, Y.M.; Aljohany, S.M.; Al Zaibag, M.; Baharoon, S.; Alothman, A.F. Antimicrobial consumption in five adult intensive care units: A 33-month surveillance study. *Antimicrob. Resist. Infect. Control* **2018**, *7*, 156. [CrossRef]
20. Silva, A.R.O.; Salgado, D.R.; Lopes, L.P.N.; Castanheira, D.; Emmerick, I.C.M.; Lima, E.C. Increased Use of Antibiotics in the Intensive Care Unit During Coronavirus Disease (COVID-19) Pandemic in a Brazilian Hospital. *Front. Pharmacol.* **2021**, *12*, 778386. [CrossRef]
21. Grau, S.; Hernández, S.; Echeverría-Esnal, D.; Almendral, A.; Ferrer, R.; Limón, E.; Horcajada, J.P.; on behalf of the Catalan Infection Control Antimicrobial Stewardship Program. Antimicrobial Consumption among 66 Acute Care Hospitals in Catalonia: Impact of the COVID-19 Pandemic. *Antibiotics* **2021**, *10*, 943. [CrossRef]
22. Satlin, M.J.; Lewis, J.S., II; Weinstein, M.P.; Patel, J.; Humphries, R.M.; Kahlmeter, G.; Giske, C.G.; Turnidge, J. Clinical and Laboratory Standards Institute and European Committee on Antimicrobial Susceptibility Testing Position Statements on Polymyxin B and Colistin Clinical Breakpoints. *Clin. Infect. Dis.* **2020**, *71*, e523–e529. [CrossRef]
23. Hindler, J.A.; Schuetz, A.N. CLSI AST News Update (1 January 2020). Available online: https://docs.google.com/viewer?url=https%3A%2F%2Fclsi.org%2Fmedia%2F3486%2Fclsi_astnewsupdate_january2020.pdf (accessed on 17 August 2022).
24. Tsuji, B.T.; Pogue, J.M.; Zavascki, A.P.; Paul, M.; Daikos, G.L.; Forrest, A.; Giacobbe, D.R.; Viscoli, C.; Giamarellou, H.; Karaiskos, I.; et al. International Consensus Guidelines for the Optimal Use of the Polymyxins: Endorsed by the American College of Clinical Pharmacy (ACCP), European Society of Clinical Microbiology and Infectious Diseases (ESCMID), Infectious Diseases Society of America (IDSA), International Society for Anti-infective Pharmacology (ISAP), Society of Critical Care Medicine (SCCM), and Society of Infectious Diseases Pharmacists (SIDP). *Pharmacother. J. Hum. Pharmacol. Drug Ther.* **2019**, *39*, 10–39. [CrossRef]
25. Kalil, A.C.; Metersky, M.L.; Klompas, M.; Muscedere, J.; Sweeney, D.A.; Palmer, L.B.; Napolitano, L.M.; O'Grady, N.P.; Bartlett, J.G.; Carratalà, J.; et al. Management of Adults with Hospital-acquired and Ventilator-associated Pneumonia: 2016 Clinical Practice Guidelines by the Infectious Diseases Society of America and the American Thoracic Society. *Clin. Infect. Dis.* **2016**, *63*, e61–e111. [CrossRef]

26. Alfonso-Sanchez, J.L.; Agurto-Ramirez, A.; Chong-Valbuena, M.A.; De-Jesús-María, I.; Julián-Paches, P.; López-Cerrillo, L.; Piedrahita-Valdés, H.; Giménez-Azagra, M.; Martín-Moreno, J.M. The Influence of Infection and Colonization on Outcomes in Inpatients With COVID-19: Are We Forgetting Something? *Front. Public Health* **2021**, *9*, 747791. [CrossRef]
27. WHO. The 2019 WHO AWaRe Classification of Antibiotics for Evaluation and Monitoring of Use. Available online: https://docs.google.com/viewer?url=https%3A%2F%2Fapps.who.int%2Firis%2Fbitstream%2Fhandle%2F10665%2F327957%2FWHO-EMP-IAU-2019.11-eng.xlsx (accessed on 11 June 2022).
28. Zhang, J.; Liu, W.; Shi, W.; Cui, X.; Liu, Y.; Lu, Z.; Xiao, W.; Hua, T.; Yang, M. A Nomogram With Six Variables Is Useful to Predict the Risk of Acquiring Carbapenem-Resistant Microorganism Infection in ICU Patients. *Front. Cell. Infect. Microbiol.* **2022**, *12*, 852761. [CrossRef]
29. Sulis, G.; Sayood, S.; Katukoori, S.; Bollam, N.; George, I.; Yaeger, L.H.; Chavez, M.A.; Tetteh, E.; Yarrabelli, S.; Pulcini, C.; et al. Exposure to World Health Organization's AWaRe antibiotics and isolation of multidrug resistant bacteria: A systematic review and meta-analysis. *Clin. Microbiol. Infect.* **2022**. [CrossRef]
30. Salmon-Rousseau, A.; Martins, C.; Blot, M.; Buisson, M.; Mahy, S.; Chavanet, P.; Piroth, L. Comparative review of imipenem/cilastatin versus meropenem. *Med. Mal. Infect.* **2020**, *50*, 316–322. [CrossRef]
31. Rhodes, A.; Evans, L.E.; Alhazzani, W.; Levy, M.M.; Antonelli, M.; Ferrer, R.; Kumar, A.; Sevransky, J.E.; Sprung, C.L.; Nunnally, M.E.; et al. Surviving Sepsis Campaign: International Guidelines for Management of Sepsis and Septic Shock: 2016. *Intensive Care Med.* **2017**, *43*, 304–377. [CrossRef]
32. Phua, J.; Weng, L.; Ling, L.; Egi, M.; Lim, C.M.; Divatia, J.V.; Shrestha, B.R.; Arabi, Y.M.; Ng, J.; Gomersall, C.D.; et al. Intensive care management of coronavirus disease 2019 (COVID-19): Challenges and recommendations. *Lancet Respir. Med.* **2020**, *8*, 506–517. [CrossRef]
33. Gauzit, R.; Pean, Y.; Alfandari, S.; Bru, J.P.; Bedos, J.P.; Rabaud, C.; Robert, J. Carbapenem use in French hospitals: A nationwide survey at the patient level. *Int. J. Antimicrob. Agents* **2015**, *46*, 707–712. [CrossRef]
34. Frencken, J.F.; Wittekamp, B.H.J.; Plantinga, N.L.; Spitoni, C.; van de Groep, K.; Cremer, O.L.; Bonten, M.J.M. Associations Between Enteral Colonization With Gram-Negative Bacteria and Intensive Care Unit–Acquired Infections and Colonization of the Respiratory Tract. *Clin. Infect. Dis.* **2017**, *66*, 497–503. [CrossRef]
35. Teysseyre, L.; Ferdynus, C.; Miltgen, G.; Lair, T.; Aujoulat, T.; Lugagne, N.; Allou, N.; Allyn, J. Derivation and validation of a simple score to predict the presence of bacteria requiring carbapenem treatment in ICU-acquired bloodstream infection and pneumonia: CarbaSCORE. *Antimicrob. Resist. Infect. Control* **2019**, *8*, 1–13. [CrossRef]
36. Barbier, F.; Pommier, C.; Essaied, W.; Garrouste-Orgeas, M.; Schwebel, C.; Ruckly, S.; Dumenil, A.S.; Lemiale, V.; Mourvillier, B.; Clec'h, C.; et al. Colonization and infection with extended-spectrum β-lactamase-producing Enterobacteriaceae in ICU patients: What impact on outcomes and carbapenem exposure? *J. Antimicrob. Chemother.* **2016**, *71*, 1088–1097. [CrossRef] [PubMed]
37. Prevel, R.; Boyer, A.; M'Zali, F.; Lasheras, A.; Zahar, J.-R.; Rogues, A.-M.; Gruson, D. Is systematic fecal carriage screening of extended-spectrum beta-lactamase-producing Enterobacteriaceae still useful in intensive care unit: A systematic review. *Crit. Care* **2019**, *23*, 170. [CrossRef] [PubMed]
38. Mohd Sazlly Lim, S.; Wong, P.L.; Sulaiman, H.; Atiya, N.; Hisham Shunmugam, R.; Liew, S.M. Clinical prediction models for ESBL-Enterobacteriaceae colonization or infection: A systematic review. *J. Hosp. Infect.* **2019**, *102*, 8–16. [CrossRef]
39. Kenaa, B.; O'Hara, L.M.; Richert, M.E.; Brown, J.P.; Shanholtz, C.; Armahizer, M.J.; Leekha, S. A qualitative assessment of the diagnosis and management of ventilator-associated pneumonia among critical care clinicians exploring opportunities for diagnostic stewardship. *Infect. Control Hosp. Epidemiol.* **2022**, *43*, 284–290. [CrossRef]
40. De Waele, J.J.; Derde, L.; Bassetti, M. Antimicrobial stewardship in ICUs during the COVID-19 pandemic: Back to the 90s? *Intensive Care Med.* **2021**, *47*, 104–106. [CrossRef]
41. Bej, T.A.; Christian, R.L.; Sims, S.V.; Wilson, B.M.; Song, S.; Akpoji, U.C.; Bonomo, R.A.; Perez, F.; Jump, R.L.P. Influence of microbiological culture results on antibiotic choices for veterans with hospital-acquired pneumonia and ventilator-associated pneumonia. *Infect. Control Hosp. Epidemiol.* **2022**, *43*, 589–596. [CrossRef]
42. Beović, B.; Doušak, M.; Ferreira-Coimbra, J.; Nadrah, K.; Rubulotta, F.; Belliato, M.; Berger-Estilita, J.; Ayoade, F.; Rello, J.; Erdem, H. Antibiotic use in patients with COVID-19: A 'snapshot' Infectious Diseases International Research Initiative (ID-IRI) survey. *J. Antimicrob. Chemother.* **2020**, *75*, 3386–3390. [CrossRef]
43. Anton-Vazquez, V.; Suarez, C.; Krishna, S.; Planche, T. Factors influencing antimicrobial prescription attitudes in bloodstream infections: Susceptibility results and beyond. An exploratory survey. *J. Hosp. Infect.* **2021**, *111*, 140–147. [CrossRef]
44. Wunderink, R.G.; Srinivasan, A.; Barie, P.S.; Chastre, J.; Dela Cruz, C.S.; Douglas, I.S.; Ecklund, M.; Evans, S.E.; Evans, S.R.; Gerlach, A.T.; et al. Antibiotic Stewardship in the Intensive Care Unit. An Official American Thoracic Society Workshop Report in Collaboration with the AACN, CHEST, CDC, and SCCM. *Ann. Am. Thorac. Soc.* **2020**, *17*, 531–540. [CrossRef]
45. Thorndike, J.; Kollef, M.H. Culture-negative sepsis. *Curr. Opin. Crit. Care* **2020**, *26*, 473–477. [CrossRef]
46. Teitelbaum, D.; Elligsen, M.; Katz, K.; Lam, P.W.; Lo, J.; MacFadden, D.; Vermeiren, C.; Daneman, N. Introducing the Escalation Antibiogram: A Simple Tool to Inform Changes in Empiric Antimicrobials in the Non-Responding Patient. *Clin. Infect. Dis.* **2022**, ciac256. [CrossRef] [PubMed]
47. Rangel, K.; Chagas, T.P.G.; De-Simone, S.G. Acinetobacter baumannii Infections in Times of COVID-19 Pandemic. *Pathogens* **2021**, *10*, 1006. [CrossRef]

48. Russo, A.; Gavaruzzi, F.; Ceccarelli, G.; Borrazzo, C.; Oliva, A.; Alessandri, F.; Magnanimi, E.; Pugliese, F.; Venditti, M. Multidrug-resistant Acinetobacter baumannii infections in COVID-19 patients hospitalized in intensive care unit. *Infection* **2022**, *50*, 83–92. [CrossRef] [PubMed]
49. Tamma, P.; Aitken, S.; Bonomo, R.; Mathers, A.; van Duin, D.; Clancy, C. Infectious Diseases Society of America Guidance on the Treatment of AmpC β-Lactamase-Producing Enterobacterales, Carbapenem-Resistant Acinetobacter baumannii, and Stenotrophomonas maltophilia Infections. *Clin. Infect. Dis.* **2022**, *74*, 2089–2114. [CrossRef]
50. Adrie, C.; Garrouste-Orgeas, M.; Ibn Essaied, W.; Schwebel, C.; Darmon, M.; Mourvillier, B.; Ruckly, S.; Dumenil, A.S.; Kallel, H.; Argaud, L.; et al. Attributable mortality of ICU-acquired bloodstream infections: Impact of the source, causative micro-organism, resistance profile and antimicrobial therapy. *J. Infect.* **2017**, *74*, 131–141. [CrossRef]
51. Chan, L.; Mat Nor, M.B.; Ibrahim, N.A.; Ling, T.L.; Tay, C.; Lin, K.T.H. *Guide to Antimicrobial Therapy in the Adult ICU*, 2nd ed.; Malaysian Society of Intensive Care: Kuala Lumpur, Malaysia, 2017; Available online: https://www.msic.org.my/download/AntibioticGuidelines.pdf (accessed on 1 April 2022).
52. Rhee, C.; Kadri, S.S.; Dekker, J.P.; Danner, R.L.; Chen, H.-C.; Fram, D.; Zhang, F.; Wang, R.; Klompas, M.; CDC Prevention Epicenters Program. Prevalence of Antibiotic-Resistant Pathogens in Culture-Proven Sepsis and Outcomes Associated With Inadequate and Broad-Spectrum Empiric Antibiotic Use. *JAMA Netw. Open* **2020**, *3*, e202899. [CrossRef]
53. Harris, P.N.; Tambyah, P.A.; Lye, D.C.; Mo, Y.; Lee, T.H.; Yilmaz, M.; Alenazi, T.H.; Arabi, Y.; Falcone, M.; Bassetti, M. Effect of piperacillin-tazobactam vs. meropenem on 30-day mortality for patients with E coli or Klebsiella pneumoniae bloodstream infection and ceftriaxone resistance: A randomized clinical trial. *JAMA* **2018**, *320*, 984–994. [CrossRef]
54. Tabah, A.; Bassetti, M.; Kollef, M.H.; Zahar, J.-R.; Paiva, J.-A.; Timsit, J.-F.; Roberts, J.A.; Schouten, J.; Giamarellou, H.; Rello, J.; et al. Antimicrobial de-escalation in critically ill patients: A position statement from a task force of the European Society of Intensive Care Medicine (ESICM) and European Society of Clinical Microbiology and Infectious Diseases (ESCMID) Critically Ill Patient. *Intensive Care Med.* **2020**, *46*, 245–265. [CrossRef]
55. Teshome, B.F.; Vouri, S.M.; Hampton, N.B.; Kollef, M.H.; Micek, S.T. Evaluation of a ceiling effect on the association of new resistance development to antipseudomonal beta-lactam exposure in the critically ill. *Infect. Control Hosp. Epidemiol.* **2020**, *41*, 484–485. [CrossRef]
56. Van Belkum, A.; Burnham, C.-A.D.; Rossen, J.W.A.; Mallard, F.; Rochas, O.; Dunne, W.M. Innovative and rapid antimicrobial susceptibility testing systems. *Nat. Rev. Microbiol.* **2020**, *18*, 299–311. [CrossRef]
57. Noster, J.; Thelen, P.; Hamprecht, A. Detection of multidrug-resistant Enterobacterales—from ESBLs to carbapenemases. *Antibiotics* **2021**, *10*, 1140. [CrossRef]
58. Banerjee, R.; Humphries, R. Rapid Antimicrobial Susceptibility Testing Methods for Blood Cultures and Their Clinical Impact. *Front. Med.* **2021**, *8*, 635831. [CrossRef]
59. Anton-Vazquez, V.; Hine, P.; Krishna, S.; Chaplin, M.; Planche, T. Rapid versus standard antimicrobial susceptibility testing to guide treatment of bloodstream infection. *Cochrane Database Syst. Rev.* **2021**, *2021*, CD013235. [CrossRef]
60. Timbrook, T.T.; Morton, J.B.; McConeghy, K.W.; Caffrey, A.R.; Mylonakis, E.; LaPlante, K.L. The Effect of Molecular Rapid Diagnostic Testing on Clinical Outcomes in Bloodstream Infections: A Systematic Review and Meta-analysis. *Clin. Infect. Dis.* **2017**, *64*, 15–23. [CrossRef] [PubMed]
61. Ransom, E.M.; Alipour, Z.; Wallace, M.A.; Burnham, C.A. Evaluation of Optimal Blood Culture Incubation Time To Maximize Clinically Relevant Results from a Contemporary Blood Culture Instrument and Media System. *J. Clin. Microbiol.* **2021**, *59*, e02459-20. [CrossRef]
62. Lambregts, M.M.C.; Bernards, A.T.; van der Beek, M.T.; Visser, L.G.; de Boer, M.G. Time to positivity of blood cultures supports early re-evaluation of empiric broad-spectrum antimicrobial therapy. *PLoS ONE* **2019**, *14*, e0208819. [CrossRef] [PubMed]
63. Christensen, I.; Haug, J.B.; Berild, D.; Bjørnholt, J.V.; Jelsness-Jørgensen, L.-P. Hospital physicians' experiences with procalcitonin—Implications for antimicrobial stewardship; a qualitative study. *BMC Infect. Dis.* **2020**, *20*, 515. [CrossRef] [PubMed]
64. Wang, X.; Long, Y.; Su, L.; Zhang, Q.; Shan, G.; He, H. Using Procalcitonin to Guide Antibiotic Escalation in Patients With Suspected Bacterial Infection: A New Application of Procalcitonin in the Intensive Care Unit. *Front. Cell. Infect. Microbiol.* **2022**, *12*, 844134. [CrossRef]
65. Schuetz, P.; Beishuizen, A.; Broyles, M.; Ferrer, R.; Gavazzi, G.; Gluck, E.H.; Castillo, J.G.d.; Jensen, J.-U.; Kanizsai, P.L.; Kwa, A.L.H.; et al. Procalcitonin (PCT)-guided antibiotic stewardship: An international experts consensus on optimized clinical use. *Clin. Chem. Lab. Med. (CCLM)* **2019**, *57*, 1308–1318. [CrossRef]
66. Hohn, A.; Balfer, N.; Heising, B.; Hertel, S.; Wiemer, J.C.; Hochreiter, M.; Schröder, S. Adherence to a procalcitonin-guided antibiotic treatment protocol in patients with severe sepsis and septic shock. *Ann. Intensive Care* **2018**, *8*, 68. [CrossRef]
67. Kooistra, E.J.; van Berkel, M.; van Kempen, N.F.; van Latum, C.R.M.; Bruse, N.; Frenzel, T.; van den Berg, M.J.W.; Schouten, J.A.; Kox, M.; Pickkers, P. Dexamethasone and tocilizumab treatment considerably reduces the value of C-reactive protein and procalcitonin to detect secondary bacterial infections in COVID-19 patients. *Crit. Care* **2021**, *25*, 281. [CrossRef]
68. Langford, B.J.; Daneman, N.; Leung, V.; Langford, D.J. Cognitive bias: How understanding its impact on antibiotic prescribing decisions can help advance antimicrobial stewardship. *JAC-Antimicrob. Resist.* **2020**, *2*, dlaa107. [CrossRef]
69. Krockow, E.M.; Colman, A.M.; Chattoe-Brown, E.; Jenkins, D.R.; Perera, N.; Mehtar, S.; Tarrant, C. Balancing the risks to individual and society: A systematic review and synthesis of qualitative research on antibiotic prescribing behaviour in hospitals. *J. Hosp. Infect.* **2019**, *101*, 428–439. [CrossRef]

70. Di Gennaro, F.; Marotta, C.; Amicone, M.; Bavaro, D.F.; Bernaudo, F.; Frisicale, E.M.; Kurotschka, P.K.; Mazzari, A.; Veronese, N.; Murri, R.; et al. Italian young doctors' knowledge, attitudes and practices on antibiotic use and resistance: A national cross-sectional survey. *J. Glob. Antimicrob. Resist.* **2020**, *23*, 167–173. [CrossRef]
71. Chiotos, K.; Tamma, P.D.; Gerber, J.S. Antibiotic stewardship in the intensive care unit: Challenges and opportunities. *Infect. Control Hosp. Epidemiol.* **2019**, *40*, 693–698. [CrossRef]
72. Warreman, E.B.; Lambregts, M.M.C.; Wouters, R.H.P.; Visser, L.G.; Staats, H.; van Dijk, E.; de Boer, M.G.J. Determinants of in-hospital antibiotic prescription behaviour: A systematic review and formation of a comprehensive framework. *Clin. Microbiol. Infect.* **2019**, *25*, 538–545. [CrossRef]
73. Trivedi, K.K.; Bartash, R.; Letourneau, A.R.; Abbo, L.; Fleisher, J.; Gagliardo, C.; Kelley, S.; Nori, P.; Rieg, G.K.; Silver, P.; et al. Opportunities to Improve Antibiotic Appropriateness in U.S. ICUs: A Multicenter Evaluation. *Crit. Care Med.* **2020**, *48*, 968–976. [CrossRef]
74. Salluh, J.I.F.; Soares, M.; Keegan, M.T. Understanding intensive care unit benchmarking. *Intensive Care Med.* **2017**, *43*, 1703–1707. [CrossRef]
75. Dalton, K.R.; Rock, C.; Carroll, K.C.; Davis, M.F. One Health in hospitals: How understanding the dynamics of people, animals, and the hospital built-environment can be used to better inform interventions for antimicrobial-resistant gram-positive infections. *Antimicrob. Resist. Infect. Control* **2020**, *9*, 78. [CrossRef]
76. WHO. Global Antimicrobial Resistance and Use Surveillance System (GLASS). Available online: https://www.who.int/initiatives/glass (accessed on 20 August 2022).
77. Trifi, A.; Abdellatif, S.; Abdennebi, C.; Daly, F.; Nasri, R.; Touil, Y.; Ben Lakhal, S. Appropriateness of empiric antimicrobial therapy with imipenem/colistin in severe septic patients: Observational cohort study. *Ann. Clin. Microbiol. Antimicrob.* **2018**, *17*, 39. [CrossRef]
78. Chiotos, K.; Tamma, P.D. Antibiotics: How can we make it as easy to stop as it is to start? *Clin. Microbiol. Infect.* **2020**, *26*, 1600–1601. [CrossRef] [PubMed]
79. Baur, D.; Gladstone, B.P.; Burkert, F.; Carrara, E.; Foschi, F.; Döbele, S.; Tacconelli, E. Effect of antibiotic stewardship on the incidence of infection and colonisation with antibiotic-resistant bacteria and Clostridium difficile infection: A systematic review and meta-analysis. *Lancet Infect. Dis.* **2017**, *17*, 990–1001. [CrossRef]
80. Manning, M.L.; Septimus, E.J.; Ashley, E.S.D.; Cosgrove, S.E.; Fakih, M.G.; Schweon, S.J.; Myers, F.E.; Moody, J.A. Antimicrobial stewardship and infection prevention—Leveraging the synergy: A position paper update. *Am. J. Infect. Control* **2018**, *46*, 364–368. [CrossRef]
81. Ministry of Health Malaysia. Clinical Management of Confirmed COVID-19 Case in Adult and Paediatric (Updated 3 May 2021). Available online: http://COVID-19.moh.gov.my/garis-kkm/Annex_2e_CLINICAL_MANAGEMENT_OF_CONFIRMED_COVID-19_CASE_IN_ADULT_AND_PEADIATRICS-03052021.pdf (accessed on 1 April 2022).
82. Deva, S.R.; Chan, L.; Ibrahim, N.A.; Ling, T.L. MSIC Consensus Statement A Clinical Guide to Decision-Making for Critically Ill COVID-19 Patients (1 March 2021). Available online: https://www.msic.org.my/download/MSIC_Statement_Clinical_Guide_to_Decision_Making.pdf (accessed on 1 April 2022).
83. Academy of Medicine of Malaysia. Malaysia Society of Anaesthesiologist CoA Malaysian Society of Intensive Care Joint Statement on Critical Care Triage during the COVID 19 Pandemic (27 July 2021). Available online: http://www.acadmed.org.my/newsmaster.cfm?&menuid=174&action=view&retrieveid=160 (accessed on 1 April 2022).
84. Ikhwan, M.; Zulaikha, N.S.; Nadia, A.; Aidalina, M. Policies on Intensive Care Unit (ICU) Admission during COVID-19 Pandemic. *Int. J. Public Health Clin. Sci.* **2021**, *8*, 1–15.
85. Deva, S.R.; Ling, T.L.; Abdul Rahim, A.H.; Weng, F.K.; Tan, I.T.M.A.; Meng, K.T.; Pheng, L.S.; Har, L.C.; Kassim, M.B.; Mohd Noor, M.R.; et al. *ICU Management Protocols*, 2nd ed.; Malaysian Society of Intensive Care: Kuala Lumpur, Malaysia, 2020. Available online: https://www.msic.org.my/download/ICU_Protocol_Management.pdf (accessed on 1 April 2022).
86. Knaus, W. APACHE II Score. Available online: https://www.mdcalc.com/calc/1868/apache-ii-score. (accessed on 30 June 2022).
87. *CLSI Supplement M100*; Performance Standards for Antimicrobial Susceptibility Testing. CLSI: Wayne, PA, USA, 2021.
88. Chiriac, U.; Frey, O.R.; Roehr, A.C.; Koeberer, A.; Gronau, P.; Fuchs, T.; Roberts, J.A.; Brinkmann, A. Personalized ß-lactam dosing in patients with coronavirus disease 2019 (COVID-19) and pneumonia: A retrospective analysis on pharmacokinetics and pharmacokinetic target attainment. *Medicine* **2021**, *100*, e26253. [CrossRef] [PubMed]
89. Sheu, C.-C.; Chang, Y.-T.; Lin, S.-Y.; Chen, Y.-H.; Hsueh, P.-R. Infections Caused by Carbapenem-Resistant Enterobacteriaceae: An Update on Therapeutic Options. *Front. Microbiol.* **2019**, *10*, 80. [CrossRef] [PubMed]
90. Carrara, E.; Pfeffer, I.; Zusman, O.; Leibovici, L.; Paul, M. Determinants of inappropriate empirical antibiotic treatment: Systematic review and meta-analysis. *Int. J. Antimicrob. Agents* **2018**, *51*, 548–553. [CrossRef] [PubMed]
91. Cardoso, T.; Almeida, M.; Friedman, N.D.; Aragão, I.; Costa-Pereira, A.; Sarmento, A.E.; Azevedo, L. Classification of healthcare-associated infection: A systematic review 10 years after the first proposal. *BMC Med.* **2014**, *12*, 40. [CrossRef]
92. Cardoso, T.; Almeida, M.; Carratalà, J.; Aragão, I.; Costa-Pereira, A.; Sarmento, A.E.; Azevedo, L. Microbiology of healthcare-associated infections and the definition accuracy to predict infection by potentially drug resistant pathogens: A systematic review. *BMC Infect. Dis.* **2015**, *15*, 565. [CrossRef]
93. Schechner, V.; Nobre, V.; Kaye, K.S.; Leshno, M.; Giladi, M.; Rohner, P.; Harbarth, S.; Anderson, D.J.; Karchmer, A.W.; Schwaber, M.J.; et al. Gram-Negative Bacteremia upon Hospital Admission: When Should Pseudomonas aeruginosa Be Suspected? *Clin. Infect. Dis.* **2009**, *48*, 580–586. [CrossRef]

94. Parasakthi, N.; Ariffin, H. *Consensus Guidelines for the Management of Infections by ESBL Producing Bacteria*; Ministry of Health; Academy of Medicine of Malaysia; Malaysian Society of Infectious Disease and Chemotherapy: Kuala Lumpur, Malaysia, 2001.
95. Ben-Ami, R.; Rodríguez-Baño, J.; Arslan, H.; Pitout, J.D.D.; Quentin, C.; Calbo, E.S.; Azap, Ö.K.; Arpin, C.; Pascual, A.; Livermore, D.M.; et al. A Multinational Survey of Risk Factors for Infection with Extended-Spectrum β-Lactamase-Producing Enterobacteriaceae in Nonhospitalized Patients. *Clin. Infect. Dis.* **2009**, *49*, 682–690. [CrossRef]

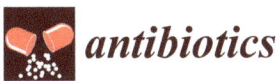

Perspective

Why We May Need Higher Doses of Beta-Lactam Antibiotics: Introducing the 'Maximum Tolerable Dose'

Sofie A. M. Dhaese [1,2,*], Eric A. Hoste [1,2] and Jan J. De Waele [1,2,*]

1. Department of Intensive Care Medicine, Ghent University Hospital, 9000 Ghent, Belgium
2. Department of Internal Medicine and Pediatrics, Ghent University Hospital, 9000 Ghent, Belgium
* Correspondence: sofie.dhaese@ugent.be (S.A.M.D.); jan.dewaele@ugent.be (J.J.D.W.)

Abstract: The surge in antimicrobial resistance and the limited availability of new antimicrobial drugs has fueled the interest in optimizing antibiotic dosing. An ideal dosing regimen leads to maximal bacterial cell kill, whilst minimizing the risk of toxicity or antimicrobial resistance. For beta-lactam antibiotics specifically, PK/PD-based considerations have led to the widespread adoption of prolonged infusion. The rationale behind prolonged infusion is increasing the percentage of time the beta-lactam antibiotic concentration remains above the minimal inhibitory concentration (%$fT_{>MIC}$). The ultimate goal of prolonged infusion of beta-lactam antibiotics is to improve the outcome of infectious diseases. However, merely increasing target attainment (or the %$fT_{>MIC}$) is unlikely to lead to improved clinical outcome for several reasons. First, the PK/PD index and target are dynamic entities. Changing the PK (as is the case if prolonged instead of intermittent infusion is used) will result in different PK/PD targets and even PK/PD indices necessary to obtain the same level of bacterial cell kill. Second, the minimal inhibitory concentration is not a good denominator to describe either the emergence of resistance or toxicity. Therefore, we believe a different approach to antibiotic dosing is necessary. In this perspective, we introduce the concept of the maximum tolerable dose (MTD). This MTD is the highest dose of an antimicrobial drug deemed safe for the patient. The goal of the MTD is to maximize bacterial cell kill and minimize the risk of antimicrobial resistance and toxicity. Unfortunately, data about what beta-lactam antibiotic levels are associated with toxicity and how beta-lactam antibiotic toxicity should be measured are limited. This perspective is, therefore, a plea to invest in research aimed at deciphering the dose–response relationship between beta-lactam antibiotic drug concentrations and toxicity. In this regard, we provide a theoretical approach of how increasing uremic toxin concentrations could be used as a quantifiable marker of beta-lactam antibiotic toxicity.

Keywords: beta-lactam antibiotics; pharmacokinetics; pharmacodynamics; ICU; critically ill

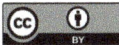

1. Introduction

Increasing drug resistance rates and the scarcity of new antibacterial drugs pose a serious threat for the clinical utility of antimicrobial drugs [1]. In response, Antimicrobial Stewardship Programs (ASP) were introduced to help preserve our antimicrobial armamentarium by interventions designed to ensure the appropriate use of antimicrobial drugs [2,3]. One of these interventions is dose-optimization, i.e., informed decision making regarding the optimal dose and dosing regimen for the individual patient [4].

The scientific advances in the field of antimicrobial dose optimization have mainly been determined by pharmacokinetic (PK) and pharmacodynamic (PD) principles. PK/PD is the science relating the effect of drug exposure (PK) to an outcome measurement (PD) [5]. For antibiotics specifically, PK/PD describes the drug exposure necessary to achieve bacterial cell kill, while limiting its side effects i.e., toxicity and antimicrobial resistance. Beta-lactam antibiotics, amongst the most commonly prescribed antimicrobial drugs in the ICU, are a present-day example of how PK/PD considerations led to the adoption of alternative modes of infusion to optimize their use [6].

In recent years, a wealth of evidence emerged, demonstrating that the PK of beta-lactam antibiotics in critically ill patients is significantly different from the beta-lactam PK observed in healthy volunteers or non-critically ill patients [7]. The patients with sepsis and septic shock may have an increased or decreased drug clearance and an increased volume of distribution. Because of their hydrophilic nature and predominantly renal elimination, changes in kidney function and the volume of distribution profoundly impact the beta-lactam antibiotic PK [7,8]. As a result, several reports have illustrated subtherapeutic antibiotic drug concentrations in critically ill patients treated with standard dosing beta-lactam antibiotic drugs [9,10].

2. How PK/PD Is Currently Used to Optimize Dosing of Beta-Lactam Antibiotics in the Critically Ill

Beta-lactam antibiotics are considered time-dependent antibiotics and the time (T) that the unbound fraction (f) of the antibiotic drug remains above the minimal inhibitory concentration (MIC) is the PK/PD index of choice ($fT_{>MIC}$) [11,12]. By convention, the magnitude of the PK/PD index necessary to achieve a certain outcome (for example a 3-log$_{10}$ reduction of colony-forming units (CFU/mL)) is called the PK/PD target [5]. Importantly, the MIC is a value determined in the laboratory under highly standardized conditions that are very different from in vivo conditions; and the MIC therefore does not represent a concentration that can be compared with an in vivo drug concentration [13].

The rationale for prolonged (i.e., both extended and continuous) infusion of beta-lactam antibiotics is extending the duration of infusion in order to increase the $\%fT_{>MIC}$ and target attainment rates (Figure 1). The ultimate goal of prolonged infusion is improving the outcome of the infection.

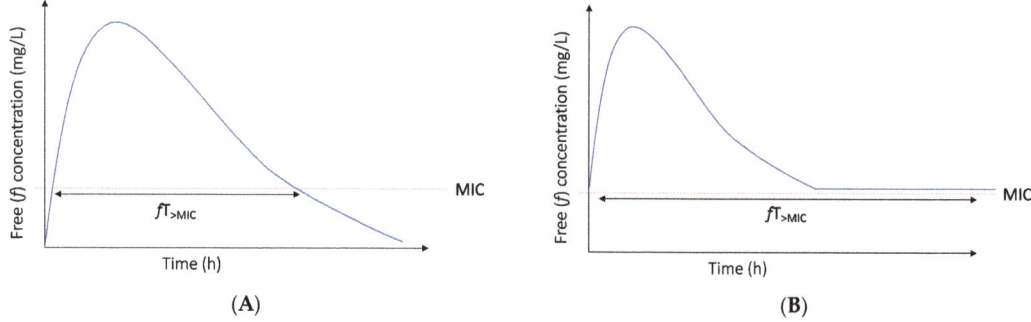

Figure 1. Time above the MIC for intermittent (**A**) and continuous (**B**) infusion with initial bolus.

The ability of prolonged infusion to increase the $\%fT_{>MIC}$ has been clearly demonstrated [14,15]. Unfortunately, the benefit of prolonged infusion in terms of reduced mortality is still a matter of debate. Indeed, many clinical studies have evaluated intermittent versus prolonged infusion of beta-lactam antibiotics, but very few have evaluated mortality as an outcome parameter. Only two randomized clinical trials (RCTs) have demonstrated a lower mortality rate with a prolonged versus intermittent infusion of beta-lactam antibiotics in critically ill patients [16,17]. Other RCTs have demonstrated improved clinical cure rates [14,18], lower costs [19,20], a faster reduction of the APACHE (Acute Physiology and Chronic Health Evaluation) II score [21], increased microbiological success rates [22] or improved target attainment rates [15,23] with prolonged infusion, albeit without an effect on mortality. Two systematic reviews and one individual patient meta-analysis demonstrated lower mortality rates with prolonged as opposed to intermittent infusion in patients with sepsis and severe sepsis [24–26]. Currently, BLING III, a large multicenter trial comparing the 90-day all-cause mortality between intermittent and continuous infusion piperacillin and meropenem has almost finished recruitment, and the results are eagerly awaited [27].

3. Why We Need to Rethink the Use of Prolonged Infusion of Beta-Lactam Antibiotics to Improve the Outcome of Infection

3.1. The PK/PD Index and Target of Choice for Beta-Lactam Antibiotics Are Not Static Entities

Prolonging the duration of infusion to increase the target attainment depends on the assumption that the PK/PD index and target by itself are static and are independent of the mode of infusion used. However, this theory has been challenged, and attaining the same PK/PD target with a different mode of infusion does not necessarily imply an equal level of bacterial cell kill [28]. For example, Felton et al. [29] published an in vitro *Pseudomonas aeruginosa* hollow-fiber infection model for piperacillin. A dosing of 3, 9 and 17 g of piperacillin, either via intermittent (0.5 h infusion duration) or extended infusion (4 h infusion duration) was simulated. The targets (in C_{min}/MIC ratios) reported for stasis, 1-, 2- and 3-$\log_{10}$ kill and the suppression of resistance for extended infusion were consistently higher compared with the targets documented for intermittent infusion (Figure 2). In addition, Sumi et al. [30] evaluated intermittent, extended and continuous infusion piperacillin/tazobactam in an in vitro dynamic hollow-fiber infection model against ceftriaxone-resistant *Klebsiella pneumoniae*. For the Kp69 strain (with an MIC of 1 mg/L), a C_{min}/MIC ratio of 1.09 with intermittent infusion was sufficient to avoid resistance development, while for the extended infusion a C_{min}/MIC ratio of 3.18 was necessary. These examples illustrate that different PK/PD targets may apply for the same reduction of CFU when different modes of infusion are used.

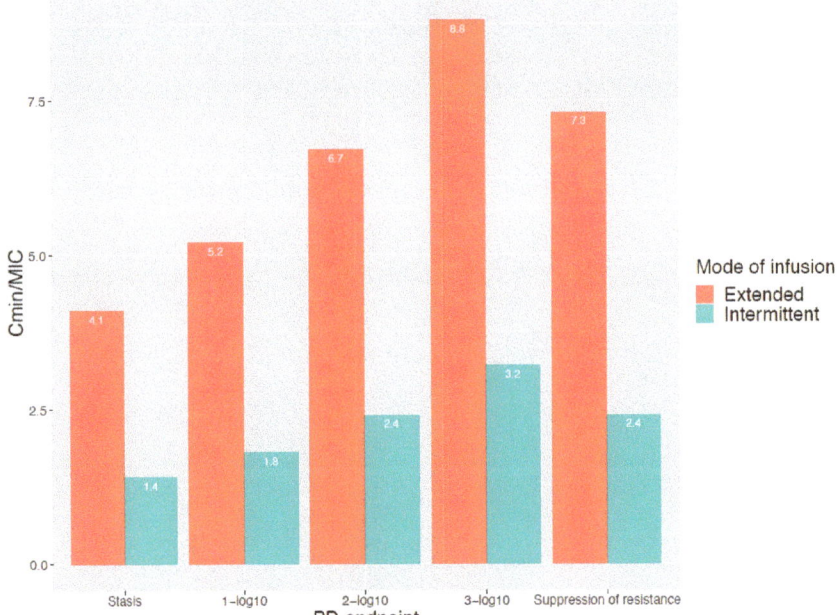

Figure 2. C_{min}/MIC ratio for different PD endpoints and for both intermittent and extended infusion. Reproduced from Felton et al. [29].

The concept of dynamic PK/PD indices and targets in terms of changing beta-lactam antibiotic concentrations have previously been described [31–34], and the idea of a dynamic PK/PD relationship, linking changing antibiotic concentrations to bacterial kill or growth over time, is well established [5,13,33,35,36]. However, we do not generally consider that, for a different mode of infusion of the same antibiotic, different indices and targets may apply. When comparing the probability of target attainment between intermittent and continuous infusion, which implies a fundamentally different concentration–time curve, it is usually assumed that the PK/PD index and target remain the same [6,28,35–37].

Intriguingly, the optimal PK/PD index is also dependent on PK, as described by Nielsen et al. [38] and Kristofferson et al. [33]. These authors argue that the choice of $fT_{>MIC}$ as the PK/PD index of beta-lactam antibiotics is related to the short half-life (and therefore the PK) of most of these drugs. In situations where the half-life is prolonged, for example in patients with kidney failure, $fAUC/MIC$ was found as the best predictor of the antibacterial effect of beta-lactam antibiotics [33]. Even more so, when other drugs (from different antibiotic classes, such as fluoroquinolones or glycopeptides) were used for simulation, with a half-life equal to the half-life of benzylpenicillin, $fT_{>MIC}$ was the PK/PD index best related to the antibacterial efficacy [38]. The fact that the PK/PD index is a summary endpoint, dependent on both PK and PD, has also been demonstrated for drugs other than beta-lactam antibiotics. For example, in a lung and thigh infection neutropenic mouse model of Craig et al. [39], $fT_{>MIC}$ is the PK/PD index of choice for amikacin in mice with a normal kidney function (half-life of 18.5–32.5 min), as opposed to $fAUC/MIC$ in mice with an impaired kidney function (half-life of 93.3–121 min).

3.2. Bacterial Cell Kill Is Not the Only Goal

An optimal dosing regimen would allow maximal antibacterial effect, whilst minimizing drug toxicity and the risk of resistance development. Nevertheless, most of our beta-lactam antibiotic dosing regimens were based upon PK/PD targets and indices for bacterial cell kill alone. However, the recent literature has illustrated that we may need different antibiotic exposures (illustrated by different PK/PD targets and indices) for the suppression of resistance, as opposed to bacterial cell kill [40,41]. Moreover, several authors have advocated for the mutant prevention concentration (MPC) instead of the MIC as the PD endpoint for the suppression of resistance [42]. The MPC is the concentration that prevents the growth of first-step resistant mutants. This concept is based on the idea that a large initial bacterial burden has a high probability of harboring a first-step mutant. The mutant selection window (MSW) is defined as a range of concentrations between the MIC and the MPC. The concentrations within the MSW are expected to promote the selection of resistance [43,44]. However, the MIC may not necessarily be correlated to the MPC or MSW, and using MIC as a PD denominator to describe the suppression of resistance might therefore not be appropriate [45]. If the MIC is not a good PD denominator to describe the risk for resistance development, increasing the $\%fT_{>MIC}$ with a prolonged infusion of beta-lactam antibiotics will be of no use when resistance development is concerned. Indeed, determinants other than the mode of infusion, such as the pathogen involved, the duration of therapy and the initial inoculum size, may be much more important for regrowth [41].

Finally, a PK/PD index or target linked to bacterial cell kill will tell us nothing about the risk of toxicity, as toxicity for a patient is not associated with susceptibility. Hence, using a PK/PD target (for example C_{ss} 10 times the MIC) to avoid toxicity is not relevant. As Lau et al. [46] and others [47–51] observed, beta-lactam drug toxicity is most likely linked to the through concentrations. This finding is especially worrisome, as prolonged infusions of beta-lactam antibiotics will, by definition, lead to higher through (or, in the case of continuous infusion, steady state) concentrations.

4. Introducing the 'Maximum Tolerable Dose' to Overcome the above Limitations

Based on the above considerations, and from a purely clinical point of view, using a 'maximum tolerable dose' could be an attractive alternative for beta-lactam dosing. It would maximize the cell kill, avoid resistance development and alleviate the need for complex dosing regimens in response to dynamic PK/PD indices and targets (of which most were derived from preclinical experiments). In addition, higher dosing will lead to higher tissue concentrations, which is important in critically ill patients, given the high variability of tissue penetration to different foci of infection [7,52]. Finally, using the MTD may also facilitate shortening the duration of the antimicrobial therapy.

Translation into practice would require knowledge of the concentrations associated with beta-lactam toxicity and, preferably, toxicity would be easily measurable [5]. To date, there is very little information available regarding beta-lactam antibiotic toxicity and dose–response relationships. Known beta-lactam adverse reactions are hypersensitivity, nephrotoxicity, myelotoxicity, neurotoxicity, hepatotoxicity and *Clostridioides difficile* infection [53]. Of these adverse reactions, the evidence for an exposure–response relationship is strongest for neurotoxicity. Several beta-lactam antibiotic concentrations have been linked to neurotoxicity (Table 1), although the beta-lactam antibiotic subclass prescribed is also an important predictor. For example, the proconvulsive effect of cefepime is estimated to be ten to fifteen times as high when compared with meropenem and piperacillin respectively [54]. Approximately 10–15% of the ICU patients receiving beta-lactam antibiotic drugs develop neurotoxicity, but this usually soon resolves after discontinuation or dose reduction [53,54]. The problem with beta-lactam antibiotic neurotoxicity, especially in critically ill patients, is the fact that it is difficult to distinguish from other causes of neurologic changes, such as brain damage, encephalopathy, sepsis, other toxic medications, delirium, etc. Unfortunately, no neurologic symptom is specific for beta-lactam-induced neurotoxicity [54].

Crystal nephropathy, which is a result of antimicrobial precipitation and crystallization in the renal tubuli has been documented with high amoxicillin concentrations, but is assumed to be very rare and a specific drug level linked to crystallization has not been defined [55,56].

Hypersensitivity is a common side-effect of beta-lactam antibiotics, but is likely not linked to the dosing regimen or drug concentration. Acute interstitial nephritis and drug-induced liver injury (DILI) are immune-mediated idiosyncratic reactions, and it is therefore assumed that these reactions are also not linked to the drug concentration. Whether or not myelotoxicity is dose-dependent is a matter of debate [57].

Table 1. Beta-lactam neurotoxicity levels.

Beta-Lactam Antibiotic	Neurotoxicity Levels Reported	References
Cefepime	20 mg/dL (II, t), 21.6 mg/dL (II, t), 22 mg/dL (II, t), 36 mg/dL (II, t), 63.2 mg/dL (CI, ss)	[49–51,58,59]
Piperacillin/tazobactam	361.4 mg/dL (II, t), 157 mg/dL (CI, ss)	[47,60]
Meropenem	64.2 mg/dL (II, t)	[47]
Flucloxacillin	125.1 mg/dL (II, t)	[47]

II: intermittent infusion; CI: continuous infusion; t: trough concentration; ss: steady state concentration.

5. What Other Options Might We Have to Assess Beta-Lactam Antibiotic Toxicity?

Not unsurprisingly, beta-lactam through concentrations are related to a decline in kidney function [47,50,51]. Indeed, beta-lactam antibiotics are predominantly renally eliminated, and reduced elimination will lead to higher serum levels [8]. However, other aspects of a decline in kidney function, such as uremic toxin accumulation, might also be relevant with regards to beta-lactam toxicity. Uremic toxins are endogenous waste products that are secreted by the kidney in healthy individuals. In patients with kidney disease, uremic toxins accumulate, leading to symptoms of uremia, such as anorexia, lethargy and altered mental function [61]. Uremic toxins are divided into small, water-soluble toxins, middle molecules and protein-bound uremic toxins (PBUTs) [62]. The clearance of PBUTs is more dependent on tubular secretion than glomerular filtration [63]. The tubular secretion of these toxins is mediated by basolateral and luminal transporters expressed on the tubular epithelial cells. More specifically, the organic anion transporter 1 (OAT1) and the organic anion transporter 3 (OAT3) are the main transporters responsible for the basolateral uptake of PBUTs from renal blood. For several β-lactam antibiotics, renal elimination is assumed to consist of both glomerular filtration, as well as tubular secretion via the basolateral OAT1 and OAT3 transporters [64–69]. It is, for example, assumed that as much as 50 to 75% of the renal elimination of piperacillin, a broad spectrum β-lactam antibiotic, is governed by tubular secretion [70]. Unlike glomerular filtration, tubular secretion is a competitive process with the potential for interactions between several drugs and/or endogenous solutes, in this case, an interaction between PBUTS and beta-lactam antibiotic concentrations [71].

With respect to the theory of the 'maximum tolerable dose', modeling beta-lactam concentrations (PK) as well as modeling uremic toxin concentrations (PD) as two dynamic parameters (pharmacokinetic/toxicodynamic modeling), analogous to the PK/PD models incorporating dynamic bacterial growth in response to changing antibiotic concentrations, may circumvent the issues we currently experience with static PK/PD indices and targets [5].

6. Conclusions

An ideal antibiotic dosing regimen maximizes bacterial cell kill, whilst minimizing drug toxicity and the risk for resistance development. In critically ill patients, the finding of low beta-lactam antibiotic concentrations due to PK variability has led to the adoption of prolonged infusion to increase target attainment. From a purely PK/PD point of view, increasing the duration of the infusion to increase the $\%fT_{>MIC}$ will not, by definition, lead to increased bacterial cell kill given that the PK/PD index and target are not static entities. Moreover, merely prolonging the duration of infusion in an attempt to increase the $\%fT_{>MIC}$ is likely irrelevant when it comes to suppression of regrowth and avoidance of toxicity. In the future, administering a maximum tolerable dose instead of a (minimum) dose that has been developed to achieve a predefined PK/PD target for efficacy only, may help preserve our antimicrobial armamentarium. Currently, the specific levels of beta-lactam drug toxicity are ill-defined and therefore research focusing on the pharmacodynamics of beta-lactam antibiotic toxicity is urgently needed. A first step in this process should be measuring the uremic toxin concentrations in patients receiving beta-lactam antibiotics. These data can then be used to develop a pharmacokinetic/toxicodynamic model, which in turn could inform clinicians on the maximum tolerable dose. The patients with advanced kidney disease are at risk of both high uremic toxin concentrations, as well as high beta-lactam antibiotic concentrations and therefore represent a study population of interest for the purpose of developing such a pharmacokinetic/toxicodynamic model.

Author Contributions: Conceptualization, S.A.M.D. and J.J.D.W.; methodology, S.A.M.D.; resources, S.A.M.D., E.A.H. and J.J.D.W.; writing—original draft preparation, S.A.M.D.; writing—review and editing, E.A.H. and J.J.D.W.; visualization, S.A.M.D., E.A.H. and J.J.D.W.; supervision, J.J.D.W.; project administration, S.A.M.D. All authors have read and agreed to the published version of the manuscript.

Funding: This research received no external funding.

Institutional Review Board Statement: Not applicable.

Informed Consent Statement: Not applicable.

Data Availability Statement: Not applicable.

Conflicts of Interest: The authors declare no conflict of interest.

References

1. Kollef, M.H.; Bassetti, M.; Francois, B.; Burnham, J.; Dimopoulos, G.; Garnacho-Montero, J.; Lipman, J.; Luyt, C.-E.; Nicolau, D.P.; Postma, M.J.; et al. The Intensive Care Medicine Research Agenda on Multidrug-Resistant Bacteria, Antibiotics, and Stewardship. *Intensive Care Med.* **2017**, *43*, 1187–1197. [CrossRef]
2. Dyar, O.J.; Huttner, B.; Schouten, J.; Pulcini, C. ESGAP (ESCMID Study Group for Antimicrobial stewardshiP) What Is Antimicrobial Stewardship? *Clin. Microbiol. Infect.* **2017**, *23*, 793–798. [CrossRef]

3. Society for Healthcare Epidemiology of America; Infectious Diseases Society of America; Pediatric Infectious Diseases Society. Policy Statement on Antimicrobial Stewardship by the Society for Healthcare Epidemiology of America (SHEA), the Infectious Diseases Society of America (IDSA), and the Pediatric Infectious Diseases Society (PIDS). *Infect. Control Hosp. Epidemiol.* **2012**, *33*, 322–327. [CrossRef]
4. Roberts, J.A.; Roger, C.; De Waele, J.J. Personalized Antibiotic Dosing for the Critically Ill. *Intensive Care Med.* **2019**, *45*, 715–718. [CrossRef]
5. Nielsen, E.I.; Friberg, L.E. Pharmacokinetic-Pharmacodynamic Modeling of Antibacterial Drugs. *Pharmacol. Rev.* **2013**, *65*, 1053–1090. [CrossRef]
6. Roberts, J.A.; Lipman, J.; Blot, S.; Rello, J. Better Outcomes through Continuous Infusion of Time-Dependent Antibiotics to Critically Ill Patients? *Curr. Opin. Crit. Care* **2008**, *14*, 390–396. [CrossRef]
7. Roberts, J.A.; Abdul-Aziz, M.H.; Lipman, J.; Mouton, J.W.; Vinks, A.A.; Felton, T.W.; Hope, W.W.; Farkas, A.; Neely, M.N.; Schentag, J.J.; et al. Individualised Antibiotic Dosing for Patients Who Are Critically Ill: Challenges and Potential Solutions. *Lancet Infect. Dis.* **2014**, *14*, 498–509. [CrossRef]
8. Veiga, R.P.; Paiva, J.-A. Pharmacokinetics–Pharmacodynamics Issues Relevant for the Clinical Use of Beta-Lactam Antibiotics in Critically Ill Patients. *Crit. Care* **2018**, *22*, 233. [CrossRef]
9. DALI: Defining Antibiotic Levels in Intensive Care Unit Patients: Are Current β-Lactam Antibiotic Doses Sufficient for Critically Ill Patients? | Clinical Infectious Diseases | Oxford Academic. Available online: https://academic.oup.com/cid/article/58/8/1072/356400?login=true (accessed on 29 March 2022).
10. Taccone, F.S.; Laterre, P.-F.; Dugernier, T.; Spapen, H.; Delattre, I.; Wittebole, X.; De Backer, D.; Layeux, B.; Wallemacq, P.; Vincent, J.-L.; et al. Insufficient β-Lactam Concentrations in the Early Phase of Severe Sepsis and Septic Shock. *Crit. Care* **2010**, *14*, R126. [CrossRef]
11. Craig, W.A. Interrelationship between Pharmacokinetics and Pharmacodynamics in Determining Dosage Regimens for Broad-Spectrum Cephalosporins. *Diagn. Microbiol. Infect. Dis.* **1995**, *22*, 89–96. [CrossRef]
12. Craig, W.A. Pharmacokinetic/Pharmacodynamic Parameters: Rationale for Antibacterial Dosing of Mice and Men. *Clin. Infect. Dis.* **1998**, *26*, 1–12. [CrossRef]
13. Mouton, J.W.; Muller, A.E.; Canton, R.; Giske, C.G.; Kahlmeter, G.; Turnidge, J. MIC-Based Dose Adjustment: Facts and Fables. *J. Antimicrob. Chemother.* **2018**, *73*, 564–568. [CrossRef]
14. Abdul-Aziz, M.H.; Sulaiman, H.; Mat-Nor, M.-B.; Rai, V.; Wong, K.K.; Hasan, M.S.; Abd Rahman, A.N.; Jamal, J.A.; Wallis, S.C.; Lipman, J.; et al. Beta-Lactam Infusion in Severe Sepsis (BLISS): A Prospective, Two-Centre, Open-Labelled Randomised Controlled Trial of Continuous versus Intermittent Beta-Lactam Infusion in Critically Ill Patients with Severe Sepsis. *Intensive Care Med.* **2016**, *42*, 1535–1545. [CrossRef]
15. Roberts, J.A.; Kirkpatrick, C.M.J.; Roberts, M.S.; Dalley, A.J.; Lipman, J. First-Dose and Steady-State Population Pharmacokinetics and Pharmacodynamics of Piperacillin by Continuous or Intermittent Dosing in Critically Ill Patients with Sepsis. *Int. J. Antimicrob. Agents* **2010**, *35*, 156–163. [CrossRef]
16. Lyu, Y.; Yang, Y.; Li, X.; Peng, M.; He, X.; Zhang, P.; Dong, S.; Wang, W.; Wang, D. Selection of Piperacillin/Tazobactam Infusion Mode Guided by SOFA Score in Cancer Patients with Hospital-Acquired Pneumonia: A Randomized Controlled Study. *Ther. Clin. Risk Manag.* **2017**, *14*, 31–37. [CrossRef]
17. Wang, Z.; Shan, T.; Liu, Y.; Ding, S.; Li, C.; Zhai, Q.; Chen, X.; Du, B.; Li, Y.; Zhang, J.; et al. Comparison of 3-hour and 30-minute infusion regimens for meropenem in patients with hospital acquired pneumonia in intensive care unit: A randomized controlled clinical trial. *Zhonghua Wei Zhong Bing Ji Jiu Yi Xue* **2014**, *26*, 644–649. [CrossRef]
18. Dulhunty, J.M.; Roberts, J.A.; Davis, J.S.; Webb, S.A.R.; Bellomo, R.; Gomersall, C.; Shirwadkar, C.; Eastwood, G.M.; Myburgh, J.; Paterson, D.L.; et al. Continuous Infusion of Beta-Lactam Antibiotics in Severe Sepsis: A Multicenter Double-Blind, Randomized Controlled Trial. *Clin. Infect. Dis.* **2013**, *56*, 236–244. [CrossRef]
19. Bao, H.; Lv, Y.; Wang, D.; Xue, J.; Yan, Z. Clinical Outcomes of Extended versus Intermittent Administration of Piperacillin/Tazobactam for the Treatment of Hospital-Acquired Pneumonia: A Randomized Controlled Trial. *Eur. J. Clin. Microbiol. Infect. Dis.* **2017**, *36*, 459–466. [CrossRef]
20. Wang, D. Experience with Extended-Infusion Meropenem in the Management of Ventilator-Associated Pneumonia Due to Multidrug-Resistant Acinetobacter Baumannii. *Int. J. Antimicrob. Agents* **2009**, *33*, 290–291. [CrossRef]
21. Rafati, M.R.; Rouini, M.R.; Mojtahedzadeh, M.; Najafi, A.; Tavakoli, H.; Gholami, K.; Fazeli, M.R. Clinical Efficacy of Continuous Infusion of Piperacillin Compared with Intermittent Dosing in Septic Critically Ill Patients. *Int. J. Antimicrob. Agents* **2006**, *28*, 122–127. [CrossRef]
22. Chytra, I.; Stepan, M.; Benes, J.; Pelnar, P.; Zidkova, A.; Bergerova, T.; Pradl, R.; Kasal, E. Clinical and Microbiological Efficacy of Continuous versus Intermittent Application of Meropenem in Critically Ill Patients: A Randomized Open-Label Controlled Trial. *Crit. Care* **2012**, *16*, R113. [CrossRef] [PubMed]
23. Georges, B.; Conil, J.M.; Cougot, P.; Decun, J.F.; Archambaud, M.; Seguin, T.; Chabanon, G.; Virenque, C.; Houin, G.; Saivin, S. Cefepime in Critically Ill Patients: Continuous Infusion vs. an Intermittent Dosing Regimen. *Int. J. Clin. Pharmacol. Ther.* **2005**, *43*, 360–369. [CrossRef] [PubMed]

24. Vardakas, K.Z.; Voulgaris, G.L.; Maliaros, A.; Samonis, G.; Falagas, M.E. Prolonged versus Short-Term Intravenous Infusion of Antipseudomonal β-Lactams for Patients with Sepsis: A Systematic Review and Meta-Analysis of Randomised Trials. *Lancet Infect. Dis.* **2018**, *18*, 108–120. [CrossRef]
25. Roberts, J.A.; Abdul-Aziz, M.-H.; Davis, J.S.; Dulhunty, J.M.; Cotta, M.O.; Myburgh, J.; Bellomo, R.; Lipman, J. Continuous versus Intermittent β-Lactam Infusion in Severe Sepsis. A Meta-Analysis of Individual Patient Data from Randomized Trials. *Am. J. Respir. Crit. Care Med.* **2016**, *194*, 681–691. [CrossRef] [PubMed]
26. Rhodes, N.J.; Liu, J.; O'Donnell, J.N.; Dulhunty, J.M.; Abdul-Aziz, M.H.; Berko, P.Y.; Nadler, B.; Lipman, J.; Roberts, J.A. Prolonged Infusion Piperacillin-Tazobactam Decreases Mortality and Improves Outcomes in Severely Ill Patients: Results of a Systematic Review and Meta-Analysis. *Crit. Care Med.* **2018**, *46*, 236–243. [CrossRef]
27. The George Institute. A Phase III Randomised Controlled Trial of Continuous Beta-Lactam Infusion Compared with Intermittent Beta-Lactam Dosing in Critically Ill Patients; clinicaltrials.gov, 2021. Available online: https://clinicaltrials.gov/ct2/show/NCT03213990 (accessed on 14 April 2022).
28. Dhaese, S.; Heffernan, A.; Liu, D.; Abdul-Aziz, M.H.; Stove, V.; Tam, V.H.; Lipman, J.; Roberts, J.A.; De Waele, J.J. Prolonged Versus Intermittent Infusion of β-Lactam Antibiotics: A Systematic Review and Meta-Regression of Bacterial Killing in Preclinical Infection Models. *Clin. Pharmacokinet.* **2020**, *59*, 1237–1250. [CrossRef]
29. Felton, T.W.; Goodwin, J.; O'Connor, L.; Sharp, A.; Gregson, L.; Livermore, J.; Howard, S.J.; Neely, M.N.; Hope, W.W. Impact of Bolus Dosing versus Continuous Infusion of Piperacillin and Tazobactam on the Development of Antimicrobial Resistance in Pseudomonas Aeruginosa. *Antimicrob. Agents Chemother.* **2013**, *57*, 5811–5819. [CrossRef]
30. Sumi, C.D.; Heffernan, A.J.; Naicker, S.; Islam, K.; Cottrell, K.; Wallis, S.C.; Lipman, J.; Harris, P.N.A.; Sime, F.B.; Roberts, J.A. Pharmacodynamic Evaluation of Intermittent versus Extended and Continuous Infusions of Piperacillin/Tazobactam in a Hollow-Fibre Infection Model against Klebsiella Pneumoniae. *J. Antimicrob. Chemother.* **2020**, *75*, 2633–2640. [CrossRef]
31. Sinnollareddy, M.G.; Roberts, M.S.; Lipman, J.; Roberts, J.A. β-Lactam Pharmacokinetics and Pharmacodynamics in Critically Ill Patients and Strategies for Dose Optimization: A Structured Review. *Clin. Exp. Pharmacol. Physiol.* **2012**, *39*, 489–496. [CrossRef]
32. Bergen, P.J.; Bulitta, J.B.; Kirkpatrick, C.M.J.; Rogers, K.E.; McGregor, M.J.; Wallis, S.C.; Paterson, D.L.; Nation, R.L.; Lipman, J.; Roberts, J.A.; et al. Substantial Impact of Altered Pharmacokinetics in Critically Ill Patients on the Antibacterial Effects of Meropenem Evaluated via the Dynamic Hollow-Fiber Infection Model. *Antimicrob. Agents Chemother.* **2017**, *61*, e02642-16. [CrossRef]
33. Kristoffersson, A.N.; David-Pierson, P.; Parrott, N.J.; Kuhlmann, O.; Lave, T.; Friberg, L.E.; Nielsen, E.I. Simulation-Based Evaluation of PK/PD Indices for Meropenem Across Patient Groups and Experimental Designs. *Pharm. Res.* **2016**, *33*, 1115–1125. [CrossRef] [PubMed]
34. Bergen, P.J.; Bulitta, J.B.; Kirkpatrick, C.M.J.; Rogers, K.E.; McGregor, M.J.; Wallis, S.C.; Paterson, D.L.; Lipman, J.; Roberts, J.A.; Landersdorfer, C.B. Effect of Different Renal Function on Antibacterial Effects of Piperacillin against Pseudomonas Aeruginosa Evaluated via the Hollow-Fibre Infection Model and Mechanism-Based Modelling. *J. Antimicrob. Chemother.* **2016**, *71*, 2509–2520. [CrossRef]
35. Sjövall, F.; Alobaid, A.S.; Wallis, S.C.; Perner, A.; Lipman, J.; Roberts, J.A. Maximally Effective Dosing Regimens of Meropenem in Patients with Septic Shock. *J. Antimicrob. Chemother.* **2018**, *73*, 191–198. [CrossRef] [PubMed]
36. Van Herendael, B.; Jeurissen, A.; Tulkens, P.M.; Vlieghe, E.; Verbrugghe, W.; Jorens, P.G.; Ieven, M. Continuous Infusion of Antibiotics in the Critically Ill: The New Holy Grail for Beta-Lactams and Vancomycin? *Ann. Intensive Care* **2012**, *2*, 22. [CrossRef] [PubMed]
37. Taccone, F.S.; Laupland, K.B.; Montravers, P. Continuous Infusion of β-Lactam Antibiotics for All Critically Ill Patients? *Intensive Care Med.* **2016**, *42*, 1604–1606. [CrossRef]
38. Nielsen, E.I.; Cars, O.; Friberg, L.E. Pharmacokinetic/Pharmacodynamic (PK/PD) Indices of Antibiotics Predicted by a Semimechanistic PKPD Model: A Step toward Model-Based Dose Optimization. *Antimicrob. Agents Chemother.* **2011**, *55*, 4619–4630. [CrossRef]
39. Craig, W.A.; Redington, J.; Ebert, S.C. Pharmacodynamics of Amikacin in Vitro and in Mouse Thigh and Lung Infections. *J. Antimicrob. Chemother.* **1991**, *27*, 29–40. [CrossRef]
40. Tam, V.H.; Schilling, A.N.; Poole, K.; Nikolaou, M. Mathematical Modelling Response of Pseudomonas Aeruginosa to Meropenem. *J. Antimicrob. Chemother.* **2007**, *60*, 1302–1309. [CrossRef]
41. Sumi, C.D.; Heffernan, A.J.; Lipman, J.; Roberts, J.A.; Sime, F.B. What Antibiotic Exposures Are Required to Suppress the Emergence of Resistance for Gram-Negative Bacteria? A Systematic Review. *Clin. Pharmacokinet.* **2019**, *58*, 1407–1443. [CrossRef]
42. Li, X.; Wang, L.; Zhang, X.-J.; Yang, Y.; Gong, W.-T.; Xu, B.; Zhu, Y.-Q.; Liu, W. Evaluation of Meropenem Regimens Suppressing Emergence of Resistance in Acinetobacter Baumannii with Human Simulated Exposure in an in Vitro Intravenous-Infusion Hollow-Fiber Infection Model. *Antimicrob. Agents Chemother.* **2014**, *58*, 6773–6781. [CrossRef]
43. Drusano, G.L.; Hope, W.; MacGowan, A.; Louie, A. Suppression of Emergence of Resistance in Pathogenic Bacteria: Keeping Our Powder Dry, Part 2. *Antimicrob. Agents Chemother.* **2015**, *60*, 1194–1201. [CrossRef]
44. Firsov, A.A.; Vostrov, S.N.; Lubenko, I.Y.; Drlica, K.; Portnoy, Y.A.; Zinner, S.H. In Vitro Pharmacodynamic Evaluation of the Mutant Selection Window Hypothesis Using Four Fluoroquinolones against Staphylococcus Aureus. *Antimicrob. Agents Chemother.* **2003**, *47*, 1604–1613. [CrossRef] [PubMed]

45. Gugel, J.; Dos Santos Pereira, A.; Pignatari, A.C.C.; Gales, A.C. Beta-Lactam MICs Correlate Poorly with Mutant Prevention Concentrations for Clinical Isolates of Acinetobacter Spp. and Pseudomonas Aeruginosa. *Antimicrob. Agents Chemother.* **2006**, *50*, 2276–2277. [CrossRef]
46. Lau, C.; Marriott, D.; Schultz, H.B.; Gould, M.; Andresen, D.; Wicha, S.G.; Alffenaar, J.-W.; Penm, J.; Reuter, S.E. Assessment of Cefepime Toxicodynamics: Comprehensive Examination of Pharmacokinetic/Pharmacodynamic Targets for Cefepime-Induced Neurotoxicity and Evaluation of Current Dosing Guidelines. *Int. J. Antimicrob. Agents* **2021**, *58*, 106443. [CrossRef] [PubMed]
47. Imani, S.; Buscher, H.; Marriott, D.; Gentili, S.; Sandaradura, I. Too Much of a Good Thing: A Retrospective Study of β-Lactam Concentration-Toxicity Relationships. *J. Antimicrob. Chemother.* **2017**, *72*, 2891–2897. [CrossRef] [PubMed]
48. Beumier, M.; Casu, G.S.; Hites, M.; Wolff, F.; Cotton, F.; Vincent, J.L.; Jacobs, F.; Taccone, F.S. Elevated β-Lactam Concentrations Associated with Neurological Deterioration in ICU Septic Patients. *Minerva Anestesiol* **2015**, *81*, 497–506. [PubMed]
49. Huwyler, T.; Lenggenhager, L.; Abbas, M.; Ing Lorenzini, K.; Hughes, S.; Huttner, B.; Karmime, A.; Uçkay, I.; von Dach, E.; Lescuyer, P.; et al. Cefepime Plasma Concentrations and Clinical Toxicity: A Retrospective Cohort Study. *Clin. Microbiol. Infect.* **2017**, *23*, 454–459. [CrossRef] [PubMed]
50. Boschung-Pasquier, L.; Atkinson, A.; Kastner, L.K.; Banholzer, S.; Haschke, M.; Buetti, N.; Furrer, D.I.; Hauser, C.; Jent, P.; Que, Y.A.; et al. Cefepime Neurotoxicity: Thresholds and Risk Factors. A Retrospective Cohort Study. *Clin. Microbiol. Infect.* **2020**, *26*, 333–339. [CrossRef]
51. Lau, C.; Marriott, D.; Gould, M.; Andresen, D.; Reuter, S.E.; Penm, J. A Retrospective Study to Determine the Cefepime-Induced Neurotoxicity Threshold in Hospitalized Patients. *J. Antimicrob. Chemother.* **2020**, *75*, 718–725. [CrossRef]
52. Lodise, T.P.; Sorgel, F.; Melnick, D.; Mason, B.; Kinzig, M.; Drusano, G.L. Penetration of Meropenem into Epithelial Lining Fluid of Patients with Ventilator-Associated Pneumonia. *Antimicrob. Agents Chemother.* **2011**, *55*, 1606–1610. [CrossRef]
53. Vardakas, K.Z.; Kalimeris, G.D.; Triarides, N.A.; Falagas, M.E. An Update on Adverse Drug Reactions Related to β-Lactam Antibiotics. *Expert Opin. Drug Saf.* **2018**, *17*, 499–508. [CrossRef] [PubMed]
54. Roger, C.; Louart, B. Beta-Lactams Toxicity in the Intensive Care Unit: An Underestimated Collateral Damage? *Microorganisms* **2021**, *9*, 1505. [CrossRef] [PubMed]
55. Mousseaux, C.; Rafat, C.; Letavernier, E.; Frochot, V.; Kerroumi, Y.; Zeller, V.; Luque, Y. Acute Kidney Injury After High Doses of Amoxicillin. *Kidney Int. Rep.* **2021**, *6*, 830–834. [CrossRef] [PubMed]
56. Demotier, S.; Limelette, A.; Charmillon, A.; Baux, E.; Parent, X.; Mestrallet, S.; Pavel, S.; Servettaz, A.; Dramé, M.; Muggeo, A.; et al. Incidence, Associated Factors, and Effect on Renal Function of Amoxicillin Crystalluria in Patients Receiving High Doses of Intravenous Amoxicillin (The CRISTAMOX Study): A Cohort Study. *eClinicalMedicine* **2022**, *45*, 101340. [CrossRef] [PubMed]
57. Barreto, E.F.; Webb, A.J.; Pais, G.M.; Rule, A.D.; Jannetto, P.J.; Scheetz, M.H. Setting the Beta-Lactam Therapeutic Range for Critically Ill Patients: Is There a Floor or Even a Ceiling? *Crit. Care Explor.* **2021**, *3*, e0446. [CrossRef]
58. Lamoth, F.; Buclin, T.; Pascual, A.; Vora, S.; Bolay, S.; Decosterd, L.A.; Calandra, T.; Marchetti, O. High Cefepime Plasma Concentrations and Neurological Toxicity in Febrile Neutropenic Patients with Mild Impairment of Renal Function. *Antimicrob. Agents Chemother.* **2010**, *54*, 4360–4367. [CrossRef]
59. Vercheval, C.; Sadzot, B.; Maes, N.; Denooz, R.; Damas, P.; Frippiat, F. Continuous Infusion of Cefepime and Neurotoxicity: A Retrospective Cohort Study. *Clin. Microbiol. Infect.* **2021**, *27*, 731–735. [CrossRef]
60. Quinton, M.-C.; Bodeau, S.; Kontar, L.; Zerbib, Y.; Maizel, J.; Slama, M.; Masmoudi, K.; Lemaire-Hurtel, A.-S.; Bennis, Y. Neurotoxic Concentration of Piperacillin during Continuous Infusion in Critically Ill Patients. *Antimicrob. Agents Chemother.* **2017**, *61*, e00654-17. [CrossRef]
61. Meyer, T.W.; Hostetter, T.H. Uremia. *N. Engl. J. Med.* **2007**, *357*, 1316–1325. [CrossRef]
62. Rosner, M.H.; Reis, T.; Husain-Syed, F.; Vanholder, R.; Hutchison, C.; Stenvinkel, P.; Blankestijn, P.J.; Cozzolino, M.; Juillard, L.; Kashani, K.; et al. Classification of Uremic Toxins and Their Role in Kidney Failure. *CJASN* **2021**, *16*, 1918–1928. [CrossRef]
63. Masereeuw, R.; Mutsaers, H.A.M.; Toyohara, T.; Abe, T.; Jhawar, S.; Sweet, D.H.; Lowenstein, J. The Kidney and Uremic Toxin Removal: Glomerulus or Tubule? *Semin. Nephrol.* **2014**, *34*, 191–208. [CrossRef] [PubMed]
64. Deguchi, T.; Kusuhara, H.; Takadate, A.; Endou, H.; Otagiri, M.; Sugiyama, Y. Characterization of Uremic Toxin Transport by Organic Anion Transporters in the Kidney. *Kidney Int.* **2004**, *65*, 162–174. [CrossRef] [PubMed]
65. Wu, W.; Bush, K.T.; Nigam, S.K. Key Role for the Organic Anion Transporters, OAT1 and OAT3, in the in Vivo Handling of Uremic Toxins and Solutes. *Sci. Rep.* **2017**, *7*, 4939. [CrossRef] [PubMed]
66. Nigam, S.K.; Wu, W.; Bush, K.T.; Hoenig, M.P.; Blantz, R.C.; Bhatnagar, V. Handling of Drugs, Metabolites, and Uremic Toxins by Kidney Proximal Tubule Drug Transporters. *Clin. J. Am. Soc. Nephrol.* **2015**, *10*, 2039–2049. [CrossRef] [PubMed]
67. Ivanyuk, A.; Livio, F.; Biollaz, J.; Buclin, T. Renal Drug Transporters and Drug Interactions. *Clin. Pharmacokinet.* **2017**, *56*, 825–892. [CrossRef]
68. Miners, J.O.; Yang, X.; Knights, K.M.; Zhang, L. The Role of the Kidney in Drug Elimination: Transport, Metabolism, and the Impact of Kidney Disease on Drug Clearance. *Clin. Pharmacol. Ther.* **2017**, *102*, 436–449. [CrossRef]
69. Wen, S.; Wang, C.; Duan, Y.; Huo, X.; Meng, Q.; Liu, Z.; Yang, S.; Zhu, Y.; Sun, H.; Ma, X.; et al. OAT1 and OAT3 Also Mediate the Drug-Drug Interaction between Piperacillin and Tazobactam. *Int. J. Pharm.* **2018**, *537*, 172–182. [CrossRef]
70. Tjandramaga, T.B.; Mullie, A.; Verbesselt, R.; De Schepper, P.J.; Verbist, L. Piperacillin: Human Pharmacokinetics after Intravenous and Intramuscular Administration. *Antimicrob. Agents Chemother.* **1978**, *14*, 829–837. [CrossRef]
71. Wang, K.; Kestenbaum, B. Proximal Tubular Secretory Clearance: A Neglected Partner of Kidney Function. *Clin. J. Am. Soc. Nephrol.* **2018**, *13*, 1291–1296. [CrossRef]

Article

Clinical Features and Outcomes of Monobacterial and Polybacterial Episodes of Ventilator-Associated Pneumonia Due to Multidrug-Resistant *Acinetobacter baumannii*

Dalia Adukauskiene [1], Ausra Ciginskiene [1,*], Agne Adukauskaite [2], Despoina Koulenti [3,4] and Jordi Rello [5,6]

1. Medical Academy, Lithuanian University of Health Sciences, 44307 Kaunas, Lithuania; daliaadu@gmail.com
2. Department of Cardiology and Angiology, University Hospital of Innsbruck, 6020 Innsbruck, Austria; agne.adukauskaite@tirol-kliniken.at
3. Second Critical Care Department, Attikon University Hospital, 12462 Athens, Greece; deskogr@yahoo.gr
4. UQ Centre for Clinical Research (UQCCR), Faculty of Medicine, The Univesrity of Queensland, Brisbane 4029, Australia
5. Vall d'Hebron Institute of Research, Vall d'Hebron Campus Hospital, 08035 Barcelona, Spain; jrello@crips.es
6. Clinical Research, CHU Nîmes, 30900 Nîmes, France
* Correspondence: ausra.ciginskiene@lsmu.lt

Abstract: Multidrug-resistant *A. baumannii* (MDRAB) VAP has high morbidity and mortality, and the rates are constantly increasing globally. Mono- and polybacterial MDRAB VAP might differ, including outcomes. We conducted a single-center, retrospective (January 2014–December 2016) study in the four ICUs (12–18–24 beds each) of a reference Lithuanian university hospital, aiming to compare the clinical features and the 30-day mortality of monobacterial and polybacterial MDRAB VAP episodes. A total of 156 MDRAB VAP episodes were analyzed: 105 (67.5%) were monomicrobial. The 30-day mortality was higher ($p < 0.05$) in monobacterial episodes: overall (57.1 vs. 37.3%), subgroup with appropriate antibiotic therapy (50.7 vs. 23.5%), and subgroup of XDR *A. baumannii* (57.3 vs. 36.4%). Monobacterial MDRAB VAP was associated ($p < 0.05$) with Charlson comorbidity index ≥ 3 (67.6 vs. 47.1%), respiratory comorbidities (19.0 vs. 5.9%), obesity (27.6 vs. 9.8%), prior hospitalization (58.1 vs. 31.4%), prior antibiotic therapy (99.0 vs. 92.2%), sepsis (88.6 vs. 76.5%), septic shock (51.9 vs. 34.6%), severe hypoxemia (23.8 vs. 7.8%), higher leukocyte count on VAP onset (median [IQR] 11.6 [8.4–16.6] vs. 10.9 [7.3–13.4]), and RRT need during ICU stay (37.1 vs. 17.6%). Patients with polybacterial VAP had a higher frequency of decreased level of consciousness ($p < 0.05$) on ICU admission (29.4 vs. 14.3%) and on VAP onset (29.4 vs. 11.4%). We concluded that monobacterial MDRAB VAP had different demographic/clinical characteristics compared to polybacterial and carried worse outcomes. These important findings need to be validated in a larger, prospective study, and the management implications to be further investigated.

Keywords: *Acinetobacter baumannii*; antibiotic optimisation; antibiotic stewardship (AMS); aspiration pneumonia; colistin; hospital-acquired pneumonia (HAP); multidrug-resistance (MDR); mortality; non-fermentative Gram-negative bacilli (GNB); polymicrobial; pneumonia resolution; ventilator-associated pneumonia (VAP)

1. Introduction

Ventilator-associated pneumonia (VAP) is the most frequent infection in the intensive care unit (ICU) with a significant impact on the morbidity and mortality of critically ill patients, as VAP development has been associated with increased duration of mechanical ventilation (MV), prolonged ICU and hospital stay, increased consumption of antibiotics, and increased health-care costs [1,2]. The reported incidence varies significantly in the relevant literature, from 1–2.5 cases per 1000 ventilator-days in the USA to 116 cases per 1000 ventilator-days in the Southeast Asian Region, and this variation might be, at least partially, attributed to differences in prevention measures, definitions used, and case mix [3,4]. It has been demonstrated that the clinical manifestation and outcomes of VAP might vary depending on the pathogen. There are multiple VAP studies on specific pathogens describing their clinical, management, and outcome-related aspects without, however, considering the mono- or polybacterial VAP origin [5,6].

The clinical importance of *Acinetobacter baumannii* (*A. baumannii*) has been steadily increasing on a worldwide level. It has established a niche in the hospital environment causing a variety of severe infections, especially in the critical care setting. It is usually a difficult-to-treat pathogen displaying a high resistance profile and has been associated with high mortality, morbidity, and health care costs [5–22]. Although some controversy exists in the relevant literature, it seems that the high mortality of infections caused by multidrug-resistant (MDR) pathogens may be related not only to the bacterial resistance but also to the severity of illness and the appropriateness and timeliness of antibacterial treatment [1,5,8–12].

Regarding VAP, *A. baumannii* is one of the most common pathogens of both mono- and polybacterial VAP [6,7]. The association between mono- and polybacterial VAP caused by MDRAB and patients' mortality has not been thoroughly investigated yet. We believe that it would be methodologically more accurate to analyze the monobacterial VAP cases separately from the polybacterial ones in order to reliably estimate the association between a pathogen and the clinical presentation and outcomes of VAP. Our hypothesis was that the mortality and clinical characteristics of patients with VAP due to MDRAB differ between mono- and polybacterial cases. Hence, the primary objective of our study was to compare the 30-day mortality between patients with mono- and polybacterial MDRAB VAP, while the secondary objective was to compare their clinical features.

2. Methods and Materials

A retrospective cohort study was conducted in the four adult ICUs (medical-surgical, neurosurgical, cardiosurgical, and coronary care; 12–18–24 beds each) of the Hospital of Lithuanian University of Health Sciences Kaunas Clinics, a reference hospital that is the largest of the country (2300 beds). The study was approved by Kaunas Regional Biomedical Research Ethics Committee (No BEC-MF-156 and No P1-BE-2-13/2016). The need for written consent was waived due to the observational nature of the study.

The medical records of all patients admitted to the ICUs over a three-year period (from January 2014 to December 2016) were reviewed. Inclusion criteria were as follows: (1) age $\geq$ 18 years and (2) the first episode of VAP due to MDRAB. Exclusion criteria were: (1) polybacterial cases with Gram-positive co-pathogens, (2) neutropenia, and (3) deceased within the first 24 h after VAP onset.

Pneumonia was considered to be ventilator-associated when it occurred 48 h or more after intubation and onset of mechanical ventilation. Clinical diagnosis of VAP was made according to 2005 American Thoracic Society/Infectious Diseases Society of America (ATS/IDSA) criteria [23]. Sepsis status was diagnosed according to Sepsis-2 criteria [24]. The severity of illness was assessed on ICU admission and on VAP diagnosis using the Sequential Organ Failure Assessment (SOFA) and Simplified Acute Physiology Score II (SAPS II) scores. The identification of *A. baumannii* isolates and antibiotic susceptibility was performed according to the European Committee on Antimicrobial Susceptibility Testing (EUCAST) guidelines [25]. *A. baumannii* isolates were defined as MDR and extensively drug-resistant (XDR) according to an international expert proposal for the interim standard definitions for acquired resistance criteria, i.e., MDR when they were non-susceptible to at least one agent in three or more antimicrobial categories, and XDR when they were non-susceptible to at least one agent in all but two or fewer antimicrobial categories [26]. XDR isolates represent a sub-group of MDRs [26].

Demographics, clinical and laboratory data for each VAP case were recorded, including: (1) data of the first MDRAB positive tracheal aspirate culture, bacterial load (moderate/heavy growth), and drug resistance of *A. baumannii* strains; (2) age, gender, type of admission (medical/surgical), and comorbidities; (3) red blood cell (RBC) transfusion, reintubation, tracheostomy, and the need for renal replacement therapy (RRT) during the ICU stay; (4) sepsis, septic shock, oxygenation, temperature, inflammatory, and acid-base status on VAP diagnosis; (5) severity of illness on ICU admission and on VAP onset; (6) the use of intravenous (IV) antibiotics within the prior 90 days; (7) outcome: discharge or death at day 30 after VAP onset. The SOFA score was used to define organ dysfunction (>0) and organ failure (>2) both on ICU admission and on VAP onset. The baseline comorbidities were assessed using the Charlson comorbidity index (CCI), and the sepsis status using SEPSIS 2 criteria. Admission was considered as surgical in patients who had undergone surgery in the preceding four weeks. Antibacterial therapy was considered appropriate when at least one antibacterial agent, to which all causative pathogens were susceptible in vitro, was administered.

The mortality was defined as all-cause mortality within 30-day period after VAP diagnosis. To rule out the potential impact of several factors on mortality, the patients were grouped based on their disease severity on VAP diagnosis (SOFA < 8 vs. SOFA > 7), antimicrobial resistance of *A. baumannii* strains (MDR vs. XDR), appropriateness (appropriate vs. inappropriate) and timeliness (less vs. more than 48 h from VAP onset) of antibacterial treatment.

Statistical Analysis

The variables were summarized as frequencies and percentages or medians and interquartile range (IQR). Mann–Whitney non-parametric test, Pearson's chi-square test, or two-tailed Fisher's exact test were performed to detect the differences between groups as appropriate. Mortality was analyzed both, as a binary outcome (survivor/non-survivor) and as survival time data. In the survival analysis, Kaplan–Meier estimates of the probability of survival were obtained, and survival curves were compared between groups using the Log Rank test. Two-sided p values of <0.01 and <0.05 were considered statistically significant for the Log Rank test and all other analyses, respectively. Statistical analysis was performed using the Statistical Package for the Social Sciences (SPSS), version 24 (SPSS, Chicago, IL, USA).

3. Results

A total of 156 VAP cases due to MDRAB were included in the analysis: 105 (67.3%) monobacterial and 51 (32.7%) polybacterial episodes, $p < 0.001$. In association with *A. baumannii*, one co-pathogen was found in 40 (25.6%), and two co-pathogens in 11 (7.1%) cases of polybacterial VAP; *Klebsiella* spp. and *P. aeruginosa* were the most frequently isolated co-pathogens. Most of *A. baumannii* strains (85.3%) were found to be of XDR profile ($p < 0.001$). All of them were susceptible to colistin, however, the vast majority (>90%) were resistant to piperacillin/tazobactam, cephalosporins, and carbapenems.

Patients with monobacterial episodes had more frequently prior antibiotic use, particularly carbapenems and antifungals, higher CCI, higher white blood cells count on VAP onset, and more frequent RRT during the ICU stay. Moreover, they had a higher respiratory SOFA score on ICU admission and more severe hypoxia on VAP onset, as depicted by the PaO_2/FiO_2 ratio (detailed comparison in Table 1).

Patients with monobacterial VAP due to MDRAB had higher mortality compared to those with polybacterial VAP, even after controlling for factors that may affect mortality. The detailed characteristics of 30-day mortality are provided in Table 2.

The time to death (censored at day 30) was also shorter in the group with monobacterial VAP due to MDRAB, $p = 0.01$ (Figure 1).

Table 1. Characteristics of mono- and polybacterial cases of VAP due to MDRAB.

Variable	VAP Origin		p Value
	Monobacterial n = 105	Polybacterial * n = 51	
Age, years, median (IQR)	63 (54–72)	59 (52–67)	0.22
Sex, male, n (%)	61 (58.1)	32 (62.7)	0.61
Prior hospitalization within 90 days, n (%)	**61 (58.1)**	16 (31.4)	**<0.01**
Disease severity on ICU admission, median (IQR):			
■ SOFA	7 (4–9)	7 (5–8)	0.64
■ SAPS II	40.5 (33.0–56.0)	44.0 (35.0–54.0)	0.66
Admission to ICU from, n (%):			
■ Community—ED	39 (37.1)	23 (45.1)	
■ Ward	37 (35.2)	15 (29.4)	0.62
■ Other ICU	29 (27.6)	13 (25.5)	
Duration of hospital stay prior to VAP onset, days, median (IQR)	13.0 (6.25–20.0)	11.0 (6.0–16.75)	1.00
Duration of ICU stay prior to VAP onset, days, median, IQR	8.5 (5.0–14.0)	9.0 (5.0–13.75)	0.26
Admission, n (%):			
■ Medical	66 (62.9)	30 (58.8)	0.73
■ Surgical	39 (37.1)	21 (41.2)	
CCI ≥ 3, n (%)	**71 (67.6)**	24 (47.1)	**0.01**
Chronic illness, n (%):	86 (81.9)	39 (76.5)	0.43
■ Cardiovascular	73 (69.5)	33 (64.7)	0.55
■ Respiratory	**20 (19.0)**	3 (5.9)	**0.03**
■ Neurological	8 (7.6)	2 (3.9)	0.50
■ Renal	22 (21.0)	7 (13.7)	0.28
■ Liver	9 (8.6)	4 (7.8)	0.89
■ DM	18 (17.1)	7 (13.7)	0.59
■ Oncology **	17 (16.2)	4 (7.8)	0.15
■ Obesity ***	**29 (27.6)**	5 (9.8)	**0.01**
Organ failure on ICU admission, n (%):			
■ SOFA respiratory ≥ 3	**75 (71.4)**	26 (50.0)	**0.01**
■ SOFA cardiovascular ≥ 3	42 (40.0)	20 (39.2)	0.93
■ SOFA neurologic ≥ 3	15 (14.3)	**15 (29.4)**	**0.03**
■ SOFA renal ≥ 3	17 (16.2)	6 (11.8)	0.47
■ SOFA liver ≥ 3	2 (1.9)	0 (0)	0.56
■ SOFA coagulation ≥ 3	6 (5.7)	3 (5.9)	0.97
■ MODS	53 (34)	22 (14.1)	0.39
Tracheostomy before VAP, n (%)	15 (14.3)	10 (19.6)	0.49
Reintubation before VAP, n (%)	13 (12.4)	4 (7.8)	0.39
RBC transfusion before VAP, n (%)	55 (51.9)	28 (57.1)	0.54
Use of IV antibiotics within 90 days, n (%):	**104 (99)**	47 (92.2)	**0.04**
■ Penicillins	44 (41.9)	16 (31.4)	0.21
■ Cephalosporins	86 (81.9)	39 (76.5)	0.43
■ Fluoroquinolones	21 (20.0)	6 (11.8)	0.20
■ Aminoglycosides	5 (4.8)	1 (2.0)	0.66
■ Carbapenems	**9 (37.1)**	9 (17.6)	**0.02**
■ Antifungal	**16 (15.2)**	1 (2.0)	**0.01**

Table 1. Cont.

Variable	VAP Origin		p Value
	Monobacterial n = 105	Polybacterial * n = 51	
Disease severity on VAP onset, median (IQR):			
▪ SAPS II score	45 (32.5–54.5)	43 (33.0–51.0)	0.40
▪ SOFA score	6 (4–10)	5 (4–8)	0.53
Organ failure on VAP onset, n (%):			
▪ SOFA respiratory ≥ 3	86 (81.9)	35 (68.6)	0.06
▪ SOFA cardiovascular ≥ 3	41 (39.0)	14 (27.5)	0.16
▪ SOFA neurological ≥ 3	12 (11.4)	**15 (29.4)**	**0.01**
▪ SOFA renal ≥ 3	18 (17.1)	6 (11.8)	0.38
▪ SOFA liver ≥ 3	4 (3.8)	0 (0)	0.30
▪ SOFA coagulation ≥ 3	9 (8.6)	2 (3.9)	0.29
▪ MODS	51 (48.6)	17 (33.3)	0.07
Sepsis on VAP onset, n (%)	**93 (88.6)**	39 (76.5)	**0.049**
Septic shock on VAP onset, n (%)	**54 (51.9)**	18 (34.6)	**0.041**
Temperature on VAP onset, n (%):			
▪ <36 °C	13 (12.4)	6 (11.8)	0.91
▪ ≥38.3 °C	48 (45.7)	22 (43.1)	0.76
Oxygenation index on VAP onset, n (%)			
▪ $PaO_2/FiO_2 \leq 300$–>200	19 (18.1)	14 (27.5)	0.18
▪ $PaO_2/FiO_2 \leq 200$–>100	62 (59.0)	34 (64.7)	0.36
▪ $PaO_2/FiO_2 \leq 100$	**24 (22.9)**	3 (5.9)	**<0.01**
Inflammatory markers on VAP onset, median (IQR):			
▪ WBC, cells × 10^9/L	**12.2 (8.7–17.9)**	10.9 (7.3–13.4)	**0.03**
▪ CRP, mg/L	172 (113–241)	172 (119–235)	0.88
Acidosis on VAP onset, metabolic, n (%)	39 (37.1)	17 (33.3)	0.64
RRT during the ICU stay, n (%)	**39 (37.1)**	9 (17.6)	**0.01**

CCI: Charlson comorbidity index; CRP: C-reactive protein; DM: diabetes mellitus; ED: emergency department; ICU: intensive care unit; IQR: interquartile range; IV: intravenous; MDRAB: multidrug-resistant *Acinetobacter baumannii*; MODS: multiple organ dysfunction syndrome; SAPS II: Simplified Acute Physiology Score II; SOFA: Sequential Organ Failure Assessment; RBC: red blood cells; RRT: renal replacement therapy; VAP: ventilator-associated pneumonia; WBC: white blood cells. * polybacterial VAP only due to Gram-negative pathogens; ** Oncology: cancer of a solid organ; *** Obesity: body mass index over 30 kg/m^2.

Table 2. The 30-day mortality of mono- and polybacterial cases of VAP due to MDRAB.

Variable	30-Day Mortality		p Value
	VAP Origin		
	Monobacterial, n/Total (%) **	Polybacterial *, n/Total (%) **	
All sample	60/105 (57.1)	19/51 (37.3)	0.02
Severity on VAP diagnosis			
▪ SOFA < 8	**28/64 (43.8)**	9/35 (25.7)	0.08
▪ SOFA > 7	32/41 (78.0)	10/16 (62.5)	0.23
Appropriateness of antibacterial treatment			
▪ Appropriate	**35/69 (50.7)**	8/34 (23.5)	**<0.01**
▪ Inappropriate	25/36 (69.4)	11/17 (64.7)	0.73

Table 2. Cont.

Variable	30-Day Mortality		p Value
	VAP Origin		
	Monobacterial, n/Total (%) **	Polybacterial *, n/Total (%) **	
Appropriate treatment and severity on VAP diagnosis			
■ SOFA < 8	18/43 (41.9)	4/21 (19.0)	0.07
■ SOFA > 7	**17/26 (65.4)**	4/13 (10.3)	**0.04**
Time of appropriate antibacterial treatment			
■ Early	26/47 (55.3)	6/18 (33.3)	0.11
■ Late	34/58 (58.6)	13/33 (39.4)	0.08
Antibacterial resistance profile of A. baumannii strains			
■ MDR	9/16 (56.3)	3/7 (42.9)	0.68
■ XDR	**51/89 (57.3)**	16/44 (36.4)	**0.02**

ICU: intensive care unit; MDR: multidrug-resistant; SOFA: Sequential Organ Failure Assessment; XDR: extensively drug resistant; VAP: ventilator-associated pneumonia. * polybacterial VAP only due to Gram-negative pathogens; ** n: number of deceased patients in the subgroup/total: total of the respective subgroup.

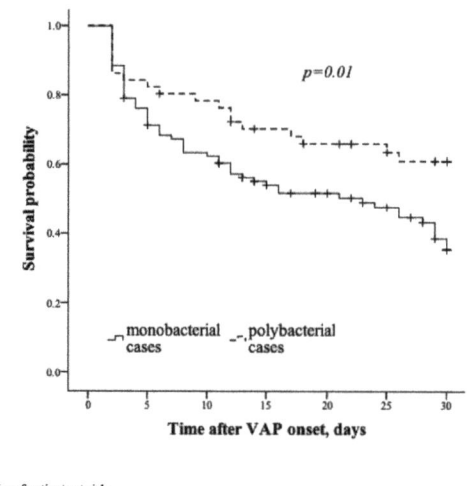

Figure 1. Kaplan–Meier survival curves for time to death in monobacterial vs. polybacterial VAP due to MDR A. baumannii (censored at 30 days).

4. Discussion

The key new finding of this analysis: the 30-day mortality rate in VAP due to MDRAB was higher in monobacterial compared to polybacterial cases. Mortality remained higher or showed the trend to be higher even after adjusting for the impact of disease severity, adequacy of treatment, timeliness of treatment, and the resistance profile of A. baumannii strains. Moreover, mono- and polybacterial cases of VAP had different demographic and clinical characteristics.

Previous studies show high all-cause mortality due to MDRAB VAP, however, it remains unclear whether, and to what degree, the poor outcomes are associated with the case mix, the underlying comorbidities, the multi-organ dysfunction, the pathogenicity and antibiotic resistance of A. baumannii strains, or other factors, such as the presence of co-pathogens in case of polybacterial infection [27–30]. The role of a specific pathogen in the disease course and outcome of polybacterial infections is difficult to be estimated due to possible positive or negative bacterial interactions. Although MDRAB is becoming one of the most common pathogens of VAP in several countries, so far, we have found no study comparing the impact of monobacterial and polybacterial origin of VAP on patient mortality. The current study adds knowledge to the field, demonstrating that the 30-day mortality was statistically significantly higher (57.1% vs. 37.3%) in the group of monobacterial VAP compared to polybacterial cases. Similarly, in the study of Brewer et al. [31] that compared mono- and polybacterial *P. aeruginosa* VAP, there was a trend for higher mortality in monobacterial cases (78.0% vs. 53.0%, $p = 0.15$). In contrast, Combes et al. [32] did not identify any differences in 30-day mortality between mono- and polybacterial VAP cases. Nevertheless, it is difficult to compare these results with ours, as they did not analyze MDRAB cases exclusively, but VAP caused by various pathogens, including Gram-positive ones, without specifying their antimicrobial susceptibility. Furthermore, in the study of Combes et al., *Acinetobacter* species accounted for less than 6% of all pathogens [32].

To assess the possible impact of confounders affecting mortality, we stratified monobacterial and polybacterial VAP cases into subgroups according to the severity of illness, appropriateness, and timeliness of antibacterial treatment, and MDR profile (MDR vs. XDR). When we controlled for the severity of illness (SOFA < 8 vs. SOFA > 7), we noted a trend for increased mortality in both sub-groups of monobacterial VAP cases. Both recent studies of Chang et al. [11] on HAP/VAP, with MDRAB as the most common pathogen, and of the ID-IRI group [9] on *A. baumannii* VAP demonstrated an association between reduced mortality and appropriate treatment. Nonetheless, these studies did not analyze whether this association persisted after assessing pneumonia's mono- vs. polybacterial origin. In our analysis, 30-day mortality was found to be significantly higher in the monobacterial cases, even in the cases with appropriate antibacterial treatment. When comparing the additional impact of both disease severity and appropriateness of treatment, we revealed higher 30-day mortality in monobacterial VAP cases in the sub-group with the more severe disease, while a trend for higher mortality was shown in the lower disease severity sub-group, too ($p = 0.07$). Early appropriate therapy was not associated with mortality differences in mono- vs. polybacterial VAP cases. On the other hand, in delayed appropriate treatment, a trend for increased 30-day mortality in monobacterial VAP cases was identified.

The fact that the monobacterial MDRAB VAP had a worse outcome compared to the polybacterial cases might be explained by possible higher pathogen virulence and, consequently, a worse disease course. There is evidence that the same pathogen in a polybacterial environment might become less virulent compared to a monobacterial setting due to pathogen competition in the process of infection [33–35]. Bacteria can form dynamic polymicrobial communities with complex interactions, either co-operative or competitive [33–35]. Competition between bacteria may be expressed in several ways, including consuming resources to limit the growth of the competitor and even production of intrinsic antimicrobial compounds [33–36]. If *A. baumannii* is the only causative agent of VAP, there is no need for an intraspecies fight, and authentic virulence is revealed. Furthermore, there is evidence in the literature that the co-existence of several pathogens may influence their physiological functions, including their susceptibility to specific antimicrobial agents [33]. Further research is needed to address pending questions regarding the molecular mechanisms behind the interactions between co-existing pathogens in terms of virulence and antimicrobial susceptibility and between co-existing pathogens and host immune responses [35].

Although it has been speculated that bacteria lose their fitness and virulence by gaining antibiotic resistance, several studies that report very high infection-related mortality contrast this speculation [30,36–38]. Almomani et al. [38] had reported mortality of 42.0% in MDRAB VAP, while the reported mortality of Choi et al. [30] in XDR *A. baumannii* VAP was 23.8%. The high mortality of monobacterial MDRAB VAP reported in our study corroborates the data that demonstrate the very aggressive nature of these bacteria.

A rapid spread of resistance of *A. baumannii* strains against most of the widely used antibiotics limits the therapeutic choices and make appropriate treatment challenging.

Although a clear and unanimous consensus on MDRAB VAP treatment is still missing, the current ATS/IDSA hospital-acquired/ventilator-associated (HAP/VAP) guidelines [39] recommend reserving colistin for cases of *A. baumannii* sensitive only to this agent. Polymyxins effectively suppress *A. baumannii* growth in vitro, however, the following factors question their safety and efficacy in clinical use: narrow therapeutic window and only bacteriostatic effect, variable PK/PDs, side effects, and not clearly determined optimal dosage [40,41]. Moreover, strong evidence is missing on whether colistin should be used as monotherapy or in combination. It has been suggested that colistin, combined with other antibiotics, such as carbapenems, leads to better outcomes due to the synergism of the different antibiotic classes [42]. Many clinical studies on MDRAB VAP treatment with colistin or its combinations have been conducted, however, most of them were retrospective and heterogeneous (diverse patient populations, *A. baumannii* phenotypes and genotypes, and different antibiotic combinations), that is why their results cannot be easily compared, generalized, or translated into clinical practice. For instance, Tsioutis et al. [6] and Gu et al. [43] did not find any statistically significant differences in patient groups treated with colistin as monotherapy compared to colistin combinations with tigecycline, carbapenems, aminoglycosides, and trimethoprim/sulfamethoxazole. On the other hand, in the meta-analysis of Wang et al. [40], the mortality trend was shown to be higher in the colistin monotherapy group. A possible explanation for worse outcomes in the colistin monotherapy group could be the phenomenon that some subpopulations of MDRAB strains, which are resistant to colistin, are able to multiply in an environment with a much higher colistin concentration than the minimum inhibitory concentration (MIC) [43,44]. What also might contribute to worse outcomes is the poor colistin penetration into the lung tissue that leads to insufficient concentration in epithelial lining fluid when administered IV in the regular recommended dose. Therefore, it has been suggested to administer colistin, not only by IV, but also by inhalation [45]. It has been hypothesized that an aerosolized route of administration may contribute to a higher local colistin concentration and lower incidence of superinfections and side effects [46]. However, the meta-analyses of Florescu et al. [46] and Gu et al. [43] that compared the treatment efficacy of colistin administered alone IV vs. a combination of IV and inhaled colistin in VAP due to Gram-negative bacilli (GNB), did not reveal any significant differences in 28-day mortality or ICU- and hospital-related mortality, even after controlling for concomitant antibiotic treatment or the dose of IV colistin. Moreover, although the meta-analysis of 16 studies conducted by Valachis et al. [47] showed that a combination treatment of IV antibiotic plus inhaled colistin reduced the infection-related mortality (OR 0.58; 95% CI, 0.34–0.96), it did not show any significant influence on all-cause mortality (OR 0.74, 95% CI, 0.54–1.01). Nonetheless, this meta-analysis included observational cohorts only, and most studies were of low/very low quality of evidence with multiple risks of bias. Another systematic review and meta-analysis of randomized clinical trials restricted to VAP did not confirm the findings of Valachis et al. and, moreover, reported that aerosolized colistin might increase respiratory complications in severely hypoxemic patients [48]. A position paper of the European Society of Clinical Microbiology and Infectious Diseases (ESCMID) [49] recommended against the use of aerosolized antibiotics in addition to IV treatment as standard clinical practice. Among VAP cases caused by resistant pathogens, replacing systemic administration by aerosolization also failed to demonstrate further efficacy but showed reduced nephrotoxicity. In addition, the role of the aerosol device and standardization of administration is a major issue [50].

Treatment of infections due to MDR GNBs using colistin alternatives—sulbactam and tigecycline combinations—has been investigated [7,51,52]. However, most of the studies that compared the outcomes of *A. baumannii* infections treated with colistin vs. other antibiotics did not find any significant differences in mortality [32,35,40,43,45–47,53–55]. On the other hand, a meta-analysis of Jung et al. [7] on critically ill patients with pneumonia due to MDR/XDR *A. baumannii* investigated treatment efficacy with colistin compared to 15 other antibiotic regiments (sulbactam, high sulbactam dose, fosfomycin + IV colistin, high tigecycline dose, and IV + inhaled colistin) and found that a cefoperazone/sulbactam combination ranked higher than IV colistin for reducing all-cause mortality. In summary, these results should be interpreted cautiously, since the studies included not only VAP cases, but other infections, as well, and not all of them were *A. baumannii*-associated. Regarding cefoperazone/sulbactam, specifically, an open-label clinical trial in a patient with MDRAB HAP/VAP suggested that a combined pharmacokinetics/pharmacodynamics (PK/PD) index for both antibiotic agents [%(T > MIC_{cpz} × T > MIC_{sul})] was more appropriate for dose optimization than for a single agent PK/PD index [56]. Due to the limited therapeutic options, minocycline, alone or in combination, has also been used for MDRAB treatment, and a recent systematic review of MDRAB infections (the majority was pneumonia cases) has reported promising results that set the ground for further research [57]. New antibiotics are needed to reinforce the limited armamentarium against MDRAB [58].

The effect of the drug resistance profile of *A. baumannii* strains on mortality remains unclear. A large study by Lakbar et al. [10] that analyzed the association between antibiotic resistance and mortality in ICU-acquired pneumonia found that higher resistance of the causative pathogens increased the risk of death. On the contrary, Paramythiotou et al. [59] did not confirm the link between higher resistance of GNBs as VAP pathogens and increased mortality. The potential differences in the in vitro and in vivo activity of the antimicrobial agents might confound the association between drug resistance profiles and mortality. In our study, a higher resistance profile of *A. baumannii* strains, i.e., XDR, was significantly associated with increased mortality in monobacterial VAP cases. This relationship could be partly explained by the fact that the more resistant the pathogen, the less likely was the administration of appropriate antibacterial treatment.

Bringing novelty to the literature, we also compared the clinical characteristics of mono- and polybacterial MDRAB VAP on ICU admission and VAP onset. On ICU admission, the main findings were the more frequent multiple comorbidities (CCI $\geq$ 3, chronic respiratory disease, and obesity) and prior hospitalization in the monobacterial sub-group, whereas, on VAP onset, the patients with monobacterial MDRAB were in more severe conditions (e.g., leukocytosis, sepsis, septic shock, hypoxemia, and organ dysfunction). Moreover, the use of IV antibiotics, particularly carbapenems and antifungals, within 90-day before VAP onset was strongly associated with the monobacterial cases. The higher frequency of prior carbapenem use might have led to less diversity of bacterial flora in the lower respiratory tract and, thus, to monobacterial MDRAB VAP. The interaction between non-fermentative bacilli in the respiratory tract and yeast has been well documented, particularly for *P. aeruginosa*. Our findings support a close relationship between microbiome and microbiota diversity and the development of monobacterial episodes, with potentially important implications for antimicrobial stewardship. Ferrer et al. [27], in a methodologically quite similar study, also demonstrated that chronic underlying diseases were more prevalent among patients with monobacterial ICU-related pneumonia, but contrary to our study, it was found that hypoxemia and inflammatory response did not differ between mono- and polybacterial cases. However, a direct comparison of our study and the one of Ferrer et al. [27] would be inaccurate since the latter included ICU-related pneumonia cases with various pathogens/resistance profiles (not only Gram-negatives/MDRs). On the other hand, an interesting finding is that neurological impairment (as depicted by higher neurological SOFA) was significantly more frequent in the polybacterial VAP subgroup. Similar to our results, in the very recent study of Natarajan et al. [60], the decreased level of consciousness at the time of intubation (Glasgow Coma Scale < 8) was the single independent predictor of polybacterial VAP. The link between impaired consciousness and polybacterial VAP might be partly attributed to the fact that neurological dysfunction increases the risk of regurgitation and aspiration of polymicrobial-laden oropharyngeal secretion and gastric contents [60–64].

Study Novelties and Limitations

To our knowledge, this is the first study to compare the mortality and the clinical characteristics of the mono- vs. the polybacterial episodes of VAP due to MDRAB. The results of our study indicate the important differences in the clinical characteristics and mortality of monobacterial vs. polybacterial MDRAB VAP. This information, along with the bacterial load (as depicted by quantitative or semi-quantitative cultures), could be taken into consideration when the results of respiratory cultures indicate polybacterial growth and we face the dilemma of whether *A. baumannii* represents a pathogen or an innocent by-stander (colonizer).

Our study also has some limitations. Although the data were collected in ICUs with a variety of case-mix in the country's largest university hospital, it is still a single-center, retrospective study, so the results might not exactly depict the situation in other hospitals in the country, and further research is required before extrapolating them. On the other hand, regional hospitals use to transfer the critically ill patients to the tertiary care ICUs where the study was conducted, that is why we think our findings should represent well the whole country's profile of VAP due to MDRAB. Furthermore, due to the quite limited size of the study cohort, some differences in the mortality of monobacterial in comparison with polybacterial episodes were found only in clinical relevance and did not reach statistical significance. Moreover, due to the limited sample size, neither sub-group analysis of MDRAB strains with different resistance profiles nor sub-group analysis of MDRAB co-infection with different pathogens could be performed. Finally, tracheobronchitis, VAP relapses, or superinfections were not recorded in our database, while the results of the respiratory cultures were not quantitative, facts that might have led to misclassification and under- or over-estimation of VAP.

5. Conclusions

Despite the limitation of being retrospective and single-centered, our study has provided important information on a field that the relevant literature is limited: whether monobacterial MDRAB VAP differs from the polybacterial one in clinical findings and mortality. Although the current study by itself, due to the limitations mentioned already, cannot inform change in practice, it can act as a platform for larger, well-designed, prospective studies that will further explore the difference between mono- and polymicrobial MDRAB VAP and their potential clinical implications, such as, whether—and to which subgroups of patients—the antimicrobial agent(s) could be withheld or discontinued when the results of the respiratory cultures depict polybacterial MDRAB VAP.

Author Contributions: Conceptualization, D.A. and J.R.; investigation D.A. and A.C.; data curation, A.C.; methodology, D.A., A.C. and J.R.; writing, A.C. and A.A.; writing—review and editing, D.A., D.K. and J.R.; visualization, A.C.; supervision, D.A. All authors have read and agreed to the published version of the manuscript.

Funding: This research received no external funding.

Institutional Review Board Statement: The study was conducted in accordance with the Declaration of Helsinki, and approved by Kaunas Regional Biomedical Research Ethics Committee (No. BEC-MF-156 and No. P1-BE-2-13/2016).

Informed Consent Statement: Not applicable.

Data Availability Statement: The data presented in this study are available on request from the corresponding author.

Conflicts of Interest: The authors declare no conflict of interest.

References

1. Rello, J.; Lisboa, T.; Koulenti, D. Respiratory infections in patients undergoing mechanical ventilation. *Lancet Respir. Med.* **2014**, *2*, 764–774. [CrossRef]
2. Kollef, M.; Hamilton, C.W.; Ernst, F.R. Economic impact of ventilator-associated pneumonia in a large matched cohort. *Infect. Control Hosp. Epidemiol.* **2012**, *3*, 250–256. [CrossRef] [PubMed]
3. Papazian, L.; Klompas, M.; Luyt, C.E. Ventilator-associated pneumonia in adults: Narrative review. *Intensive Care Med.* **2020**, *46*, 888–906. [CrossRef] [PubMed]

4. Kharel, S.; Bist, A.; Mishra, S.M. Ventilator-associated pneumonia among ICU patients in WHO Southeast Asian region: A systematic review. *PLoS ONE* **2021**, *16*, e0247832. [CrossRef] [PubMed]
5. Inchai, J.; Pothirat, C.; Bumroongkit, C.; Limsukon, A.; Khositsakulchai, W.; Liwsrisakun, C. Prognostic factors associated with mortality of drug-resistant Acinetobacter baumannii ventilator-associated pneumonia. *J. Intensive Care* **2015**, *3*, 9. [CrossRef] [PubMed]
6. Tsioutis, C.; Kritsotakis, E.I.; Karageorgos, S.A.; Stratakou, S.; Psarologakis, C.; Kokkini, S.; Gikas, A. Clinical epidemiology, treatment and prognostic factors of extensively drug-resistant Acinetobacter baumannii ventilator-associated pneumonia in critically ill patients. *Int. J. Antimicrob. Agents* **2016**, *48*, 492–497. [CrossRef] [PubMed]
7. Jung, S.Y.; Lee, S.H.; Lee, S.Y.; Yang, S.; Noh, H.; Chung, E.K.; Lee, J.I. Antimicrobials for the treatment of drug-resistant Acinetobacter baumannii pneumonia in critically ill patients: A systemic review and Bayesian network meta-analysis. *Crit. Care* **2017**, *21*, 319. [CrossRef]
8. Melsen, W.G.; Rovers, M.M.; Groenwold, R.H.; Bergmans, D.C.; Camus, C.; Bauer, T.T.; Hanisch, E.W.; Klarin, B.; Koeman, M.; Krueger, W.A.; et al. Attributable mortality of ventilator-associated pneumonia: A meta-analysis of individual patient data from randomised prevention studies. *Lancet Infect. Dis.* **2013**, *13*, 665–671. [CrossRef]
9. Erdem, H.; Cag, Y.; Gencer, S.; Uysal, S.; Karakurt, Z.; Harman, R.; Aslan, A.; Mutlu-Yilmaz, E.; Karabay, O.; Uygun, Y.; et al. Treatment of ventilator-associated pneumonia (VAP) caused by Acinetobacter: Results of perspective and multicenter ID-IRI study. *Eur. J. Clin. Microbiol. Infect. Dis.* **2020**, *39*, 45–52. [CrossRef]
10. Lakbar, I.; Medam, S.; Ronfle, R.; Cassir, N.; Delamerre, L.; Hammad, E.; Lopez, A.; Lepape, A.; Machut, A.; Boucekine, M.; et al. REA RAISIN Study Group. Association between mortality and highly antimicrobial-resistant bacteria in intensive care unit-acquired pneumonia. *Sci. Rep.* **2021**, *11*, 16487. [CrossRef]
11. Chang, Y.; Jeon, K.; Lee, S.M.; Cho, Y.J.; Kim, Y.S.; Chong, Y.P.; Hong, S.B. The Distribution of Multidrug-resistant Microorganisms and Treatment Status of Hospital-acquired Pneumonia/Ventilator-associated Pneumonia in Adults Intensive Care Units: A Prospective Cohort Observational Study. *J. Korean Med. Sci.* **2021**, *36*, e251. [CrossRef] [PubMed]
12. Amaral, A.C.K.B.; Holder, M.W. Timing of antimicrobial therapy after identification of ventilator-associated condition is not associated with mortality in patients with ventilator-associated pneumonia: A cohort study. *PLoS ONE* **2014**, *9*, e97575. [CrossRef]
13. Joseph, N.M.; Sistla, S.; Dutta, T.K.; Badhe, A.S.; Rasitha, D.; Parija, S.C. Outcome of ventilator-associated pneumonia: Impact of antibiotic therapy and other factors. *Australas. Med. J.* **2012**, *5*, 135–140. [CrossRef]
14. Nowak, J.; Zander, E.; Stefanik, D.; Higgins, P.G.; Roca, I.; Vila, J.; McConnell, M.J.; Cisneros, J.M.; Seifert, H.; MagicBullet Working Group WP4. High incidence of pandrug-resistant Acinetobacter baumannii isolates collected from patients with ventilator-associated pneumonia in Greece, Italy and Spain as part of the MagicBullet clinical trial. *J. Antimicrob. Chemother.* **2017**, *72*, 3277–3282. [CrossRef] [PubMed]
15. Papathanakos, G.; Andrianopoulos, I.; Papathanasiou, A.; Priavali, E.; Koulenti, D.; Koulouras, V. Colistin-resistant *Acinetobacter baumannii* bacteremia: A serious threat for critically ill patients. *Microorganisms* **2020**, *8*, 287. [CrossRef] [PubMed]
16. Papathanakos, G.; Andrianopoulos, I.; Papathanasiou, A.; Koulenti, D.; Gartzonika, K.; Koulouras, V. Pandrug-resistant Acinetobacter baumannii treatment: Still a debatable topic with no definite solutions. *J. Antimicrob. Chemother.* **2020**, *75*, 3081. [CrossRef]
17. Čiginskienė, A.; Dambrauskienė, A.; Rello, J.; Adukauskienė, D. Ventilator-Associated Pneumonia due to Drug-Resistant *Acinetobacter baumannii*: Risk Factors and Mortality Relation with Resistance Profiles, and Independent Predictors of In-Hospital Mortality. *Medicina* **2019**, *55*, 49. [CrossRef] [PubMed]
18. Karakonstantis, S.; Ioannou, P.; Samonis, G.; Kofteridis, D.P. Systematic Review of Antimicrobial Combination Options for Pandrug-Resistant *Acinetobacter baumannii*. *Antibiotics* **2021**, *10*, 1344. [CrossRef]
19. Kumar, S.; Anwer, R.; Azzi, A. Virulence potential and treatment options of multidrug-resistant (MDR) *Acinetobacter baumannii*. *Microorganisms* **2021**, *9*, 2104. [CrossRef]
20. Rello, J.; Ulldemolins, M.; Lisboa, T.; Koulenti, D.; Mañez, R.; Martin-Loeches, I.; De Waele, J.J.; Putensen, C.; Guven, M.; Deja, M.; et al. EU-VAP/CAP Study Group. Determinants of prescription and choice of empirical therapy for hospital-acquired and ventilator-associated pneumonia. *Eur. Respir. J.* **2011**, *37*, 1332–1339. [CrossRef]
21. Koulenti, D.; Tsigou, E.; Rello, J. Nosocomial pneumonia in 27 ICUs in Europe: Perspectives from the EU-VAP/CAP study. *Eur. J. Clin. Microbiol. Infect. Dis.* **2017**, *36*, 1999–2006. [CrossRef] [PubMed]
22. Xu, E.; Pérez-Torres, D.; Fragkou, P.C.; Zahar, J.R.; Koulenti, D. Nosocomial pneumonia in the era of multidrug-resistance: Updates in diagnosis and management. *Microorganisms* **2021**, *9*, 534. [CrossRef] [PubMed]
23. Guidelines for the management of adults with hospital-acquired, ventilator-associated, and healthcare-associated pneumonia. *Am. J. Respir. Crit. Care Med.* **2005**, *171*, 388–416. [CrossRef] [PubMed]
24. Dellinger, R.F.; Levy, M.M.; Rhodes, A.; Annane, D.; Gerlach, H.; Opal, S.M.; Sevransky, J.E.; Sprung, C.L.; Douglas, I.S.; Jaeschke, R.; et al. Surviving Sepsis Campaign: International guidelines for management of sepsis and septic shock: 2012. *Crit. Care Med.* **2013**, *41*, 580–637. [CrossRef] [PubMed]
25. The European Committee on Antimicrobial Susceptibility Testing. Breakpoint Tables for Interpretation of MICs and Zone Diameters. Version 6.0. 2016. Available online: http://www.eucast.org (accessed on 18 May 2021).

26. Magiorakos, A.P.; Srinivasan, A.; Carey, R.B.; Carmeli, Y.; Falagas, M.E.; Giske, C.G.; Harbarth, S.; Hindler, J.F.; Kahlmeter, G.; Ollson-Liljequist, B.; et al. Multidrug-resistant, extensively drug-resistant and pandrug-resistant bacteria: An international expert proposal for interim standard definitions for acquired resistance. *Clin. Microbiol. Infect.* **2012**, *18*, 268–281. [CrossRef] [PubMed]
27. Ferrer, M.; Difrancesco, L.F.; Liapikou, A.; Rinaudo, M.; Carbonara, M.; Li Bassi, G.; Gabarrus, A.; Torres, A. Polymicrobial intensive care unit-acquired pneumonia: Prevalence, microbiology and outcome. *Crit. Care* **2015**, *19*, 450. [CrossRef]
28. Sarda, C.; Fazal, F.; Rello, J. Management of ventilator-associated pneumonia (VAP) caused by resistant gram-negative bacteria: Which is the best strategy to treat? *Expert Rev. Respir. Med.* **2019**, *13*, 789–798. [CrossRef]
29. Vardakas, K.Z.; Rafailidis, P.I.; Konstantelias, A.A.; Falagas, M.E. Predictors of mortality in patients with infections due to multi-drug resistant Gram negative bacteria: The study, the patient, the bug or the drug? *J. Infect.* **2013**, *66*, 401–414. [CrossRef] [PubMed]
30. Choi, I.S.; Lee, Y.J.; Wi, Y.M.; Kwan, B.S.; Jung, K.H.; Hong, W.P.; Kim, J.M. Predictors of mortality in patients with extensively drug-resistant Acinetobacter baumannii pneumonia receiving colistin therapy. *Int. J. Antimicrob. Agents* **2016**, *48*, 175–180. [CrossRef] [PubMed]
31. Brewer, S.C.; Wunderink, R.G.; Jones, C.B.; Leeper, K.V. Ventilator-associated pneumonia due to Pseudomonas Aeruginosa. *Chest* **1996**, *109*, 1019–1029. [CrossRef] [PubMed]
32. Combes, A.; Figliolini, C.; Trouillet, J.L.; Kassis, N.; Wolff, M.; Gibert, C.; Chastre, J. Incidence and outcomes of polymicrobial ventilator-associated pneumonia. *Chest* **2002**, *121*, 1618–1623. [CrossRef] [PubMed]
33. Lasa, I.; Solano, C. Polymicrobial infections: Do bacteria behave differently depending on their neighbours? *Virulence* **2018**, *9*, 895–897. [CrossRef] [PubMed]
34. García-Pérez, A.N.; de Jong, A.; Junker, S.; Becher, D.; Chlebowicz, M.A.; Duipmans, J.C.; Jonkman, M.F.; van Dijl, J.M. From the wound to the bench: Exoproteome interplay between wound-colonizing Staphylococcus aureus strains and co-existing bacteria. *Virulence* **2018**, *9*, 363–378. [CrossRef]
35. Short, F.L.; Murdoch, S.L.; Ryan, R.P. Polybacterial human disease: The ills of social networking. *Trends Microbiol.* **2014**, *32*, 508–516. [CrossRef] [PubMed]
36. Fields, F.R.; Lee, S.W.; McConnell, M.J. Using bacterial genomes and essential genes for the development of new antibiotics. *Biochem. Pharmacol.* **2017**, *134*, 74–86. [CrossRef]
37. Butler, D.A.; Biagi, M.; Tan, X.; Qasmieh, S.; Bulman, Z.P.; Wenzler, E. Multidrug Resistant Acinetobacter baumannii: Resistance by Any Other Name Would Still be Hard to Treat. *Curr. Infect. Dis. Rep.* **2019**, *21*, 46. [CrossRef]
38. Almomani, B.A.; McCullough, A.; Gharaibeh, R.; Samrah, S.; Mahasneh, F. Incidence and predictors of 14-day mortality in multidrug-resistant Acinetobacter baumannii in ventilator-associated pneumonia. *J. Infect. Dev. Ctries.* **2015**, *9*, 1323–1330. [CrossRef]
39. Kalil, A.C.; Metersky, M.L.; Klompas, M.; Muscedere, J.; Sweeney, D.A.; Palmer, L.B.; Napolitano, L.M.; O'Grady, N.P.; Bartlet, J.; Carratala, J.; et al. Management of Adults With Hospital-acquired and Ventilator-associated Pneumonia: 2016 Clinical Practice Guidelines by the Infectious Diseases Society of America and the American Thoracic Society. *Clin. Infect. Dis.* **2016**, *63*, e61–e111. [CrossRef]
40. Wang, J.; Niu, H.; Wang, R.; Cai, Y. Safety and efficacy of colistin alone or in combination in adults with Acinetobacter baumannii infection: A systematic review and meta-analysis. *Int. J. Antimicrob. Agents* **2019**, *53*, 383–400. [CrossRef]
41. Isler, B.; Doi, Y.; Bonomo, R.A.; Paterson, D.L. New treatment options against carbapenem-resistant Acinetobacter baumannii infections. *Antimicrob. Agents Chemother.* **2019**, *63*, e01110-18. [CrossRef]
42. Gurjar, M. Colistin for lung infection: An update. *J. Intensive Care* **2015**, *3*, 3. [CrossRef] [PubMed]
43. Gu, W.J.; Wang, F.; Tang, L.; Bakker, J.; Liu, J.C. Colistin for the treatment of ventilator-associated pneumonia caused by multidrug-resistant Gram-negative bacteria: A systematic review and meta-analysis. *Int. J. Antimicrob. Agents* **2014**, *44*, 477–485. [CrossRef] [PubMed]
44. Thet, K.T.; Lunha, K.; Srisrattakarn, A.; Lulitanond, A.; Tavichakorntrakool, R.; Kuwatjanakul, W.; Charoensri, N.; Chanawong, A. Colistin heteroresistance in carbapenem-resistant Acinetobacter baumannii isolates from a Thai university hospital. *World. J. Microbiol. Biotechnol.* **2020**, *36*, 102. [CrossRef] [PubMed]
45. Biagi, M.; Butler, D.; Tan, X.; Qasmieh, S.; Wenzler, E. A Breath of Fresh Air in the Fog of Antimicrobial Resistance: Inhaled Polymyxins for Gram-Negative Pneumonia. *Antibiotics* **2019**, *8*, 27. [CrossRef] [PubMed]
46. Florescu, D.F.; Qiu, F.; McCartan, M.A.; Mindru, C.; Fey, P.D.; Kalil, A.C. What is the efficacy and safety of colistin for the treatment of ventilator-associated pneumonia? A systematic review and meta-regression. *Clin. Infect. Dis.* **2012**, *54*, 670–680. [CrossRef] [PubMed]
47. Valachis, A.; Samonis, G.; Kofteridis, D.P. The role of aerosolized colistin in the treatment of ventilator-associated pneumonia: A systematic review and metaanalysis. *Crit. Care Med.* **2015**, *43*, 527–533. [CrossRef]
48. Sole-Lleonart, C.; Rouby, J.J.; Blot, S.; Poulakou, G.; Chastre, J.; Palmer, L.B.; Bassetti, M.; Luyt, C.E.; Pereira, J.M.; Riera, J.; et al. Nebulization of antiinfective agents in invasively mechanically ventilated adults: A systematic review and meta-analysis. *Anesthesiology* **2017**, *126*, 890–908. [CrossRef]
49. Rello, J.; Solé-Lleonart, C.; Rouby, J.J.; Chastre, J.; Blot, S.; Poulakou, G.; Luyt, C.E.; Riera, J.; Palmer, L.B.; Pereira, J.M.; et al. Use of nebulized antimicrobials for the treatment of respiratory infections in invasively mechanically ventilated adults: A position paper from the European Society of Clinical Microbiology and Infectious Diseases. *Clin. Microbiol. Infect.* **2017**, *23*, 629–639. [CrossRef]

50. Rello, J.; Rouby, J.J.; Sole-Lleonart, C.; Chastre, J.; Blot, S.; Luyt, C.E.; Riera, J.; Vos, M.C.; Monsel, A.; Dhanani, J.; et al. Key considerations on nebulization of antimicrobial agents to mechanically ventilated patients. *Clin. Microbiol. Infect.* 2017, 23, 640–646. [CrossRef]
51. Mei, H.; Yang, T.; Wang, J.; Wang, R.; Cai, Y. Efficacy and safety of tigecycline in treatment of pneumonia caused by MDR *Acinetobacter baumannii*: A systematic review and meta-analysis. *J. Antimicrob. Chemother.* 2019, 74, 3423–3431. [CrossRef]
52. Liu, J.; Shu, Y.; Zhu, F.; Feng, B.; Zhang, Z.; Liu, L.; Wang, G. Comparative efficacy and safety of combination therapy with high-dose sulbactam or colistin with additional antibacterial agents for multiple drug-resistant and extensively drug-resistant *Acinetobacter baumannii* infections: A systematic review and network meta-analysis. *J. Glob. Antimicrob. Resist.* 2021, 24, 136–147. [CrossRef] [PubMed]
53. Zalts, R.; Neuberger, A.; Hussein, K.; Raz-Pasteur, A.; Geffen, Y.; Mashiach, T.; Finkelstein, R. Treatment of carbapenem-resistant *Acinetobacter baumannii* ventilator-associated pneumonia: Retrospective comparison between intravenous colistin and intravenous ampicillin-sulbactam. *Am. J. Ther.* 2016, 23, e78–e85. [CrossRef] [PubMed]
54. Cisneros, J.M.; Rosso-Fernández, C.M.; Roca-Oporto, C.; De Pascale, G.; Jiménez-Jorge, S.; Fernández-Hinojosa, E.; Matthaiou, D.K.; Ramírez, P.; Díaz-Miguel, R.O.; Estella, A.; et al. Colistin versus meropenem in the empirical treatment of ventilator-associated pneumonia (Magic Bullet study): An investigator-driven, open-label, randomized, noninferiority controlled trial. *Crit. Care* 2019, 23, 383. [CrossRef] [PubMed]
55. Salloju, V.; Venapally, S.; Putti, N.; Priyanka, A. Safety and effectiveness of colistin compared with non-colistin combinations in the treatment of multi drug resistant bacterial infections. *Int. J. Basic. Clin. Pharmacol.* 2017, 6, 1137. [CrossRef]
56. Zhou, Y.; Zhang, J.; Chen, Y.; Wu, J.; Guo, B.; Wu, X.; Zhang, Y.; Wang, M.; Ya, R.; Huang, H. Combined PK/PD Index May Be a More Appropriate PK/PD Index for Cefoperazone/Sulbactam against *Acinetobacter baumannii* in Patients with Hospital-Acquired Pneumonia. *Antibiotics* 2022, 11, 703. [CrossRef]
57. Fragkou, P.C.; Poulakou, G.; Blizou, A.; Blizou, M.; Rapti, V.; Karageorgopoulos, D.E.; Koulenti, D.; Papadopoulos, A.; Matthaiou, D.K.; Tsiodras, S. The Role of Minocycline in the Treatment of Nosocomial Infections Caused by Multidrug, Extensively Drug and Pandrug Resistant *Acinetobacter baumannii*: A Systematic Review of Clinical Evidence. *Microorganisms* 2019, 7, 159. [CrossRef]
58. Koulenti, D.; Song, A.; Ellingboe, A.; Abdul-Aziz, M.H.; Harris, P.; Gavey, E.; Lipman, J. Infections by multidrug-resistant Gram-negative Bacteria: What's new in our arsenal and what's in the pipeline? *Int. J. Antimicrob. Agents* 2019, 53, 211–224. [CrossRef]
59. Paramythiotou, E.; Routsi, C. Association between infections caused by multidrug-resistant gram-negative bacteria and mortality in critically ill patients. *World. J. Crit. Care Med.* 2016, 5, 111–120. [CrossRef]
60. Natarajan, R.; Ramanathan, V.; Sistla, S. Poor sensorium at the time of intubation predicts polymicrobial ventilator associated pneumonia. *Ther. Clin. Risk Manag.* 2022, 18, 125–133. [CrossRef]
61. Ketter, P.; Yu, J.; Guentzel, M.; May, H.; Gupta, R.; Eppinger, M.; Klose, K.E.; Seshu, J.; Chambers, J.P.; Cap, A.P.; et al. Acinetobacter baumannii gastrointestinal colonization is facilitated by secretory IgA which is reductively dissociated by bacterial thioredoxin A. *MBio* 2018, 9, e01298-18. [CrossRef]
62. Hernandez, G.; Rico, P.; Diaz, E.; Rello, J. Nosocomial lung infections in adult intensive care units. *Microbes Infect.* 2004, 6, 1004–1014. [CrossRef] [PubMed]
63. Mandell, L.; Niederman, M.S. Aspiration pneumonia. *N. Engl. J. Med.* 2019, 380, 651–663. [CrossRef] [PubMed]
64. Marin-Corral, J.; Pascual-Guardia, S.; Amati, F.; Aliberti, S.; Masclans, J.R.; Soni, N.; Rodriguez, A.; Sibila, O.; Sanz, F.; Sotgiu, N.; et al. Aspiration risk factors, microbiology, and empiric antibiotics for patients hospitalized with community-acquired pneumonia. *Chest* 2021, 159, 58–72. [CrossRef] [PubMed]

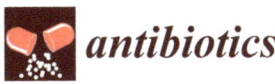

Article

Epidemiology of Candidemia and Fluconazole Resistance in an ICU before and during the COVID-19 Pandemic Era

Christina Routsi [1,*], Joseph Meletiadis [2], Efstratia Charitidou [1], Aikaterini Gkoufa [1], Stelios Kokkoris [1], Stavros Karageorgiou [1], Charalampos Giannopoulos [1], Despoina Koulenti [3], Petros Andrikogiannopoulos [4], Efstathia Perivolioti [4], Athina Argyropoulou [4], Ioannis Vasileiadis [1], Georgia Vrioni [5] and Elizabeth Paramythiotou [3]

1. First Department of Intensive Care, School of Medicine, National and Kapodistrian University of Athens, Evangelismos Hospital, 10676 Athens, Greece; ef.charitidou@gmail.com (E.C.); katergouf@yahoo.gr (A.G.); skokkoris2003@yahoo.gr (S.K.); stavros99k@gmail.com (S.K.); harry.giannopoulos@gmail.com (C.G.); ioannisvmed@yahoo.gr (I.V.)
2. Clinical Microbiology Laboratory, School of Medicine, National and Kapodistrian University of Athens, Attikon University Hospital, 12461 Athens, Greece; jmeletiadis@med.uoa.gr
3. Second Department of Intensive Care, School of Medicine, National and Kapodistrian University of Athens, Attikon University Hospital, 12461 Athens, Greece; d.koulenti@uq.edu.au (D.K.); lparamyth61@hotmail.com (E.P.)
4. Department of Clinical Microbiology, Evangelismos Hospital, 10676 Athens, Greece; velavalton@hotmail.gr (P.A.); perivolioti@yahoo.gr (E.P.); athina.argyropoulou@gmail.com (A.A.)
5. Department of Microbiology, School of Medicine, National and Kapodistrian University of Athens, 11527 Athens, Greece; gvrioni@med.uoa.gr
* Correspondence: chroutsi@med.uoa.gr; Tel.: +30-213204-3314; Fax: +30-213204-3307

Abstract: The objectives of this study were to investigate the incidence of candidemia, as well as the factors associated with *Candida* species distribution and fluconazole resistance, among patients admitted to the intensive care unit (ICU) during the COVID-19 pandemic, as compared to two pre-pandemic periods. All patients admitted to the ICU due to COVID-19 from March 2020 to October 2021, as well as during two pre-pandemic periods (2005–2008 and 2012–2015), who developed candidemia, were included. During the COVID-19 study period, the incidence of candidemia was 10.2%, significantly higher compared with 3.2% and 4.2% in the two pre-pandemic periods, respectively. The proportion of non-*albicans Candida* species increased (from 60.6% to 62.3% and 75.8%, respectively), with a predominance of *C. parapsilosis*. A marked increase in fluconazole resistance (from 31% to 37.7% and 48.4%, respectively) was also observed. Regarding the total patient population with candidemia ($n = 205$), fluconazole resistance was independently associated with ICU length of stay (LOS) before candidemia (OR 1.03; CI: 1.01–1.06, $p = 0.003$), whereas the presence of shock at candidemia onset was associated with *C. albicans* (OR 6.89; CI: 2.2–25, $p = 0.001$), and with fluconazole-susceptible species (OR 0.23; CI: 0.07–0.64, $p = 0.006$). In conclusion, substantial increases in the incidence of candidemia, in non-*albicans Candida* species, and in fluconazole resistance were found in patients admitted to the ICU due to COVID-19, compared to pre-pandemic periods. At candidemia onset, prolonged ICU LOS was associated with fluconazole-resistant and the presence of shock with fluconazole-susceptible species.

Keywords: candidemia; ICU; incidence; epidemiology; *Candida* species; non-*albicans Candida* species; fluconazole resistance; COVID-19; critically ill

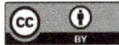

1. Introduction

Coronavirus disease 2019 (COVID-19), caused by the severe acute respiratory syndrome coronavirus 2 (SARS-CoV-2), being declared a pandemic by the World Health Organization on 11 March 2020 [1], spread rapidly around the world, causing a global health emergency [2]. Severe forms are complicated by hypoxemic acute respiratory failure requiring intensive care unit (ICU) admission [3,4]. In these patients, secondary infections, both bacterial and fungal, have been increasingly reported [5–9], resulting in the widespread use of antibiotics for the empirical treatment of suspected as well as of microbiologically confirmed infections, hence contributing to an increase in multidrug-resistant bacteria and fungi and increased costs of care [10].

Regarding fungal infections, a growing number of studies have mainly focused on *Aspergillus* superinfections in mechanically ventilated patients admitted to the ICU due to COVID-19, whereas bloodstream infections due to *Candida* species have been less studied thus far [11–16]. On the other hand, candidemia's incidence, often cited as the fourth most common bloodstream infection in the ICU [17], is increasing, particularly in ICU patients [18,19]. In addition, the epidemiology of candidemia may change over time and can vary significantly across different geographic regions and hospitals. Furthermore, emerging azole resistance displays major challenges for therapeutic strategies [20,21]. Information on the epidemiology of candidemia in the ICU remains limited in the context of the ongoing COVID-19 pandemic. The objectives of the present study were to investigate the incidence of candidemia, as well as the factors associated with *Candida* species distribution and fluconazole resistance, among patients admitted to the intensive care unit (ICU) during the COVID-19 pandemic, as compared to two pre-pandemic periods.

2. Methods

2.1. Study Setting and Design

All patients with SARS-CoV-2 infection confirmed by reverse transcription polymerase chain reaction on nasopharyngeal swabs, and acute respiratory failure, admitted to the COVID-19 ICUs of 'Evangelismos' Hospital, a tertiary-care medical center, from March 2020 to October 2021, who developed candidemia during their ICU stay, constituted the COVID-19 candidemia cohort. Candidemia cases were identified through the electronic system. Approval for the use of the de-identified data was obtained from the ethics committee of the hospital (approval number 116/03-2021). Demographics, dates of hospital and ICU admissions, date of candidemia, detected *Candida* species, admission diagnosis classified as medical or surgical, main co-morbidities including diabetes mellitus and current malignancy, illness severity, length of stay (LOS) in ICU and ICU clinical outcome were recorded. The severity of acute illness was evaluated by the Acute Physiology and Chronic Health Evaluation (APACHE) II score [22] on ICU admission. The severity of organ dysfunction was assessed by the Sequential Organ Failure Assessment (SOFA) score [23], calculated on the first day of ICU admission and, additionally, on the day of candidemia. The difference (Delta) in the SOFA score, defined as the SOFA score on the ICU day that the positive blood culture for *Candida* species was collected minus the SOFA score on ICU admission, was also calculated. For the management and therapy of the ICU patients with COVID-19, international recommendations were followed [24]. For the treatment of candidemia, recommendations for application in non-immunocompromised critically ill patients were followed [25]. Accordingly, after candidemia diagnosis, antifungal treatment, mainly an echinocandin, was given, with the exception of three patients who died because of the severity of their acute illness before blood culture results were available. After the susceptibility results became available, the initial treatment could be modified by the attending intensivists.

Characteristics of COVID-19 patients who developed candidemia were compared with those of two historical candidemia cohorts from our ICU before the COVID-19 pandemic—in particular, an earlier cohort including all ICU patients who developed candidemia from 2005 to 2008 (n = 66) and a later one comprising all ICU patients who developed candidemia from 2012 to 2015 (n = 77).

2.2. Definitions

ICU-acquired candidemia was defined as the presence of at least one positive blood culture for any *Candida* species in the blood specimen collected more than 48 h after ICU admission. Blood cultures were performed in the presence of signs and symptoms of sepsis or when infection was suspected on clinical rounds. The onset of candidemia was defined as the specimen collection date for the positive *Candida* blood culture.

2.3. Species Identification and Antifungal Susceptibility Testing

The BD Bactec (Becton Dickinson, Sparks, MD, USA) automated blood culture system was used for monitoring blood culture bottles. Fungal isolates were identified at species level by using the VitekMS (BioMeriéux, Marcy l'Etoile, France) device and MALDI-TOF MS method. Antifungal susceptibility was evaluated with the Vitek2 (BioMeriéux, Marcy l'Etoile, France) automated system. The phenotypic susceptibility profile for each fungal isolate was interpreted according to the EUCAST standard (European Committee on Antimicrobial Susceptibility Testing Breakpoint tables for interpretation of MICs for antifungal agents, Version 10.0, valid from 4 February 2020). In addition, for the period of March 2020 to October 2021, directly from the signal-positive blood culture vials with yeasts in Gram staining, a multiplex syndromic approach was applied, namely the FilmArray Blood Culture Identification 2 panel (BCID2 assay, BioMeriéux, Marcy l'Etoile, France), for the early detection of the emerging species *Candida auris*.

2.4. Statistical Analysis

Statistical data analysis was performed using the R software, Version 4.1.1 (R Foundation for Statistics, Vienna, Austria). Data are described as mean ± SD or median and interquartile range (IQR) in case of variables with non-normal distribution, and as number and percentage (%) in case of categorical variables. In order to compare the distributions of numerical variables between two groups of patients, we used the two-sample t-test, or, alternatively, the Mann–Whitney U test in case of variables with non-normal distribution, whereas associations between qualitative factors were appropriately investigated via the chi-squared (X^2) statistic or Fisher's exact test. Incidence between the various cohorts was also compared via the statistical test of proportions. Univariate and multivariate binary logistic regression models were built for the determination of risk factors for bloodstream infection with *albicans* versus non-*albicans Candida* species and for potentially fluconazole-resistant species, reporting odds ratios (OR) and corresponding 95% confidence intervals (CI) in relation to the model covariates. The level of statistical significance was set at 0.05.

3. Results

3.1. COVID-19 Candidemia Cohort

In the 18-month study period during the pandemic, among 600 patients who were admitted to the ICU due to COVID-19, 62 patients developed candidemia during the ICU stay, accounting for an incidence of 10.2%. The median [IQR] age of the patients with candidemia was 69 [15.8] years, and 72.4% were males. Admission APACHE II and SOFA scores were 15 [7] and 8 [3], respectively.

The median [IQR] time between hospital and ICU admission and positive *Candida* culture was 28.5 [19.5] days and 22 [18.2] days, respectively. Non-*albicans Candida* species predominated (in 47 out of 62 patients, 77%). Among the non-*albicans* species, the most frequently isolated was *C. parapsilosis* (31 patients, 50%), followed by *C. auris* (9 patients, 14%) and *C. glabrata* (6 patients, 9.7%).

3.2. Comparison between COVID-19 Candidemia Cohort and the Pre-COVID-19 Cohorts

Baseline characteristics of the ICU patients with candidemia development, stratified according to the time period of ICU admission, are presented in Table 1. Compared with patients without COVID-19, patients with COVID-19 were older and had lower illness severity as expressed by APACHE II and SOFA scores on ICU admission. However, on candidemia day, they were more likely to present circulatory shock and they had a higher SOFA score. As a result, the Delta SOFA score was significantly higher in COVID-19 patients than in the non-COVID-19 ones (3 (6) versus 0 (4) and −1 (3.5), respectively, $p < 0.001$).

As expected, patients with COVID-19 were less likely to have a surgical diagnosis on ICU admission. Patients with and without COVID-19 had similar hospital and ICU LOS before candidemia development. While the incidence of candidemia did not change significantly between 2005–2008 and 2012–2015, a significant increase was observed in the COVID-19 cohort compared to the two pre-pandemic cohorts (10.2% (62/600) versus 3.8% (66/1737) and 4.2% (77/1833), respectively, $p < 0.001$). All-cause ICU mortality was 47.8% for *C. albicans* and 59% for non-*albicans* Candida. There were no differences in mortality rates among the three periods; see Table 1.

Table 1. Characteristics of ICU patients with candidemia in the three candidemia cohorts.

Variables	Pre-COVID-19 Cohorts		COVID-19 Cohort	p-Value
	2005–2008 n = 66	2012–2015 n = 77	2019–2021 n = 62	
Age, median (IQR)	67 (21)	63 (31)	69 (15.8)	0.001
males, n (%)	45 (68.1)	46 (59.7)	45 (72.4)	0.27
APACHE II score on ICU admission, median (IQR)	19 (8.8)	20 (10)	15 (7)	<0.001
SOFA score on ICU admission, median (IQR)	9 (4)	10 (5)	8 (3)	0.001
SOFA score on candidemia day, median (IQR)	8.5 (6)	7 (5)	11 (6)	0.001
Delta SOFA score, median (IQR)	0 (4)	−1 (3.5)	3 (6)	<0.001
ICU admission diagnosis Medical, n (%) Surgical, n (%)	22 (33) 44 (66.7)	40 (53.3) 35 (46.7)	62 (100) 0 (0)	<0.001
Co-morbidities Diabetes mellitus, n (%) Current malignancy, n (%)	5 (7.6) 6 (9.1)	3 (3.9) 5 (6.5)	16 (25.8) 5 (8.1)	<0.001 0.99
Hospital stay before candidemia onset, days, median (IQR)	24 (18)	30 (41.8)	28.5 (19.5)	0.15
ICU stay before candidemia onset, days, median (IQR)	15.5 (19.8)	25 (34.5)	22 (18.2)	0.69
ICU length of stay, days, median (IQR)	35.5 (34.5)	49 (51)	34.5 (39.8)	0.029
Presence of shock on candidemia day, n (%)	34 (52.3)	30 (46.1)	45 (75)	0.001
Incidence of candidemia, (%)	3.8	4.2	10.3	<0.001
Mortality, n (%)	42 (63.6)	35 (46.7)	35 (56.5)	0.92

ICU, intensive care unit; IQR, interquartile range; APACHE, Acute Physiology and Chronic Health Evaluation; SOFA, Sequential Organ Failure Assessment; Delta SOFA, SOFA score on candidemia day minus SOFA score on ICU admission.

3.3. Candida Species Distribution and Fluconazole Resistance

The distribution of *Candida* species and the antifungal susceptibility during the three study periods are shown in Table 2. Non-*albicans* Candida species predominated in all cohorts, with *C. parapsilosis* being the most commonly isolated. Considerable differences in *Candida* species distributions were observed over the years. In particular, a gradual decrease in the incidence of *C. albicans* was observed in the COVID-19 pandemic cohort (from 39.4% in 2005–2008 and 37.7% in 2012–2015 to 24.2% in COVID-19 cohort), accompanied by a corresponding increase in non-*albicans* Candida species, including the emergence of *C. auris*; see Figure 1.

During the COVID-19 period, fluconazole resistance occurred in 30 (48.4%) candidemia cases: 2/15 in *C. albicans*, 17/31 in *C. parapsilosis*, 3/6 in *C. glabrata*, 9/9 in *C. auris*; see Table 2. Fluconazole resistance considerably increased over the three time periods, from 31.8% in 2005–2008, to 37.7% in 2012–2015, and to 48.4% in the COVID-19 period, $p = 0.098$; see Table 2 and Figure 1.

Table 2. *Candida* species and fluconazole resistance in the three candidemia cohorts.

	Pre-COVID-19 Cohorts		COVID-19 Cohort	p
	2005–2008 n = 66	2012–2015 n = 77	2020–2021 n = 62	
Candida species				
C. albicans, n (%)	26 (39.4)	29 (37.7)	15 (24.2)	0.069
non-albicans Candida, n (%)	40 (60.6)	48 (62.3)	47 (75.8)	0.069
C. parapsilosis	28 (70)	36 (75)	31 (66)	0.16
C. glabrata	8 (20)	6 (12.5)	5 (10.6)	1
C. tropicalis	2 (5)	3 (6.3)	1 (2)	0.77
C. krusei	0 (0)	1 (2)	0 (0)	1
C. auris	0 (0)	0 (0)	9 (19)	<0.001
other Candida species	2 (5)	2		1
Fluconazole resistance				
Fluconazole-resistant, n (%)	21 (31.8)	29 (37.7)	30/62 (48.4)	0.098
C. albicans	4/26 (15.4)	1/29 (3.4)	2/15 (13.3)	
C. parapsilosis	10/28 (35.7)	20/36 (55.6)	17/31 (48.6)	
C. glabrata	7/8 (87.5)	2/6 (33.3)	2/5 (40)	
C. tropicalis	0/2 (0)	0/3 (0)	0/1 (0)	
C. krusei	NA	1/1 (100)	NA	
C. auris	NA	NA	9/9 (100)	

NA: non-applicable.

Regarding the susceptibility tests for other antifungal agents, we did not observe resistance of the aforementioned *Candida* species to amphotericin B, echinocandins and voriconazole.

3.4. Factors Associated with Non-Albicans Candidemia

Regarding the entire cohort of patients who developed candidemia during the three time periods (n = 205), factors associated with non-*albicans Candida* species, according to univariate and multivariate models, are shown in Table 3.

Table 3. Factors associated with candidemia development due to *Candida albicans* versus non-*albicans Candida* species in the overall study population: univariate and multivariate models. OR (95% CI) takes non-*albicans Candida* as the reference group.

	Patients with Candidemia, n = 205			
	Candida albicans Species, n = 70	Non-*albicans Candida* Species, n = 135	OR (95% CI)	p-Value
Univariate analysis				
Age (years) ‡	63.0 (22.0)	67.0 (21.0)	0.98 (0.97–1.01) [b]	0.19
Gender (Female), n (%)	24 (34.3%)	45 (33.3%)	1.04 (0.56–1.91)	0.89
ICU stay before candidaemia onset, days ‡	15.0 (19.2)	23.0 (24.5)	0.98 (0.9–1.00) [c]	0.08
Hospital stay before candidaemia onset, days ‡	23 (25)	29.5 (24)	0.99 (0.98–1.01) [c]	0.17
Delta SOFA	−0.32 ± 4.07	1.10 ± 4.15	0.91 (0.84–0.98) [d]	0.03

Table 3. Cont.

	Patients with Candidemia, n = 205			
	Candida albicans Species, n = 70	Non-*albicans Candida* Species, n = 135	OR (95% CI)	*p*-Value
ICU length of stay, days ‡	39.0 (36.5)	38.0 (37.0)	0.99 (0.99–1.01) [c]	0.90
Diagnosis (surgical), n (%)	30 (43.5%)	49 (36.6%)	1.33 (0.73–2.41)	0.33
Presence of shock on candidemia day, n (%)	36 (54.5%)	73 (58.9%)	0.83 (0.45–1.53)	0.56
COVID-19	15 (24.2%)	47 (75.8%)	0.51 (0.25–0.98)	**0.049**
Multivariate analysis [a]				
ICU stay before candidemia onset, days			0.97 (0.95–1.00) [c]	0.08
Delta SOFA			0.74 (0.60–0.89) [d]	**0.002**
Presence of shock on candidemia day			6.89 (2.2–25.0)	**0.001**

‡: Median (IQR) for skewed parameters; OR: odds ratio; CI: confidence interval. [a] Significant results adjusted for other variables in the model; [b] per each year increase; [c] per each day increase; [d] per each unit increase; ICU, intensive care unit; SOFA, Sequential Organ Failure Assessment; Delta SOFA, SOFA score on candidemia day minus SOFA score on ICU admission.

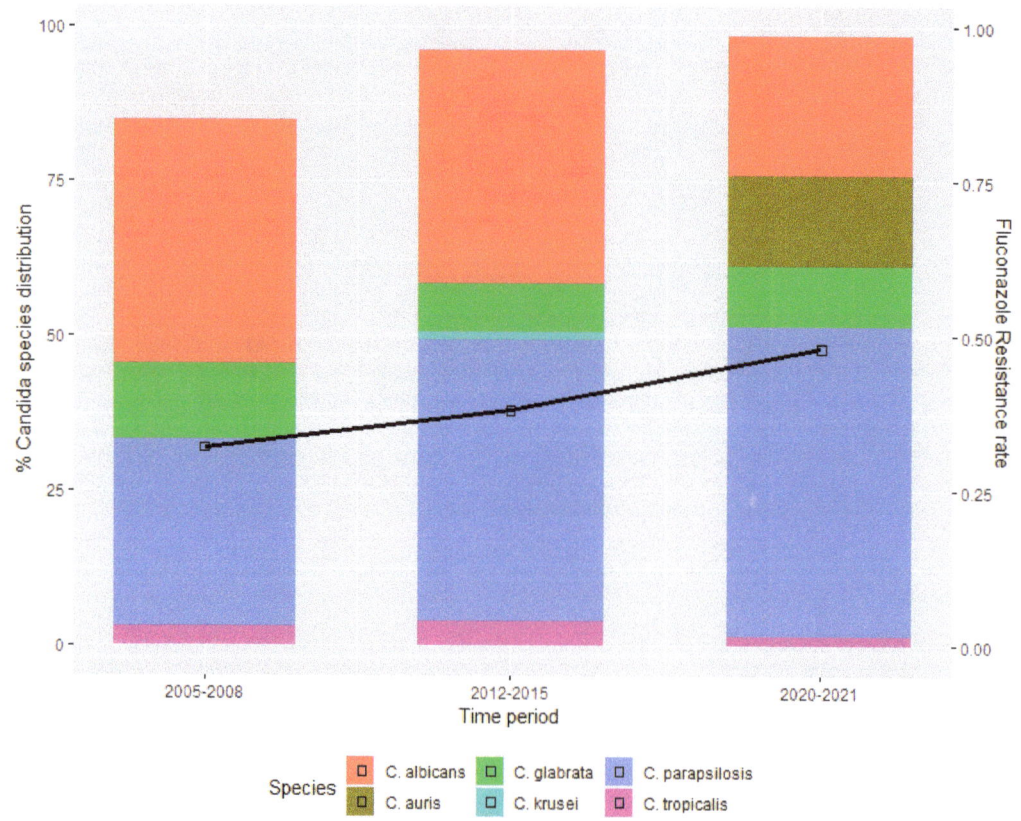

Figure 1. Species distribution of *Candida* bloodstream isolates and fluconazole resistance before and during the COVID-19 pandemic era.

Multivariate logistic regression analysis revealed that an increased SOFA score on candidemia day (compared to that on ICU admission) was independently associated with candidemia due to *Candida albicans*, whereas the presence of shock on candidemia day was independently associated with candidemia due to non-*albicans Candida* species; see Table 3.

3.5. Factors Associated with Fluconazole Resistance

Resistance to fluconazole was significantly associated with non-*albicans Candida* species (54.8% versus 8.6%, in non-*albicans Candida* species and *C. albicans*, respectively, $p < 0.001$); see Figure 2. Factors associated with fluconazole resistance are shown in Table 4. Compared to patients who developed candidemia due to fluconazole-susceptible *Candida* species, patients with fluconazole-resistant strains had longer hospital and ICU LOS before the onset of candidemia (33 (27) versus 23 (22.8) days, $p = 0.03$, and 26 (22.5) versus 16 (21) days, $p = 0.003$, respectively). Multivariate analysis showed that prolonged ICU LOS before candidemia onset was significantly associated with the development of candidemia due to fluconazole-resistant *Candida* species (OR 1.03, CI: 1.01–1.06, $p = 0.003$), whereas the presence of shock at candidemia onset was independently associated with candidemia due to fluconazole-susceptible *Candida* species (OR 0.23, CI: 0.07–0.64, $p = 0.006$); see Table 4.

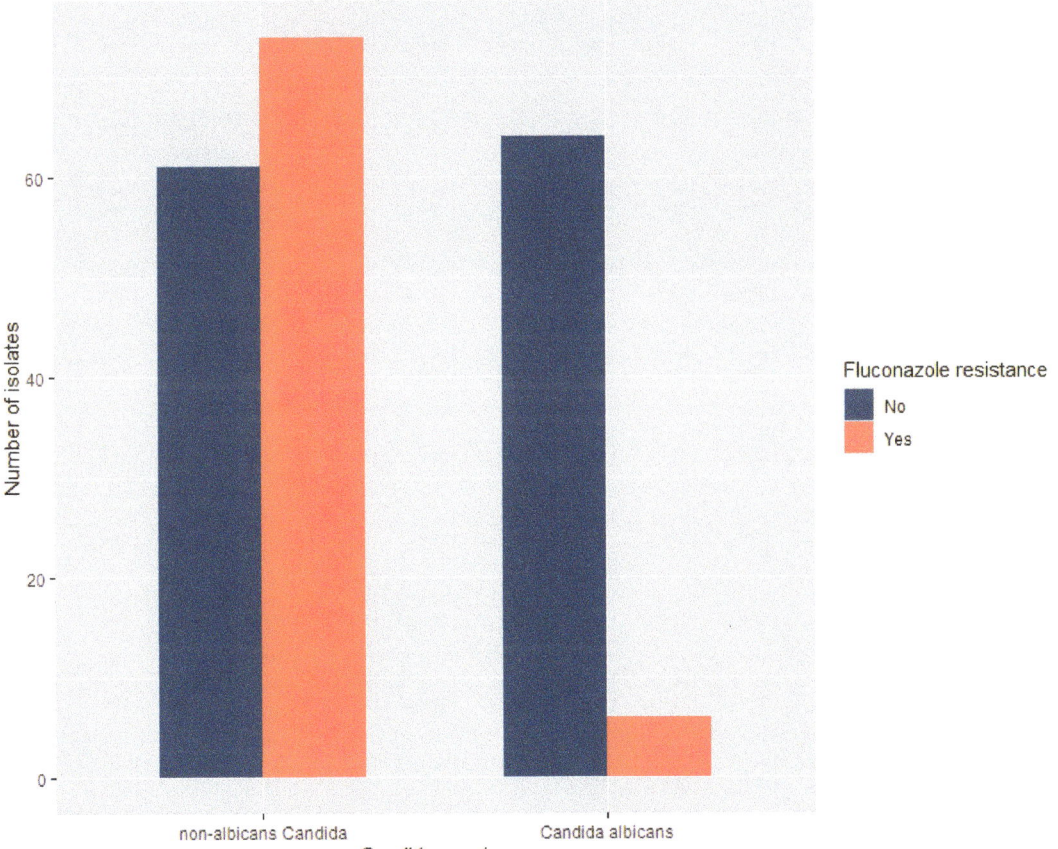

Figure 2. Fluconazole resistance in all ($n = 205$) bloodstream-isolated *Candida albicans* and non-*albicans Candida* species.

Table 4. Factors associated with candidemia development due to fluconazole-resistant *Candida* species in the overall patient population: univariate and multivariate models. OR (95% CI) takes fluconazole-susceptible as the reference group.

	Patients with Candidemia, n = 205			
	Fluconazole-Resistant Species, n = 80	Fluconazole-Susceptible Species, n = 125	OR (95% CI)	p-Value
Univariate analysis				
Age (years) ‡	67.0 (20.8)	65.5 (22.5)	1.01 (0.98–1.03) [b]	0.22
Gender (Female), n (%)	29 (36.2%)	40 (32.0%)	1.20 (0.66–2.17)	0.53
ICU stay before candidemia onset, days ‡	26.0 (22.5)	16 (21.0)	**1.02 (1.01–1.04)** [c]	**0.003**
Hospital stay before candidemia onset, days ‡	33.0 (27.0)	23.0 (22.8)	**1.01 (1.00–1.03)** [c]	**0.03**
Delta SOFA	0.49 ± 4.64	0.68 ± 3.87	0.98 (0.91–1.06) [d]	0.76
ICU length of stay, days ‡	43.0 (48.0)	36.0 (37.0)	1.01 (0.99–1.02) [c]	0.09
Diagnosis (surgical), n (%)	30 (38.0%)	49 (39.5%)	0.93 (0.52–1.66)	0.82
Presence of shock on candidemia day, n (%)	37 (52.9%)	72 (60.0%)	0.74 (0.41–1.35)	0.33
COVID-19	30 (48.4%)	32 (51.6%)	1.74 (0.95–3.20)	0.07
Multivariate analysis [a]				
ICU stay before candidemia onset			1.03 (1.01–1.06)	**0.003**
Presence of shock on candidemia day			0.23 (0.07–0.64)	**0.006**

‡: Median (IQR) for skewed parameters; OR: odds ratio; CI: confidence interval. [a] Significant results adjusted for other variables in the model; [b] per each year increase; [c] per each day increase; [d] compared to Day 0; ICU, intensive care unit; SOFA, Sequential Organ Failure Assessment; Delta SOFA, SOFA score on candidemia day minus SOFA score on ICU admission.

4. Discussion

This study investigated the incidence and epidemiology of candidemia in patients admitted to the ICU due to COVID-19, compared to two previous non-COVID-19 ICU candidemia cohorts. The main findings are the following: (i) candidemia incidence was 10%, more than two-fold higher compared to the pre-pandemic era; (ii) there was an epidemiological shift to non-*albicans Candida* species from 60.6% to 75.8% with a predominance of *C. parapsilosis* and (iii) there was a considerable increase in the rate of fluconazole resistance from 31.8% to 48.4%. In addition, for the whole cohort of patients with candidemia, fluconazole resistance was independently associated with ICU LOS before candidemia onset, whereas fluconazole susceptibility was independently associated with the presence of shock at candidemia onset.

The increase in the incidence of candidemia shown in our study during the ongoing pandemic is striking, though consistent with initial findings from our ICU in the first pandemic wave [8], as well as with findings of other institutions in different geographic regions [6,11,14,16,26–28]. In particular, in studies comparing patients with and without COVID-19, a two-fold increase in the incidence of candidemia in COVID-19 compared to non-COVID-19 patients was observed in two ICUs in India [29], whereas a nearly five-fold increase has been reported in Brazil [16], and a 10-fold rise in another report [27]. Similarly, in another case series from Italy, a higher incidence of candidemia in COVID-19 patients compared with a historical control has been reported [11], though, in the latter two studies, information about patients' hospital location (i.e., ICU or ward) was not reported.

There was no difference in the incidence of candidemia in our ICU between the two pre-pandemic periods. This is in accordance with nationwide data from Germany showing that there was no increase in the ICU-acquired candidemia incidence during the period from 2006 to 2011 [30]. However, an increasing incidence of candidemia has been reported in internal medicine wards in our country, possibly associated with the financial crisis [20]; the present study shows that COVID-19 has further accelerated the phenomenon.

In fact, the above findings are not surprising since critically ill patients with COVID-19 have similar risk factors for candidemia development with the other, non-neutropenic ICU patients and they also received corticosteroid treatment, as recommended after the first pandemic wave [31], which might have been an additional risk factor, as already commented elsewhere [27]. Furthermore, over-occupancy of the ICU, along with the higher workload of healthcare workers and the subsequent relaxation in compliance with the infection control measures, might be additional causes [28].

The increased incidence of non-*albicans Candida* species detected in our study is consistent with comparable data previously reported from our ICU [32] and elsewhere [19], as well as with recent data demonstrating an increasing incidence of candidemia in a nationwide study from Greece, with a species shift towards *C. parapsilosis* [33]. The increased incidence of non-*albicans Candida* species is in accordance with an epidemiological shift across the globe, including the emergence of non-*albicans Candida* species. Indicatively, in a recent study [27], non-*albicans Candida* collectively constituted the majority of isolates in candidemic patients, considering non-COVID-19 and COVID-19 cases together. Similarly, in another study from India during the current pandemic [30], 64% of candidemia cases were due to non-*albicans Candida* species. On the contrary, *C. albicans* remains the predominant pathogen of candidemia in COVID-19 patients in Europe [11,13,34–36], as well as in the pre-pandemic era, according to German data for candidemia in the ICUs [31].

Introduced in the early 1990s, fluconazole is an often-preferred treatment for many systemic *Candida* infections as it is inexpensive and exhibits limited toxicity; it is implicated, however, in the subsequent resistance acquisition due to its extensive use over the years [19,37].

According to our results, concomitantly to the increase in non-*albicans Candida* species, a worrisome increase in the rate of fluconazole resistance was observed, from around 32% in the pre-COVID-19 era to 48% in the COVID-19 period. Although not surprising, since fluconazole resistance is closely associated with non-*albicans Candida* species, such an increase in fluconazole-resistant *Candida* species is of major concern. Notably, among the various isolated species, *C. parapsilosis* presented the highest proportion of resistance of around 50% across all three time periods, with the exception of *C. auris*, which has expected fluconazole resistance as a potential multidrug-resistant yeast. All-cause mortality did not differ significantly among the three study periods.

In our analysis, at candidemia onset, the SOFA score was significantly higher and the presence of shock was more frequent in patients with COVID-19 compared to those in the pre-pandemic periods, indicating an excess severity of the multi-organ dysfunction in those patients, though without a significant increase in mortality.

Interestingly, considering non-COVID-19 and COVID-19 cases together, the results of multivariate analyses revealed that the presence of shock at candidemia onset was independently associated with the isolation of *Candida albicans* and with fluconazole-susceptible species. This is a novel finding, possibly suggesting a more virulent capacity of the *Candida albicans* compared to non-*albicans* species. Although this finding is consistent with recent experimental data [38], it deserves further research.

Certain limitations of the present study should be pointed out. The first is the absence of a contemporaneous group to the COVID-19 pandemic cohort, i.e., critically ill patients admitted to the non-COVID-19 ICUs during the current pandemic; thus, the comparisons have been made with pre-pandemic cohorts. In fact, such a design was not feasible since the majority of our ICU beds were dedicated entirely to the admission of COVID-19 patients. However, thanks to the availability of data from the two historical non-COVID-19 cohorts, the trends in the incidence and epidemiology of candidemia in our ICU have been shown. Secondly, consumption of antifungal drugs, namely fluconazole, at the individual patient level before the onset of candidemia has not been recorded. However, in our ICU, there was no routine prophylactic use of antifungals, as has already been reported [31]; therefore, pre-exposure to fluconazole is less likely to have influenced these results.

Finally, comparisons between patients with and without candidemia during the study periods were not available, since only patients who developed candidemia have been included in the analysis. However, despite the above limitations, the present study highlights the importance for the critical care teams to be aware of the increased incidence of candidemia and of fluconazole resistance in COVID-19 ICU patients, in order to recognize cases early and treat them accordingly, as well as the urgent need to integrate antimicrobial stewardship activities in the pandemic response.

5. Conclusions

In summary, the present study provides temporal trends for candidemia in an ICU setting. The incidence of candidemia was significantly increased during the COVID-19 pandemic compared to previous non-COVID-19 periods. Additionally, a substantial increase in the incidence of non-*albicans Candida* and in fluconazole-resistant species was observed during the COVID-19 era. Prolonged ICU LOS was associated with fluconazole-resistant and the presence of shock with flunonazole-susceptible species. Further study is needed to clarify the reasons for the increased incidence of candidemia and of fluconazole resistance in the COVID-19 ICU patients. Meanwhile, the present findings underscore the urgent need for increased awareness, as well as for the implementation of antimicrobial and antifungal stewardship programs in order to diminish the incidence of candidemia and fluconazole resistance rates.

Author Contributions: Conceptualization and writing, C.R., J.M., E.P. (Elizabeth Paramythiotou) and E.P. (Efstathia Perivolioti); statistical analysis, E.C. and S.K. (Stelios Kokkoris); data collection, C.R., A.G., S.K. (Stavros Karageorgiou), C.G. and D.K.; microbiological data, E.P. (Efstathia Perivolioti), P.A. and A.A.; review and editing, S.K. (Stelios Kokkoris), I.V. and G.V. All authors have read and agreed to the published version of the manuscript.

Funding: This research received no external funding.

Institutional Review Board Statement: The ethics committee of the hospital approved this study (Protocol 116/03-2021).

Informed Consent Statement: Informed consent was waived as the data were anonymized and retrospectively obtained.

Data Availability Statement: Data supporting the results can be provided from the corresponding author on request.

Conflicts of Interest: The authors declare no conflict of interest.

References

1. World Health Organization. Coronavirus Disease 2019 (COVID-19) Situation Report–51. Available online: https://www.who.int/docs/default-source/coronaviruse/situation-reports/20200311-sitrep-51-covid-19.pdf?sfvrsn=1ba62e57_10 (accessed on 30 January 2022).
2. World Health Organization. Coronavirus Disease (COVID-19) Pandemic. 2021. Available online: https://www.who.int/emergencies/diseases/novel-coronavirus-2019?gclid=Cj0KCQiAhs79BRD0ARIsAC6XpaXhxHeN64r7-j5rvv0ZDtNGxNkA0e2EWCAUr8QWWj-qi_PPrXOljroaAjXBEALw_wcB (accessed on 30 January 2022).
3. Grasselli, G.; Greco, M.; Zanella, A.; Albano, G.; Antonelli, M.; Bellani, G.; Bonanomi, E.; Cabrini, L.; Carlesso, E.; Castelli, G.; et al. Risk Factors Associated With Mortality Among Patients With COVID-19 in Intensive Care Units in Lombardy, Italy. *JAMA Intern. Med.* **2020**, *180*, 1345–1355. [CrossRef] [PubMed]
4. Zhou, F.; Yu, T.; Du, R.; Fan, G.; Liu, Y.; Liu, Z.; Xiang, J.; Wang, Y.; Song, B.; Gu, X.; et al. Clinical course and risk factors for mortality of adult inpatients with COVID-19 in Wuhan, China: A retrospective cohort study. *Lancet* **2020**, *395*, 1054–1062. [CrossRef]
5. Giacobbe, D.R.; Battaglini, D.; Ball, L.; Brunetti, I.; Bruzzone, B.; Codda, G.; Crea, F.; De Maria, A.; Dentone, C.; Di Biagio, A.; et al. Bloodstream infections in critically ill patients with COVID-19. *Eur. J. Clin. Investig.* **2020**, *50*, e13319. [CrossRef] [PubMed]
6. Shukla, B.S.; Warde, P.R.; Knott, E.; Arenas, S.; Pronty, D.; Ramirez, D.; Rego, A.; Levy, M.; Zak, M.; Parekh, D.J.; et al. Bloodstream infection risk, incidence, and deaths for hospitalized patients during coronavirus disease pandemic. *Emerg. Infect. Dis.* **2021**, *27*, 2588–2594. [CrossRef] [PubMed]

7. Patel, P.R.; Weiner-Lastinger, L.M.; Dudeck, M.A.; Fike, L.V.; Kuhar, D.T.; Edwards, J.R.; Pollock, D.; Benin, A. Impact of COVID-19 pandemic on central-line-associated bloodstream infections during the early months of 2020, National Healthcare Safety Network. *Infect. Control. Hosp. Epidemiol.* **2021**, *15*, 1–4. [CrossRef] [PubMed]
8. Kokkoris, S.; Papachatzakis, I.; Gavrielatou, E.; Ntaidou, T.; Ischaki, E.; Malachias, S.; Vrettou, C.; Nichlos, C.; Kanavou, A.; Zervakis, D.; et al. ICU-acquired bloodstream infections in critically ill patients with COVID-19. *J. Hosp. Infect.* **2021**, *107*, 95–97. [CrossRef] [PubMed]
9. Cona, A.; Tavelli, A.; Renzelli, A.; Varisco, B.; Bai, F.; Tesoro, D.; Za, A.; Biassoni, C.; Battaglioli, L.; Allegrini, M.; et al. Incidence, risk factors and impact on clinical outcomes of bloodstream infections in patients hospitalised with COVID-19: A prospective cohort study. *Antibiotics* **2021**, *10*, 1031. [CrossRef]
10. Segala, F.V.; Bavaro, D.F.; Di Gennaro, F.; Salvati, F.; Marotta, C.; Saracino, A.; Murri, R.; Fantoni, M. Impact of SARS-CoV-2 Epidemic on Antimicrobial Resistance: A Literature Review. *Viruses* **2021**, *13*, 2110. [CrossRef]
11. Mastrangelo, A.; Germinario, N.; Ferrante, M.; Frangi, C.; Voti, R.L.; Muccini, C.; Ripa1, M.; On behalf of COVID-BioB Study Group. Candidemia in COVID-19 patients: Incidence and characteristics in a prospective cohort compared to historical non-COVID-19 controls. *Clin. Infect. Dis.* **2021**, *73*, e2838–e2839. [CrossRef]
12. Rawson, T.M.; Moore, L.S.P.; Zhu, N.; Ranganathan, N.; Skolimowska, K.; Gilchrist, M.; Satta, G.; Cooke, G.; Holmes, A. Bacterial and fungal co-infection in individuals with coronavirus: A rapid review to support COVID-19 antimicrobial prescribing. *Clin. Infect. Dis.* **2020**, *71*, 2459–2468. [CrossRef]
13. White, P.L.; Dhillon, R.; Cordey, A. A national strategy to diagnose COVID-19 associated invasive fungal disease in the ICU. *Clin. Infect. Dis.* **2021**, *73*, e1634–e1644. [CrossRef] [PubMed]
14. Seagle, E.E.; Jackson, B.R.; Lockhart, S.R.; Georgacopoulos, O.; Nunnally, N.S.; Roland, J.; Barter, D.M.; Johnston, H.L.; Czaja, C.A.; Kayalioglu, H.; et al. The landscape of candidemia during the COVID-19 pandemic. *Clin. Infect. Dis.* **2022**, *74*, 802–811. [CrossRef] [PubMed]
15. Bishburg, E.; Okoh, A.; Nagarakanti, S.R.; Lindner, M.; Migliore, C.; Patel, P. Fungemia in COVID-19 ICU patients, a single medical center experience. *J. Med. Virol.* **2021**, *93*, 2810–2814. [CrossRef] [PubMed]
16. Nucci, M.; Barreiros, G.; Guimaraes, L.F.; Deriquehem, V.A.S.; Castineiras, A.C.; Nouer, S.A. Increased incidence of candidemia in a tertiary care hospital with the COVID-19 pandemic. *Mycoses* **2021**, *64*, 152–156. [CrossRef]
17. Wisplinghoff, H.; Bischoff, T.; Tallent, S.M.; Seifert, H.; Wenzel, R.P.; Edmond, M.B. Nosocomial bloodstream infections in US hospitals: Analysis of 24,179 cases from a prospective nationwide surveillance study. *Clin. Infect. Dis.* **2004**, *39*, 309–317. [CrossRef]
18. Lortholary, O.; Renaudat, C.; Sitbon, K.; Madec, Y.; Denoeud-Ndam, L.; Wolff, M.; Fontanet, A.; Bretagne, S.; Dromer, F.; Dromer, F. Worrisome trends in incidence and mortality of candidemia in intensive care units (Paris area, 2002–2010). *Intensive Care Med.* **2014**, *40*, 1303–1312. [CrossRef]
19. Goemaere, B.; Becker, P.; Van Wijngaerden, E.; Maertens, J.; Spriet, I.; Hendrickx, M.; Lagrou, K. Increasing candidaemia incidence from 2004 to 2015 with a shift in epidemiology in patients preexposed to antifungals. *Mycoses* **2018**, *61*, 127–133. [CrossRef]
20. Siopi, M.; Tarpatzi, A.; Kalogeropoulou, E.; Damianidou, S.; Vasilakopoulou, A.; Vourli, S.; Pournaras, S.; Meletiadis, J. Epidemiological trends of fungemia in Greece with a focus on candidemia during the recent financial crisis: A 10-year survey in a tertiary care academic hospital and review of literature. *Antimicrob. Agents Chemother.* **2020**, *64*, e01516–e01519. [CrossRef]
21. Guinea, J. Global trends in the distribution of *Candida* species causing candidemia. *Clin. Microbiol. Infect.* **2014**, *20*, 5–10. [CrossRef]
22. Knaus, W.; Draper, E.; Wagner, D.P.; Zimmerman, J.E. APACHE II: A severity of disease classification system. *Crit. Care Med.* **1985**, *13*, 818–829. [CrossRef]
23. Vincent, J.L.; de Mendonça, A.; Cantraine, F.; Moreno, R.; Takala, J.; Suter, P.; Sprung, C.; Colardyn, F.; Serge, B. Use of the SOFA score to assess the incidence of organ dysfunction/failure in intensive care units: Results of a multicenter, prospective study. *Crit. Care Med.* **1998**, *26*, 1793–1800. [CrossRef] [PubMed]
24. Alhazzani, W.; Evans, L.; Alshamsi, F.; Møller, M.H.; Ostermann, M.; Prescott, H.C.; Arabi, Y.M.; Loeb, M.; Ng Gong, M.; Fan, E.; et al. Surviving Sepsis Campaign Guidelines on the Management of Adults With Coronavirus Disease 2019 (COVID-19) in the ICU: First Update. *Crit. Care Med.* **2021**, *49*, e219–e234. [CrossRef]
25. Martin-Loeches, I.; Antonelli, M.; Cuenca-Estrella, M.; Dimopoulos, G.; Einav, S.; De Waele, J.; Garnacho-Montero, J.; Kanj, S.S.; Machado, F.R.; Montravers, P.; et al. ESICM/ESCMID task force on practical management of invasive candidiasis in critically ill patients. *Intensive Care Med.* **2019**, *45*, 789–805. [CrossRef] [PubMed]
26. Macauley, P.; Epelbaum, O. Epidemiology and mycology of Candidaemia in non-oncological medical intensive care unit patients in a tertiary center in the United States: Overall analysis and comparison between non-COVID-19 and COVID-19 cases. *Mycoses* **2021**, *64*, 634–640. [CrossRef] [PubMed]
27. Riche, C.V.W.; Cassol, R.; Pasqualotto, A.C. Is the frequency of candidemia increasing in COVID-19 patients receiving corticosteroids? *J. Fungi* **2020**, *6*, 286. [CrossRef]
28. Mulet Bayona, J.V.; Tormo Palop, N.; Salvador García, C.; Fuster Escrivá, B.; Chanzá Aviñó, M.; Ortega García, P.; Gimeno Cardona, C. Impact of the SARS-CoV-2 pandemic in candidaemia, invasive aspergillosis and antifungal consumption in a tertiary hospital. *J. Fungi* **2021**, *7*, 440. [CrossRef]

29. Rajni, E.; Singh, A.; Tarai, B.; Jain, K.; Shankar, R.; Pawar, K.; Mamoria, V.; Chowdhary, A. A high frequency of Candida auris blood stream infections in Coronavirus disease 2019 patients admitted to intensive care units, Northwestern India: A Case Control Study. *Open Forum Infect. Dis.* **2021**, *8*, ofab452. [CrossRef]
30. Meyer, E.; Geffers, C.; Gastmeier, P.; Schwab, F. No increase in primary nosocomial candidemia in 682 German intensive care units during 2006 to 2011. *Eurosurveillance* **2013**, *18*, 20505. Available online: http://www.eurosurveillance.org/ViewArticle.aspx?ArticleId=20505 (accessed on 30 January 2022). [CrossRef]
31. The Recovery Collaborative Group. Dexamethazone in hospitalized patients with COVID-19. *N. Engl. J. Med.* **2021**, *384*, 693–704. [CrossRef]
32. Pratikaki, M.; Platsouka, E.; Sotiropoulou, C.; Douka, E.; Paramythiotou, E.; Kaltsas, P.; Kotanidou, A.; Paniara, O.; Roussos, C.; Routsi, C. Epidemiology, risk factors for and outcome of candidaemia among non-neutropenic patients in a Greek intensive care unit. *Mycoses* **2011**, *54*, 154–161. [CrossRef]
33. Mamali, V.; Siopi, M.; Charpantidis, S.; Samonis, G.; Tsakris, A.; Vrioni, G. On Behalf of the Candi-Candi network.increasing incidence and shifting epidemiology of candidemia in Greece: Results from the first nationwide 10-year survey. *J. Fungi* **2022**, *8*, 116. [CrossRef] [PubMed]
34. Hughes, S.; Troise, O.; Donaldson, H.; Mughal, N.; Moore, L.S.P. Bacterial and fungal coinfection among hospitalized patients with COVID-19: A retrospective cohort study in a UK secondary-care setting. *Clin. Microbiol. Infect.* **2020**, *26*, 1395–1399. [CrossRef] [PubMed]
35. Bardi, T.; Pintado, V.; Gomez-Rojo, M.; Escudero-Sanchez, R.; Azzam Lopez, A.; Diez-Remesal, Y.; Castro, N.M.; Ruiz-Garbajosa, P.; Pestaña, D. Nosocomial infections associated to COVID-19 in the intensive care unit: Clinical characteristics and outcome. *Eur. J. Clin. Microbiol. Infect. Dis.* **2021**, *40*, 495–502. [CrossRef] [PubMed]
36. Agrifoglio, A.; Cachafeiro, L.; Figueira, J.C.; Añón, J.M.; de Lorenzo, A.G. Critically ill patients with COVID-19 and candidaemia: We must keep this in mind. *J. Mycol. Med.* **2020**, *30*, 10101. [CrossRef]
37. Berrouane, Y.F.; Herwaldt, L.A.; Pfaller, M.A. Trends in antifungal use and epidemiology of nosocomial yeast infections in a university hospital. *J. Clin. Microbiol.* **1999**, *37*, 531–537. [CrossRef] [PubMed]
38. Hirayama, T.; Miyazaki, T.; Ito, Y.; Wakayama, M.; Shibuya, K.; Yamashita, K.; Takazono, T.; Saijo, T.; Shimamura, S.; Yamamoto, K.; et al. Virulence assessment of six major pathogenic Candida species in the mouse model of invasive candidiasis caused by fungal translocation. *Sci. Rep.* **2020**, *10*, 3814. [CrossRef] [PubMed]

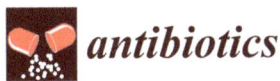

Article

ICU-Associated Gram-Negative Bloodstream Infection: Risk Factors Affecting the Outcome Following the Emergence of Colistin-Resistant Isolates in a Regional Greek Hospital

Marios Karvouniaris [1,*], Garyphallia Poulakou [2], Konstantinos Tsiakos [2], Maria Chatzimichail [3], Panagiotis Papamichalis [3], Anna Katsiaflaka [4], Katerina Oikonomou [3], Antonios Katsioulis [5], Eleni Palli [6] and Apostolos Komnos [3]

[1] Intensive Care Unit, AHEPA University Hospital, 54636 Thessaloniki, Greece
[2] Third Department of Internal Medicine, School of Medicine, Sotiria General Hospital, National and Kapodistrian University, 11527 Athens, Greece; gpoulakou@gmail.com (G.P.); konstantinostsiakos@gmail.com (K.T.)
[3] Intensive Care Unit, General Hospital of Larissa, 41221 Larissa, Greece; hatzimihail_m@yahoo.gr (M.C.); ppapanih@uth.gr (P.P.); kgoikonomou@hotmail.com (K.O.); komnosapo@gmail.com (A.K.)
[4] Department of Microbiology, General Hospital of Larissa, 41221 Larissa, Greece; akatsaf@med.uth.gr
[5] School of Nursing, University of Thessaly, 41500 Larissa, Greece; akatsioul@med.uth.gr
[6] Intensive Care Unit, General University Hospital of Larissa, 41110 Larissa, Greece; kimnef@yahoo.gr
* Correspondence: karvmarevg@hotmail.com; Tel.: +30-697-2994869

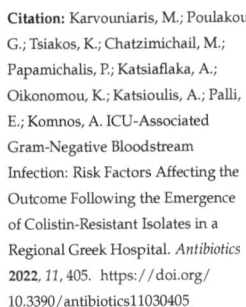

Citation: Karvouniaris, M.; Poulakou, G.; Tsiakos, K.; Chatzimichail, M.; Papamichalis, P.; Katsiaflaka, A.; Oikonomou, K.; Katsioulis, A.; Palli, E.; Komnos, A. ICU-Associated Gram-Negative Bloodstream Infection: Risk Factors Affecting the Outcome Following the Emergence of Colistin-Resistant Isolates in a Regional Greek Hospital. *Antibiotics* 2022, 11, 405. https://doi.org/10.3390/antibiotics11030405

Academic Editors: Elizabeth Paramythiotou, Christina Routsi and Antoine Andremont

Received: 17 February 2022
Accepted: 15 March 2022
Published: 17 March 2022

Publisher's Note: MDPI stays neutral with regard to jurisdictional claims in published maps and institutional affiliations.

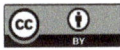

Copyright: © 2022 by the authors. Licensee MDPI, Basel, Switzerland. This article is an open access article distributed under the terms and conditions of the Creative Commons Attribution (CC BY) license (https://creativecommons.org/licenses/by/4.0/).

Abstract: Intensive care unit patients may present infections by difficult-to-treat-resistant Gram-negative microorganisms. Colistin resurfaced as a last resort antibiotic for the treatment of multi-drug-resistant Gram-negative bacteria. However, colistin might not improve survival, particularly after the emergence of colistin-resistant isolates. We aimed to (1) examine the first Gram-negative-associated-bloodstream infection (GN-BSI) effect on 28-day mortality and (2) distinguish mortality risk factors. From 1 January 2018 to 31 December 2019, we retrospectively studied all adult patients admitted for more than 48 h in the critical care department of a regional Greek hospital, with prevalent difficult-to-treat Gram-negative pathogens. We examined the patient records for the first GN-BSI. The local laboratory used broth microdilution to evaluate bacterial susceptibility to colistin. Seventy-eight patients fulfilled the entry criteria: adult and first GN-BSI. They developed GN-BSI on day 10 (6–18), while the overall mortality was 26.9%. Thirty-two and 46 individuals comprised the respective colistin-resistant and colistin-sensitive groups. The admission Acute Physiology Assessment and Chronic Health Evaluation II score was associated with acquiring colistin-resistant GN-BSI in the multivariable logistic regression analysis (odds ratio (CI), 1.11 (1.03–1.21)). Regarding mortality, the index day sequential organ failure assessment score was solely associated with the outcome (hazard-ratio (CI), 1.23 (1.03–1.48), Cox proportional hazard analysis). GN-BSI was often caused by colistin-resistant bacteria. Concerning our data, sepsis severity was the independent predictor of mortality regardless of the colistin-resistance phenotype or empirical colistin treatment.

Keywords: APACHE II score; bacteremia; bloodstream infection; broth microdilution; colistin; colistin-resistant; Gram-negative; intensive care unit; mortality; SOFA score

1. Introduction

Intensive care unit patients are predisposed to bacterial infection, as they are exposed to invasive devices and the critical illness might impair their immune response. A large worldwide point prevalence study of infections in the intensive care unit (ICU) found that 15.1% of the infected patients had bacteremia [1]. Another multicenter study highlighted that multi-drug-resistant Gram-negative (MDR-GN) bacteria are responsible for most bacteremic episodes and are associated with increased mortality [2]. Polymyxin E (colistin) is a drug of last resort to deal with these difficult-to-treat, often carbapenem-resistant, microorganisms [3]. Colistin is a polycationic peptide that disrupts the bacterial cell by binding to its anionic lipid A (endotoxin) part of the outer lipopolysaccharide membrane. The drug also possesses in vivo anti-endotoxin activity, and free radical generation through its passage via the outer bacterial membrane [4,5].

However, empirical colistin treatment may fail to demonstrate efficacy against carbapenem-resistant bacteria [6,7]. Meanwhile, acquired resistance to this drug has spread globally, following its increased use in agriculture and medicine. Bacteria present various genetic determinants of colistin resistance, either chromosomal or plasmid-related. Notably, the latter, transferrable plasmid-mediated resistance genes, can spread fast through the food chain. At the time being, their expanding list requires vigilant epidemiological surveillance [8]. Regarding resistance mechanisms, modification of the lipid A component of the outer bacterial membrane, via the chromosomal modulation of PmrAB and PhoPQ two-component systems, can lead to a decreased negative membrane charge, and, thus, to lower detergent action of the drug [4,5]. Moreover, bacteria may shed capsular polysaccharides that bind to colistin and decrease its availability to interact with the membrane molecules or may possess efflux pumps [4,5,9]. The increasing colistin-resistance prevalence can be particularly challenging in countries with an overall heavy MDR burden, infection control challenges, and submarginal antimicrobial stewardship [10]. Additionally, heteroresistance to colistin, i.e., a resistant subpopulation that co-exists as part of an otherwise sensitive population, may not allow the correct classification of the MDR-GN bacteria, regarding colistin susceptibility status [4]. Finally, the clinical interpretation of colistin resistance has been jeopardized by methodological issues on susceptibility testing. The European Committee On Antimicrobial Susceptibility Testing (EUCAST) recently issued guidelines (second version) for the detection of resistance mechanisms; the document advises laboratories to invariably use broth microdilution in the process of distinguishing colistin-resistant microorganisms to avoid major errors in the interpretation of susceptibility [11].

Although bloodstream infections (BSI) occur less often than lower respiratory tract infections [1], the isolation of a microorganism in a blood sample is solid evidence of infection compared to an isolate recovered from the tracheal secretions, which may represent colonization [12].

We aimed to explore the impact of a first episode of GN bacteremia on the primary outcome of 28-day all-cause mortality and other secondary endpoints. Additionally, we aimed to identify risk factors for (1) a colistin-resistant (CR) bacteremic episode and (2) 28-day mortality in an area of prevalent and endemic multi-drug resistance, after the adoption of EUCAST recommendations concerning colistin's susceptibility testing.

2. Materials and Methods

Our current study results were presented in part at the 40th International Symposium on Intensive Care and Emergency Medicine.

2.1. Study Design, Setting, and Selection Criteria

The study setting was a 16-bed mixed ICU in a regional hospital with 400 admissions per year. It is one of the largest ICUs in central Greece, an area populated by one million people.

From 1 January 2018 to 31 December 2019, all adult patients with an ICU stay >48 h had their data retrospectively examined for the presence of a GN-BSI.

The infection control policy comprises a hand hygiene protocol and widely recommended bundles concerning ventilator-associated pneumonia and catheter-related BSI prevention [13,14]. More specifically, to prevent CVC-related BSI, the bundle included the following measures: (1) meticulous hand hygiene, (2) insertion of CVC through echocardiographic guidance and with full-barrier precautions, (3) skin disinfection with chlorhexidine, (4) avoiding the femoral vein as a CVC placement site, and (5) disposal of nonessential CVCs. Whenever the CVC catheter had remained in place for more than 48 h and there was a suspicion of infection without an evident focus, it was removed.

The protocol for culturing includes: (1) avoidance of routine culturing, (2) culturing whenever there is a suspicion of infection or sepsis, (3) at a minimum, we draw two sets of blood cultures, one from the central venous catheter if present and the other through venipuncture, (4) a single positive blood culture suffices for the diagnosis of GN-BSI, (5) the CVC tip is cultured after its withdrawal, and (6) routine lower respiratory tract culturing is performed through endotracheal aspirate sampling, to validate infection or once weekly for surveillance reasons.

Regarding colistin administration, the individuals with normal renal function received 4.5 million units twice daily; otherwise, the dose was modified accordingly [15]. Patients in need of continuous renal replacement therapy were given a higher colistin dose of 6 million units bis in die [15].

This hospital's microbiology department had adopted broth microdilution for colistin susceptibility assessment since October 2017 [16].

The patients enrolled in this study fulfilled the following criteria: adult, first bloodstream infection due to a GN pathogen. We excluded non-bacteremic patients, individuals with Gram-positive or fungal BSI, and those with an incomplete data file.

The handling of individual patient data followed the Declaration of Helsinki and the current Health Insurance Portability and Accountability Act regulations [17]. No informed consent was required, as we used anonymized hospital data. We reported our results based on the Statement on Strengthening the Reporting of Observational Studies in Epidemiology [18]. The ethics committee of the hospital approved this study (Protocol 187/4-11-2019).

2.2. Variables

Variables of interest on admission were: age, sex, Charlson Comorbidity Index [19], prior ICU stay during the previous 12 months, medical or surgical admission category, infectious disease status, presence o-immunosuppression, and receipt of antibiotic therapy in the last three months. Moreover, we evaluated the clinical severity on the day of admission with the Acute Physiology Chronic Health Evaluation II score (APACHE II) and the Sequential Organ Failure Assessment (SOFA) score [20,21]. Before the event, we reported the CVC status (CVC for at least 48 h) and antibiotic treatment with activity against Gram-negative bacteria. We documented the day of the BSI event, its timing (<48 h or $\geq$48 h from admission), the bacteremia source, and whether it was controlled within 24 h following the episode. Finally, on the index day, we recorded the Pitt bacteremia score and the fever or hypothermia status [22]. We assessed the severity of the index event with the SOFA score every 48 h from day 2 before the event until day 10 after the episode. We also recorded the maximum body temperature, white blood cell count, C-reactive protein, and procalcitonin at the aforementioned 48 h intervals.

2.3. Definitions

We defined GN-BSI whenever there was a positive blood culture for a GN microorganism, and the patient presented clinical and laboratory indices of infection. Index day was the day of collecting the first positive blood culture (index culture) that recovered a GN isolate. ICU-associated GN-BSI was further defined as the first bacteremic episode under two circumstances: (1) When the index culture was collected after two days in the ICU [23]; (2) We also included earlier onset events if the patients had been treated in an ICU during the previous year, as they likely continued to carry bacteria having similar resistance profiles [24]. In the case of a prior ICU stay, the patient should have been discharged from the ICU at least one month before the current readmission to be considered a first bacteremia event. Therefore, it was less likely to misclassify a bacteremia recurrence as a first event. We defined recurrent bacteremia, sepsis, and septic shock accordingly [25,26]. We examined only the first GN bloodstream infection.

The local laboratory categorized the bacteria isolated for susceptibility according to EUCAST criteria (version 7.0; 2017, EUCAST) [16]. Colistin-resistance was considered a minimal inhibitory concentration higher than 2 ng/mL, in line with EUCAST reports [16]. In the case of a polymicrobial BSI, we considered an event as colistin-resistant if at least one GN isolate was resistant to the drug. A minimal inhibitory concentration $\geq$8 ng/mL defined carbapenem (meropenem) resistance according to the EUCAST clinical breakpoints [16].

Primary BSI, source control, and CVC-related BSI have been defined accordingly [27,28]. The empirical treatment delivered to an infected patient was considered appropriate if the drug(s) was (were) active in vitro to the isolate (or both isolates, if present) [29]. We defined immunosuppression in keeping with predefined criteria [21]. Renal failure was characterized as risk, injury, failure, loss, and end-stage kidney disease (RIFLE) stage $\geq$3 (with a 3-fold rise in the serum creatinine, urine volume less than 0.3 mL/kg/h for 24 h, or no urine output for 12 h, or the use of renal replacement treatment) [30].

2.4. Outcome

The primary study outcome was 28-day mortality after the event. Secondary outcomes were 14-day mortality post-event, overall ICU mortality, hospital mortality, ICU stay post-event, overall ICU stay. More secondary outcomes included recurrent bacteremia, secondary bacteremia, mechanical ventilation days post-event, overall mechanical ventilation days, renal failure-free days, renal SOFA at 7 and 14 days, and continuous renal replacement therapy at 7 and 14 days following the index day.

2.5. Statistical Analysis

We used the median with interquartile range (IQR) and number with percentage (%) to describe quantitative data and qualitative data, where appropriate. Fisher's exact (or Chi-squared test) and Mann–Whitney test (or t-test) were used to compare qualitative and quantitative variables. Statistical significance was set at a p-value of <0.05.

Missing data, concerning only laboratory values, were handled in keeping with a reported algorithm [31]. Specifically, we imputed missing numerical values with the respective median if the percentage of not-available numbers was <10%. However, we added the values derived from multivariate imputation, with the predictive mean matching method, if the total non-available variable values were less than 50%. Otherwise, we excluded the variables implicated.

The longitudinal variables were analyzed by comparing their means with the Tukey test and the alternative method "less".

Regarding multivariable regression analyses [32], at first, we considered the clinical value of a variable before its inclusion into the model, regardless of the univariate comparison. Despite any significant difference, we have not included variables that did not convey unique information in the models assessed (i.e., immunosuppression status is included in the APACHE II score, the index day temperature is part of the Pitt bacteremia score, and event day septic shock status adds 4 points to the index day SOFA score). Secondly, we included any variable presenting a p-value of $\leq$0.10. Finally, we tested multicollinearity using a variance inflation factor score before inserting any variables in the model.

Overall, the optimal cutoffs of quantitative explanatory variables were assessed with the Youden criterion.

We performed multivariable logistic regression analysis to evaluate risk factors for developing colistin-resistant BSI. The initial full model for CR phenotype was comprised of age, admission due to infection, Charlson Comorbidity Index, and the APACHE II and SOFA scores on admission. The final model was selected in a backward, stepwise method following a bootstrap resampling of the original data. The derived variables then entered the final model.

Regarding 28-day mortality, we used Kaplan–Meier survival analysis and log-rank test to assess the association between colistin susceptibility and mortality [33]. We also performed Cox proportional hazard analysis to evaluate time to 28-day mortality [33]. The initial, full model included age, Charlson Comorbidity Index, APACHE II, Pitt Bacteremia score, index day SOFA score, CR status, and empirical receipt of colistin for 5 days. The full model variables were examined for violation of proportionality assumption via the global Schoenfeld test and the visual inspection of the covariate Cox model plots. Any violating variable was used as a stratification variable. Afterward, the qualifying variables were regularized by the Least Absolute Shrinkage and Selection Operator to select the explanatory variables of the final model. Finally, the discriminative power of the final Cox proportional hazard model was evaluated with the concordance index.

We also conducted three more statistical sensitivity studies: (1) regarding a threshold of colistin sensitivity at a minimal inhibitory concentration of 0.5 ng/mL instead of the recommended 2 ng/mL, (2) data were reanalyzed after exclusion of eleven patients who presented early BSI, before a 48 h stay in the ICU, and (3) finally, dividing the patients into two groups by the median SOFA score at the index day (the sicker group had a score ≥ 7).

We analyzed data with R version 4.0.3 (R Core Team, Vienna, Austria) [34].

3. Results

3.1. Population

During the study period (Figure 1, flowchart), seventy-eight patients fulfilled the entry criteria: eleven (14.1%) received BSI diagnosis during the first two days of admission and the rest afterward. The colistin-resistant (CRG) and the colistin-sensitive groups (CSG) comprised thirty-two and forty-six patients, respectively. The baseline patient characteristics are shown in Table 1. Notably, most patients had received antibiotics in the three months before the admission, and a third had been treated in an ICU during the previous year. Before the event, 80% of the study participants had had a CVC in place and had received antibiotics.

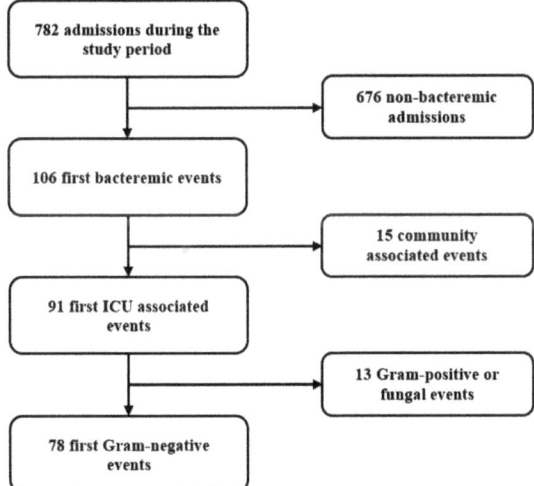

Figure 1. Study flowchart.

3.2. Infection

Bloodstream infection occurred on day 10 (IQR 6–18), and it was most often primary or related to intravascular catheter use (Table 1). Most isolates (73.1%) were carbapenem-resistant. Eight episodes were polymicrobial (including two GN isolates). The culprit isolates differed between groups; of note, the CRG included pathogens endogenously resistant to colistin (*Serratia* and *Providencia* spp.), and no *Pseudomonas* isolates, in contrast to the CSG (Table 2).

Table 1. Patient characteristics on admission, before the bloodstream infection, and on the day of the event.

	Overall (n = 78)	Colistin-Resistant (n = 32)	Colistin-Sensitive (n = 46)	p-Value **	Odds Ratio (95% CI) ##
On admission					
Age, years	66 (50.2–76)	72 (59–78)	62.5 (47.7–74.5)	0.07	
Male	51 (65.4)	22 (68.7)	29 (63)	0.64	
Charlson Comorbidity Index	3 (1–5)	4 (2–5)	2.5 (1–5)	0.25	
APACHE II	19 (13–24)	21.5 (15.2–25)	17.5 (10.7–21)	**0.01**	1.11 (1.03–1.21)
SOFA score	8 (5–10)	9 (6.2–10)	7 (3.5–10.5)	0.15	
Prior ICU stay, previous year	27 (34.6)	12 (37.5)	15 (32.6)	0.80	
Medical patients	48 (61.5)	23 (71.9)	25 (54.3)	0.16	
Immunosuppression	9 (11.5)	6 (18.7)	3 (6.5)	0.14	
Admission due to infection	21 (26.9)	6 (18.7)	15 (32.6)	0.20	0.35 (0.1–1.07)
Antibiotics in the previous 3 months	48 (61.5)	19 (59.4)	29 (63)	0.64	
Before the event					
CVC for at least 48 h	61 (78.2)	25 (78.1)	36 (78.3)	>0.99	
Antibiotics in the ICU	61 (78.2)	24 (75)	37 (80.4)	0.59	
Maximum number of drugs with AGNA at any time				0.29	
None given	17 (21.8)	8 (25)	9 (19.6)		
Single	31 (39.7)	9 (28.1)	22 (47.8)		
Two	9 (11.6)	3 (9.4)	6 (13)		
Three	10 (12.8)	5 (15.6)	5 (10.9)		
Four	11 (14.1)	7 (21.9)	4 (8.7)		
Antibiotic classes/class members *					
Third & fourth generation cephalosporins	26 (33.3)	11 (34.4)	15 (32.6)		
Colistin	28 (35.9)	14 (43.8)	14 (30.4)		
Tigecycline	24 (30.8)	13 (40.7)	11 (23.9)		
Carbapenems	33 (42.3)	14 (43.8)	19 (41.3)		
Aminoglycosides	10 (12.8)	5 (15.6)	5 (10.9)		
Quinolones	13 (16.7)	10 (31.2)	3 (6.5)		
Ampicillin/sulbactam	15 (19.2)	8 (25)	7 (15.2)		
Piperacillin/tazobactam	9 (11.5)	4 (12.5)	5 (10.9)		
Ceftazidime/avibactam	7 (9)	4 (12.5)	3 (6.5)		
Index day					NA
Event, days	10 (6–18)	12 (5.2–21.5)	9.5 (6–17.2)	0.66	
Timing of the event				0.34	
>48 h stay	67 (85.9)	26 (81.3)	41 (89.1)		
<48 h stay	11 (14.1)	6 (18.7)	5 (10.9)		
Source				0.73	
Primary	32 (41)	13 (40.6)	19 (41.3)		

Table 1. Cont.

	Overall (n = 78)	Colistin-Resistant (n = 32)	Colistin-Sensitive (n = 46)	p-Value **	Odds Ratio (95% CI) ##
Catheter-related #	25 (32.1)	12 (37.5)	13 (28.3)		
Urinary	5 (6.4)	3 (9.4)	2 (4.3)		
Intraabdominal	5 (6.4)	1 (3.1)	4 (8.7)		
Surgical site infection	5 (6.4)	1 (3.1)	4 (8.7)		
Lung/pleural empyema	4 (5.1)	1 (3.1)	3 (6.5)		
Bone/joint	2 (2.6)	1 (3.1)	1 (2.2)		
Source control performed	30 (38.5)	15 (46.9)	15 (32.6)	0.24	
Pitt bacteremia score	3 (1–4)	4 (2–4.7)	3 (1–4.2)	0.25	
Septic shock	43 (55.1)	18 (56.2)	25 (54.3)	>0.99	
Temperature max, °C	38.5 (37.9–39)	38.5 (37.9–39)	38.5 (37.7–39)	0.97	
Fever	49 (62.8)	22 (68.7)	32 (69.6)	>0.99	
Hypothermia	4 (5.1)	0 (0)	4 (8.7)	0.14	
SOFA score	6.5 (3.8–11)	8 (5–12.7)	5 (3–11)	0.07	-
White Blood Cells /mm^3, ×1000	13.4 (9.5–18.1)	13.94 (11.47–19.63)	12.97 (9.25–16.83)	0.69	
Leucopenia	2 (2.6)	1 (3.1)	1 (2.2)	>0.99	
CRP, mg/L	121 (62.7–155)	125 (58–204)	119 (63.2–141)	0.34	
Procalcitonin, µg/L	1.23 (0.34–2.08)	1.51 (0.51–2.94)	1.01 (0.22–2.16)	0.19	
Final model's accuracy, AUC (95% CI)					0.71 (0.59–0.83)

Abbreviations: AGNA, anti-Gram-negative activity; APACHE II, Acute Physiology Assessment and Chronic Health Evaluation; AUC, area under the curve; CI, confidence intervals; CRP, C-reactive protein; ICU, intensive care unit; NA, not applicable; SOFA, sequential organ failure assessment. Apart from the cells where it is otherwise stated, all values are in median (IQR) and n (%). * Often two or more combined antibiotics; only antibiotics with Gram-negative activity included. No comparison is feasible as patients were usually receiving more than a single antibiotic; # 24 central venous catheters and 1 peripherally inserted central catheter are included; ** Values in bold represent variables that entered the initial, full multivariate models with response variable the development of colistin-resistant bacteremia; ## Final logistic model for a colistin-resistant event. The explanatory variables included APACHE II score and admission due to infection.

Concerning the colistin susceptibility phenotype, patients of the CRG were older and presented increased APACHE II score on the day of admission compared to the CSG; however, in the final multivariable logistic regression model, only the APACHE II score remained independently associated with the development of CR-GN-BSI (Table 1, Supplementary Tables S1 and S2).

The estimated optimal cutoff value of the APACHE II score for discriminating CR from CS events was 20, with an AUC (95% CI) of 0.67 (0.55–0.79), a sensitivity of 59.4%, and a specificity of 69.6%.

The clinical and laboratory parameters on the index day are displayed in Table 1; there were no significant differences between the two groups. Overall, septic shock was evident in 55.1% of cases. The presence of septic shock and the sepsis rate of the CRG, indicated by the SOFA score, were similar to the CSG (Supplementary Materials Figure S1).

The temporal evolution of the SOFA score, the maximum daily temperature, white blood cell count, C-reactive protein, and procalcitonin unveiled a limited, though steady decline (Supplementary Materials Table S1, $p = 0.01$). In the vast majority of measured values, there was no difference as to colistin susceptibility status (Supplementary Materials Table S3).

Table 2. Microbiology of index culture.

	Overall	Colistin-Resistant Group	Colistin-Sensitive Group
		Pathogen *	
Acinetobacter baumannii	29	12	17
Klebsiella pneumoniae	24	8	16
Pseudomonas aeruginosa	10	0	10
Proteus mirabilis	6	6	0
Enterobacter cloace	4	0	4
Providencia stuartii	4	4	0
Serratia marcescens	2	2	0
Carbapenem-resistant	57	24	33
Event > 48 h	47	19	28
Event < 48 h	10	5	5
Colistin MIC (ng/mL) #			
=2	-	-	8
=1	-	-	4
≤0.5	-	-	34

* $p < 0.01$ (chi-square test); Other pathogens include: *Elizabethkingia meningoseptica, E. coli, Ochrobactrum anthropi, Pseudomonas putida, Stenotrophomonas maltophilia,* Sphingomonas paucimobilis. # Plausible only in the presence of colistin susceptibility.

3.3. Sensitivity Analyses for the Occurrence of the Colistin-Resistant Phenotype

We re-explored the data by lowering the susceptibility threshold to a minimal inhibitory concentration to colistin of 0.5 ng/mL and confirmed the significance of the admission APACHE II score. Moreover, we found that ICU admission due to infection was found more often in the optimal colistin-sensitive group (Supplementary Materials Table S1).

We also repeated the analysis after the exclusion of eleven patients who presented early BSI, before a 48 h stay in the ICU. The reanalysis showed that the APACHE score was the sole independent variable associated with the presence of colistin BSI phenotype (Supplementary Materials Table S2).

3.4. Treatment

The infection was empirically, appropriately treated in less than half the cases (Supplementary Materials Table S4). The most commonly administered antibiotics, possessing anti-Gram-negative activity and used for the treatment of various infections before the BSI diagnosis, were: carbapenems in 33 (42.3%), colistin in 28 (35.9%), cephalosporins in 26 (33.3%), tigecycline in 24 (30.8%), and ampicillin-sulbactam in 15 (19.2%) patients. Colistin has already been given for a median of 12.5 days before the event (IQR 5–15.5 days).

Thirty patients (45.5%) received combined targeted treatment for the GN-BSI event. The most frequently prescribed antimicrobial was colistin (30/67), followed by tigecycline (22/67), carbapenems (18/67), and aminoglycosides (16/67).

Overall, colistin was extensively used, usually in combination with other drugs (Supplementary Materials Table S4). There was no difference between the two groups regarding treatment aspects; of note, at least five-day colistin administration in the CRG started as an empirical antimicrobial regimen was similar to the CSG. However, the CR individuals tended to receive delayed targeted therapy than the CSG (on day three vs. day 0).

3.5. Outcomes

The study outcomes are displayed in Supplementary Materials Table S5.

Twenty-eight-day mortality post-event was overall 26.9%, and the Kaplan–Meier curves did not reveal any difference between the colistin-sensitive and the colistin-resistant groups (log-rank test, $p = 0.57$) (Figure 2). The corresponding 28-day mortality of the carbapenem-resistant *Acinetobacter baumannii* and *Klebsiella pneumoniae* infected patients was 34.5% and 28.6%.

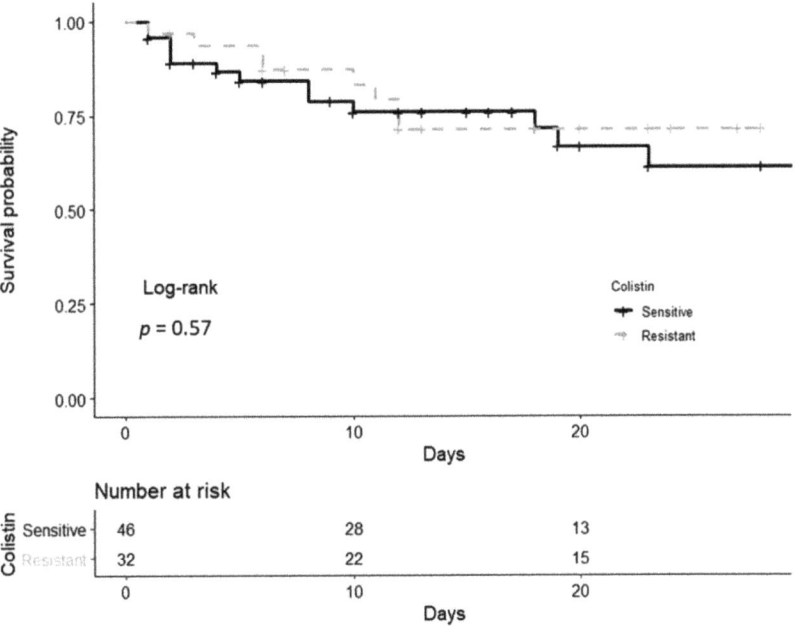

Figure 2. Kaplan–Meier survival curve of both colistin-resistant and colistin-sensitive groups until day 28 post-event.

Regarding 28-day mortality, univariate analysis and the hazard ratios of the multivariable Cox proportional hazard analysis are presented in Table 3. The SOFA score on the index day was independently associated with higher mortality (Table 3 and Supplementary Materials Table S5). The optimal discriminative cutoff value for the index day SOFA score was 11 (AUC (95% CI) 0.871 (0.77–0.97)), while the respective sensitivity and specificity were 76% and 88%.

Concerning sepsis evaluation, analysis of the data by using the median SOFA score threshold, which is valued at 7 in this dataset, the high SOFA score group had similar CR-BSI incidence compared to the lower SOFA score group. Of interest, the individuals with the higher score had independently had a prior ICU admission, increased Charlson Comorbidity Index, and Pitt bacteremia score on the event day (Supplementary Materials Table S7).

Recurrent bacteremia occurred on 8 (6–12) and secondary BSI on 12 (7–18) days following the index culture (Supplementary Materials Table S6). Secondary isolates were mostly Gram-negative (89%); the latter were often colistin-resistant (41.2%). Neither the primary analysis nor the alternative, using a strict, 0.5 ng/mL, the threshold for susceptibility to the drug, have revealed significant differences in the secondary study outcomes (Supplementary Materials Tables S5 and S8).

Table 3. Factors associated with 28-day mortality.

	Dead (n = 21)	Alive (n = 57)	p-Value #	Hazard Ratio (95% CI) ##
Age	75 (67–79)	62 (47–73)	**<0.01**	
Male	12 (57.1)	39 (68.4)	0.42	
APACHE II	20 (19–25)	17 (12–22)	**0.04**	
CCI	4 (4–5)	2 (1–4)	**0.01**	
SOFA Admission	10 (8–12.2)	7 (4–10)	0.01 **	
Prior ICU admission *	8 (38.1)	19 (33.3)	0.79	
Infectious admission	7 (33.3)	14 (24.6)	0.57	
Medical admission	10 (47.6)	38 (66.7)	0.19	
Immunosuppression	2 (9.5)	7 (14)	>0.99	
Source control	10 (47.6)	20 (35.1)	0.43	
Pitt bacteremia score	4 (4–6)	3 (1–4)	**<0.01**	
Septic shock	20 (95.2)	23 (40.4)	**<0.01**	
Colistin-resistance status			0.80	
-Colistin-resistant	8 (38.1)	24 (42.1)		
-Colistin-sensitive	13 (61.9)	33 (57.9)		
Colistin MIC $\leq$ 0.5	12 (57.1)	32 (56.1)	>0.99	
Empirical colistin for at least 3 days	8 (38.1)	25 (43.9)	0.80	
SOFA index day	13 (11–16)	5 (3–9)	**<0.01** **	1.23 (1.03–1.48)
Temperature index day, °C	38 (36.8–38.5)	38.7 (38.1–39.2)	0.01	
WBC index day, $10^3/mm^3$, ×1000	13.63 (10.44–17.88)	13.43 (9.31–18.14)	0.99	
CRP index day, mg/L	109.4 (71.83–136.25)	126 (61.08–154.5)	0.53	
Procalcitonin index day, ng/mL	1.33 (1.13–5.63)	0.84 (0.32–1.94)	0.20	
Five-day empirical treatment with colistin	6 (28.6)	20 (35.1)	0.79	
Ten-day colistin treatment, post-event	5 (23.8)	16 (28.1)	0.58	
One appropriate drug within 24 h post-event	7 (33.3)	21 (36.8)	>0.99	
One appropriate drug within 48 h post-event	8 (38.1)	25 (43.9)	0.80	
Two appropriate drugs within 24 h post-event	3 (14.3)	7 (12.3)	>0.99	
Two appropriate drugs within 48 h post-event	3 (14.3)	11 (19.3)	0.75	

All values are in median (IQR) and n (%). APACHE II, Acute Physiology Assessment and Chronic Health Evaluation; CCI: Charlson comorbidity index; CI, confidence intervals; CRP, C-reactive protein; ICU, intensive care unit; MIC, minimal inhibitory concentration; SOFA, sequential organ failure assessment; WBC; white blood cell count. * 2–12 months before the index admission; # Values in bold represent variables that entered the initial, full multivariate Cox model. ** We considered the index SOFA score as it was more recent and clinically more relevant than the admission score. ## Final Cox proportional hazard model for 28-day mortality. The final model, stratified for age, included one explanatory variable, the index day SOFA score; the concordance index was 0.83 (se = 0.128).

4. Discussion

The present study reports on a population of critically ill patients with GN-BSI presenting overall 28-day mortality of 26.9%. The occurrence of the colistin-resistant phenotype was independently associated with the patients' clinical severity status on ICU admission, evaluated by an increased APACHE II score, and not with the antimicrobials administered. Similarly, the sepsis severity status of the patient on the index day, as assessed by the SOFA score, was associated with worse 28-day mortality; however, we could not link the colistin susceptibility status or administration of colistin to the outcome.

In other studies, regarding CR, *K. pneumoniae*, and *A. baumannii*, infections had not presented increased admission severity in the non-susceptible group. However, their participants were often not critically ill and not exclusively bloodstream-infected [7,35]. Apart from the worse admission status, the CRG's event SOFA score was higher, though not significantly, than the respective CSG's value ($p = 0.07$). Re-analyzing the data by the index day SOFA value, the sicker patients (score ≥ 7) had independently had a prior ICU admission (Supplementary Materials Table S7), which is in line with a CDC-affiliated study showing that prior hospitalization with broad-spectrum antimicrobials' exposure increases sepsis risk [36].

A recent ICU study showed that combined *A. baumannii* CR-BSI and septic shock were always fatal [37]. Only half of our population presented septic shock, and the corresponding mortality was in comparison lower, at 34.5%. However, according to the above, a higher event SOFA score was independently associated with 28-day mortality regardless of the CR phenotype (Table 3). Notably, a re-analysis of *A. baumannii*-infected patients unexpectedly found that the CR individuals presented less mortality than their CS counterparts [7]. Regarding combined carbapenem-resistant and CR *K. pneumoniae* infections, we observed a fatality rate of 28.6%, contrary to recent literature, which had exhibited increased mortality, over 50%, before ceftazidime-avibactam's inception [35,38]. In this study, carbapenem-resistant *K. pneumoniae*-associated BSI patients often received ceftazidime-avibactam, as part of empirical or targeted treatment (data not shown), a drug with superior efficacy compared to colistin [39].

Colistin has recently re-emerged as therapy for the difficult-to-treat GN pathogens [3,40]. Regardless of the susceptibility status, colistin's BSI treatment failed to add any survival benefit despite its extensive empirical use and its recommended dosing [14]. However, antimicrobial coverage's appropriateness throughout the study groups was less than 50% in the first 48 h post-event (Supplementary Materials Table S4). Many CRG patients regularly received colistin as an empirical regimen, and they would likely have survived regardless of an ineffective antibiotic scheme. Unfortunately, similar to other investigators [6], we could not demonstrate any benefit from the empirical regimen. The reasons for the lack of colistin's therapeutic efficacy could be the gloomy evolution of high-level resistance, leaving little room for efficacious antibiotic therapy, or the insufficient activity of the drugs delivered, notably colistin, or even the decreased fitness—virulence of the CR bacteria [41,42]. A final issue could be the possible antagonistic rather than synergistic effects of colistin with other antimicrobials, which may have influenced the outcome [40].

Nonetheless, there are in vitro data that seem promising for the development of future therapeutic strategies. At first, *Enterobacterales* bacterial strains that expressed the mobilized colistin-resistant gene-1 were tested for resistance to several antibiotics; these strains remained susceptible to eravacycline, which can be studied in vivo for the treatment of CR bacteria [43]. Analysis of the secondary resistome, i.e., genes that are not known resistance determinants, of *K. pneumoniae* has found a conditionally essential gene for the CR phenotype (only in the presence of colistin) [44]. That chromosomal gene encodes a DedA family membrane transporter protein, which can restore sensitivity to the drug if depolarized [45].

The study's strength lies in the adoption of broth microdilution, a robust methodology concerning colistin susceptibility. The routine use of the recommended laboratory method minimizes bacterial misclassification and enables between-study comparison. Moreover, we dosed colistin according to the latest pharmacokinetic data [15]. Notably, we also included very early infections in those patients who had previously been cared for in an ICU. These patients probably remain critically ill, viewed from a microbiological viewpoint, as they carry resistant microbiota, which may evolve to even more resistant phenotypes through rehospitalizations [24,46].

The single-center study design limits its generalizability. Moreover, the investigation setting presents extreme multi-drug-resistant GN flora that renders the results plausible only to critical care departments with isolates of similar susceptibility patterns. In addition, we do not have local data regarding the molecular determinants of colistin resistance; however, it is likely to represent similar mutations as those reported from other Greek hospitals [47,48]. Another drawback is that the hospital laboratory had not performed assays to evaluate colistin's synergy with other antibiotics; however, such assays are complex and of questionable predictive value for therapeutic efficacy [49].

5. Conclusions

ICU-associated Gram-negative bloodstream infection in a setting of limited treatment options can adversely impact outcomes. The colistin-resistant phenotype was more common in association with a high APACHE II score on admission. The higher SOFA score on the BSI index day was associated with increased 28-day mortality, contrary to the isolate's susceptibility status to colistin or treatment of the episode with colistin, which were unassociated with this outcome. However, due to the study's retrospective design, these observations should be re-evaluated in a future prospective study.

Supplementary Materials: The following are available online at https://www.mdpi.com/article/10.3390/antibiotics11030405/s1, Figure S1: The evolution of the median SOFA score of both study groups every two days, starting from two days before the index day until day 10 post-event, Table S1: Patient characteristics regarding the 0.5 ng/mL threshold for colistin resistance, Table S2: Patients' characteristics regarding bacteremia acquisition >48 h after the present ICU admission., Table S3: Evolution of clinical and laboratory indices at 48 h intervals, Table S4: Antibiotic treatment, Table S5: Outcomes, Table S6: Factors associated with 28-day mortality in patients with bacteremia acquisition >48 h after ICU admission, Table S7: Patient characteristics in relation to SOFA score on the index day, Table S8: Outcomes of bloodstream infections regarding a 0.5 ng/mL threshold for colistin resistance.

Author Contributions: M.K.: conceptualization, data collection, methodology, software, formal analysis, original draft preparation; G.P., conceptualization, methodology, software, review and editing; K.T., methodology, software, formal analysis, review and editing; M.C., data collection, software; P.P., data collection, software; A.K. (Anna Katsiaflaka), data collection, software; K.O., data collection, software; A.K. (Antonios Katsioulis), data collection, software; E.P., formal analysis, review and editing; A.K. (Apostolos Komnos), conceptualization, supervision, review and editing. All authors have read and agreed to the published version of the manuscript.

Funding: This research received no external funding.

Institutional Review Board Statement: The ethics committee of the hospital approved this study (Protocol 187/4-11-2019).

Informed Consent Statement: Informed consent was waived as the data were anonymized and retrospectively obtained.

Data Availability Statement: Data supporting the results can be provided from the corresponding author on request. The data are not publicly available due to privacy policy of the hospital.

Conflicts of Interest: The authors declare no conflict of interest.

Abbreviations

APACHE II	Acute Physiology Assessment and Chronic Health Evaluation
AUC	area under the curve
BSI	bloodstream infection
CI	confidence interval
CR	colistin-resistant
CRG	colistin-resistant group

CSG	colistin-sensitive group
CVC	central venous catheter
EUCAST	European Committee On Antimicrobial Susceptibility Testing
GN	Gram-negative
ICU	intensive care unit
IQR	interquartile range
MDR	multi-drug-resistant
SOFA	sequential organ failure assessment

References

1. Vincent, J.L.; Rello, J.; Marshall, J.; Silva, E.; Anzueto, A.; Martin, C.D.; Moreno, R.; Lipman, J.; Gomersall, C.; Sakr, Y.; et al. International study of the prevalence and outcomes of infection in intensive care units. *JAMA* **2009**, *302*, 2323–2329. [CrossRef] [PubMed]
2. Tabah, A.; Koulenti, D.; Laupland, K.; Misset, B.; Valles, J.; Bruzzi de Carvalho, F.; Paiva, J.A.; Cakar, N.; Ma, X.; Eggimann, P.; et al. Characteristics and determinants of outcome of hospital-acquired bloodstream infections in intensive care units: The EUROBACT International Cohort Study. *Intensive Care Med.* **2012**, *38*, 1930–1945. [CrossRef] [PubMed]
3. Kadri, S.S.; Adjemian, J.; Lai, Y.L.; Spaulding, A.B.; Ricotta, E.; Prevots, D.R.; Palmore, T.N.; Rhee, C.; Klompas, M.; Dekker, J.P.; et al. Difficult-to-Treat Resistance in Gram-negative Bacteremia at 173 US Hospitals: Retrospective Cohort Analysis of Prevalence, Predictors, and Outcome of Resistance to All First-line Agents. *Clin. Infect. Dis.* **2018**, *67*, 1803–1814. [CrossRef] [PubMed]
4. Sherry, N.; Howden, B. Emerging Gram-negative resistance to last-line antimicrobial agents fosfomycin, colistin and ceftazidime-avibactam-epidemiology, laboratory detection and treatment implications. *Expert Rev. Anti-Infect. Ther.* **2018**, *16*, 289–306. [CrossRef] [PubMed]
5. Olaitan, A.O.; Morand, S.; Rolain, J.-M. Mechanisms of polymyxin resistance: Acquired and intrinsic resistance in bacteria. *Front. Microbiol.* **2014**, *5*, 643. [CrossRef]
6. Zak-Doron, Y.; Dishon Benattar, Y.; Pfeffer, I.; Daikos, G.L.; Skiada, A.; Antoniadou, A.; Durante-Mangoni, E.; Andini, R.; Cavezza, G.; Leibovici, L.; et al. The Association between Empirical Antibiotic Treatment and Mortality in Severe Infections Caused by Carbapenem-resistant Gram-negative Bacteria: A Prospective Study. *Clin. Infect. Dis.* **2018**, *67*, 1815–1823. [CrossRef]
7. Dickstein, Y.; Lellouche, J.; Ben Dalak Amar, M.; Schwartz, D.; Nutman, A.; Daitch, V.; Yahav, D.; Leibovici, L.; Skiada, A.; Antoniadou, A.; et al. Treatment Outcomes of Colistin- and Carbapenem-resistant *Acinetobacter baumannii* Infections: An Exploratory Subgroup Analysis of a Randomized Clinical Trial. *Clin. Infect. Dis.* **2019**, *69*, 769–776. [CrossRef] [PubMed]
8. Xavier, B.B.; Lammens, C.; Ruhak, R.; Kumar-Singh, S.; Butaye, P.; Goossens, H.; Malhotra-Kumar, S. Identification of a novel plasmid-mediated colistin-resistance gene, *mcr-2*, in *Escherichia coli*, Belgium, June 2016. *Eurosurveillance* **2016**, *21*, 30280. [CrossRef]
9. Ni, W.; Li, Y.; Guan, J.; Zhao, J.; Cui, J.; Wang, R.; Liu, Y. Effects of Efflux Pump Inhibitors on Colistin Resistance in Multidrug-Resistant Gram-Negative Bacteria. *Antimicrob. Agents Chemother.* **2016**, *60*, 3215–3218. [CrossRef]
10. Miyakis, S.; Pefanis, A.; Tsakris, A. The challenges of antimicrobial drug resistance in Greece. *Clin. Infect. Dis.* **2011**, *53*, 177–184. [CrossRef]
11. European Committee on Antimicrobial Susceptibility Testing. Antimicrobial Susceptibility Testing of Colistin-Problems Detected with Several Commercially Available Products. 2016. Available online: http://www.eucast.org (accessed on 15 December 2017).
12. Kalil, A.; Meterski, M.L.; Klompas, M.; Muscedere, J.; Sweeney, D.A.; Palmer, L.B.; Napolitano, L.M.; O'Grady, N.P.; Bartlett, J.G.; Carratalà, J.; et al. Management of Adults with Hospital-acquired and Ventilator-associated Pneumonia: 2016 Clinical Practice Guidelines by the Infectious Diseases Society of America and the American Thoracic Society. *Clin. Infect. Dis.* **2016**, *63*, e61–e111. [CrossRef]
13. Pronovost, P.; Needham, D.; Berenholtz, S.; Sinopoli, D.; Chu, H.; Cosgrove, S.; Sexton, B.; Hyzy, R.; Welsh, R.; Roth, G.; et al. An Intervention to Decrease Catheter-Related Bloodstream Infections in the ICU. *N. Engl. J. Med.* **2006**, *355*, 2725–2732. [CrossRef] [PubMed]
14. Institute for Healthcare Improvement. How-to Guide: Prevent Ventilator-Associated Pneumonia. Available online: http://www.ihi.org (accessed on 10 May 2018).
15. Nation, R.L.; Garonzik, S.M.; Thamlikitkul, V.; Giamarellos-Bourboulis, E.J.; Forrest, A.; Paterson, D.L.; Li, J.; Silveira, F.P. Dosing Guidance for Intravenous Colistin in Critically Ill Patients. *Clin. Infect. Dis.* **2017**, *64*, 565–571. [CrossRef]
16. European Committee on Antimicrobial Susceptibility Testing. Breakpoint Tables for Interpretation of MICs and Zone Diameters Version 7.0. Available online: http://www.eucast.org (accessed on 10 December 2017).
17. World Medical Association Declaration of Helsinki—Ethical Principles for Medical Research Involving Human Subjects. Available online: http://www.wma.net (accessed on 15 December 2018).
18. Vandenbroucke, J.P.; von Elm, E.; Altman, D.G.; Gøtzsche, P.C.; Mulrow, C.D.; Pocock, S.J.; Poole, C.; Schlesselman, J.J.; Egger, M. For the STROBE Initiative Strengthening the Reporting of Observational Studies in Epidemiology (STROBE): Explanation and Elaboration. *PLoS Med.* **2007**, *4*, e296. [CrossRef] [PubMed]
19. Charlson, M.E.; Pompei, P.; Ales, K.L.; MacKenzie, C.R. A new method of classifying prognostic comorbidity in longitudinal studies: Development and validation. *J. Chronic Dis.* **1987**, *40*, 373–383. [CrossRef]

20. Knaus, W.A.; Draper, E.A.; Wagner, D.P.; Zimmerman, J.E. APACHE II: A severity of disease classification system. *Crit. Care Med.* **1985**, *13*, 818–829. [CrossRef]
21. Vincent, J.L.; Moreno, R.; Takala, J.; Willatts, S.; De Mendonça, A.; Bruining, H.; Reinhart, C.K.; Suter, P.M.; Thijs, L.G. The SOFA (Sepsis-related Organ Failure Assessment) score to describe organ dysfunction/failure. *Intensive Care Med.* **1996**, *22*, 707–710. [CrossRef]
22. Korvick, J.A.; Bryan, C.S.; Farber, B.; Beam, T.R., Jr.; Schenfeld, L.; Muder, R.R.; Weinbaum, D.; Lumish, R.; Gerding, D.N.; Wagener, M.M. Prospective observational study of Klebsiella bacteremia in 230 patients: Outcome for antibiotic combinations versus monotherapy. *Antimicrob. Agents Chemother.* **1992**, *36*, 2639–2644. [CrossRef]
23. Lambert, M.-L.; Suetens, C.; Savey, A.; Palomar, M.; Hiesmayr, M.; Morales, I.; Agodi, A.; Frank, U.; Mertens, K.; Schumacher, M.; et al. Clinical outcomes of health-care-associated infections and antimicrobial resistance in patients admitted to European intensive-care units: A cohort study. *Lancet Infect. Dis.* **2011**, *11*, 30–38. [CrossRef]
24. Haverkate, M.R.; Derde, L.P.G.; Brun-Buisson, C.; Bonten, M.J.M.; Bootsma, M.C.J. Duration of colonization with antimicrobial-resistant bacteria after ICU discharge. *Intensive Care Med.* **2014**, *40*, 564–571. [CrossRef]
25. Woudt, S.H.S.; de Greeff, S.C.; Schoffelen, A.F.; Vlek, A.L.M.; Bonten, M.J.M. Antibiotic Resistance and the Risk of Recurrent Bacteremia. *Clin. Infect. Dis.* **2018**, *66*, 1651–1657. [CrossRef] [PubMed]
26. Rhodes, A.; Evans, L.E.; Alhazzani, W.; Levy, M.M.; Antonelli, M.; Ferrer, R.; Kumar, A.; Sevransky, J.E.; Sprung, C.L.; Nunnally, M.E.; et al. Surviving Sepsis Campaign: International Guidelines for Management of Sepsis and Septic Shock: 2016. *Intensive Care Med.* **2017**, *43*, 304–377. [CrossRef] [PubMed]
27. Falcone, M.; Russo, A.; Iacovelli, A.; Restuccia, G.; Ceccarelli, G.; Giordano, A.; Farcomeni, A.; Morelli, A.; Venditti, M. Predictors of outcome in ICU patients with septic shock caused by *Klebsiella pneumoniae* carbapenemase–producing *K. pneumoniae*. *Clin. Microbiol. Infect.* **2016**, *22*, 444–450. [CrossRef] [PubMed]
28. Mermel, L.A.; Allon, M.; Bouza, E.; Craven, D.E.; Flynn, P.; O'Grady, N.P.; Raad, I.I.; Rijnders, B.J.A.; Sherertz, R.J.; Warren, D.K. Clinical Practice Guidelines for the Diagnosis and Management of Intravascular Catheter-Related Infection: 2009 Update by the Infectious Diseases Society of America. *Clin. Infect. Dis.* **2009**, *49*, 1–45. [CrossRef]
29. Girometti, N.; Lewis, R.E.; Giannella, M.; Ambretti, S.; Bartoletti, M.; Tedeschi, S.; Tumietto, F.; Cristini, F.; Trapani, F.; Gaibani, P.; et al. *Klebsiella pneumoniae* Bloodstream Infection Epidemiology and Impact of Inappropriate Empirical Therapy. *Medicine* **2014**, *93*, 298–308. [CrossRef] [PubMed]
30. Ong, D.S.Y.; Frencken, J.F.; Klein Klouwenberg, P.M.C.; Juffermans, N.; van der Poll, T.; Bonten, M.J.M.; Cremer, O.L.; MARS Consortium. Short-Course Adjunctive Gentamicin as Empirical Therapy in Patients with Severe Sepsis and Septic Shock: A Prospective Observational Cohort Study. *Clin. Infect. Dis.* **2017**, *64*, 1731–1736. [CrossRef]
31. Vesin, A.; Azoulay, E.; Ruckly, S.; Vignoud, L.; Rusinovà, K.; Benoit, D.; Soares, M.; Azeivedo-Maia, P.; Abroug, F.; Benbenishty, J.; et al. Reporting and handling missing values in clinical studies in intensive care units. *Intensive Care Med.* **2013**, *39*, 1396–1404. [CrossRef]
32. Nunez, E.; Steyerberg, E.W.; Nunez, J. Regression Modeling Strategies. *Rev. Esp. Cardiol.* **2011**, *64*, 501–507.
33. The R Project for Statistical Computing. Available online: http://www.r-project.org (accessed on 15 April 2021).
34. Rohas, L.J.; Salim, M.; Cober, E.; Richter, S.S.; Perez, F.; Salata, R.A.; Kalayjian, R.C.; Watkins, R.R.; Marshall, S.; Rudin, S.D.; et al. Colistin Resistance in Carbapenem-Resistant *Klebsiella pneumoniae*: Laboratory Detection and Impact on Mortality. *Clin. Infect. Dis.* **2017**, *64*, 711–718.
35. Baggs, J.; Jernigan, J.A.; Laufer Halpin, A.; Epstein, L.; Hatfield, K.M.; McDonald, L.C. Risk of Subsequent Sepsis within 90 Days after a Hospital Stay by Type of Antibiotic Exposure. *Clin. Infect. Dis.* **2018**, *66*, 1004–1012. [CrossRef]
36. Papathanakos, G.; Andrianopoulos, I.; Papathanasiou, A.; Priavali, E.; Koulenti, D.; Koulouras, V. Colistin-Resistant Acinetobacter Baumannii Bacteremia: A Serious Threat for Critically Ill Patients. *Microorganisms* **2020**, *8*, 287. [CrossRef]
37. Giacobbe, D.R.; Del Bono, V.; Trecarichi, E.M.; De Rosa, F.G.; Giannella, M.; Bassetti, M.; Bartoloni, A.; Losito, A.R.; Corcione, C.; Bartoletti, M.; et al. Risk factors for bloodstream infections due to colistin-resistant KPC-producing *Klebsiella pneumoniae*: Results from a multicenter case–control–control study. *Clin. Microbiol. Infect.* **2015**, *21*, 1106.e1–1106.e8. [CrossRef]
38. van Duin, D.; Lok, J.J.; Earley, M.; Cober, E.; Richter, S.S.; Perez, F.; Salata, R.A.; Kalayjian, R.C.; Watkins, R.R.; Doi, Y.; et al. Colistin versus Ceftazidime-Avibactam in the Treatment of Infections Due to Carbapenem-Resistant Enterobacteriaceae. *Clin. Infect. Dis.* **2018**, *66*, 163–171. [CrossRef] [PubMed]
39. Karaiskos, I.; Lagou, S.; Pontikis, K.; Rapti, V.; Poulakou, G. The "Old" and the "New" Antibiotics for MDR Gram-Negative Pathogens: For Whom, When, and How. *Front. Public Health* **2019**, *7*, 151. [CrossRef] [PubMed]
40. Bassetti, M.; Poulakou, G.; Ruppe, E.; Bouza, E.; Van Hal, S.J.; Brink, A. Antimicrobial resistance in the next 30 years, humankind, bugs and drugs: A visionary approach. *Intensive Care Med.* **2017**, *43*, 1464–1475. [CrossRef] [PubMed]
41. Beseiro, A.; Moreno, A.; Fernandez, N.; Vallejo, J.A.; Aranda, J.; Adler, B.; Harper, M.; Boyce, J.D.; Bou, G. Biological Cost of Different Mechanisms of Colistin Resistance and Their Impact on Virulence in *Acinetobacter baumannii*. *Antimicrob. Agents Chemother.* **2014**, *58*, 518–526. [CrossRef]
42. Liu, E.; Jia, P.; Li, X.; Zhou, M.; Kudinha, T.; Wu, C.; Xu, Y.; Yang, Q. In vitro and in vivo Effect of Antimicrobial Agent Combinations against Carbapenem-Resistant *Klebsiella pneumoniae* with Different Resistance Mechanisms in China. *Infect. Drug Resist.* **2021**, *14*, 917–928. [CrossRef]

43. Fyfe, C.; LeBlanc, G.; Close, B.; Nordmann, P.; Dumas, J.; Grossman, T.H. Eravacycline Is Active against Bacterial Isolates Expressing the Polymyxin Resistance Gene *mcr-1*. *Antimicrob. Agents Chemother.* **2016**, *60*, 6989–6990. [CrossRef] [PubMed]
44. Jana, B.; Cain, A.K.; Doerrler, W.T.; Boinett, C.J.; Fookes, M.C.; Parkhill, J.; Guardabassi, L. The secondary resistome of multidrug-resistant *Klebsiella pneumoniae*. *Sci. Rep.* **2017**, *7*, 42483. [CrossRef]
45. Panta, P.R.; Kumar, S.; Stafford, S.F.; Billiot, C.E.; Douglass, M.V.; Herrera, C.M.; Trent, M.S.; Doerrler, W.T. A DedA Family Membrane Protein Is Required for *Burkholderia thailandensis* Colistin Resistance. *Front. Microbiol.* **2019**, *10*, 2532. [CrossRef]
46. Jousset, A.B.; Bonnin, R.A.; Rosinski-Chupin, I.; Girlich, D.; Cuzon, G.; Cabanel, N.; Frech, H.; Farfour, E.; Dortet, L.; Glaser, P.; et al. A 4.5-Year Within-Patient Evolution of a Colistin-Resistant *Klebsiella pneumoniae* Carbapenemase–Producing, *K. pneumoniae* Sequence Type 258. *Clin. Infect. Dis.* **2018**, *67*, 1388–1394. [CrossRef]
47. Mattia Palmieri, M.; D'Andrea, M.M.; Pelegrin, A.C.; Perrot, N.; Mirande, C.; Blanc, B.; Legakis, N.; Goossens, H.; Rossolini, G.M.; van Belkum, A. Abundance of Colistin-Resistant, OXA-23- and ArmA-Producing *Acinetobacter baumannii* Belonging to International Clone 2 in Greece. *Front. Microbiol.* **2020**, *11*, 294.
48. Mavroidi, A.; Katsiari, M.; Likousi, S.; Palla, E.; Roussou, Z.; Nikolaou, C.; Maguina, A.; Platsouka, E.D. Characterization of ST258 Colistin-Resistant, blaKPC-Producing *Klebsiella pneumoniae* in a Greek Hospital. *Microb. Drug Resist.* **2016**, *22*, 392–398. [CrossRef]
49. Brennan-Krohn, T.; Kirby, J.E. When One Drug Is Not Enough: Context, Methodology, and Future Prospects in Antibacterial Synergy Testing. *Clin. Lab. Med.* **2019**, *39*, 345–358. [CrossRef] [PubMed]

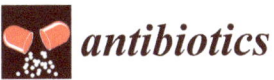

Review

Antimicrobial Stewardship Using Biomarkers: Accumulating Evidence for the Critically Ill

Evdoxia Kyriazopoulou [1] and Evangelos J. Giamarellos-Bourboulis [2,*]

[1] 2nd Department of Critical Care Medicine, National and Kapodistrian University of Athens, 12462 Athens, Greece; ekyri@med.uoa.gr
[2] 4th Department of Internal Medicine, National and Kapodistrian University of Athens, 12462 Athens, Greece
* Correspondence: egiamarel@med.uoa.gr; Tel.: +30-210-5831994

Abstract: This review aims to summarize current progress in the management of critically ill, using biomarkers as guidance for antimicrobial treatment with a focus on antimicrobial stewardship. Accumulated evidence from randomized clinical trials (RCTs) and observational studies in adults for the biomarker-guided antimicrobial treatment of critically ill (mainly sepsis and COVID-19 patients) has been extensively searched and is provided. Procalcitonin (PCT) is the best studied biomarker; in the majority of randomized clinical trials an algorithm of discontinuation of antibiotics with decreasing PCT over serial measurements has been proven safe and effective to reduce length of antimicrobial treatment, antibiotic-associated adverse events and long-term infectious complications like infections by multidrug-resistant organisms and *Clostridioides difficile*. Other biomarkers, such as C-reactive protein and presepsin, are already being tested as guidance for shorter antimicrobial treatment, but more research is needed. Current evidence suggests that biomarkers, mainly procalcitonin, should be implemented in antimicrobial stewardship programs even in the COVID-19 era, when, although bacterial coinfection rate is low, antimicrobial overconsumption remains high.

Keywords: antimicrobial stewardship; sepsis; COVID-19; ICU; procalcitonin; C-reactive protein; presepsin; infection; biomarker; guided antimicrobial therapy

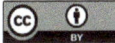

1. Introduction

Early and appropriate antimicrobial treatment remains key for sepsis management [1]. It is, however, sometimes difficult even for the most experienced physician to rule-out an infection in the critically ill and withhold antibiotics. The appropriate duration of treatment for severe infections is also not fully described. Current sepsis guidelines recommend a shorter rather than longer duration of antimicrobial treatment, but the definite duration remains at the discretion of the treating physician [2]. Doubts and fear for relapse have led to injudicious broad-spectrum and unnecessarily long antimicrobial treatment adding up to the emergence of antimicrobial resistance. In 2019, about 5 million deaths have been associated with bacterial antimicrobial resistance, underlying the urgent need for tight infection control and robust antimicrobial stewardship programs [3].

A biomarker should be easily measured and interpreted as an indicator of biological or pharmacologic responses to a therapeutic intervention [4]. The optimal sepsis biomarker should be sensitive and specific enough to rule in/out diagnosis, predict unfavorable outcomes and evaluate the host's response to treatment in order to encourage escalation or de-escalation; this is a strategy called "biomarker-guided treatment" [5]. More than one hundred biomarkers have been studied for sepsis management [6]. However, the only biomarker developed to guide antimicrobial treatment based on evidence coming from randomized clinical trials (RCTs) is procalcitonin (PCT). PCT is a precursor of the thyroid gland hormone calcitonin, and it is increased in the circulation during bacterial infection as a product of cells of mesenchymal origin. This review aims to present cumulative evidence from clinical trials, mainly RCTs, on the use of PCT-guidance in promoting antimicrobial stewardship for the critically-ill by restriction of injudicious antimicrobial treatment. Brief reference is also done to other biomarkers that are under consideration.

2. Results and Discussion

2.1. Antimicrobial Stewardship through PCT-Guidance for Lower Respiratory Tract Infections

PCT is the best studied biomarker to guide antimicrobial treatment in lower respiratory tract infections (LRTI). The majority of these RCTs shared a common design comparing an algorithm to start or discontinue antibiotics based on measurements of PCT, with standard-of-care (SOC); SOC was defined as start, continuation, or stop of antibiotics at the discretion of the treating physician and in accordance with local and international guidelines [7–29]. Available trials of PCT-guidance versus SOC are summarized in Table 1. Participants have a wide spectrum of symptoms, ranging from acute exacerbation of asthma and chronic obstructive pulmonary disease admitted in the Emergency Department, to severe community- or hospital-acquired pneumonia necessitating admission in medical wards or in the Intensive Care Unit (ICU). The common finding of all studies is the reduction of antimicrobial treatment duration with PCT-guidance. This reduction of antimicrobial treatment did not generate any safety signal as far as infection relapse, new infection, adverse events, or mortality are concerned. The ProHOSP trial studied the efficacy of PCT guidance directed to both start and stop of antibiotics. More precisely, 671 patients with LRTI received PCT-guided treatment and 688 received SOC [12]. For the PCT group, physicians were advised to start antibiotics when serum PCT was more than 0.25 ng/mL. Measurements were repeated on days 3, 5 and, 7 and stop of treatment was encouraged when levels decreased to more than 80% from the baseline. PCT-guidance led to a shorter antimicrobial treatment compared to SOC (5.7 versus 8.7 days, $p < 0.05$). However, the ProACT trial conducted in the USA a decade later, failed to show a similar effect. In the ProACT trial, mean duration of treatment for the 826 patients randomized in the PCT group was 4.2 days compared to that of 4.3 days for the 830 patients allocated in the SOC group (p: 0.87) [24]. One explanation for this lack of effect is the already reduced SOC duration of treatment in patients following local guidelines which does not allow any further benefit from the intervention to be shown. The majority of the first trials evaluating PCT-guidance provided such promising results that led to a switch in the current guidelines to a shorter duration of antimicrobial treatment for pneumonia [30] and to the approval of PCT guidance by the US Food and Drug Administration [31].

Table 1. Summary of randomized trials evaluating Procalcitonin (PCT)-guided antimicrobial treatment in patients with infections outside the Intensive Care Unit (ICU).

Ref	Trial Setting	PCT Algorithm Applied	N of Patients	Main Results
[7]	LRTI—ED Single-center—Switzerland	Initiation-cessation	PCT: 124 SOC: 119	Prescription of antimicrobials: 44% vs. 83%, $p < 0.0001$ LOT: 10.3 vs. 12.8 days, $p < 0.0001$ Decreased cost
[8]	CAP (requiring hospitalization) Single-center—Switzerland	Initiation-cessation	PCT: 151 SOC: 151	Prescription of antimicrobials: 85% vs. 99%, $p < 0.0001$ LOT: 5.8 vs. 12.9 days, $p < 0.0001$ Decreased cost
[9]	COPD exacerbation—ED Single-center—Switzerland	Initiation-cessation	PCT: 113 SOC: 113	Prescription of antimicrobials: 40% vs. 72%, $p < 0.0001$
[10]	Symptoms compatible with respiratory (upper/lower) infection—prehospital Multicenter—Switzerland	Initiation-cessation	PCT: 230 SOC: 223	Restriction in activity at day 14: 0.14 (95% CI: −0.53 to 0.81) Prescription of antimicrobials: decrease 72% (95% CI: 66–78)
[11]	CAP (requiring hospitalization) Multicenter—Denmark	Initiation with PCT > 0.25 ng/mL	PCT: 103 SOC: 107	LOT: 5.1 vs. 6.8 days, $p = 0.007$
[12]	CAP (requiring hospitalization) Multicenter—Switzerland	Initiation-cessation	PCT: 687 SOC: 694	Total adverse outcomes: 15.4% vs. 18.9%, OR −3.5 (95% CI: −7.6 to 0.4) LOT: 5.7 vs. 8.7 days, $p < 0.05$ AE due to antimicrobials: 19.8% vs. 28.1%, $p < 0.05$
[13]	Symptoms compatible with respiratory (upper/lower) infection—prehospital	Initiation-cessation	PCT: 275 SOC: 275	Restriction in activity at day 14: 0.04 (95% CI: 0.73 to 0.81) Prescription of antimicrobials: 21.5% vs. 36.7%, $p < 0.0005$
[14]	CAP (requiring hospitalization) Single-center—Shanghai	Initiation-cessation	PCT: 81 SOC: 81	Prescription of antimicrobials: 84.4% vs. 97.5%, $p = 0.004$ LOT: 5 vs. 7 days, $p < 0.001$
[15]	Acute asthma exacerbation Single-center—Shanghai	Initiation	PCT: 132 SOC: 133	Prescription of antimicrobials: 46.1% vs. 74.8%, $p < 0.01$
[16]	Aspiration pneumonia Single-center—Japan	If initial PCT < 0.5 ng/mL treat 3 days; if 0.5–1.0 treat for 5 days; if >1.0 treat for 7 days; stop with decrease ≥90%	PCT: 53 SOC: 52	Relapse (30 days): 25% vs. 37.5%, $p = 0.19$ LOT: 5 vs. 8 days, $p < 0.0001$
[17]	Acute asthma exacerbation Single-center—Shanghai	Initiation	PCT: 90 SOC: 90	Prescription of antimicrobials: 48.9% vs. 87.8%, $p < 0.001$ LOT: 6 vs. 6 days, $p = 0.198$ Exacerbation (1 year): 78.8% vs. 82.1%, $p = 0.586$
[18]	COPD exacerbation Multicenter—Italy	Stop after 3 days if PCT < 0.25 ng/mL; if not treat for 10 days	PCT: 88 SOC: 90	Exacerbation rate difference (6 months): 4.04% (90% CI: −7.23 to 15.31)
[19]	LRTI (requiring hospitalization)—ED Single-center—USA	Initiation, combined with multiplex PCR	PCT: 151 SOC: 149	LOT: 3 vs. 4 days, $p = 0.42$ Duration of symptoms: 16 vs. 20 days, $p = 0.03$

Table 1. Cont.

Ref	Trial Setting	PCT Algorithm Applied	N of Patients	Main Results
[20]	COPD exacerbation Single-center—Denmark	Initiation-cessation	PCT: 62 SOC: 58	LOT: 3.5 vs. 8.5 days, $p = 0.0169$ Patients (%) under treatment ≥ 5 days: 41.9 vs. 67.2, $p = 0.006$
[21]	After stroke Multicenter—International	Initiation	PCT: 112 SOC: 115	modified Rankin Scale (3 months): 4 vs. 4, $p = 0.452$ Prescription of antimicrobials: 63% vs. 45%, $p = 0.01$
[22] *	COPD exacerbation Single-center—USA	Initiation	Before:139 After: 166	LOT: 3 vs. 5.3 days, $p = 0.01$ Length of hospital stay: 2.9 vs. 4.1 days, $p = 0.01$ Rehospitalization (30 days): 16.6% vs. 14.5%, $p = 0.25$
[23]	COPD exacerbation Multicenter—France	Initiation-cessation	PCT: 151 SOC: 151	Mortality (3 months): 20% vs. 14%, LOT: no difference
[24]	LRTI—ED Multicenter—USA	Initiation-cessation	PCT: 826 SOC: 830	LOT: 4.2 vs. 4.3 days, difference -0.05 (95% CI -0.6 to 0.5) Prescription of antimicrobials (30 days): 57% vs. 61.8% Length of hospital stay: 4.7 vs. 5.0 days
[25]	Fever $\geq 38.2\,^\circ\text{C}$—ED (main infection [40% respiratory]) Two-center—Netherlands	Initiation	PCT: 275 SOC: 276	Prescription of antimicrobials: 73% vs. 77%, $p = 0.28$ Readmission at ED (14 days): 7% vs. 10%, $p = 0.20$ Hospitalization: 74% vs. 81%, $p = 0.10$ Mortality (30 days): 2% vs. 4%, $p = 0.11$
[26] **	LRTI (requiring hospitalization)—ED Single-center—USA	Initiation-cessation	After: 174 Before: 200	LOT: 5 vs. 6 days, $p = 0.052$ LOT-pneumonia: 6 vs. 7 days, $p = 0.045$ LOT-COPD exacerbation: 3 vs. 4 days, $p = 0.01$
[27]	CAP—ED Multicenter—France	Initiation-cessation	PCT: 142 SOC: 143	LOT:10 vs. 9 days, $p = 0.21$ AE: 15% vs. 20%, difference 5% (95% CI: -4 to 14%) Mortality (30 days): 1% vs. 2%, $p > 0.05$
[28] ***	CAP and/or HCAP Single-center—Japan	Cessation cutoff 0.2 ng/mL	PCT: 116 SOC: 116	LOT: 8 vs. 11 days, $p < 0.001$ Relapse (30 days): 4.3% vs. 6.0%, $p = 0.5541$
[29]	Symptoms of acute heart failure—ED Multicenter—International	Initiation cutoff 0.2 ng/mL	PCT: 370 SOC: 372	Mortality (90 days): 10.3% vs. 8.2%, $p = 0.316$ Mortality (30 days): 6.8% vs. 4.3%, $p = 0.152$ Prescription of antimicrobials: 18% vs. 14%, $p = 0.145$ Rehospitalization (30 days): 17.3 vs. 9.7%, $p = 0.004$

* retrospective before–after study; ** prospective before–after study; *** patient-historical control study. Abbreviations: CAP—community-acquired pneumonia; COPD—chronic obstructive pulmonary disease; CI—confidence interval; ED—emergency department; HCAP—healthcare-associated pneumonia; ICU—intensive care unit; LOT—length of therapy; LRTI—lower respiratory tract infection; PCT—procalcitonin; SOC—standard-of-care.

2.2. Antimicrobial Stewardship through PCT-Guidance in Sepsis

Critically ill and sepsis patients are the next most commonly studied population for benefit following PCT-guidance [32–51]. The efficacy of existing trials is summarized in Table 2. The majority of participants suffered from LRTI and intra-abdominal or urinary infections were less common. The majority of RCTs were conducted before Sepsis-3 implementation. One concern is that specific subgroups of patients, like pregnant and immunosuppressed, have been excluded from participation. Most of trials conclude that a PCT strategy reduces antimicrobial treatment duration without increase in adverse events and unfavorable outcomes.

The PRORATA trial was the first large study evaluating PCT-guidance in ICU patients with suspicion of bacterial infection [36]. Three hundred and seven patients were randomized to PCT-guided treatment and 314 to SOC. For those in the PCT group, an algorithm of both initiation and cessation of antimicrobials was applied. When serum PCT was 0.5 ng/mL or more, physicians were encouraged to start antimicrobials and continue treatment until levels became less than 0.5 ng/mL in serial measurements or they decreased by at least 80% of the baseline value. The same algorithm was followed for every secondary infection episode until day 28 or discharge. The trial ended in a significant decrease in antimicrobial treatment duration from 14.3 days in SOC to 11.6 in PCT group ($p < 0.0001$). Mortality, relapse, and re-infection rate was similar between the two groups. There was however a trend for higher mortality with PCT-guidance after 60 days.

The largest SAPS trial so far incorporated this knowledge and was designed to evaluate a stopping algorithm based on serial PCT measurements [44]. In the PCT group, physicians were encouraged to stop antimicrobials when PCT was less than 0.5 ng/mL on two consecutive days or PCT decreased by at least 80% of the baseline value. Mean antimicrobial duration was 5 days for 761 patients allocated to PCT group compared to 7 days for 785 patients allocated to SOC ($p < 0.0001$). Surprisingly, SAPS investigators came across a novel, interesting finding; PCT-guidance reduced both 28-day (19.6% vs. 25%, p: 0.0122) and 1-year mortality (34.8% vs. 40.9%, p: 0.0158).

The recently published PROGRESS trial was the first trial conducted after the introduction of the Sepsis-3 definitions using the same stopping rule for antimicrobials as the SAPS trial [48]. PROGRESS was designed to provide an explanation of the findings of the SAPS trial on mortality. As a consequence, the primary endpoint of PROGRESS was the effect of long-term infectious complications in the critically ill, i.e., the incidence of new infection by multi-drug resistant organisms (MDRO) and *Clostridioides difficile* and mortality associated with baseline infection by MDRO or *C. difficile*. The incidence of these long-term complications after six months was 7.2% in the PCT and 15.3% in the SOC group (p: 0.045). Alongside this benefit, PCT guidance, decreased the length of antimicrobial treatment (5 vs. 7 days; $p < 0.0001$); and decreased 28-day mortality (15.2% vs. 28.2%; p: 0.02) among the 125 patients allocated in the PCT group compared to 131 patients allocated in the SOC group. The incidence of antibiotic-associated adverse events was strikingly decreased using PCT-guidance, in particular diarrhea and acute kidney injury (AKI); in the SOC arm, 36.6% of patients presented diarrhea and 17.6% AKI, compared to 19.2% (p: 0.002) and 7.2% (p: 0.01) in the PCT-guidance arm, respectively. Interestingly, the incidence of gut colonization by MDRO and *C. difficile* was similar between the two groups but the risk for clinical infection was significantly higher in colonized patients in the SOC but not in the PCT arm. These results indicate that long-term antibiotic exposure in the SOC arm could either affect the integrity of the mucosal barrier or modulate the composition of the gut microbiota resulting in the increased incidence of infections by MDRO and *C. difficile*.

Two trials similar in design to PROGRESS, are ongoing in France. The MultiCov trial (NCT04334850) is randomizing patients with severe COVID-19 into PCT-guided treatment or SOC. PCT-guidance is accompanied by sampling of respiratory secretions with multiplex PCR to identify bacterial pathogens [52]. The main aim of the study is to show a reduction in antibiotic exposure in the era of COVID-19 having as primary endpoint the number of antibiotic-free days until day 28 and among secondary outcomes the rate of colonization and/or infection by MDRO or *C. difficile* [53]. The MULTI-CAP trial randomizes patients with severe community-acquired pneumonia in the ICU to a combined PCT/multiplex respiratory PCR arm versus SOC; primary endpoint is antibiotic-free days until day 28.

The benefit disclosed by the larger ProHOSP and SAPS trial was further corroborated by smaller studies from developing countries [49–51] and meta-analyses [54–62]. A first meta-analysis was published in 2018 including a total of 4482 ICU patients and sub-analyzing patients meeting Sepsis-3 criteria [58]. PCT-guidance reduced 28-day mortality (OR 0.89; 95% CI: 0.80–0.99; p: 0.03) and mean duration of antibiotic treatment (−1.19 days; 95% CI: −1.73 to −0.66; $p < 0.0001$). Meta-analyses also confirmed reduction of antimicrobial treatment by PCT-guidance in special populations, such as patients with bacteremia [63], renal failure [64], or among the elderly [65]. Interestingly, some meta-analyses support that PCT-guidance is associated with decreased antimicrobial consumption and mortality only if cessation algorithms are applied [58]. A summary of published meta-analyses evaluating PCT-guidance is presented in Table 3 [54–66].

Table 2. Summary of randomized trials evaluating Procalcitonin (PCT)-guided antimicrobial treatment in critically ill patients with severe infection/sepsis in the Intensive Care Unit (ICU).

Ref	Trial Setting	PCT Algorithm Applied	N of Patients	Main Results
[32]	Severe sepsis and septic shock (65% respiratory infections) Single-center—Switzerland	Cessation if ≥90% decrease or PCT < 0.25 ng/mL	PCT: 31 SOC: 37	LOT: 3.5 vs. 6 days, $p = 0.15$ (ITT) 6 vs. 10 days, $p = 0.003$ (PP) Length of ICU stay: 4 vs. 7 days, $p = 0.02$
[33]	Severe sepsis after intraabdominal surgery Single-center—Germany	Cessation if PCT < 1 ng/mL for 3 consecutive days	PCT: 14 SOC: 13	LOT: 6.6 vs. 8.3 days, $p < 0.001$
[34]	Sepsis Single-center—Germany	Cessation if PCT < 1 ng/mL or ≥65% decrease for 3 serial days	PCT: 57 SOC: 53	LOT: 5.9 vs. 7.9 days, $p < 0.001$ Length of ICU stay: 15.5 vs. 17.7 days, $p = 0.046$
[35]	VAP Multicenter—Switzerland and USA	Initiation-cessation	PCT: 50 SOC: 51	LOT: 7 vs. 11 days, $p = 0.044$
[36]	Sepsis (mainly [70%] respiratory infections) Multicenter—France	Initiation-cessation	PCT: 307 SOC: 314	LOT: 6.1 vs. 9.9 days, $p < 0.0001$ Relapse: absolute difference 1.4% Reinfection: absolute difference 3.6%
[37]	Suspected infection Multicenter—Denmark	Up-escalation when PCT > 1.0 ng/mL	PCT: 604 SOC: 596	Significantly higher antimicrobial consumption in PCT group
[38]	Suspected infection (60% respiratory infections) Single-center—Belgium	Initiation	PCT: 258 SOC: 251	Antimicrobial consumption (% days in ICU): 62.6 vs. 57.7, $p = 0.11$
[39]	Acute pancreatitis Single-center—China	Initiation-cessation PCT cutoff: 0.5 ng/mL	PCT: 35 SOC: 36	LOT: 10.89 vs. 16.06 days, $p < 0.001$ Length of stay: 16.66 vs. 23.81 days, $p < 0.001$
[40]	Sepsis Single-center—Brazil	Cessation if PCT < 0.5 ng/mL or ≥90% decrease	PCT: 42 SOC: 39	LOT: 10 vs. 11 days, $p = 0.44$ (ITT) 9 vs. 13 days, $p = 0.008$ (PP)
[41]	Sepsis (60% respiratory infections) Two-center—Brazil	Cessation PCT < 0.1 ng/mL or ≥90% from baseline CRP < 25 mg/L or ≥50% decrease from baseline	PCT: 50 CRP: 47	LOT: 7 vs. 6 days, $p = 0.06$ Mortality: 32.7% vs. 33.3%, $p = 1.000$
[42]	Sepsis Multicenter—France	Initiation-cessation	PCT: 27 SOC: 26	Patients (%) under treatment at day 5: 67 vs. 81, $p = 0.24$
[43]	Suspected sepsis Multicenter—Australia	Initiation-cessation Cessation when PCT < 0.10 ng/mL or ≥90% decrease from baseline	PCT: 196 SOC: 198	LOT: 9 vs. 11 days, $p = 0.58$ Total doses of antimicrobials: 1200 vs. 1500, $p = 0.001$

Table 2. Cont.

Ref	Trial Setting	PCT Algorithm Applied	N of Patients	Main Results
[44]	Sepsis Multicenter—Netherlands	Cessation if PCT < 0.5 ng/mL or ≥80% from baseline for 2 serial days	PCT: 761 SOC: 785	LOT: 5 vs. 7 days, $p < 0.0001$ Mortality (28 days):19.6% vs. 25%, $p = 0.0122$ Mortality (1 year): 34.8% vs. 40.9%, $p = 0.0158$
[45]	Sepsis Multicenter—Germany	Cessation if PCT < 1.0 ng/mL or ≥50% decrease	PCT: 552 SOC: 537	Mortality: 25.6% vs. 28.2%, $p = 0.34$ Antimicrobials/1000 ICU days: 823 vs. 862, decrease 4.5%, $p = 0.02$
[46]	Severe sepsis and/or septic shock Multicenter—Korea	Cessation if PCT < 0.5 ng/mL or ≥90% from baseline	PCT: 23 SOC: 29	LOT:10 vs. 13 days, $p = 0.078$ (ITT), 8 vs. 14 days, $p < 0.001$ (PP) Mortality (28 days): 17% vs. 21%, $p = 0.709$
[47] *	VAP Multicenter—France	Initiation-cessation	PCT: 76 No-PCT: 81	LOT: 8 vs. 9.5 days, $p = 0.02$ Death and/or relapse: 51.3% vs. 46.9%, $p = 0.47$
[48]	Sepsis-3 Multicenter—Greece	Cessation if PCT < 0.5 ng/mL or ≥80% decrease from baseline	PCT: 125 SOC: 131	LOT: 5 vs. 10 days; $p < 0.001$ Mortality (28 days): 15.2% vs. 28.2%, $p = 0.02$
[49] **	Surgical trauma Single center—South Africa	Cessation if PCT < 0.5 ng/mL or ≥80% from baseline	PCT: 40 SOC: 40	LOT: 9.3 vs. 10.9 days, $p = 0.10$ Mortality: 15% vs. 30%, $p = 0.045$
[50]	VAP Single center—Malaysia	Cessation if PCT < 0.5 ng/mL or ≥80% from baseline	PCT: 43 SOC: 42	LOT: 10.28 vs. 11.52 days, difference −1.25 (95%CI −2.48 to 0.01), $p = 0.049$
[51]	Sepsis and septic shock Single center—India	Cessation if PCT < 0.01 ng/mL or ≥80% from baseline	PCT: 45 SOC: 45	LOT: 4.98 vs. 7.73 days, $p < 0.001$ Length of ICU stay: 5.98 vs. 8.80 days, $p < 0.001$ Secondary infections: 4.4% vs. 26.7%, $p = 0.014$ Mortality: 8.9% vs. 15.6%, $p = 0.522$ Readmission: no difference

* prospective observational trial; ** prospective two-period cross-over trial. Abbreviations: CI—confidence interval; ICU—intensive care unit; ITT—intention to treat; LOT—length of therapy; PCT—procalcitonin; PP—per protocol; SOC—standard-of-care; VAP—ventilator-associated pneumonia.

Table 3. Summary of meta-analyses evaluating Procalcitonin (PCT)-guided antimicrobial treatment in critically ill patients.

Ref	N of Trials	N of Patients	Focus of Interest	Main Results
[54]	10	1215	NA	Antibiotic duration (days): −1.28 days (95% CI −1.95 to −0.61) Mortality: RR 0.81 (95% CI 0.65 to 1.01)
[55]	13	5136	Antibiotic Initiation, Cessation, or Mixed Strategies	Antibiotic duration (days): −1.66 (95% CI −2.36 to −0.96) Mortality: RR 0.87 (95% CI 0.76 to 0.98)
[56]	26	6708	Acute respiratory infections	Antibiotic duration (days): −2.4 (95% CI −2.71 to −2.15) Mortality: OR 0.83 (95% CI 0.70 to 0.99) Antibiotic-related side-effects: OR 0.68 (95% CI 0.57 to 0.82)
[57]	11	4482	Subgroup of sepsis-3	Antibiotic duration (days): −1.19 (95% CI −1.73 to −0.66) Mortality: OR 0.89 (95% CI 0.80 to 0.99) Sepsis-3, OR 0.86 (95% CI 0.76 to 0.98)
[58]	15		Antibiotic Initiation, Cessation, or Mixed Strategies	Antibiotic duration (days): −1.26 ($p < 0.001$) and −3.10 ($p = 0.04$) for cessation and mixed strategies, respectively Mortality: OR 1.00 (95% CI 0.86 to 1.15), 0.87 (95% CI 0.77 to 0.98), and 1.01 (95% CI 0.80 to 1.29) for the initiation, cessation, and mixed procalcitonin strategies, respectively
[59]	10	3489	Suspected or confirmed sepsis	Antibiotic duration (days): −1.49 (95% CI −2.27 to −0.71) Mortality: RR 0.90 (95% CI 0.79 to 1.03)
[60]	16	5158	Subgroup (5 trials) with high algorithm adherence	Mortality: RR 0.89 (95% CI 0.83 to 0.97) In high algorithm adherence, RR 0.93 (95% CI 0.71 to 1.22)
[61]	16	6452	NA	Antibiotic duration (days): −0.99 (95% CI −1.85 to −0.13), $p = 0.02$ Mortality: OR 0.90 (95% CI 0.80 to 1.01)

Table 3. Cont.

Ref	N of Trials	N of Patients	Focus of Interest	Main Results
[62]	14	4744	NA	Antibiotic duration (days): −1.23 (95% CI −1.61 to −0.85) Mortality: OR 0.91 (95% CI 0.82 to 1.01)
[63]	13	523 (IPD)	Positive blood culture	Antibiotic duration (days): −2.86 (95% CI −4.88 to −0.84) Mortality: 16.6% vs. 20.0%, $p = 0.263$
[64]	15	5002 (IPD)	Kidney function (3 groups: GFR > 90, GFR 15–89 and GFR < 15)	Antibiotic duration (days): −2.06 (95% CI −2.87 to −1.25), −1.72 (95% CI −2.29 to −1.16), −2.49 (95% CI −3.59 to −1.40), $p_{interaction} = 0.336$. Overall, −2.01 (95% CI −2.45 to −1.58) Mortality: OR 1.08 (95% CI 0.79 to 1.49), 0.74 (95% CI 0.63 to 0.87), 1.03 (95% CI 0.83 to 1.29), $p_{interaction} = 0.888$. Overall, 0.88 (95% CI 0.78 to 0.98)
[65]	28	9421 (IPD)	Age (4 groups: <75, 75–80, 81–85 and >85 years)	Antibiotic duration per age group (days): Less than 75 years: −1.99 (95% CI −2.36 to −1.62); 75–80 years: −1.98 (95% CI −2.94 to −1.02); 81–85 years: −2.20 (95% CI −3.15 to −1.25), more than 85 years: −2.10 (95% CI −3.29 to −0.91), $p_{interaction} = 0.654$. Overall, −2.01 (95% CI −2.32 to −1.69) Mortality: Less than 75 years: OR 0.87 (95% CI 0.76 to 1.00); 75–80 years 0.86 (95% CI 0.67 to 1.10); 81–85 years 1.19 (95% CI 0.76 to 1.06), $p_{interaction} = 0.891$. Overall, 0.90 (95% CI 0.81 to 1.00)
[66]	12	42,921	NA	Antibiotic duration (days): 1.98 days (95% CI: −2.76, −1.21) Mortality: RR 0.89 (95% CI 0.79 to 0.99) ICU-length of stay (days): −1.21 (95% CI −4.16 to 1.74)

Abbreviations: CI—confidence interval; GFR—glomerular filtration rate; IPD—individual patient data; NA—non applicable; OR—odds ratio; PCT—procalcitonin; RR—risk ratio.

2.3. Real-World Data

Evidence supporting PCT-guidance for antimicrobial stewardship in critically ill patients, as already discussed, is from RCTs with different degrees of compliance to the PCT rule applied in each RCT, ranging from 44% up to 97%. It has not yet been clear if low adherence to PCT algorithms interferes with results and affects antimicrobial duration and mortality. Results of RCTs may not be in alignment with real-world data. Treating physicians participating in a RCT are influenced in decision making as they may feel under observation from the Sponsor or trial coordinators; this is namely the "Hawthorne effect" [67]. With this in mind, real-world evidence is mandatory. Soon after ProHOSP trial has been published, real world data supported compliance of physicians with the suggested algorithm as high as 72.5% [68].

Several implementation trials have investigated the effect of PCT-guidance in antimicrobial stewardship programs [69–77]. Main conclusions of these trials include (i) reduction in antimicrobial consumption; (ii) reduction in length of stay; (iii) reduction in hospitalization cost; and (iv) no difference in infection-relapse of rehospitalization rate. Best implementation of the biomarker in real-world settings requires constant education of treating physicians for rightful use [78,79].

2.4. Antimicrobial Stewardship through Other Biomarkers

Other biomarkers have been also tested in antibiotic stewardship programs like serum C-reactive protein (CRP), serum presepsin, and interleukin (IL)-1β/IL-18 in bronchoalveolar lavage (BAL).

In a former trial, CRP was compared to PCT for the early stop of antibiotics. Discontinuation of antibiotics in the PCT arm was advised by more than 90% baseline decreases (n = 49) and in the CRP arm by more than 50% baseline decreases or values less than 25 mg/L (n = 45) [41]. Both strategies were non-inferior in terms of length of treatment, relapse rate, and ICU length of stay. A recent trial compared in a 1:1:1 randomization pattern, the clinical effectiveness of CRP-guided stop of antibiotics with fixed 7- and 14-day antibiotic durations in 504 hospitalized patients with gram-negative bacteremia [80]. Median antibiotic duration in the CRP group was seven days; clinical failure between the three arms of treatment was non-inferior. In another open-label RCT, CRP-guided antimicrobial treatment was compared to SOC in 130 ICU patients with sepsis and/or septic shock [81]. In the CRP arm, the biomarker was measured after five days from start of antibiotics and antibiotics were stopped when CRP decrease more than 50% or when it was found less than 35 mg/L. This strategy did reduce antibiotic duration or 28-day mortality.

Presepsin is the soluble form of CD14 (sCD14), an anchored glycoprotein expressed on monocytes and macrophages, serving as a receptor for bacterial lipopolysaccharide (LPS) [82]. Compared to CRP and PCT, presepsin appears advantageous in sepsis diagnosis, as it rises early, already in the first two hours after an infection. Recently, Xiao et al., conducted a prospective, multicenter, not randomized trial in China, comparing presepsin-guidance to SOC in sepsis [83]. In the presepsin group, physicians were advised to stop the antibiotics by serum concentrations lower than 350 pg/mL or any baseline decrease more than 80%. Antibiotic adjustment was encouraged when the blood presepsin concentration did not decline. Although the primary outcome (days without antibiotics at day 28) was achieved, mortality did not differ between treatment arms.

In a recent trial conducted in the United Kingdom, 210 ICU patients with suspicion of ventilator-associated pneumonia (VAP) were allocated to a biomarker-guided approach (n: 104) or SOC (n: 106) [84]. In the biomarker-guided recommendation group measurements of IL-1β and IL-18 were performed in the bronchoalveolar lavage (BAL), and if concentrations were below a previously validated cutoff, clinicians were advised that VAP was unlikely and withheld antibiotics. The primary outcome was antibiotic-free days in the seven days following BAL; the trial did not achieve this endpoint.

2.5. Antimicrobial Stewardship Using Biomarkers in the COVID-19 Era

In December 2019, a novel coronavirus, namely SARS-CoV-2, spread rapidly around the globe causing millions of cases of pneumonia leading to a rapid increase in hospitalizations and deaths. Patients presenting with COVID-19 pneumonia share common features with bacterial pneumonia (fever, cough, dyspnea, infiltrates in chest X-ray, and elevated inflammation markers) making the differential diagnosis troublesome. In severe cases, COVID-19 may resemble bacterial sepsis leading to multiorgan failure and requiring organ support in the ICU [85]. Although data are very heterogenous, unlike other viral respiratory diseases, bacterial co-infection at the time of hospital admission is rare in COVID-19; this may occur during hospital and/or ICU stay. A recent systematic review reports a rate of 8% of COVID-19 bacterial coinfection; surprisingly, the proportion of patients receiving antimicrobials is as high as 72% [86]. In such case, biomarkers, mainly PCT, may be useful in reducing unnecessary antimicrobial consumption.

A number of small case-series support that PCT is not elevated in COVID-19 patients, in contrast to other inflammation markers like CRP and ferritin [87–89]. The largest of these observational studies, conducted in New York, reports that only 16.9% of patients have PCT levels 0.5 ng/mL or more at hospital admission [90] and such high levels are associated with development of critical disease, admission in the ICU and increased risk for death [91–93]. A recent meta-analysis of 10 cohort studies including a total of 7716 patients estimated a pooled risk of 1.77 (95% CI, 1.38 to 2.29) for severe and critical COVID-19 by elevated PCT levels at admission, although results are highly heterogenous (I^2:85.6%) [94]. Similarly, rise in PCT is associated with secondary bacterial infections, such as VAP and bacteremia [91,95–97]. PCT levels less than 0.25 ng/mL have been suggested as an optimal cut-off to rule out bacterial co-infection (negative predictive value 81%) and levels more than 1 ng/mL as optimal cutoff to rule in bacterial co-infection (positive predictive value 93%) [95].

It is questionable if pre-treatment with dexamethasone and tocilizumab in these patients is limiting the diagnostic performance of biomarkers. Kooistra et al. studied 190 ICU patients with COVID-19 having received different immunomodulatory agents and concluded that after treatment with dexamethasone and/or tocilizumab, CRP levels remain suppressed in case of a secondary bacterial infection but that the kinetics of PCT were not affected [98]. Thus, it is reasonable that CRP, which is elevated by the COVID-19-driven hyperinflammation and is suppressed by the immunomodulatory treatment does not represent the optimal biomarker to screen for bacterial complications in critically ill COVID-19. In contrast, PCT may inform about the early diagnosis of bacterial superinfection.

Real world data of PCT-guidance in COVID-19 support its use for a judicious antimicrobial approach. In a small retrospective cohort of 48 patients, median duration of antimicrobials was shorter if at least one PCT measurement was performed [99]. Similar results were also reported by Calderon et al. [100]. Williams et al. implemented a PCT guideline in the first 48 h after hospital admission of COVID-19 patients to withhold antibiotics with PCT less than 25 ng/mL [101]. Adherence to the guideline was high (77%). This strategy ended in lower defined daily doses (DDDs) per day alive, lower 28-day mortality, lower intubation, and ICU-admission rate. Staub et al. reported an increase in the antimicrobial usage during the COVID-19 pandemic compared with the pre-COVID era, but this usage decreased again after implementation of a guidance team using biomarkers [102]. A summary of PCT trials in COVID-19 patients is provided in Table 4.

Table 4. Summary of trials evaluating Procalcitonin (PCT) in COVID-19 patients.

Ref	Type and Setting of Study	N of Patients	Severity of COVID-19	Main Results
[87]	Observational February-March 2020 Single-center, USA	21	Critical ICU patients	Median PCT 1.8 (0.12–9.56)
[88]	January-February 2020 Single-center, Wuhan China	138	Hospitalized Both critical/non-critical	PCT ≥ 0.05 ng/mL in 35.5% of patients Higher levels in patients requiring ICU
[90]	Retrospective case series March 2020 Two-center, USA	393	Hospitalized Both critical/non-critical	PCT ≥ 0.05 ng/mL in 16.9% of patients Higher levels in patients requiring intubation
[91]	Retrospective observational March-April 2020 Single-center, USA	324	Hospitalized Both critical/non-critical	PCT for prediction of bacteremia, AUC 0.81 (0.64–0.98) PCT for prediction of bacterial pneumonia, AUC 0.75 (0.64–0.86)
[92]	Retrospective observational March-April 2020 Multicenter, UK	224	Hospitalized Both critical/non-critical	PCT > 0.5 ng/mL in 16.5% of patients PCT associated with increased risk of death ($p = 0.0004$)
[93]	Retrospective observational March-June 2020 Multicenter, Spain	777	Critical ICU patients	PCT 0.64 (0.17–1.44) ng/mL in non-survivors compared to 0.23 (0.11–0.60) ng/mi in survivors, $p < 0.01$
[95]	Observational Single-center, Netherlands	66	Critical ICU patients	PCT > 1.00 ng/mL at admission rule in secondary bacterial infection PCT < 0.25 ng/mL at admission rule out secondary bacterial infection
[96]	Retrospective observational March-June 2020 Single-center, UK	65	Critical ICU patients	PCT rise in 81.5% of patients PCT rise in 97% of patients with confirmed VAT/VAP and/or BSI
[97]	Retrospective observational March-October 2020 Single-center, Germany	99	Hospitalized Both critical/non-critical	PCT of patients with secondary bacterial infection 0.4 ng/mL versus 0.1 of those without, $p = 0.016$ cut-off 0.55 ng/mL: sensitivity 91%, specificity 81% for bacterial infection

Abbreviations: AUC—area under the curve; BSI—bloodstream infection; ICU—intensive care unit; PCT—procalcitonin; VAT—ventilator-associated tracheobronchitis; VAP—ventilator-associated pneumonia.

In contrast with a plethora of RCTs evaluating PCT-guidance in sepsis, such high-quality data are missing for COVID-19. MultiCov is an ongoing RCT in France, evaluating PCT-guided treatment in combination with FilmArray syndromic diagnostics compared to SOC to prove a benefit in the number of antibiotic-free days, mortality, rate of bacterial superinfection and rate of colonization/infection by MDRO and/or *C. difficile* (NCT04334850) [52]. Results of the trial will be of great interest to guide appropriate antimicrobial administration in the COVID-19 era.

3. Materials and Methods

To address the aim of this review and to present recent evidence in biomarker-guidance in the critically ill with emphasis on antimicrobial stewardship, the authors searched independently "Pubmed" and the database "clinicaltrials.gov" under the terms: "sepsis", "COVID-19", "infection", "critically ill", "intensive care unit", "biomarker guidance", "guided treatment", "procalcitonin", and "c-reactive protein" about randomized clinical trials and observational studies conducted in humans aged equal to or older than 18 years old, published in English, with emphasis on trials published in the last decade (2012–2022). The literature search yielded 11,791 records; after removal of duplicates and records with irrelevant titles, 611 were screened in full-text by the reviewers. After applying exclusion criteria, 102 studies were finally analyzed (Figure 1).

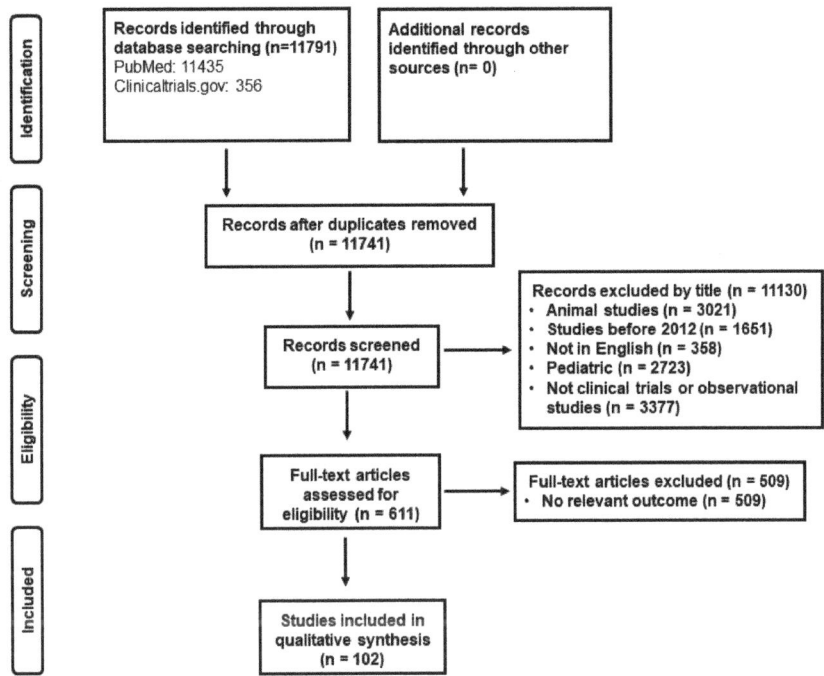

Figure 1. Study selection.

4. Conclusions

Biomarkers, mainly procalcitonin, may guide antimicrobial treatment with safety in two directions; (i) improve patient outcomes by reduction in antibiotic-associated adverse events and (ii) globally reduce the high burden of antimicrobial resistance. Procalcitonin-guidance of antimicrobial treatment for the critically ill decreases the length of antimicrobial treatment, the length of stay (Hospital/ICU), and the cost of hospitalization and in parallel, the strategy improves both short- and long-term outcomes including mortality and rate of secondary infections by MDRO and *C. difficile*. In the COVID-19 era, data suggest a crucial role of the biomarker to reduce unnecessary antimicrobial overuse. Thus, biomarkers should be incorporated in antimicrobial stewardship programs and physicians' education is key for their appropriate application in every day clinical practice.

Author Contributions: E.K. drafted the first version of the manuscript and E.J.G.-B. critically revised for intellectual content. All authors have read and agreed to the published version of the manuscript.

Funding: This study was funded by the Hellenic Institute for the Study of Sepsis.

Data Availability Statement: All data are presented throughout the manuscript.

Conflicts of Interest: E.J.G.-B. has received honoraria from Abbott CH, bioMérieux, Brahms GmbH, GSK, InflaRx GmbH, Sobi and XBiotech Inc; independent educational grants from Abbott CH, AxisShield, bioMérieux Inc, InflaRx GmbH, Johnson & Johnson, MSD, Sobi and XBiotech Inc.; and funding from the Horizon2020 Marie-Curie Project European Sepsis Academy (granted to the National and Kapodistrian University of Athens), and the Horizon 2020 European Grants ImmunoSep and RISCinCOVID (granted to the Hellenic Institute for the Study of Sepsis). E.K. reports no conflicts of interest.

References

1. Kumar, A.; Roberts, D.; Wood, K.E.; Light, B.; Parrillo, J.E.; Sharma, S.; Suppes, R.; Feinstein, D.; Zanotti, S.; Taiberg, L.; et al. Duration of hypotension before initiation of effective antimicrobial therapy is the critical determinant of survival in human septic shock. *Crit. Care Med.* **2006**, *34*, 1589–1596. [CrossRef]
2. Evans, L.; Rhodes, A.; Alhazzani, W.; Antonelli, M.; Coopersmith, C.M.; French, C.; Machado, F.R.; Mcintyre, L.; Ostermann, M.; Prescott, H.C.; et al. Surviving sepsis campaign: International guidelines for management of sepsis and septic shock 2021. *Intensive Care Med.* **2021**, *47*, 1181–1247. [CrossRef]
3. Antimicrobial Resistance Collaborators. Global burden of bacterial antimicrobial resistance in 2019: A systematic analysis. *Lancet* **2022**, *399*, 629–655. [CrossRef]
4. The Biomarker Definitions Working Group. Biomarkers and surrogate endpoints: Preferred definitions and conceptual framework. *Clin. Pharmacol. Ther.* **2001**, *69*, 89–95. [CrossRef]
5. Sankar, V.; Webster, N.R. Clinical application of sepsis biomarkers. *J. Anesth.* **2013**, *27*, 269–283. [CrossRef]
6. Pierrakos, C.; Vincent, J.L. Sepsis biomarkers: A review. *Crit. Care* **2010**, *14*, R15. [CrossRef]
7. Christ-Crain, M.; Jaccard-Stolz, D.; Bingisser, R.; Gencay, M.M.; Huber, P.R.; Tamm, M.; Müller, B. Effect of procalcitonin-guided treatment on antibiotic use and outcome in lower respiratory tract infections: Cluster-randomised, single-blinded intervention trial. *Lancet* **2004**, *363*, 600–607. [CrossRef]
8. Christ-Crain, M.; Stolz, D.; Bingisser, R.; Muller, C.; Miedinger, D.; Huber, P.R.; Zimmerli, W.; Harbarth, S.; Tamm, M.; Muller, B. Procalcitonin guidance of antibiotic therapy in community-acquired pneumonia: A randomized trial. *Am. J. Respir. Crit. Care Med.* **2006**, *174*, 84–93. [CrossRef]
9. Stolz, D.; Christ-Crain, M.; Bingisser, R.; Leuppi, J.; Miedinger, D.; Müller, C.; Huber, P.; Müller, B.; Tamm, M. Antibiotic treatment of exacerbations of COPD: A randomized, controlled trial comparing procalcitonin-guidance with standard therapy. *Chest* **2007**, *131*, 9–19. [CrossRef]
10. Briel, M.; Schuetz, P.; Mueller, B.; Young, J.; Schild, U.; Nusbaumer, C.; Périat, P.; Bucher, H.C.; Christ-Crain, M. Procalcitonin-guided antibiotic use vs a standard approach for acute respiratory tract infections in primary care. *Arch. Intern. Med.* **2008**, *168*, 2000–2008. [CrossRef]
11. Kristoffersen, K.; Søgaard, O.; Wejse, C.; Black, F.; Greve, T.; Tarp, B.; Storgaard, M.; Sodemann, M. Antibiotic treatment interruption of suspected lower respiratory tract infections based on a single procalcitonin measurement at hospital admission—A randomized trial. *Clin. Microbiol. Infect.* **2009**, *15*, 481–487. [CrossRef]
12. Schuetz, P.; Christ-Crain, M.; Thomann, R.; Falconnier, C.; Wolbers, M.; Widmer, I.; Neidert, S.; Fricker, T.; Blum, C.; Schild, U.; et al. Effect of procalcitonin-based guidelines vs standard guidelines on antibiotic use in lower respiratory tract infections: The ProHOSP randomized controlled trial. *JAMA* **2009**, *302*, 1059–1066. [CrossRef]
13. Burkhardt, O.; Ewig, S.; Haagen, U.; Giersdorf, S.; Hartmann, O.; Wegscheider, K.; Hummers-Pradier, E.; Welte, T. Procalcitonin guidance and reduction of antibiotic use in acute respiratory tract infection. *Eur. Respir. J.* **2010**, *36*, 601–607. [CrossRef]
14. Long, W.; Deng, X.; Zhang, Y.; Lu, G.; Xie, J.; Tang, J. Procalcitonin guidance for reduction of antibiotic use in low-risk outpatients with community-acquired pneumonia. *Respirology* **2011**, *16*, 819–824. [CrossRef]
15. Tang, J.; Long, W.; Yan, L.; Zhang, Y.; Xie, J.; Lu, G.; Yang, C. Procalcitonin guided antibiotic therapy of acute exacerbations of asthma: A randomized controlled trial. *BMC Infect. Dis.* **2013**, *13*, 596. [CrossRef]
16. Ogasawara, T.; Umezawa, H.; Naito, Y.; Takeuchi, T.; Kato, S.; Yano, T.; Kasamatsu, N.; Hashizume, I. Procalcitonin-guided antibiotic therapy in aspiration pneumonia and an assessment of the continuation of oral intake. *Respir. Investig.* **2014**, *52*, 107–113. [CrossRef]
17. Long, W.; Li, L.-J.; Huang, G.-Z.; Zhang, X.-M.; Zhang, Y.-C.; Tang, J.-G.; Zhang, Y.; Lu, G. Procalcitonin guidance for reduction of antibiotic use in patients hospitalized with severe acute exacerbations of asthma: A randomized controlled study with 12-month follow-up. *Crit. Care* **2014**, *18*, 471. [CrossRef]
18. Verduri, A.; Luppi, F.; D'amico, R.; Balduzzi, S.; Vicini, R.; Liverani, A.; Ruggieri, V.; Plebani, M.; Barbaro, M.P.F.; Spanevello, A.; et al. Antibiotic treatment of severe exacerbations of chronic obstructive pulmonary disease with procalcitonin: A randomized noninferiority trial. *PLoS ONE* **2015**, *10*, e0118241. [CrossRef]
19. Branche, A.R.; Walsh, E.E.; Vargas, R.; Hulbert, B.; Formica, M.A.; Baran, A.; Peterson, D.R.; Falsey, A.R. Serum procalcitonin measurement and viral testing to guide antibiotic use for respiratory infections in hospitalized adults: A randomized controlled trial. *J. Infect. Dis.* **2015**, *212*, 1692–1700. [CrossRef]

20. Corti, C.; Fally, M.; Fabricius-Bjerre, A.; Mortensen, K.; Jensen, B.N.; Andreassen, H.; Porsbjerg, C.; Knudsen, J.D.; Jensen, J.-U. Point-of-care procalcitonin test to reduce antibiotic exposure in patients hospitalized with acute exacerbation of COPD. *Int. J. Chronic Obstr. Pulm. Dis.* **2016**, *11*, 1381–1389. [CrossRef]
21. Ulm, L.; Hoffmann, S.; Nabavi, D.; Hermans, M.; Mackert, B.-M.; Hamilton, F.; Schmehl, I.; Jungehuelsing, G.-J.; Montaner, J.; Bustamante, A.; et al. The randomized controlled STRAWINSKI trial: Procalcitonin-guided antibiotic therapy after stroke. *Front. Neurol.* **2017**, *8*, 153. [CrossRef]
22. Bremmer, D.N.; DiSilvio, B.E.; Hammer, C.; Beg, M.; Vishwanathan, S.; Speredelozzi, D.; Moffa, M.A.; Hu, K.; Abdulmassih, R.; Makadia, J.T.; et al. Impact of procalcitonin guidance on management of adults hospitalized with chronic obstructive pulmonary disease exacerbations. *J. Gen. Intern. Med.* **2018**, *33*, 692–697. [CrossRef]
23. Daubin, C.; Valette, X.; Thiollière, F.; Mira, J.P.; Hazera, P.; Annane, D.; Labbe, V.; Floccard, B.; Fournel, F.; Terzi, N.; et al. Procalcitonin algorithm to guide initial antibiotic therapy in acute exacerbations of COPD admitted to the ICU: A randomized multicenter study. *Intensive Care Med.* **2018**, *44*, 428–437. [CrossRef]
24. Huang, D.T.; Yealy, D.M.; Filbin, M.R.; Brown, A.M.; Chang, C.-C.H.; Doi, Y.; Donnino, M.W.; Fine, J.; Fine, M.J.; Fischer, M.A.; et al. Procalcitonin-guided use of antibiotics for lower respiratory tract infection. *N. Engl. J. Med.* **2018**, *379*, 236–249. [CrossRef]
25. van der Does, Y.; Limper, M.; Jie, K.E.; Schuit, S.C.E.; Jansen, H.; Pernot, N.; van Rosmalen, J.; Poley, M.J.; Ramakers, C.; Patka, P.; et al. Procalcitonin-guided antibiotic therapy in patients with fever in a general emergency department population: A multicentre non-inferiority randomized clinical trial (HiTEMP study). *Clin. Microbiol. Infect.* **2018**, *24*, 1282–1289. [CrossRef]
26. Townsend, J.; Adams, V.; Galiatsatos, P.; Pearse, D.; Pantle, H.; Masterson, M.; Kisuule, F.; Jacob, E.; Kiruthi, C.; Ortiz, P.; et al. Procalcitonin-guided antibiotic therapy reduces antibiotic use for lower respiratory tract infections in a united states medical center: Results of a clinical trial. *Open Forum Infect. Dis.* **2018**, *5*, ofy327. [CrossRef]
27. Montassier, E.; Javaudin, F.; Moustafa, F.; Nandjou, D.; Maignan, M.; Hardouin, J.-B.; Annoot, C.; Ogielska, M.; Orer, P.-L.; Schotté, T.; et al. Guideline-based clinical assessment versus procalcitonin-guided antibiotic use in pneumonia: A pragmatic randomized trial. *Ann. Emerg. Med.* **2019**, *74*, 580–591. [CrossRef]
28. Akagi, T.; Nagata, N.; Wakamatsu, K.; Harada, T.; Miyazaki, H.; Takeda, S.; Ushijima, S.; Aoyama, T.; Yoshida, Y.; Yatsugi, H.; et al. Procalcitonin-guided antibiotic discontinuation might shorten the duration of antibiotic treatment without increasing pneumonia recurrence. *Am. J. Med. Sci.* **2019**, *358*, 33–44. [CrossRef]
29. Möckel, M.; De Boer, R.A.; Slagman, A.; Von Haehling, S.; Schou, M.; Vollert, J.O.; Wiemer, J.C.; Ebmeyer, S.; Martín-Sánchez, F.J.; Maisel, A.S.; et al. Improve management of acute heart failure with ProcAlCiTonin in EUrope: Results of the randomized clinical trial IMPACT EU Biomarkers in Cardiology (BIC)18. *Eur. J. Heart Fail.* **2020**, *22*, 267–275. [CrossRef]
30. Metlay, J.P.; Waterer, G.W.; Long, A.C.; Anzueto, A.; Brozek, J.; Crothers, K.; Cooley, L.A.; Dean, N.C.; Fine, M.J.; Flanders, S.A.; et al. Diagnosis and treatment of adults with community-acquired pneumonia, an official clinical practice guideline of the American thoracic society and infectious diseases society of America. *Am. J. Respir. Crit. Care Med.* **2019**, *200*, e45–e67. [CrossRef]
31. U.S. Food & Drug Administration. FDA News Release: FDA Clears Test to Help Manage Antibiotic Treatment for Lower Respiratory Tract Infections and Sepsis. 2017. Available online: https://www.fda.gov/news-events/press-announcements/fda-clears-test-help-manage-antibiotic-treatment-lower-respiratory-tract-infections-and-sepsis (accessed on 29 January 2022).
32. Nobre, V.; Harbarth, S.; Graf, J.D.; Rohner, P.; Pugin, J. Use of procalcitonin to shorten antibiotic treatment duration in septic patients: A randomized trial. *Am. J. Respir. Crit. Care Med.* **2008**, *177*, 498–505. [CrossRef]
33. Schroeder, S.; Hochreiter, M.; Koehler, T.; Schweiger, A.-M.; Bein, B.; Keck, F.S.; Von Spiegel, T. Procalcitonin (PCT)-guided algorithm reduces length of antibiotic treatment in surgical intensive care patients with severe sepsis: Results of a prospective randomized study. *Langenbecks Arch. Surg.* **2009**, *394*, 221–226. [CrossRef]
34. Hochreiter, M.; Köhler, T.; Schweiger, A.M.; Keck, F.S.; Bein, B.; Von Spiegel, T.; Schroeder, S. Procalcitonin to guide duration of antibiotic therapy in intensive care patients: A randomized prospective controlled trial. *Crit. Care* **2009**, *13*, R83. [CrossRef]
35. Stolz, D.; Smyrnios, N.; Eggimann, P.; Pargger, H.; Thakkar, N.; Siegemund, M.; Marsch, S.; Azzola, A.; Rakic, J.; Mueller, B.; et al. Procalcitonin for reduced antibiotic exposure in ventilator-associated pneumonia: A randomised study. *Eur. Respir. J.* **2009**, *34*, 1364–1375. [CrossRef]
36. Bouadma, L.; Luyt, C.-E.; Tubach, F.; Cracco, C.; Alvarez, A.; Schwebel, C.; Schortgen, F.; Lasocki, S.; Veber, B.; Dehoux, M.; et al. Use of procalcitonin to reduce patients' exposure to antibiotics in intensive care units (PRORATA trial): A multicentre randomised controlled trial. *Lancet* **2010**, *375*, 463–474. [CrossRef]
37. Jensen, J.U.; Hein, L.; Lundgren, B.; Bestle, M.H.; Mohr, T.T.; Andersen, M.H.; Thornberg, K.J.; Løken, J.; Steensen, M.; Fox, Z.; et al. Procalcitonin-guided interventions against infections to increase early appropriate antibiotics and improve survival in the intensive care unit: A randomized trial. *Crit. Care Med.* **2011**, *39*, 2048–2058. [CrossRef]
38. Layios, N.; Lambermont, B.; Canivet, J.-L.; Morimont, P.; Preiser, J.-C.; Garweg, C.; LeDoux, D.; Frippiat, F.; Piret, S.; Giot, J.-B.; et al. Procalcitonin usefulness for the initiation of antibiotic treatment in intensive care unit patients. *Crit. Care Med.* **2012**, *40*, 2304–2309. [CrossRef]
39. Qu, R.; Ji, Y.; Ling, Y.; Ye, C.Y.; Yang, S.M.; Liu, Y.Y.; Yang, R.Y.; Luo, Y.F.; Guo, Z. Procalcitonin is a good tool to guide duration of antibiotic therapy in patients with severe acute pancreatitis. A randomized prospective single-center controlled trial. *Saudi Med. J.* **2012**, *33*, 382–387.

40. Deliberato, R.O.; Marra, A.R.; Sanches, P.R.; Martino, M.D.V.; Ferreira, C.E.D.S.; Pasternak, J.; Paes, A.T.; Pinto, L.M.; dos Santos, O.F.P.; Edmond, M. Clinical and economic impact of procalcitonin to shorten antimicrobial therapy in septic patients with proven bacterial infection in an intensive care setting. *Diagn. Microbiol. Infect. Dis.* **2013**, *76*, 266–271. [CrossRef]
41. Oliveira, C.F.; Botoni, F.A.; Oliveira, C.R.; Silva, C.B.; Pereira, H.A.; Serufo, J.C.; Nobre, V. Procalcitonin versus C-reactive protein for guiding antibiotic therapy in sepsis: A randomized trial. *Crit. Care Med.* **2013**, *41*, 2336–2343. [CrossRef]
42. Annane, D.; Maxime, V.; Faller, J.P.; Mezher, C.; Clec'h, C.; Martel, P.; Gonzales, H.; Feissel, M.; Cohen, Y.; Capellier, G.; et al. Procalcitonin levels to guide antibiotic therapy in adults with non-microbiologically proven apparent severe sepsis: A randomised controlled trial. *BMJ Open* **2013**, *3*, e002186. [CrossRef]
43. Shehabi, Y.; Sterba, M.; Garrett, P.M.; Rachakonda, K.S.; Stephens, D.; Harrigan, P.; Walker, A.; Bailey, M.; Johnson, B.; Millis, D.; et al. Procalcitonin algorithm in critically ill adults with undifferentiated infection or suspected sepsis. A randomized controlled trial. *Am. J. Respir. Crit. Care Med.* **2014**, *190*, 1102–1110. [CrossRef]
44. de Jong, E.; van Oers, J.A.; Beishuizen, A.; Vos, P.; Vermeijden, W.J.; Haas, L.E.; Loef, B.G.; Dormans, T.; van Melsen, G.C.; Kluiters, Y.C.; et al. Efficacy and safety of procalcitonin guidance in reducing the duration of antibiotic treatment in critically ill patients: A randomised, controlled, open-label trial. *Lancet Infect. Dis.* **2016**, *16*, 819–827. [CrossRef]
45. Bloos, F.; Trips, E.; Nierhaus, A.; Briegel, J.; Heyland, D.K.; Jaschinski, U.; Moerer, O.; Weyland, A.; Marx, G.; Gründling, M.; et al. Effect of sodium selenite administration and procalcitonin-guided therapy on mortality in patients with severe sepsis or septic shock: A randomized clinical trial. *JAMA Intern. Med.* **2016**, *176*, 1266–1276. [CrossRef]
46. Jeon, K.; Suh, J.K.; Jang, E.J.; Cho, S.; Ryu, H.G.; Na, S.; Hong, S.B.; Lee, H.J.; Kim, J.Y.; Lee, S.M. Procalcitonin-guided treatment on duration of antibiotic therapy and cost in septic patients (PRODA): A multi-center randomized controlled trial. *J. Korean Med. Sci.* **2019**, *34*, e110. [CrossRef]
47. Beye, F.; Vigneron, C.; Dargent, A.; Prin, S.; Andreu, P.; Large, A.; Quenot, J.P.; Bador, J.; Bruyere, R.; Charles, P.E. Adhering to the procalcitonin algorithm allows antibiotic therapy to be shortened in patients with ventilator-associated pneumonia. *J. Crit. Care* **2019**, *53*, 125–131. [CrossRef]
48. Kyriazopoulou, E.; Liaskou-Antoniou, L.; Adamis, G.; Panagaki, A.; Melachroinopoulos, N.; Drakou, E.; Marousis, K.; Chrysos, G.; Spyrou, A.; Alexiou, N.; et al. Procalcitonin to reduce long-term infection-associated adverse events in sepsis. A randomized trial. *Am. J. Respir. Crit. Care Med.* **2021**, *203*, 202–210. [CrossRef]
49. Chomba, R.N.; Moeng, M.S.; Lowman, W. Procalcitonin-guided antibiotic therapy for suspected and confirmed sepsis of patients in a surgical trauma ICU: A prospective, two period cross-over, interventional study. *S. Afr. J. Surg.* **2020**, *5*, 143–149. [CrossRef]
50. Mazlan, M.Z.; Ismail, M.A.; Ali, S.; Salmuna, Z.N.; Shukeri, W.F.W.M.; Omar, M. Efficacy and safety of the point-of-care procalcitonin test for determining the antibiotic treatment duration in patients with ventilator-associated pneumonia in the intensive care unit: A randomised controlled trial. *Anaesthesiol. Intensive Ther.* **2021**, *53*, 207–214. [CrossRef]
51. Vishalashi, S.G.; Gupta, P.; Verma, P.K. Serum procalcitonin as a biomarker to determine the duration of antibiotic therapy in adult patients with sepsis and septic shock in intensive care units: A prospective study. *Indian J. Crit. Care Med.* **2021**, *25*, 507–511.
52. Use of a Respiratory Multiplex PCR and Procalcitonin to Reduce Antibiotics Exposure in Patients with Severe Confirmed COVID-19 Pneumonia (MultiCov). Available online: https://clinicaltrials.gov/ct2/show/NCT04334850 (accessed on 29 January 2022).
53. Voiriot, G.; Fartoukh, M.; Durand-Zaleski, I.; Berard, L.; Rousseau, A.; Armand-Lefevre, L.; Verdet, C.; Argaud, L.; Klouche, K.; Megarbane, B.; et al. Combined use of a broad-panel respiratory multiplex PCR and procalcitonin to reduce duration of antibiotics exposure in patients with severe community-acquired pneumonia (MULTI-CAP): A multicentre, parallel-group, open-label, individual randomised trial conducted in French intensive care units. *BMJ Open* **2021**, *11*, e048187.
54. Andriolo, B.N.; Andriolo, R.B.; Salomão, R.; Atallah, Á.N. Effectiveness and safety of procalcitonin evaluation for reducing mortality in adults with sepsis, severe sepsis or septic shock. *Cochrane Database Syst. Rev.* **2017**, *1*, CD010959. [CrossRef]
55. Huang, H.B.; Peng, J.M.; Weng, L.; Wang, C.Y.; Jiang, W.; Du, B. Procalcitonin-guided antibiotic therapy in intensive care unit patients: A systematic review and meta-analysis. *Ann. Intensive Care* **2017**, *7*, 114. [CrossRef]
56. Schuetz, P.; Wirz, Y.; Sager, R.; Christ-Crain, M.; Stolz, D.; Tamm, M.; Bouadma, L.; Luyt, C.E.; Wolff, M.; Chastre, J.; et al. Effect of procalcitonin-guided antibiotic treatment on mortality in acute respiratory infections: A patient level meta-analysis. *Lancet Infect. Dis.* **2018**, *18*, 95–107. [CrossRef]
57. Wirz, Y.; Meier, M.A.; Bouadma, L.; Luyt, C.E.; Wolff, M.; Chastre, J.; Tubach, F.; Schroeder, S.; Nobre, V.; Annane, D.; et al. Effect of procalcitonin-guided antibiotic treatment on clinical outcomes in intensive care unit patients with infection and sepsis patients: A patient-level meta-analysis of randomized trials. *Crit. Care* **2018**, *22*, 191. [CrossRef]
58. Lam, S.W.; Bauer, S.R.; Fowler, R.; Duggal, A. Systematic review and meta-analysis of procalcitonin-guidance versus usual care for antimicrobial management in critically ill patients: Focus on subgroups based on antibiotic initiation, cessation, or mixed strategies. *Crit. Care Med.* **2018**, *46*, 684–690. [CrossRef]
59. Iankova, I.; Thompson-Leduc, P.; Kirson, N.Y.; Rice, B.; Hey, J.; Krause, A.; Schonfeld, S.A.; DeBrase, C.R.; Bozzette, S.; Schuetz, P. Efficacy and safety of procalcitonin guidance in patients with suspected or confirmed sepsis: A systematic review and meta-analysis. *Crit. Care Med.* **2018**, *46*, 691–698. [CrossRef]
60. Pepper, D.J.; Sun, J.; Rhee, C.; Welsh, J.; Powers, J.H., III; Danner, R.L.; Kadri, S.S. Procalcitonin-guided antibiotic discontinuation and mortality in critically ill adults: A systematic review and meta-analysis. *Chest* **2019**, *155*, 1109–1118. [CrossRef]
61. Peng, F.; Chang, W.; Xie, J.F.; Sun, Q.; Qiu, H.B.; Yang, Y. Ineffectiveness of procalcitonin-guided antibiotic therapy in severely critically ill patients: A meta-analysis. *Int. J. Infect. Dis.* **2019**, *85*, 158–166. [CrossRef]

62. Arulkumaran, N.; Khpal, M.; Tam, K.; Baheerathan, A.; Corredor, C.; Singer, M. Effect of antibiotic discontinuation strategies on mortality and infectious complications in critically ill septic patients: A meta-analysis and trial sequential analysis. *Crit. Care Med.* **2020**, *48*, 757–764. [CrossRef]
63. Meier, M.A.; Branche, A.; Neeser, O.L.; Wirz, Y.; Haubitz, S.; Bouadma, L.; Wolff, M.; Luyt, C.E.; Chastre, J.; Tubach, F.; et al. Procalcitonin-guided antibiotic treatment in patients with positive blood cultures: A patient-level meta-analysis of randomized trials. *Clin. Infect. Dis.* **2019**, *69*, 388–396. [CrossRef]
64. Heilmann, E.; Gregoriano, C.; Wirz, Y.; Luyt, C.E.; Wolff, M.; Chastre, J.; Tubach, F.; Christ-Crain, M.; Bouadma, L.; Annane, D.; et al. Association of kidney function with effectiveness of procalcitonin-guided antibiotic treatment: A patient-level meta-analysis from randomized controlled trials. *Clin. Chem. Lab. Med.* **2020**, *59*, 441–453. [CrossRef]
65. Heilmann, E.; Gregoriano, C.; Annane, D.; Reinhart, K.; Bouadma, L.; Wolff, M.; Chastre, J.; Luyt, C.-E.; Tubach, F.; Branche, A.R.; et al. Duration of antibiotic treatment using procalcitonin-guided treatment algorithms in older patients: A patient-level meta-analysis from randomized controlled trials. *Age Ageing* **2021**, *50*, 1546–1556. [CrossRef]
66. Gutiérrez-Pizarraya, A.; León-García, M.D.C.; De Juan-Idígoras, R.; Garnacho-Montero, J. Clinical impact of procalcitonin-based algorithms for duration of antibiotic treatment in critically ill adult patients with sepsis: A meta-analysis of randomized clinical trials. *Expert Rev. Anti-Infect. Ther.* **2022**, *20*, 103–112. [CrossRef]
67. Schuetz, P.; Wahl, P.M. Additional real-world evidence supporting procalcitonin as an effective tool to improve antibiotic management and cost of the critically ill patient. *Chest* **2017**, *151*, 6–8. [CrossRef]
68. Schuetz, P.; Batschwaroff, M.; Dusemund, F.; Albrich, W.; Bürgi, U.; Maurer, M.; Brutsche, M.; Huber, A.R.; Müller, B. Effectiveness of a procalcitonin algorithm to guide antibiotic therapy in respiratory tract infections outside of study conditions: A post-study survey. *Eur. J. Clin. Microbiol. Infect. Dis.* **2010**, *29*, 269–277. [CrossRef]
69. Hohn, A.; Heising, B.; Hertel, S.; Baumgarten, G.; Hochreiter, M.; Schroeder, S. Antibiotic consumption after implementation of a procalcitonin-guided antimicrobial stewardship programme in surgical patients admitted to an intensive care unit: A retrospective before-and-after analysis. *Infection* **2015**, *43*, 405–412. [CrossRef]
70. Walsh, T.L.; DiSilvio, B.E.; Hammer, C.; Beg, M.; Vishwanathan, S.; Speredelozzi, D.; Moffa, M.A.; Hu, K.; Abdulmassih, R.; Makadia, J.T.; et al. Impact of procalcitonin guidance with an educational program on management of adults hospitalized with pneumonia. *Am. J. Med.* **2018**, *131*, 201.e1–201.e8. [CrossRef]
71. Balk, R.A.; Kadri, S.S.; Cao, Z.; Robinson, S.B.; Lipkin, C.; Bozzette, S.A. Effect of procalcitonin testing on health-care utilization and costs in critically ill patients in the United States. *Chest* **2017**, *151*, 23–33. [CrossRef]
72. Newton, J.A.; Robinson, S.; Ling, C.L.L.; Zimmer, L.; Kuper, K.; Trivedi, K.K. Impact of procalcitonin levels combined with active intervention on antimicrobial stewardship in a community hospital. *Open Forum Infect. Dis.* **2019**, *6*, ofz355. [CrossRef]
73. Collins, C.D.; Brockhaus, K.; Sim, T.; Suneja, A.; Malani, A.N. Analysis to determine cost-effectiveness of procalcitonin-guided antibiotic use in adult patients with suspected bacterial infection and sepsis. *Am. J. Health Syst. Pharm.* **2019**, *76*, 1219–1225. [CrossRef]
74. Westwood, M.; Ramaekers, B.; Whiting, P.; Tomini, F.; Joore, M.; Armstrong, N.; Ryder, S.; Stirk, L.; Severens, H.; Kleijnen, J. Procalcitonin testing to guide antibiotic therapy for the treatment of sepsis in intensive care settings and for suspected bacterial infection in emergency department settings: A systematic review and cost-effectiveness analysis. *Health Technol. Assess.* **2015**, *19*, 3–236. [CrossRef]
75. Langford, B.J.; Beriault, D.; Schwartz, K.L.; Seah, J.; Pasic, M.D.; Cirone, R.; Chan, A.; Downing, M. A real-world assessment of procalcitonin combined with antimicrobial stewardship in a community ICU. *J. Crit. Care* **2020**, *57*, 130–133. [CrossRef]
76. Broyles, M.R. Impact of procalcitonin-guided antibiotic management on antibiotic exposure and outcomes: Real-world evidence. *Open Forum Infect. Dis.* **2017**, *4*, ofx213. [CrossRef]
77. Gluck, E.; Nguyen, H.B.; Yalamanchili, K.; McCusker, M.; Madala, J.; Corvino, F.A.; Zhu, X.; Balk, R. Real-world use of procalcitonin and other biomarkers among sepsis hospitalizations in the United States: A retrospective, observational study. *PLoS ONE* **2018**, *13*, e0205924. [CrossRef]
78. Chambliss, A.B. Embracing procalcitonin for antimicrobial stewardship. *J. Appl. Lab. Med.* **2019**, *3*, 712–715. [CrossRef]
79. Christensen, I.; Haug, J.B.; Berild, D.; Bjørnholt, J.V.; Jelsness-Jørgensen, L.P. Hospital physicians' experiences with procalcitonin—Implications for antimicrobial stewardship; a qualitative study. *BMC Infect. Dis.* **2020**, *20*, 515. [CrossRef]
80. von Dach, E.; Albrich, W.C.; Brunel, A.S.; Prendki, V.; Cuvelier, C.; Flury, D.; Gayet-Ageron, A.; Huttner, B.; Kohler, P.; Lemmenmeier, E.; et al. Effect of C-reactive protein-guided antibiotic treatment duration, 7-day treatment, or 14-day treatment on 30-day clinical failure rate in patients with uncomplicated gram-negative bacteremia: A randomized clinical trial. *JAMA* **2020**, *323*, 2160–2169. [CrossRef]
81. Borges, I.; Carneiro, R.; Bergo, R.; Martins, L.; Colosimo, E.; Oliveira, C.; Saturnino, S.; Andrade, M.V.; Ravetti, C.; Nobre, V. Duration of antibiotic therapy in critically ill patients: A randomized controlled trial of a clinical and C-reactive protein-based protocol versus an evidence-based best practice strategy without biomarkers. *Crit. Care* **2020**, *24*, 281. [CrossRef]
82. Shozushima, T.; Takahashi, G.; Matsumoto, N.; Kojika, M.; Okamura, Y.; Endo, S. Usefulness of presepsin (sCD14-ST) measurements as a marker for the diagnosis and severity of sepsis that satisfied diagnostic criteria of systemic inflammatory response syndrome. *J. Infect. Chemother.* **2011**, *17*, 764–769. [CrossRef]

83. Xiao, H.; Wang, G.; Wang, Y.; Tan, Z.; Sun, X.; Zhou, J.; Duan, M.; Zhi, D.; Tang, Z.; Hang, C.; et al. Potential value of presepsin guidance in shortening antibiotic therapy in septic patients: A multicenter, prospective cohort trial. *Shock* **2022**, *57*, 63–71. [CrossRef]
84. Hellyer, T.P.; McAuley, D.F.; Walsh, T.S.; Anderson, N.; Morris, A.C.; Singh, S.; Dark, P.; Roy, A.I.; Perkins, G.D.; McMullan, R.; et al. Biomarker-guided antibiotic stewardship in suspected ventilator-associated pneumonia (VAPrapid2): A randomised controlled trial and process evaluation. *Lancet Respir. Med.* **2020**, *8*, 182–191. [CrossRef]
85. Karakike, E.; Giamarellos-Bourboulis, E.J.; Kyprianou, M.; Fleischmann-Struzek, C.; Pletz, M.W.; Netea, M.G.; Reinhart, K.; Kyriazopoulou, E. Coronavirus disease 2019 as cause of viral sepsis: A systematic review and meta-analysis. *Crit. Care Med.* **2021**, *49*, 2042–2057. [CrossRef]
86. Rawson, T.M.; Moore, L.S.P.; Zhu, N.; Ranganathan, N.; Skolimowska, K.; Gilchrist, M.; Satta, G.; Cooke, G.; Holmes, A.H. Bacterial and fungal coinfection in individuals with coronavirus: A rapid review to support COVID-19 antimicrobial prescribing. *Clin. Infect. Dis.* **2020**, *71*, 2459–2468. [CrossRef]
87. Arentz, M.; Yim, E.; Klaff, L.; Lokhandwala, S.; Riedo, F.X.; Chong, M.; Lee, M. Characteristics and outcomes of 21 critically ill patients with COVID-19 in Washington state. *JAMA* **2020**, *323*, 1612–1614. [CrossRef]
88. Wang, D.; Hu, B.; Hu, C.; Zhu, F.; Liu, X.; Zhang, J.; Wang, B.; Xiang, H.; Cheng, Z.; Xiong, Y.; et al. Clinical characteristics of 138 hospitalized patients with 2019 Novel coronavirus-infected pneumonia in Wuhan, China. *JAMA* **2020**, *323*, 1061–1069. [CrossRef]
89. Zhou, F.; Yu, T.; Du, R.; Fan, G.; Liu, Y.; Liu, Z.; Xiang, J.; Wang, Y.; Song, B.; Gu, X.; et al. Clinical course and risk factors for mortality of adult inpatients with COVID-19 in Wuhan, China: A retrospective cohort study. *Lancet* **2020**, *395*, 1054–1062. [CrossRef]
90. Goyal, P.; Choi, J.J.; Pinheiro, L.C.; Schenck, E.J.; Chen, R.; Jabri, A.; Satlin, M.J.; Campion, T.R., Jr.; Nahid, M.; Ringel, J.B.; et al. Clinical characteristics of Covid-19 in New York city. *N. Engl. J. Med.* **2020**, *382*, 2372–2374. [CrossRef]
91. Atallah, N.J.; Warren, H.M.; Roberts, M.B.; Elshaboury, R.H.; Bidell, M.R.; Gandhi, R.G.; Adamsick, M.; Ibrahim, M.K.; Sood, R.; Eddine, S.B.Z.; et al. Baseline procalcitonin as a predictor of bacterial infection and clinical outcomes in COVID-19: A case-control study. *PLoS ONE* **2022**, *17*, e0262342. [CrossRef]
92. Houghton, R.; Moore, N.; Williams, R.; El-Bakri, F.; Peters, J.; Mori, M.; Vernet, G.; Lynch, J.; Lewis, H.; Tavener, M.; et al. C-reactive protein-guided use of procalcitonin in COVID-19. *JAC Antimicrob. Resist.* **2021**, *3*, dlab180. [CrossRef]
93. Zattera, L.; Veliziotis, I.; Benitez-Cano, A.; Ramos, I.; Larrañaga, L.; Nuñez, M.; Román, L.; Adalid, I.; Ferrando, C.; Muñoz, G.; et al. Early procalcitonin to predict mortality in critically ill COVID-19 patients: A multicentric cohort study. *Minerva Anestesiol.* **2022**. [CrossRef] [PubMed]
94. Shen, Y.; Cheng, C.; Zheng, X.; Jin, Y.; Duan, G.; Chen, M.; Chen, S. Elevated procalcitonin is positively associated with the severity of COVID-19: A meta-analysis based on 10 cohort studies. *Medicina* **2021**, *57*, 594. [CrossRef] [PubMed]
95. Van Berkel, M.; Kox, M.; Frenzel, T.; Pickkers, P.; Schouten, J. Biomarkers for antimicrobial stewardship: A reappraisal in COVID-19 times? *Crit. Care* **2020**, *24*, 600. [CrossRef] [PubMed]
96. Richards, O.; Pallmann, P.; King, C.; Cheema, Y.; Killick, C.; Thomas-Jones, E.; Harris, J.; Bailey, C.; Szakmany, T. Procalcitonin increase is associated with the development of critical care-acquired infections in COVID-19 ARDS. *Antibiotics* **2021**, *10*, 1425. [CrossRef] [PubMed]
97. Pink, I.; Raupach, D.; Fuge, J.; Vonberg, R.-P.; Hoeper, M.M.; Welte, T.; Rademacher, J. C-reactive protein and procalcitonin for antimicrobial stewardship in COVID-19. *Infection* **2021**, *49*, 935–943. [CrossRef] [PubMed]
98. Kooistra, E.J.; van Berkel, M.; van Kempen, N.F.; van Latum, C.R.; Bruse, N.; Frenzel, T.; van den Berg, M.J.; Schouten, J.A.; Kox, M.; Pickkers, P. Dexamethasone and tocilizumab treatment considerably reduces the value of C-reactive protein and procalcitonin to detect secondary bacterial infections in COVID-19 patients. *Crit. Care* **2021**, *25*, 281. [CrossRef]
99. Moseley, P.; Jackson, N.; Omar, A.; Eldoadoa, M.; Samaras, C.; Birk, R.; Ahmed, F.; Chakrabarti, P. Single-centre experience of using procalcitonin to guide antibiotic therapy in COVID-19 intensive care patients. *J. Hosp. Infect.* **2022**, *119*, 194–195. [CrossRef]
100. Calderon, M.; Li, A.; Bazo-Alvarez, J.C.; Dennis, J.; Baker, K.F.; van der Loeff, I.S.; Hanrath, A.T.; Capstick, R.; Payne, B.A.I.; Weiand, D.; et al. Evaluation of procalcitonin-guided antimicrobial stewardship in patients admitted to hospital with COVID-19 pneumonia. *JAC Antimicrob. Resist.* **2021**, *3*, dlab133. [CrossRef]
101. Williams, E.J.; Mair, L.; de Silva, T.I.; Green, D.J.; House, P.; Cawthron, K.; Gillies, C.; Wigfull, J.; Parsons, H.; Partridge, D.G. Evaluation of procalcitonin as a contribution to antimicrobial stewardship in SARS-CoV-2 infection: A retrospective cohort study. *J. Hosp. Infect.* **2021**, *110*, 103–107. [CrossRef]
102. Staub, M.B.; Ouedraogo, Y.; Evans, C.D.; Katz, S.E.; Talley, P.P.; Kainer, M.A.; Nelson, G.E. Analysis of a high-prescribing state's 2016 outpatient antibiotic prescriptions: Implications for outpatient antimicrobial stewardship interventions. *Infect. Control Hosp. Epidemiol.* **2020**, *41*, 135–142. [CrossRef]

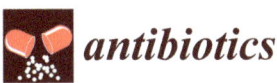

Review

Empiric Treatment in HAP/VAP: "Don't You Want to Take a Leap of Faith?"

Khalil Chaïbi [1,2], Gauthier Péan de Ponfilly [3,4], Laurent Dortet [5,6], Jean-Ralph Zahar [7] and Benoît Pilmis [4,8,*]

1. Département de Réanimation Médico-Chirurgicale, AP-HP Hôpital Avicenne, Université Sorbonne Paris Nord, 93000 Bobigny, France; khalil.chaibi@aphp.fr
2. Common and Rare Kidney Diseases, Sorbonne Université, INSERM, UMR-S 1155, 75020 Paris, France
3. Service de Microbiologie Clinique, Groupe Hospitalier Paris Saint-Joseph, 75014 Paris, France; gpeandeponfilly@ghpsj.fr
4. Institut Micalis, Unité Mixte de Recherche 1319, Université Paris-Saclay, INRAe, AgroParisTech, 92290 Châtenay Malabry, France
5. Service de Bactériologie-Hygiène, CHU de Bicêtre, Assistance Publique des Hôpitaux de Paris, Centre National de Référence de la Résistance aux Antibiotiques, 94270 Le Kremlin-Bicêtre, France; laurent.dortet@aphp.fr
6. INSERM UMR1184, Resist Unit, Université Paris-Saclay, 94270 Le Kremlin-Bicêtre, France
7. Infection Control Unit, AP-HP Hôpital Avicenne, Université Sorbonne Paris Nord, 93000 Bobigny, France; jean-ralph.zahar@aphp.fr
8. Équipe Mobile de Microbiologie Clinique, Groupe Hospitalier Paris Saint-Joseph, 75014 Paris, France
* Correspondence: bpilmis@ghpsj.fr; Tel.: +33-(1)-4412-7820; Fax: +33-(1)-4412-3684

Abstract: Ventilator-associated pneumonia is a frequent cause of ICU-acquired infections. These infections are associated with high morbidity and mortality. The increase in antibiotic resistance, particularly among Gram-negative bacilli, makes the choice of empiric antibiotic therapy complex for physicians. Multidrug-resistant organisms (MDROs) related infections are associated with a high risk of initial therapeutic inadequacy. It is, therefore, necessary to quickly identify the bacterial species involved and their susceptibility to antibiotics. New diagnostic tools have recently been commercialized to assist in the management of these infections. Moreover, the recent enrichment of the therapeutic arsenal effective on Gram-negative bacilli raises the question of their place in the therapeutic management of these infections. Most national and international guidelines recommend limiting their use to microbiologically documented infections. However, many clinical situations and, in particular, the knowledge of digestive or respiratory carriage by MDROs should lead to the discussion of the use of these new molecules, especially the new combinations with beta-lactamase inhibitors in empirical therapy. In this review, we present the current epidemiological data, particularly in terms of MDRO, as well as the clinical and microbiological elements that may be taken into account in the discussion of empirical antibiotic therapy for patients managed for ventilator-associated pneumonia.

Keywords: antibiotic choices; HAP; VAP; colonization; antibiotic pressure

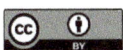

1. Introduction

Ventilator-associated pneumonia (VAP) is one of the most frequent causes of intensive care unit (ICU)-acquired infections [1]. In French ICUs, 8% of patients developed hospital-acquired pneumonia in 2016, and 88.7% among them were ventilator-associated pneumonia [2].

For more than a decade, we have been confronted with the spread of multi-resistant bacteria in hospitals [3–5] and the community [6–8].

The increasing prevalence of resistance among bacteria, particularly gram-negative bacilli (GNB) and especially *Enterobacterales*, makes harder the choice of antibiotics, in case of infection. Several factors seem to be associated with a higher risk of infection related to multidrug-resistant organisms (MDRO), such as the local prevalence, previous antibiotic therapy, time of occurrence of the infection, and previous MDRO colonization.

In our clinical practice, the spread of MDRO resistance leads to a higher risk of antibiotic inadequation. Indeed, there are two opposing risks when choosing an empirical antibiotic therapy. On one side is the individual level, reflected by the risk to choose a narrow spectrum antibiotic with potentially important consequences in terms of mortality and morbidity. On the other side is the collective level, reflected by the choice of a broad-spectrum antibiotic which could contribute to the amplification of resistance.

In the last four years, medical research has been driven by the discovery of new beta-lactamase inhibitors and the marketing of new antibiotics with broad-spectrum activity.

Numerous authors suggest and encourage rational use of these new antibiotics out of fear of the emergence of new resistance mechanisms. However, certain clinical situations require empirical choices. It, therefore, seemed important to assess relevant factors and variables at the time of prescribing in order to choose the most appropriate molecule, both in terms of spectrum and possible ecological effects.

2. HCAP, HAP, VAP: Clinical Concepts and Historical Perspective

From the first consensus conference in 1996 until now, the history of concepts and definitions around nosocomial pneumonia has never been a long calm river. Its evolution is intrinsically linked to epidemiological, diagnostic, and therapeutic advances in the context of precision medicine [9]. A remarkable example would be the path of the Healthcare-Associated Pneumonia (HCAP) category in guidelines. If the term was initially defined in the 2005 ATS recommendations [10] in order to avoid inappropriate empiric antimicrobial therapy after the emergence of the "golden hours" concept in the intensive care unit (ICU) [11], it has finally proved to be irrelevant. By HCAP, it was meant "any patient who was hospitalized in an acute care hospital for 2 or more days within 90 days of the infection". This categorization resulted in the increasing usage of broad-spectrum antibiotics in a population which eventually appeared to be no more infected with MDRO pathogens than patients with community-acquired pneumonia (CAP) [12]. Furthermore, this category failed to predict mortality [13]. The starting point was a retrospective cohort study based on more than 4000 patients with proven bacterial pneumonia within the 48 h following admission and transfer from a healthcare facility which showed an incidence of a quarter of admitted patients with Methicillin-Resistant *Staphylococcus aureus* (MRSA) infection, with the same incidence for *Pseudomonas aeruginosa* (PA) [14]. These findings, which led to treating CAP with risk factors of MDRO organisms carriage the same way as ventilator-associated pneumonia (VAP) regardless of the severity status, were later largely overruled [15]. Indeed, recent studies found no major difference in terms of bacterial epidemiology between CAP and HCAP [16], and antibiotic-resistant organisms were found to be rare whatever population at risk of carriage was analyzed [17].

Then, a deeper knowledge of bacterial epidemiology stood out as the key challenge of nosocomial pneumonia management for future years.

3. Definitions and Issues of Nosocomial Pneumonia

Hospital-Acquired Pneumonia (HAP) is defined as new pneumonia (a lower respiratory tract infection verified by the presence of a new pulmonary infiltrate on imaging) in non-intubated patients, that develops more than 48 h after admission. When it develops after 48 h of endotracheal intubation, it is categorized as a VAP. In the ICU, VAPs are the most present entity, with an overwhelming majority (more than 95%) of reported cases of pneumonia [18].

VAP is a major problem in the ICU due to its frequency and short-term consequences. It is the main source of healthcare-associated infections (HAI) in these departments, with an incidence reaching 40% of patients with up to 16 episodes per 1000 days of mechanical ventilation [19]. It is associated with significant morbidity since it is complicated in 30 to 50% of cases by septic shock, in 10 to 15% of cases by acute respiratory distress syndrome

(ARDS), and in 10 to 15% of cases by multi-organ failure (MOF) [20–24]. It also has an impact on the duration of mechanical ventilation (increased from 7 to 11 days), the length of hospital stay (increased from 11 to 13 days), and health economics (EUR 30,000 to 40,000/per episode) [25–27]. Finally, the overall mortality of patients who experienced a VAP in the ICU is considerable (20 to 40% depending on the series), with an average attributable mortality (to the VAP episode alone) of 13% [28].

4. Epidemiology

HAP and VAP may be caused by a variety of pathogens and can be polymicrobial. Common pathogens include aerobic GNB (e.g., *Escherichia coli*, *Klebsiella pneumoniae*, *Enterobacter* spp., PA, *Acinetobacter* spp.) and Gram-positive cocci (e.g., *Staphylococcus aureus*, including MRSA, *Streptococcus* spp.) [29,30]. Furthermore, there is increasing recognition that a substantial fraction of nosocomial pneumonia may be due to viruses [29].

Among 8474 cases of VAP reported in the United States Centers for Disease Control and Prevention, the distribution of pathogens associated were *Staphylococcus aureus*, *Pseudomonas aeruginosa*, *Klebsiella* species, *Enterobacter* species, *Acinetobacter baumannii*, and *E. coli* in, respectively, 24.1%, 16.6%, 10.1%, 8.6%, 6.6%, and 5.9% of cases [31]. In a prospective observational study evaluating 158,519 patients admitted to the University of North Carolina Hospital over a 4-year period, a total of 282 episodes of documented VAP and 190 episodes of documented HAP in non-ventilated patients were identified (Table 1) [32].

Table 1. Frequency of isolation of pathogens from patients with Ventilator-Associated Pneumonia (VAP) and non-ventilated patients with Hospital-Acquired Pneumonia (HAP) [32].

	Ventilator-Associated Pneumonia	Healthcare-Associated Pneumonia
Gram-positive cocci	39.3%	55.8%
Staphylococcus aureus (SA)	36.8%	47.9%
Methicillin Resistant SA	24.4%	28.9%
Methicillin Susceptible SA	12.4%	19%
Streptococcus pneumoniae	2.5%	7.9%
Gram-negative bacilli	60.7%	44.2%
Enterobacter sp.	3.2%	4.3%
Escherichia coli	3.5%	4.3%
Klebsiella pneumoniae	2.1%	6.8%
Serratia marcescens	2.8%	2.6%
Pseudomonas aeruginosa	21.3%	13.1%
Stenotrophomonas maltophilia	8.8%	1.6%
Acinetobacter spp.	10.4%	4.7%
Other species	8.6%	6.8%

These findings are similar to those observed in a meta-analysis of 24 studies performed during the development of the 2016 Infectious Disease Society of America guidelines [33].

The etiology of HAP and VAP depends largely upon whether the patient has risk factors for MDRO pathogens [33]. The frequency of specific MDRO pathogens varies among hospitals, within hospitals, and between different patient populations. One of the major problems lies in the spread of MDROs and, specifically, extended-spectrum beta-lactamase-producing *Enterobacterales* (ESBLEs) in the community. This diffusion has consequences in hospitals and in intensive care units where, among hospitalized patients, between 5 and 25% are ESBL producing *Enterobacterales* carriers [34–36].

4.1. Bacterial Epidemiology: A Practical Approach in ICU

Choosing the right antibiotic lies in anticipating both the species and the resistance mechanisms that will be involved in the infection (Figure 1). If the local epidemiology weighs heavily on the species involved, it remains that certain clinical situations and data specific to the medical history of the patient must lead to considering certain species.

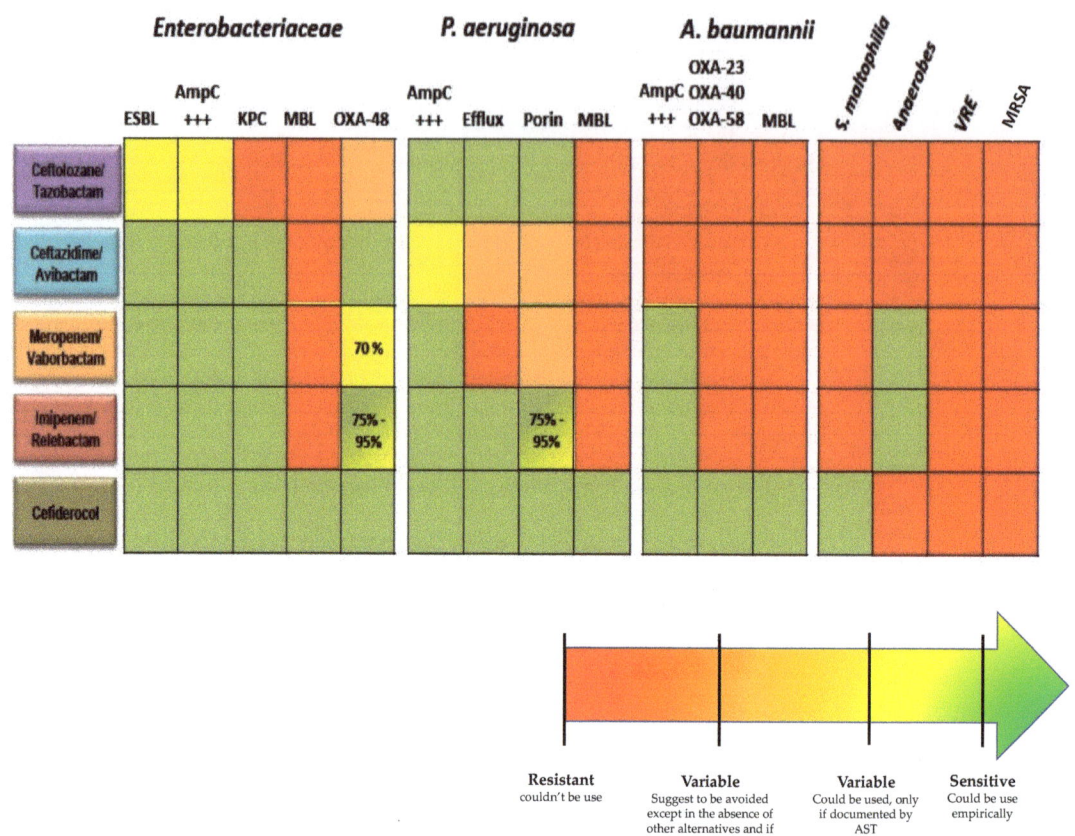

Figure 1. Spectrum of activity of new antibiotics. AST: Antibiotic susceptibility test, ESBL: Extended-spectrum beta-lactamase, AmpC: Cephalosporinase, KPC: *Klebsiella pneumoniae* carbapenemase, MBL: metallo-betalactamase, VRE: vancomycin resistant Enterococci, MRSA: Methicillin-resistant *Staphylococcus aureus*.

4.2. Profiling Bacterial Species in Pneumonia: Born to Be Wild

4.2.1. Methicillin Susceptible *Staphylococcus aureus* (MSSA)

Among the population, 30 to 50% are permanently or intermittently colonized with *Staphylococcus aureus* species. Moreover, the risk of secondary infection seems to be higher among previously colonized patients [37–39]. Indeed, in 2017 post-hoc analysis of two cohort studies of more than 9000 critically ill patients found that patients colonized with *Staphylococcus aureus* at ICU admission had an up to 15 times increased risk for developing this outcome compared with non-colonized patients [40]. *Staphylococcus aureus* should be considered in the case of HAP that complicates influenza infection or in the case of early HAP in patients known to be previously colonized with MSSA. Several authors suggested a higher risk in a specific population, such as traumatic and non-traumatic brain injury patients [41]. Indeed, the authors suggested that MSSA is most frequent in this specific population, accounting for up to 40–50% of VAP. In a recent study focusing specifically on bacteriological aspects of *Staphylococcus aureus* VAP, the authors highlighted that nearly 74% of the patients had severe head trauma or a *priori* history of coma [41,42].

4.2.2. Enterobacterales

Enterobacterales remain the most frequent species found in HAP and VAP patients. These species must be systematically considered in the choice of antibiotics, whatever the circumstances. The only question that should be asked is if the antibiotic spectrum should include resistant bacteria. In this perspective, the time of occurrence of the event should be addressed as major information. Indeed, early HAP and VAP seem to be related to sensitive species, whereas the duration of hospitalization and previous antibiotic therapy seem to be associated with more resistant species [43].

4.2.3. Pseudomonas aeruginosa

Assessing the specific risk of PA infection is highly relevant since the mortality attributable to this GNB seems more important than others (both because of the multi-resistant nature of the germ inducing a delay in appropriate antibiotic therapy and because it more often affects more severe patients) [44]. *Pseudomonas aeruginosa* colonization remains rare even in critically ill patients in the ICU. Indeed, in developed countries, the PA colonization rate at ICU admission is close to 10% in several studies [45–47]. However, PA is a highly prevalent causative pathogen in HAP and VAP. An experience of the French national surveillance, REA-RAISIN, found that a higher probability of PA-VAP is regularly associated with higher age, length of mechanical ventilation before pneumonia, antibiotics at admission, and admission in a ward with a higher incidence of patients with PA infection. Interestingly, transfer from a medical unit or ICU was also found to be associated with a higher probability of PA-VAP (45). Hospital admission should thus be considered a turning point in the colonization pressure experienced by the patient (and not only the admission in ICU). Lower probability of PA pneumonia was associated with traumatism and, as expected, with admission in a ward with higher patient turnover. Some populations seem to be more at risk, such as patients with COPD, cystic fibrosis, or bronchiectasis. Old studies suggested a higher prevalence of late VAP [48]. Indeed, as PA is a saprophytic species specifically linked to water, acquisition requires a contaminated environment and selection pressure.

4.2.4. Acinetobacter baumannii

Although found with a low worldwide prevalence, *Acinetobacter baumannii* is one of the most antibiotic-resistant pathogens, with 50% of carbapenem-resistant isolates in US intensive care units, including a vast majority of extreme drug-resistant (XDR) strains [49]. Moreover, the survival of Acinetobacter baumanii in the biofilm makes their treatment difficult [50,51].

Acinetobacter are ubiquitous organisms recovered from soil or surface water. *Acinetobacter* are rarely found in the microbiota of patients in the northern hemisphere. Indeed, several studies suggested a low rate of *Acinetobacter baumannii* carriage in the communities in Germany and France [52], even in the population of patients admitted to the intensive care unit [53]. However, authors highlighted higher carriage rates in other parts of the globe, such as Hong Kong, the Asia-Pacific region, and other countries with hot and humid climates. In these locations, *Acinetobacter baumannii* has emerged as a cause of severe community-acquired infections [54]. Classically-found risk factors for *Acinetobacter baumannii* infection are tropical or sub-tropical climate, excessive alcohol consumption, smoking, or having an underlying health condition (diabetes mellitus or chronic lung disease) with a different weight of each risk depending on the location [55]. In the ICU, a difference must be made according to the epidemiological data. Whereas *Acinetobacter baumannii* is associated with early-onset HAP/VAP in southern countries, it seems rarely isolated in northern countries and is usually associated with several risk factors. Indeed, factors independently associated with *Acinetobacter baumannii* infection are commonly found to be immunosuppression, previous antimicrobial therapy, previous sepsis in the ICU, and a history of recent invasive procedures [56].

4.2.5. Stenotrophomonas maltophilia

HAP or VAP related to *Stenotrophomonas maltophilia* (SM) are rare [30]. SM is an environmental bacterium found in aqueous habitats, including plant rhizospheres, animals, foods, and water sources. It is not a highly virulent pathogen, but it has emerged as an important nosocomial pathogen. The incidence of SM hospital-acquired infections (HAI) is increasing, particularly in the immunocompromised patient population [57,58]. Risk factors for this infection include chronic respiratory diseases (especially cystic fibrosis), hematologic malignancy, chemotherapy-induced neutropenia, organ transplant patients, human immunodeficiency virus (HIV) infection, hemodialysis patients, and neonates [59]. Furthermore, hospital settings, prolonged intensive care unit stays, mechanical ventilation, tracheostomies, central venous catheters, severe traumatic injuries, significant burns, mucositis or mucosal barrier damaging factors, and the use of broad-spectrum antibiotic courses were shown to increase the risk of infection [60,61].

4.3. Risk Factors Associated with MDRO

As highlighted before, three main factors seem to be associated with MDRO-related pulmonary infection. Firstly, previous antibiotic therapy is one of the major risk factors as it is the source of selecting/inducing MDRO, and it paves the field of acquisition of resistant bacteria from the environment. Thus, before considering a species or a particular resistance mechanism, it is essential to trace the history of specific antibiotic exposure that can help the practitioner assess the risk of dealing with a specific species or resistance mechanism (Figure 2). For instance, carbapenem exposure and exposure to β-lactams inactive against *Pseudomonas aeruginosa* have been strongly correlated to the emergence of Carbapenem-Resistant *Pseudomonas aeruginosa* isolation, due to the repression or inactivation of the OprD gene encoding porin OprD2 [62,63]. As for species, *Stenotrophomas maltophilia*-related pneumonia has been found to be associated with previous exposure to Meropenem [64,65] and *Enterococcus* with previous exposure to third-generation cephalosporins [66].

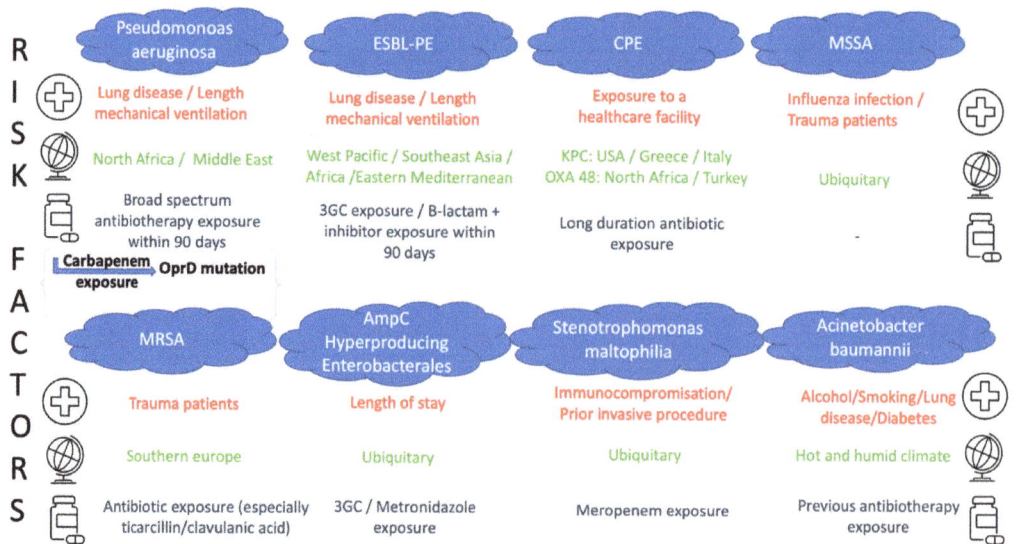

Figure 2. Risk factors for MDRO-related infections.

Secondly, the length of hospitalization seems to be an important risk factor as it corresponds to a duration of exposure to a particular (bacterial) environment, responsible for the modification of the patients' microbiota [67]. Indeed, several authors suggested [68,69] that duration of hospitalization and antibiotic therapy were the two main factors associated with MDRO-related pneumonia.

Thirdly, prior colonization with MDROs seems to be an indispensable prerequisite for the occurrence of MDRO infection [37,70,71]. In light of the spread of MDRO and the increase in the number of colonized patients [35], it seems more and more difficult to interpret the weight of MDRO colonization as a risk factor for MDRO infection. Several authors suggested that rare are the patients infected with MDRO among carriers [72,73]. In a prospective study among carriers, only 6% developed ICU-acquired pneumonia related to ESBL producing *Enterobacterales*.

A large study conducted in a French ICU suggested that the first infection episode rates in EBSL-PE carriers vary from 10% to 42% [70,74–76]. Whereas, the rate of the second episode rises from 10% to 30% [73]. *Klebsiella pneumoniae* carriage has also been found to carry a specific risk of colonization/infection transition in a surgical population of liver transplanted patients [77]. As for antibiotic use, a carbapenem exposure within the preceding three days has been reported to have a protective effect on ESBL PE VAP in one study [78]. Finally, a retrospective cohort study of more than 500 ICU patients with suspected VAP analyzed sensitivity and specificity of prior ESBL-PE colonization as a predictor of ESBL-PE-VAP and found, respectively, 85.0% and 95.7%. The positive and negative predictive values were 41.5% and 99.4%, respectively, with a positive likelihood ratio of 19.8. Moreover, no data support an impact of ESBL carriage on mortality which is a supplementary argument in favor of a "wait and see" strategy [79].

It, therefore, seems necessary to be able to identify among patients carrying multidrug-resistant bacteria those at risk of infection. Studies that occurred outside the ICU [80] and in the ICU [81,82] have suggested that relative abundance was the main risk factor associated with secondary bacteremia and VAP. Besides the risk due to the significant biomass of multidrug-resistant bacteria, it seems that colonization with non-*E. coli* species was associated with a higher risk of secondary infection [82]. Indeed, it has been shown that a high relative fecal abundance of ESBL-producing *Enterobacterales* is associated with a higher risk of ESBL-producing *Enterobacterales* associated VAP [81]. One study showed that in ICU patients colonized with ESBL-producing *Enterobacterales*, the onset of ESBL-producing *Enterobacterales* throat carriage preceded the occurrence of ESBL-producing *Enterobacterales* associated VAP [82].

4.4. Extended-Spectrum Beta-Lactamase-Producing Enterobacterales (ESBL-PE)

A recent meta-analysis found an overall prevalence of ESBL-producing *Enterobacterales* in a community of 14% among healthy individuals with an increasing annual rate of approximately 5%. The most impacted locations were in the West Pacific, Southeast Asia, Africa, and the eastern Mediterranean [83]. In Europe, Italy has a particularly high rate of ESBL, with 26% of *Escherichia coli* displaying resistance to the third-generation cephalosporins in 2013 [84]. Within a country, the prevalence can be very different from one region to another; in some locations, we observed the endemic situation in the community [35], whereas others were scarcely affected [35]. A 2012 French prospective study in a medical ICU showed a 15% ESBL-producing *Enterobacterales* carriage rate, mostly of *Escherichia coli* (62%). Transfer from another ICU, previous hospital admission in another country, surgery within the past year, prior neurologic disease, and prior administration of third-generation cephalosporin (within 3–12 months before ICU admission) have been found to be risk factors of ESBL-producing *Enterobacterales* carriage at ICU admission. Furthermore, advanced age, male gender, colonization pressure (defined as the sum of the daily proportion of patients in the unit colonized with ESBL-PE during the days preceding acquisition or ICU discharge), 3GC within the past three months, and B-lactam + inhibitor within three months were associated with the ESBL-PE-acquired carriage in the ICU in the same study [73].

4.5. AmpC Hyperproducing Enterobacterales (AHE)

In a retrospective study of more than a thousand ICU patients, the prevalence of intestinal colonization with AHE evolved from 2% at admission to 30% in patients with lengths of stay (LOS) exceeding four weeks. Metronidazole, cephalosporin use, and the LOS were found to be independently associated with acquired carriage in ICU patients [85]. It has been known for over 50 years that commensal anaerobes confer protection against exogenous pathogens, which may explain why metronidazole, by its impact on colonization resistance, favors the emergence of such mutants from subdominant, wild-type *Enterobacterales* populations. Therefore, AHE community prevalence could be considered insignificant, whereas its emergence in the ICU should not. Currently, information on the digestive carriage of AHE is not systematically provided to the clinician and differs from one center to another, even though studies have shown the value of this information for initial therapeutic adequacy in the case of sepsis [86].

4.6. Carbapenemase-Producing Enterobacterales (CPE)

The distribution of the different types of CPE is very heterogeneous on a global scale [87]. In communities, *Klebsiella*-producing Carbapenemase (KPC) is widespread in the United States and endemic in some European countries, such as Greece and Italy [88]. Among the metallo-β-lactamases (MBL), New Delhi metallo-β-lactamase (NDM), Verona integron-encoded metallo-β-lactamase (VIM), and imipenemase metallo-β-lactamase (IMP) enzymes are the most frequently identified worldwide [89]. IMP producing Gram-negative bacteria are mainly located in eastern Asia and Australia, mostly in *Acinetobacter baumannii*. VIM producers are most often found in Italy and Greece (*Enterobacterales*) and in Russia (*Pseudomonas aeruginosa*) [90,91]. OXA-48–producing *Enterobacterales* are endemic in Turkey and are frequently encountered in several European countries and across North Africa [92]. Reported risk factors for community carriage of CPE are, as expected, geographical location and recent antibiotic use. In the ICU, the prevalence of CPE varies from 6% to 37%, depending on the unit location [93,94]. A recent five-year case control study found the length of hospital admission >20 days, hospital admission within the previous year, exposure to a healthcare facility in a country with high carbapenem-resistant *Enterobacterales* prevalence 3 months before admission, and the use of antibiotics longer than 10 days to be independent predictors of CPE carriage.

4.7. Methicillin-Resistant Staphylococcus aureus (MRSA)

Several risk factors of MRSA acquisition during a hospital stay have been described as LOS, presence of patients colonized with MRSA in the same ICU at the same time, previous antibiotic use (especially ticarcillin/clavulanic acid), central venous catheter insertion, and period of nurse understaffing [95,96]. Interestingly, the specific population of trauma patients have been found to be particularly at risk of MRSA acquisition. In this very population, road traffic accident victims were at greater risk of acquiring MRSA than patients who had suffered other mechanisms of injury, probably because of more skin defects, such as open versus closed fractures, or more surgical procedures [97].

5. When to Use Broad-Spectrum Antibiotics, What Tools to Guide Us?

Colonization of the upper respiratory tract is a precondition to VAP in almost all patients [98]. However, prior colonization is not systematically responsible for the infection. Carriage should be interpreted solely as a risk factor as it could not be responsible for an infection on its own [99,100]. It is important to emphasize this point, considering the fact that knowledge of colonization misleads physicians in an overprescribing path [101].

5.1. Moving from an Empirical to Oriented Antimicrobial Choices

The conventional microbiological approach for HAP-VAP diagnosis consisted of cultures coupled with antimicrobial susceptibility testing, requiring approximately 48 h to 72 h from sampling to results delivery to physicians. It is important to notice that the implementation of MALDI-TOF MS in microbiology laboratories has already shown an impact on HAP-VAP management [102].

New strategies need to be implemented to reduce the pathogen identification time and MDRO-genes because of frequently unappropriated empirical therapy. Molecular techniques, such as syndromic m-PCR panels, have introduced a considerable change in antibiomicrobial stewardship intervention, accelerating targeted therapy in different conditions such as HAP-VAP.

Among these, the BioFire® FilmArray® Pneumonia Panel (FA-PN) (bioMérieux SA, Marcy-l'Étoile, France) is the widely used one. It is a Food and Drug Administration (FDA) syndromic m-PCR that simultaneously identifies 33 targets: 15 typical and 3 atypical bacterial pathogens, 8 respiratory viruses and 7 resistance genes in BAL/mini-BAL, tracheal aspirates (ETA), and sputum specimens.

Two recent multicentric studies on performance evaluation demonstrated excellent positive percentage agreement and negative percentage agreement values when compared with conventional culture methods [103,104]. In all these studies, it is important that the prevalence of bacteria off-panel is non-negligible and should be kept in mind by physicians and laboratory staff.

Many prospective and retrospective studies, so-called "real-life studies", have been published to evaluate the clinical impact of this approach. Caméléna et al. showed a considerably reduced sample-to-result time compared to conventional approach (5.5 h vs. 25.9 h for cultures ($p < 0.001$) and 57 h for AST ($p < 0.001$), respectively) [105]. During the COVID-19 pandemic, Maataaoui et al. revealed in a prospective cohort of 112 episodes (104 HAP-VAP) an early empirical therapeutic change in 34% of HAP-VAP episodes (of which 46.3% were withdrawn) when this panel was performed [106]. Another recent prospective study showed among COVID-19 ICU patients that antibiotics were initiated in 87 (72.5%) of 120 pneumonia episodes and were not administered in 80 (87.0%) of 92 non-pneumonia episodes based on FA results [107].

Because of the high cost of this approach, some studies suggested scores to rationalize performing such a test. A comprehensive study suggested that both clinical (temperature and Clinical Pulmonary Infection Score) and biological parameters (WBC BAL count and % of PMNs) were correlated with FA-PN with or without conventional culture results [108]. In some cases, interpretation of results remains a challenge for physicians and laboratory staff. Based on a retrospective non-interventional study, Novy et al. designed an algorithm helping antimicrobial stewardship prescription with FA-PN results in cases of HAP-VAP suspicion and confirmed the poor reliability of ETA samples because of over-detection of the microbial and viral genome [109].

Other panels exist, such as the syndromic m-PCR panel for HAP-VAP developed by Curetis (Curetis GmbH, Holzgerlingen, Germany) with The Unyvero P55 Pneumonia panel, capable of identifying 20 pathogens of lower respiratory tract infections (LRTI) and 19 resistance genes. With a longer turn-around time of 5 h, performances seemed to be lower than previously described panels. However, a non-interventional study recently showed that this test could have led to modifications of empirical therapy in 60% (57/95) of HAP-VAP episodes [110]. "In-house" multiplex PCRs have been customized by several laboratories, such as the custom-designed multi-pathogen TaqMan Array Cards (TAC; Thermo Fisher Scientific, Waltham, MA, USA) in a UK center with good analytical performance [111].

This kind of approach has the advantage of identifying multiple pathogens with a shorter turn-around time, including those which are fastidious and pathogens that cannot be retrieved by conventional cultures. This remains particularly true when antimicrobials have already been started before sampling.

However, the reliance on the presence of resistance genes should be interpreted with caution. Importantly, these methods can only detect antibiotic resistance genes which have been chosen by industrials, and the limits of these assays need to be well known by physicians and microbiology labs. Conventional culture methods shall be continued because of the significant prevalence of uncovered pathogens.

5.2. How to Choose the Empirical Antibiotic: "Because It Was Him, Because It Was Me"

The ICU carries multiple specificities making the choice of empiric antimicrobial therapy a singular decision for each patient. Indeed, multiple parameters must be considered for critically ill patients, including the severity of illness, the seriousness of the situation, the certainty of the diagnosis, the local microbial ecology, and MDR prevalence in the unit. However, once these parameters are settled, the first legitimate question would be: does the treatment have to be empirical?

5.3. Rusher or Dragger?

Delayed initiation of antibiotic therapy has often been cited as a major risk factor for excess mortality, supporting the idea that "a large antimicrobial spectrum" should be provided to ICU patients. As the global rise of MDR incidence has become more widely known among practitioners, a "structural" tension has arisen between the need not to delay antibiotic therapy and the need to choose the right one. The idea that all ICU patients should be started on antibiotics as soon as possible implies that all patients admitted in those units have the same level of severity which is obviously inaccurate [112]. Studies have shown that this increased risk of mortality due to delayed initiation of antibiotic therapy was effective, especially for the most severe patients [113]. It would, therefore, seem appropriate, when the patient's condition allows it, to wait for the germ identification and antibiogram.

5.4. Under Pressure

Local epidemiological knowledge is crucial. As seen previously, there is a heterogeneity in the distribution of MDRs, which suggests different considerations when choosing antibiotics, depending on the unit location [114]. If MDR carriage does not mandate any antibiotic therapy, it is well documented that it is a necessary step prior to infection [115]. Hence, each practitioner should be aware of the bacterial epidemiology of the hospital and unit in which they work [33].

Colonization pressure described in 1994 by Bonten et al. [116] is a fundamental concept that needs to be addressed in order to choose an adequate antibiotic. A study led by Trouillet et al. in 1998 was the first trial to link the changing bacterial epidemiology according to mechanical ventilation (MV) duration and previous antibiotic therapy. Firstly, it showed that patients who were not exposed to antibiotics and who underwent MV for less than seven days (in other terms, patients who had very low colonization pressure) were infected with the "usual" germs present in oropharyngeal and respiratory microbiota (*Streptococcus*, *Haemophilus influenzae*, Enterobacterales). On the other hand, when they underwent MV for more than seven days and had greater antibiotic exposure, non-fermenting gram-negative bacilli (PA, *Stenotrophomonas*, *Acinetobacter*) were more frequent. Multiple lessons could be drawn from this study with a remarkable reproducibility in the following years. It showed the importance of colonization pressure in VAP bacterial epidemiology and raised awareness about the fundamtental importance of selection pressure, which has been later confirmed in other studies [117]. MDR prevalence and antibiotic usage have risen in the 20 years since this historical study. If the "five days after ICU admission cut off" is since then usually used to materialize the risk of resistance [111,118], shifting the clinical and epidemiological reasoning in time could be an appropriate current adaptation. Indeed, according to geographical locations and hospital epidemiological situations, the patient admitted to the ICU or already in the ICU and undergoing MV could have experienced colonization and selection pressure for several days before. Thus, considering this pressure from the first contact with the healthcare facility (Emergency Room, medical ward, ICU), the question "what antibiotic should I use for this VAP?" as a continuum might be more relevant.

In conclusion, the reasoned choice of antibiotics to treat HAP/VAP requires the consideration of many variables ranging from local epidemiological data to the patient's personal history, including prior antibiotic therapy and length of stay (Figure 3). The new microbiological diagnostic methods make it possible to move from an empirical prescription to an oriented prescription, reducing the delay for adequate antibiotic therapy.

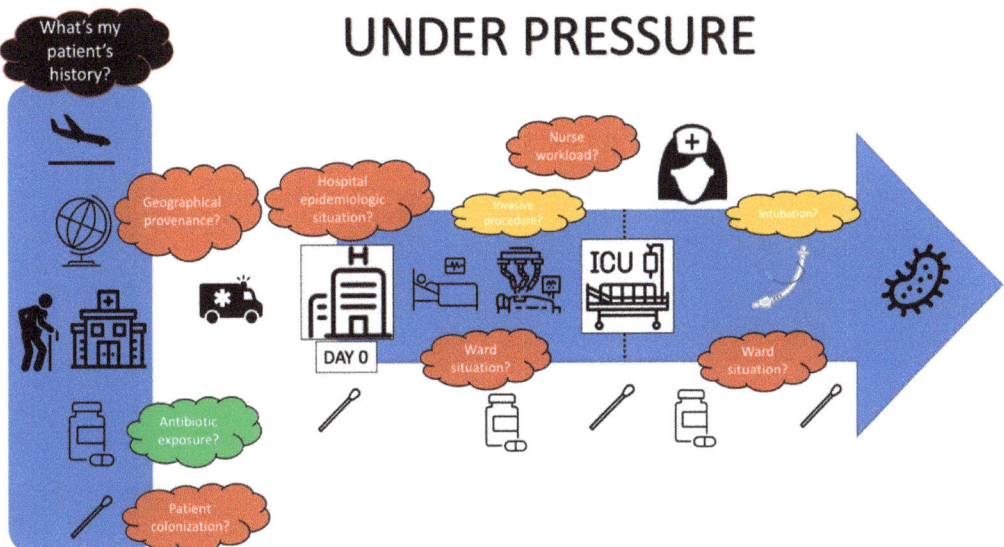

Figure 3. Under pressure.

Author Contributions: Conceptualization: K.C., G.P.d.P., J.-R.Z., B.P.; Writing original draft: K.C., G.P.d.P., B.P.; Writing review and editing: K.C., G.P.d.P., L.D., J.-R.Z., B.P. All authors have read and agreed to the published version of the manuscript.

Funding: This research received no external funding.

Conflicts of Interest: The authors declare no conflict of interest.

References

1. Torres, A.; Niederman, M.S.; Chastre, J.; Ewig, S.; Fernandez-Vandellos, P.; Hanberger, H.; Kollef, M.; Li Bassi, G.; Luna, C.M.; Martin-Loeches, I.; et al. International ERS/ESICM/ESCMID/ALAT guidelines for the management of hospital-acquired pneumonia and ventilator-associated pneumonia: Guidelines for the management of hospital-acquired pneumonia (HAP)/ventilator-associated pneumonia (VAP) of the European Respiratory Society (ERS), European Society of Intensive Care Medicine (ESICM), European Society of Clinical Microbiology and Infectious Diseases (ESCMID) and Asociación Latinoamericana del Tórax (ALAT). *Eur. Respir. J.* **2017**, *50*, 1700582. [CrossRef]
2. Rello, J.; Vidaur, L.; Sandiumenge, A.; Rodríguez, A.; Gualis, B.; Boque, C.; Diaz, E. De-escalation therapy in ventilator-associated pneumonia. *Crit. Care Med.* **2004**, *32*, 2183–2190. [CrossRef] [PubMed]
3. Bhargava, A.; Hayakawa, K.; Silverman, E.; Haider, S.; Alluri, K.C.; Datla, S.; Diviti, S.; Kuchipudi, V.; Muppavarapu, K.S.; Lephart, P.R.; et al. Risk factors for colonization due to carbapenem-resistant Enterobacteriaceae among patients exposed to long-term acute care and acute care facilities. *Infect. Control Hosp. Epidemiol.* **2014**, *35*, 398–405. [CrossRef] [PubMed]
4. Jean, S.-S.; Chang, Y.-C.; Lin, W.-C.; Lee, W.-S.; Hsueh, P.-R.; Hsu, C.-W. Epidemiology, Treatment, and Prevention of Nosocomial Bacterial Pneumonia. *J. Clin. Med.* **2020**, *9*, 275. [CrossRef] [PubMed]
5. Schwaber, M.J.; Carmeli, Y. Carbapenem-resistant Enterobacteriaceae: A potential threat. *JAMA* **2008**, *300*, 2911–2913. [CrossRef]
6. Kelly, A.M.; Mathema, B.; Larson, E.L. Carbapenem-resistant Enterobacteriaceae in the community: A scoping review. *Int. J. Antimicrob. Agents* **2017**, *50*, 127–134. [CrossRef]
7. Pitout, J.D.D. Enterobacteriaceae that produce extended-spectrum β-lactamases and AmpC β-lactamases in the community: The tip of the iceberg? *Curr. Pharm. Des.* **2013**, *19*, 257–263. [CrossRef]
8. van Duin, D.; Paterson, D.L. Multidrug-Resistant Bacteria in the Community. *Infect. Dis. Clin. North Am.* **2020**, *34*, 709–722. [CrossRef]
9. Ladner, J.T.; Grubaugh, N.D.; Pybus, O.G.; Andersen, K.G. Precision epidemiology for infectious disease control. *Nat. Med.* **2019**, *25*, 206–211. [CrossRef]

10. American Thoracic Society; Infectious Diseases Society of America Guidelines for the management of adults with hospital-acquired, ventilator-associated, and healthcare-associated pneumonia. *Am. J. Respir. Crit. Care Med.* **2005**, *171*, 388–416. [CrossRef]
11. Rivers, E.; Nguyen, B.; Havstad, S.; Ressler, J.; Muzzin, A.; Knoblich, B.; Peterson, E.; Tomlanovich, M. Early Goal-Directed Therapy in the Treatment of Severe Sepsis and Septic Shock. *N. Engl. J. Med.* **2001**, *345*, 1368–1377. [CrossRef] [PubMed]
12. Jones, B.E.; Jones, M.M.; Huttner, B.; Stoddard, G.; Brown, K.A.; Stevens, V.W.; Greene, T.; Sauer, B.; Madaras-Kelly, K.; Rubin, M.; et al. Trends in Antibiotic Use and Nosocomial Pathogens in Hospitalized Veterans With Pneumonia at 128 Medical Centers, 2006-2010. *Clin. Infect. Dis. Off. Publ. Infect. Dis. Soc. Am.* **2015**, *61*, 1403–1410. [CrossRef] [PubMed]
13. Chalmers, J.D.; Rother, C.; Salih, W.; Ewig, S. Healthcare-associated pneumonia does not accurately identify potentially resistant pathogens: A systematic review and meta-analysis. *Clin. Infect. Dis. Off. Publ. Infect. Dis. Soc. Am.* **2014**, *58*, 330–339. [CrossRef] [PubMed]
14. Kollef, M.H.; Shorr, A.; Tabak, Y.P.; Gupta, V.; Liu, L.Z.; Johannes, R.S. Epidemiology and outcomes of health-care-associated pneumonia: Results from a large US database of culture-positive pneumonia. *Chest* **2005**, *128*, 3854–3862. [CrossRef]
15. Shindo, Y.; Ito, R.; Kobayashi, D.; Ando, M.; Ichikawa, M.; Shiraki, A.; Goto, Y.; Fukui, Y.; Iwaki, M.; Okumura, J.; et al. Risk factors for drug-resistant pathogens in community-acquired and healthcare-associated pneumonia. *Am. J. Respir. Crit. Care Med.* **2013**, *188*, 985–995. [CrossRef]
16. Schweitzer, V.A.; van Werkhoven, C.H.; van Heijl, I.; Smits, R.F.; Boel, C.H.E.; Bonten, M.J.M.; Postma, D.F.; Oosterheert, J.J. Relevance of healthcare-associated pneumonia for empirical antibiotic therapy in the Netherlands. *Neth. J. Med.* **2018**, *76*, 389–396. [PubMed]
17. Garcia-Vidal, C.; Viasus, D.; Roset, A.; Adamuz, J.; Verdaguer, R.; Dorca, J.; Gudiol, F.; Carratalà, J. Low incidence of multidrug-resistant organisms in patients with healthcare-associated pneumonia requiring hospitalization. *Clin. Microbiol. Infect.* **2011**, *17*, 1659–1665. [CrossRef]
18. Healthcare-associated infections in intensive care units—Annual Epidemiological Report for 2017. Available online: https://www.ecdc.europa.eu/en/publications-data/healthcare-associated-infections-intensive-care-units-annual-epidemiological-1 (accessed on 10 September 2021).
19. Papazian, L.; Klompas, M.; Luyt, C.-E. Ventilator-associated pneumonia in adults: A narrative review. *Intensiv. Care Med.* **2020**, *46*, 888–906. [CrossRef]
20. Di Pasquale, M.; Ferrer, M.; Esperatti, M.; Crisafulli, E.; Giunta, V.; Li Bassi, G.; Rinaudo, M.; Blasi, F.; Niederman, M.; Torres, A. Assessment of severity of ICU-acquired pneumonia and association with etiology. *Crit. Care Med.* **2014**, *42*, 303–312. [CrossRef]
21. Arvanitis, M.; Anagnostou, T.; Kourkoumpetis, T.K.; Ziakas, P.D.; Desalermos, A.; Mylonakis, E. The Impact of Antimicrobial Resistance and Aging in VAP Outcomes: Experience from a Large Tertiary Care Center. *PLoS ONE* **2014**, *9*, e89984. [CrossRef]
22. Blot, S.; Koulenti, D.; Dimopoulos, G.; Martin, C.; Komnos, A.; Krueger, W.A.; Spina, G.; Armaganidis, A.; Rello, J. EU-VAP Study Investigators Prevalence, risk factors, and mortality for ventilator-associated pneumonia in middle-aged, old, and very old critically ill patients*. *Crit. Care Med.* **2014**, *42*, 601–609. [CrossRef]
23. Martin-Loeches, I.; Torres, A.; Rinaudo, M.; Terraneo, S.; de Rosa, F.; Ramirez, P.; Diaz, E.; Fernández-Barat, L.; Li Bassi, G.L.; Ferrer, M. Resistance patterns and outcomes in intensive care unit (ICU)-acquired pneumonia. Validation of European Centre for Disease Prevention and Control (ECDC) and the Centers for Disease Control and Prevention (CDC) classification of multidrug resistant organisms. *J. Infect.* **2015**, *70*, 213–222. [CrossRef]
24. Franchineau, G.; Luyt, C.E.; Combes, A.; Schmidt, M. Ventilator-associated pneumonia in extracorporeal membrane oxygenation-assisted patients. *Ann. Transl. Med.* **2018**, *6*, 427. [CrossRef]
25. Muscedere, J.G.; Day, A.; Heyland, D.K. Mortality, attributable mortality, and clinical events as end points for clinical trials of ventilator-associated pneumonia and hospital-acquired pneumonia. *Clin. Infect. Dis.* **2010**, *51* (Suppl. S1), S120–S125. [CrossRef]
26. Kollef, M.H.; Hamilton, C.W.; Ernst, F.R. Economic impact of ventilator-associated pneumonia in a large matched cohort. *Infect. Control Hosp. Epidemiol.* **2012**, *33*, 250–256. [CrossRef]
27. Zimlichman, E.; Henderson, D.; Tamir, O.; Franz, C.; Song, P.; Yamin, C.K.; Keohane, C.; Denham, C.R.; Bates, D.W. Health care-associated infections: A meta-analysis of costs and financial impact on the US health care system. *JAMA Intern. Med.* **2013**, *173*, 2039–2046. [CrossRef]
28. Melsen, W.G.; Rovers, M.M.; Groenwold, R.H.H.; Bergmans, D.C.J.J.; Camus, C.; Bauer, T.T.; Hanisch, E.W.; Klarin, B.; Koeman, M.; Krueger, W.A.; et al. Attributable mortality of ventilator-associated pneumonia: A meta-analysis of individual patient data from randomised prevention studies. *Lancet Infect. Dis.* **2013**, *13*, 665–671. [CrossRef]
29. Weiner, L.M.; Webb, A.K.; Limbago, B.; Dudeck, M.A.; Patel, J.; Kallen, A.J.; Edwards, J.R.; Sievert, D.M. Antimicrobial-Resistant Pathogens Associated With Healthcare-Associated Infections: Summary of Data Reported to the National Healthcare Safety Network at the Centers for Disease Control and Prevention, 2011–2014. *Infect. Control Hosp. Epidemiol.* **2016**, *37*, 1288–1301. [CrossRef]
30. Jones, R.N. Microbial etiologies of hospital-acquired bacterial pneumonia and ventilator-associated bacterial pneumonia. *Clin. Infect. Dis.* **2010**, *51* (Suppl. S1), S81–S87. [CrossRef]

31. Sievert, D.M.; Ricks, P.; Edwards, J.R.; Schneider, A.; Patel, J.; Srinivasan, A.; Kallen, A.; Limbago, B.; Fridkin, S. National Healthcare Safety Network (NHSN) Team and Participating NHSN Facilities Antimicrobial-resistant pathogens associated with healthcare-associated infections: Summary of data reported to the National Healthcare Safety Network at the Centers for Disease Control and Prevention, 2009–2010. *Infect. Control Hosp. Epidemiol.* **2013**, *34*, 1–14. [CrossRef]
32. Weber, D.J.; Rutala, W.A.; Sickbert-Bennett, E.E.; Samsa, G.P.; Brown, V.; Niederman, M.S. Microbiology of ventilator-associated pneumonia compared with that of hospital-acquired pneumonia. *Infect. Control Hosp. Epidemiol.* **2007**, *28*, 825–831. [CrossRef] [PubMed]
33. Kalil, A.C.; Metersky, M.L.; Klompas, M.; Muscedere, J.; Sweeney, D.A.; Palmer, L.B.; Napolitano, L.M.; O'Grady, N.P.; Bartlett, J.G.; Carratalà, J.; et al. Management of Adults With Hospital-acquired and Ventilator-associated Pneumonia: 2016 Clinical Practice Guidelines by the Infectious Diseases Society of America and the American Thoracic Society. *Clin. Infect. Dis.* **2016**, *63*, e61–e111. [CrossRef] [PubMed]
34. Derde, L.P.G.; Cooper, B.S.; Goossens, H.; Malhotra-Kumar, S.; Willems, R.J.L.; Gniadkowski, M.; Hryniewicz, W.; Empel, J.; Dautzenberg, M.J.D.; Annane, D.; et al. Interventions to reduce colonisation and transmission of antimicrobial-resistant bacteria in intensive care units: An interrupted time series study and cluster randomised trial. *Lancet Infect. Dis.* **2014**, *14*, 31–39. [CrossRef]
35. Pilmis, B.; Cattoir, V.; Lecointe, D.; Limelette, A.; Grall, I.; Mizrahi, A.; Marcade, G.; Poilane, I.; Guillard, T.; Bourgeois Nicolaos, N.; et al. Carriage of ESBL-producing Enterobacteriaceae in French hospitals: The PORTABLSE study. *J. Hosp. Infect.* **2018**, *98*, 247–252. [CrossRef] [PubMed]
36. Zahar, J.-R.; Blot, S.; Nordmann, P.; Martischang, R.; Timsit, J.-F.; Harbarth, S.; Barbier, F. Screening for Intestinal Carriage of Extended-spectrum Beta-lactamase-producing Enterobacteriaceae in Critically Ill Patients: Expected Benefits and Evidence-based Controversies. *Clin. Infect. Dis.* **2019**, *68*, 2125–2130. [CrossRef] [PubMed]
37. Wertheim, H.F.L.; Vos, M.C.; Ott, A.; van Belkum, A.; Voss, A.; Kluytmans, J.A.J.W.; van Keulen, P.H.J.; Vandenbroucke-Grauls, C.M.J.E.; Meester, M.H.M.; Verbrugh, H.A. Risk and outcome of nosocomial Staphylococcus aureus bacteraemia in nasal carriers versus non-carriers. *Lancet Lond. Engl.* **2004**, *364*, 703–705. [CrossRef]
38. Wertheim, H.F.L.; Melles, D.C.; Vos, M.C.; van Leeuwen, W.; van Belkum, A.; Verbrugh, H.A.; Nouwen, J.L. The role of nasal carriage in Staphylococcus aureus infections. *Lancet Infect. Dis.* **2005**, *5*, 751–762. [CrossRef]
39. Wertheim, H.F.L.; Verbrugh, H.A. Global prevalence of meticillin-resistant Staphylococcus aureus. *Lancet Lond. Engl.* **2006**, *368*, 1866. [CrossRef]
40. Paling, F.P.; Wolkewitz, M.; Bode, L.G.M.; Klein Klouwenberg, P.M.C.; Ong, D.S.Y.; Depuydt, P.; de Bus, L.; Sifakis, F.; Bonten, M.J.M.; Kluytmans, J.A.J.W. *Staphylococcus aureus* colonization at ICU admission as a risk factor for developing *S. aureus* ICU pneumonia. *Clin. Microbiol. Infect.* **2017**, *23*, e9–e49. [CrossRef]
41. Launey, Y.; Asehnoune, K.; Lasocki, S.; Dahyot-Fizelier, C.; Huet, O.; Le Pabic, E.; Malejac, B.; Seguin, P. AtlanRéa Group Risk factors for ventilator-associated pneumonia due to Staphylococcus aureus in patients with severe brain injury: A multicentre retrospective cohort study. *Anaesth. Crit. Care Pain Med.* **2021**, *40*, 100785. [CrossRef]
42. Tilouche, L.; Ben Dhia, R.; Boughattas, S.; Ketata, S.; Bouallegue, O.; Chaouch, C.; Boujaafar, N. Staphylococcus aureus Ventilator-Associated Pneumonia: A Study of Bacterio-Epidemiological Profile and Virulence Factors. *Curr. Microbiol.* **2021**, *78*, 2556–2562. [CrossRef]
43. Zahar, J.-R.; Lesprit, P.; Ruckly, S.; Eden, A.; Hikombo, H.; Bernard, L.; Harbarth, S.; Timsit, J.-F.; Brun-Buisson, C. BacterCom Study Group Predominance of healthcare-associated cases among episodes of community-onset bacteraemia due to extended-spectrum β-lactamase-producing Enterobacteriaceae. *Int. J. Antimicrob. Agents* **2017**, *49*, 67–73. [CrossRef]
44. Cillóniz, C.; Gabarrús, A.; Ferrer, M.; Puig de la Bellacasa, J.; Rinaudo, M.; Mensa, J.; Niederman, M.S.; Torres, A. Community-Acquired Pneumonia Due to Multidrug- and Non-Multidrug-Resistant Pseudomonas aeruginosa. *Chest* **2016**, *150*, 415–425. [CrossRef]
45. Venier, A.G.; Gruson, D.; Lavigne, T.; Jarno, P.; L'hériteau, F.; Coignard, B.; Savey, A.; Rogues, A.M. REA-RAISIN group Identifying new risk factors for Pseudomonas aeruginosa pneumonia in intensive care units: Experience of the French national surveillance, REA-RAISIN. *J. Hosp. Infect.* **2011**, *79*, 44–48. [CrossRef]
46. Paling, F.P.; Wolkewitz, M.; Depuydt, P.; de Bus, L.; Sifakis, F.; Bonten, M.J.M.; Kluytmans, J.A.J.W. *P. aeruginosa* colonization at ICU admission as a risk factor for developing *P. aeruginosa* ICU pneumonia. *Antimicrob. Resist. Infect. Control* **2017**, *6*, 38. [CrossRef]
47. Harris, A.D.; Jackson, S.S.; Robinson, G.; Pineles, L.; Leekha, S.; Thom, K.A.; Wang, Y.; Doll, M.; Pettigrew, M.M.; Johnson, J.K. Pseudomonas aeruginosa Colonization in the Intensive Care Unit: Prevalence, Risk Factors, and Clinical Outcomes. *Infect. Control Hosp. Epidemiol.* **2016**, *37*, 544–548. [CrossRef]
48. Craven, D.E.; Steger, K.A. Nosocomial pneumonia in mechanically ventilated adult patients: Epidemiology and prevention in 1996. *Semin. Respir. Infect.* **1996**, *11*, 32–53.
49. Spellberg, B.; Bonomo, R.A. Combination Therapy for Extreme Drug Resistant (XDR) Acinetobacter baumannii: Ready for Prime-Time? *Crit. Care Med.* **2015**, *43*, 1332–1334. [CrossRef]
50. Sarshar, M.; Behzadi, P.; Scribano, D.; Palamara, A.T.; Ambrosi, C. Acinetobacter baumannii: An Ancient Commensal with Weapons of a Pathogen. *Pathogens* **2021**, *10*, 387. [CrossRef]
51. Zeighami, H.; Valadkhani, F.; Shapouri, R.; Samadi, E.; Haghi, F. Virulence characteristics of multidrug resistant biofilm forming Acinetobacter baumannii isolated from intensive care unit patients. *BMC Infect. Dis.* **2019**, *19*, 629. [CrossRef]

52. Dijkshoorn, L.; van Aken, E.; Shunburne, L.; van der Reijden, T.J.K.; Bernards, A.T.; Nemec, A.; Towner, K.J. Prevalence of Acinetobacter baumannii and other Acinetobacter spp. in faecal samples from non-hospitalised individuals. *Clin. Microbiol. Infect.* **2005**, *11*, 329–332. [CrossRef]
53. Chatellier, D.; Burucoa, C.; Pinsard, M.; Frat, J.-P.; Robert, R. Prevalence of Acinetobacter baumannii carriage in patients of 53 French intensive care units on a given day. *Med. Mal. Infect.* **2007**, *37*, 112–117. [CrossRef] [PubMed]
54. Chen, M.Z.; Hsueh, P.R.; Lee, L.N.; Yu, C.J.; Yang, P.C.; Luh, K.T. Severe community-acquired pneumonia due to Acinetobacter baumannii. *Chest* **2001**, *120*, 1072–1077. [CrossRef] [PubMed]
55. Dexter, C.; Murray, G.L.; Paulsen, I.T.; Peleg, A.Y. Community-acquired Acinetobacter baumannii: Clinical characteristics, epidemiology and pathogenesis. *Expert Rev. Anti Infect. Ther.* **2015**, *13*, 567–573. [CrossRef]
56. García-Garmendia, J.-L.; Ortiz-Leyba, C.; Garnacho-Montero, J.; Jiménez-Jiménez, F.-J.; Pérez-Paredes, C.; Barrero-Almodóvar, A.E.; Miner, M.G. Risk Factors for Acinetobacter baumannii Nosocomial Bacteremia in Critically Ill Patients: A Cohort Study. *Clin. Infect. Dis.* **2001**, *33*, 939–946. [CrossRef]
57. Lee, M.-R.; Wang, H.-C.; Yang, C.-Y.; Lin, C.-K.; Kuo, H.-Y.; Ko, J.-C.; Sheng, W.-H.; Lee, L.-N.; Yu, C.-J.; Hsueh, P.-R. Clinical characteristics and outcomes of patients with pleural infections due to Stenotrophomonas maltophilia at a medical center in Taiwan, 2004–2012. *Eur. J. Clin. Microbiol.* **2014**, *33*, 1143–1148. [CrossRef]
58. Kim, E.J.; Kim, Y.C.; Ahn, J.Y.; Jeong, S.J.; Ku, N.S.; Choi, J.Y.; Yeom, J.-S.; Song, Y.G. Risk factors for mortality in patients with Stenotrophomonas maltophilia bacteremia and clinical impact of quinolone-resistant strains. *BMC Infect. Dis.* **2019**, *19*, 754. [CrossRef]
59. Ibn Saied, W.; Merceron, S.; Schwebel, C.; Le Monnier, A.; Oziel, J.; Garrouste-Orgeas, M.; Marcotte, G.; Ruckly, S.; Souweine, B.; Darmon, M.; et al. Ventilator-associated pneumonia due to Stenotrophomonas maltophilia: Risk factors and outcome. *J. Infect.* **2020**, *80*, 279–285. [CrossRef]
60. Guerci, P.; Bellut, H.; Mokhtari, M.; Gaudefroy, J.; Mongardon, N.; Charpentier, C.; Louis, G.; Tashk, P.; Dubost, C.; Ledochowski, S.; et al. Outcomes of Stenotrophomonas maltophilia hospital-acquired pneumonia in intensive care unit: A nationwide retrospective study. *Crit. Care Lond. Engl.* **2019**, *23*, 371. [CrossRef]
61. Jeon, Y.D.; Jeong, W.Y.; Kim, M.H.; Jung, I.Y.; Ahn, M.Y.; Ann, H.W.; Ahn, J.Y.; Han, S.H.; Choi, J.Y.; Song, Y.G.; et al. Risk factors for mortality in patients with Stenotrophomonas maltophilia bacteremia. *Medicine* **2016**, *95*, e4375. [CrossRef]
62. Coppry, M.; Jeanne-Leroyer, C.; Noize, P.; Dumartin, C.; Boyer, A.; Bertrand, X.; Dubois, V.; Rogues, A.-M. Antibiotics associated with acquisition of carbapenem-resistant Pseudomonas aeruginosa in ICUs: A multicentre nested case-case-control study. *J. Antimicrob. Chemother.* **2019**, *74*, 503–510. [CrossRef]
63. Paramythiotou, E.; Lucet, J.-C.; Timsit, J.-F.; Vanjak, D.; Paugam-Burtz, C.; Trouillet, J.-L.; Belloc, S.; Kassis, N.; Karabinis, A.; Andremont, A. Acquisition of multidrug-resistant Pseudomonas aeruginosa in patients in intensive care units: Role of antibiotics with antipseudomonal activity. *Clin. Infect. Dis.* **2004**, *38*, 670–677. [CrossRef]
64. Dewart, C.M.; Hebert, C.; Pancholi, P.; Stevenson, K. 482. Time Series Analysis of Antimicrobial Consumption and Pseudomonas aeruginosa Resistance in an Academic Medical Center in the United States (2013–2018). *Open Forum Infect. Dis.* **2019**, *6*, S236. [CrossRef]
65. Hotta, G.; Matsumura, Y.; Kato, K.; Nakano, S.; Yunoki, T.; Yamamoto, M.; Nagao, M.; Ito, Y.; Takakura, S.; Ichiyama, S. Risk factors and outcomes of Stenotrophomonas maltophilia bacteraemia: A comparison with bacteraemia caused by Pseudomonas aeruginosa and Acinetobacter species. *PLoS ONE* **2014**, *9*, e112208. [CrossRef]
66. Pallares, R.; Pujol, M.; Peña, C.; Ariza, J.; Martin, R.; Gudiol, F. Cephalosporins as risk factor for nosocomial Enterococcus faecalis bacteremia. A matched case-control study. *Arch. Intern. Med.* **1993**, *153*, 1581–1586. [CrossRef]
67. Planquette, B.; Timsit, J.-F.; Misset, B.Y.; Schwebel, C.; Azoulay, E.; Adrie, C.; Vesin, A.; Jamali, S.; Zahar, J.-R.; Allaouchiche, B.; et al. Pseudomonas aeruginosa ventilator-associated pneumonia. predictive factors of treatment failure. *Am. J. Respir. Crit. Care Med.* **2013**, *188*, 69–76. [CrossRef]
68. Pettigrew, M.M.; Gent, J.F.; Kong, Y.; Halpin, A.L.; Pineles, L.; Harris, A.D.; Johnson, J.K. Gastrointestinal Microbiota Disruption and Risk of Colonization With Carbapenem-resistant Pseudomonas aeruginosa in Intensive Care Unit Patients. *Clin. Infect. Dis.* **2019**, *69*, 604–613. [CrossRef]
69. Ravi, A.; Halstead, F.D.; Bamford, A.; Casey, A.; Thomson, N.M.; van Schaik, W.; Snelson, C.; Goulden, R.; Foster-Nyarko, E.; Savva, G.M.; et al. Loss of microbial diversity and pathogen domination of the gut microbiota in critically ill patients. *Microb. Genomics* **2019**, *5*. [CrossRef]
70. Bruyère, R.; Vigneron, C.; Bador, J.; Aho, S.; Toitot, A.; Quenot, J.-P.; Prin, S.; Emmanuel Charles, P. Significance of Prior Digestive Colonization With Extended-Spectrum β-Lactamase–Producing Enterobacteriaceae in Patients With Ventilator-Associated Pneumonia. *Crit. Care Med.* **2016**, *44*, 699–706. [CrossRef]
71. Dubinsky-Pertzov, B.; Temkin, E.; Harbarth, S.; Fankhauser-Rodriguez, C.; Carevic, B.; Radovanovic, I.; Ris, F.; Kariv, Y.; Buchs, N.C.; Schiffer, E.; et al. Carriage of extended-spectrum beta-lactamase-producing Enterobacteriaceae and the risk of surgical site infection after colorectal surgery: A prospective cohort study. *Clin. Infect. Dis.* **2018**, *68*, 1699–1704. [CrossRef]
72. Razazi, K.; Mekontso Dessap, A.; Carteaux, G.; Jansen, C.; Decousser, J.-W.; de Prost, N.; Brun-Buisson, C. Frequency, associated factors and outcome of multi-drug-resistant intensive care unit-acquired pneumonia among patients colonized with extended-spectrum β-lactamase-producing Enterobacteriaceae. *Ann. Intensiv. Care* **2017**, *7*, 61. [CrossRef] [PubMed]

73. Razazi, K.; Derde, L.P.G.; Verachten, M.; Legrand, P.; Lesprit, P.; Brun-Buisson, C. Clinical impact and risk factors for colonization with extended-spectrum β-lactamase-producing bacteria in the intensive care unit. *Intensiv. Care Med.* **2012**, *38*, 1769–1778. [CrossRef] [PubMed]
74. Barbier, F.; Pommier, C.; Essaied, W.; Garrouste-Orgeas, M.; Schwebel, C.; Ruckly, S.; Dumenil, A.-S.; Lemiale, V.; Mourvillier, B.; Clec'h, C.; et al. Colonization and infection with extended-spectrum β-lactamase-producing Enterobacteriaceae in ICU patients: What impact on outcomes and carbapenem exposure? *J. Antimicrob. Chemother.* **2016**, *71*, 1088–1097. [CrossRef]
75. Jalalzaï, W.; Boutrot, M.; Guinard, J.; Guigon, A.; Bret, L.; Poisson, D.-M.; Boulain, T.; Barbier, F. Cessation of screening for intestinal carriage of extended-spectrum β-lactamase-producing Enterobacteriaceae in a low-endemicity intensive care unit with universal contact precautions. *Clin. Microbiol. Infect.* **2018**, *24*, 429.e7–429.e12. [CrossRef]
76. Vodovar, D.; Marcadé, G.; Rousseau, H.; Raskine, L.; Vicaut, E.; Deye, N.; Baud, F.J.; Mégarbane, B. Predictive factors for extended-spectrum beta-lactamase producing Enterobacteriaceae causing infection among intensive care unit patients with prior colonization. *Infection* **2014**, *42*, 743–748. [CrossRef]
77. Logre, E.; Bert, F.; Khoy-Ear, L.; Janny, S.; Giabicani, M.; Grigoresco, B.; Toussaint, A.; Dondero, F.; Dokmak, S.; Roux, O.; et al. Risk Factors and Impact of Perioperative Prophylaxis on the Risk of Extended-spectrum β-Lactamase-producing Enterobacteriaceae-related Infection Among Carriers Following Liver Transplantation. *Transplantation* **2021**, *105*, 338–345. [CrossRef]
78. Barbier, F.; Bailly, S.; Schwebel, C.; Papazian, L.; Azoulay, É.; Kallel, H.; Siami, S.; Argaud, L.; Marcotte, G.; Misset, B.; et al. Infection-related ventilator-associated complications in ICU patients colonised with extended-spectrum β-lactamase-producing Enterobacteriaceae. *Intensiv. Care Med.* **2018**, *44*, 616–626. [CrossRef]
79. Repessé, X.; Artiguenave, M.; Paktoris-Papine, S.; Espinasse, F.; Dinh, A.; Charron, C.; El Sayed, F.; Geri, G.; Vieillard-Baron, A. Epidemiology of extended-spectrum beta-lactamase-producing Enterobacteriaceae in an intensive care unit with no single rooms. *Ann. Intensiv. Care* **2017**, *7*, 73. [CrossRef]
80. Ruppé, E.; Lixandru, B.; Cojocaru, R.; Büke, C.; Paramythiotou, E.; Angebault, C.; Visseaux, C.; Djuikoue, I.; Erdem, E.; Burduniuc, O.; et al. Relative fecal abundance of extended-spectrum-β-lactamase-producing Escherichia coli strains and their occurrence in urinary tract infections in women. *Antimicrob. Agents Chemother.* **2013**, *57*, 4512–4517. [CrossRef]
81. Pilmis, B.; Mizrahi, A.; Péan de Ponfilly, G.; Philippart, F.; Bruel, C.; Zahar, J.-R.; Le Monnier, A. Relative faecal abundance of extended-spectrum β-lactamase-producing Enterobacterales and its impact on infections among intensive care unit patients: A pilot study. *J. Hosp. Infect.* **2021**, *112*, 92–95. [CrossRef]
82. Andremont, O.; Armand-Lefevre, L.; Dupuis, C.; de Montmollin, E.; Ruckly, S.; Lucet, J.-C.; Smonig, R.; Magalhaes, E.; Ruppé, E.; Mourvillier, B.; et al. Semi-quantitative cultures of throat and rectal swabs are efficient tests to predict ESBL-Enterobacterales ventilator-associated pneumonia in mechanically ventilated ESBL carriers. *Intensiv. Care Med.* **2020**, *46*, 1232–1242. [CrossRef] [PubMed]
83. Karanika, S.; Karantanos, T.; Arvanitis, M.; Grigoras, C.; Mylonakis, E. Fecal Colonization With Extended-spectrum Beta-lactamase–Producing Enterobacteriaceae and Risk Factors Among Healthy Individuals: A Systematic Review and Metaanalysis. *Clin. Infect. Dis.* **2016**, *63*, 310–318. [CrossRef] [PubMed]
84. Mondain, V.; Secondo, G.; Guttmann, R.; Ferrea, G.; Dusi, A.; Giacomini, M.; Courjon, J.; Pradier, C. A toolkit for the management of infection or colonization by extended-spectrum beta-lactamase producing Enterobacteriaceae in Italy: Implementation and outcome of a European project. *Eur. J. Clin. Microbiol.* **2018**, *37*, 987–992. [CrossRef] [PubMed]
85. Poignant, S.; Guinard, J.; Guigon, A.; Bret, L.; Poisson, D.-M.; Boulain, T.; Barbier, F. Risk Factors and Outcomes for Intestinal Carriage of AmpC-Hyperproducing Enterobacteriaceae in Intensive Care Unit Patients. *Antimicrob. Agents Chemother.* **2015**, *60*, 1883–1887. [CrossRef]
86. Manquat, E.; Le Dorze, M.; Pean De Ponfilly, G.; Benmansour, H.; Amarsy, R.; Cambau, E.; Soyer, B.; Chousterman, B.G.; Jacquier, H. Impact of systematic screening for AmpC-hyperproducing Enterobacterales intestinal carriage in intensive care unit patients. *Ann. Intensiv. Care* **2020**, *10*, 149. [CrossRef]
87. Bonomo, R.A.; Burd, E.M.; Conly, J.; Limbago, B.M.; Poirel, L.; Segre, J.A.; Westblade, L.F. Carbapenemase-Producing Organisms: A Global Scourge. *Clin. Infect. Dis.* **2018**, *66*, 1290–1297. [CrossRef]
88. Munoz-Price, L.S.; Poirel, L.; Bonomo, R.A.; Schwaber, M.J.; Daikos, G.L.; Cormican, M.; Cornaglia, G.; Garau, J.; Gniadkowski, M.; Hayden, M.K.; et al. Clinical epidemiology of the global expansion of Klebsiella pneumoniae carbapenemases. *Lancet Infect. Dis.* **2013**, *13*, 785–796. [CrossRef]
89. Palzkill, T. Metallo-β-lactamase structure and function. *Ann. N. Y. Acad. Sci.* **2013**, *1277*, 91–104. [CrossRef]
90. Edelstein, M.V.; Skleenova, E.N.; Shevchenko, O.V.; D'souza, J.W.; Tapalski, D.V.; Azizov, I.S.; Sukhorukova, M.V.; Pavlukov, R.A.; Kozlov, R.S.; Toleman, M.A.; et al. Spread of extensively resistant VIM-2-positive ST235 Pseudomonas aeruginosa in Belarus, Kazakhstan, and Russia: A longitudinal epidemiological and clinical study. *Lancet Infect. Dis.* **2013**, *13*, 867–876. [CrossRef]
91. Walsh, T.R.; Toleman, M.A.; Poirel, L.; Nordmann, P. Metallo-beta-lactamases: The quiet before the storm? *Clin. Microbiol. Rev.* **2005**, *18*, 306–325. [CrossRef]
92. Potron, A.; Poirel, L.; Dortet, L.; Nordmann, P. Characterisation of OXA-244, a chromosomally-encoded OXA-48-like β-lactamase from Escherichia coli. *Int. J. Antimicrob. Agents* **2016**, *47*, 102–103. [CrossRef] [PubMed]
93. Soria-Segarra, C.; Soria-Segarra, C.; Catagua-González, A.; Gutiérrez-Fernández, J. Carbapenemase producing Enterobacteriaceae in intensive care units in Ecuador: Results from a multicenter study. *J. Infect. Public Health* **2020**, *13*, 80–88. [CrossRef] [PubMed]

94. Ahn, J.Y.; Song, J.E.; Kim, M.H.; Choi, H.; Kim, J.K.; Ann, H.W.; Kim, J.H.; Jeon, Y.; Jeong, S.J.; Kim, S.B.; et al. Risk factors for the acquisition of carbapenem-resistant Escherichia coli at a tertiary care center in South Korea: A matched case-control study. *Am. J. Infect. Control* **2014**, *42*, 621–625. [CrossRef]
95. Oztoprak, N.; Cevik, M.A.; Akinci, E.; Korkmaz, M.; Erbay, A.; Eren, S.S.; Balaban, N.; Bodur, H. Risk factors for ICU-acquired methicillin-resistant Staphylococcus aureus infections. *Am. J. Infect. Control* **2006**, *34*, 1–5. [CrossRef]
96. Dancer, S.J.; Coyne, M.; Speekenbrink, A.; Samavedam, S.; Kennedy, J.; Wallace, P.G.M. MRSA acquisition in an intensive care unit. *Am. J. Infect. Control* **2006**, *34*, 10–17. [CrossRef]
97. Marshall, C.; Wolfe, R.; Kossmann, T.; Wesselingh, S.; Harrington, G.; Spelman, D. Risk factors for acquisition of methicillin-resistant Staphylococcus aureus (MRSA) by trauma patients in the intensive care unit. *J. Hosp. Infect.* **2004**, *57*, 245–252. [CrossRef] [PubMed]
98. Bonten, M.J.; Bergmans, D.C.; Ambergen, A.W.; de Leeuw, P.W.; van der Geest, S.; Stobberingh, E.E.; Gaillard, C.A. Risk factors for pneumonia, and colonization of respiratory tract and stomach in mechanically ventilated ICU patients. *Am. J. Respir. Crit. Care Med.* **1996**, *154*, 1339–1346. [CrossRef] [PubMed]
99. Rottier, W.C.; Bamberg, Y.R.P.; Dorigo-Zetsma, J.W.; van der Linden, P.D.; Ammerlaan, H.S.M.; Bonten, M.J.M. Predictive value of prior colonization and antibiotic use for third-generation cephalosporin-resistant enterobacteriaceae bacteremia in patients with sepsis. *Clin. Infect. Dis.* **2015**, *60*, 1622–1630. [CrossRef]
100. Hagel, S.; Makarewicz, O.; Hartung, A.; Weiß, D.; Stein, C.; Brandt, C.; Schumacher, U.; Ehricht, R.; Patchev, V.; Pletz, M.W. ESBL colonization and acquisition in a hospital population: The molecular epidemiology and transmission of resistance genes. *PLoS ONE* **2019**, *14*, e0208505. [CrossRef]
101. Hayon, J.; Figliolini, C.; Combes, A.; Trouillet, J.-L.; Kassis, N.; Dombret, M.C.; Gibert, C.; Chastre, J. Role of serial routine microbiologic culture results in the initial management of ventilator-associated pneumonia. *Am. J. Respir. Crit. Care Med.* **2002**, *165*, 41–46. [CrossRef]
102. Mok, J.H.; Eom, J.S.; Jo, E.J.; Kim, M.H.; Lee, K.; Kim, K.U.; Park, H.-K.; Yi, J.; Lee, M.K. Clinical utility of rapid pathogen identification using matrix-assisted laser desorption/ionization time-of-flight mass spectrometry in ventilated patients with pneumonia: A pilot study. *Respirol. Carlton Vic* **2016**, *21*, 321–328. [CrossRef] [PubMed]
103. Gastli, N.; Loubinoux, J.; Daragon, M.; Lavigne, J.-P.; Saint-Sardos, P.; Pailhoriès, H.; Lemarié, C.; Benmansour, H.; d'Humières, C.; Broutin, L.; et al. Multicentric evaluation of BioFire FilmArray Pneumonia Panel for rapid bacteriological documentation of pneumonia. *Clin. Microbiol. Infect.* **2021**, *27*, 1308–1314. [CrossRef] [PubMed]
104. Ginocchio, C.C.; Garcia-Mondragon, C.; Mauerhofer, B.; Rindlisbacher, C.; The EME Evaluation Program Collaborative. Multi-national evaluation of the BioFire® FilmArray® Pneumonia plus Panel as compared to standard of care testing. *Eur. J. Clin. Microbiol. Infect. Dis. Off. Publ. Eur. Soc. Clin. Microbiol.* **2021**, *40*, 1609–1622. [CrossRef] [PubMed]
105. Caméléna, F.; Moy, A.-C.; Dudoignon, E.; Poncin, T.; Deniau, B.; Guillemet, L.; Le Goff, J.; Budoo, M.; Benyamina, M.; Chaussard, M.; et al. Performance of a multiplex polymerase chain reaction panel for identifying bacterial pathogens causing pneumonia in critically ill patients with COVID-19. *Diagn. Microbiol. Infect. Dis.* **2021**, *99*, 115183. [CrossRef]
106. Maataoui, N.; Chemali, L.; Patrier, J.; Tran Dinh, A.; Le Fèvre, L.; Lortat-Jacob, B.; Marzouk, M.; d'Humières, C.; Rondinaud, E.; Ruppé, E.; et al. Impact of rapid multiplex PCR on management of antibiotic therapy in COVID-19-positive patients hospitalized in intensive care unit. *Eur. J. Clin. Microbiol.* **2021**, *40*, 2227–2234. [CrossRef]
107. Posteraro, B.; Cortazzo, V.; Liotti, F.M.; Menchinelli, G.; Ippoliti, C.; De Angelis, G.; La Sorda, M.; Capalbo, G.; Vargas, J.; Antonelli, M.; et al. Diagnosis and Treatment of Bacterial Pneumonia in Critically Ill Patients with COVID-19 Using a Multiplex PCR Assay: A Large Italian Hospital's Five-Month Experience. *Microbiol. Spectr.* **2021**, *9*, e0069521. [CrossRef]
108. Rand, K.H.; Beal, S.G.; Cherabuddi, K.; Houck, H.; Lessard, K.; Tremblay, E.E.; Couturier, B.; Lingenfelter, B.; Rindlisbacher, C.; Jones, J. Relationship of Multiplex Molecular Pneumonia Panel Results With Hospital Outcomes and Clinical Variables. *Open Forum Infect. Dis.* **2021**, *8*, ofab368. [CrossRef]
109. Novy, E.; Goury, A.; Thivilier, C.; Guillard, T.; Alauzet, C. Algorithm for rational use of Film Array Pneumonia Panel in bacterial coinfections of critically ill ventilated COVID-19 patients. *Diagn. Microbiol. Infect. Dis.* **2021**, *101*, 115507. [CrossRef]
110. Peiffer-Smadja, N.; Bouadma, L.; Mathy, V.; Allouche, K.; Patrier, J.; Reboul, M.; Montravers, P.; Timsit, J.-F.; Armand-Lefevre, L. Performance and impact of a multiplex PCR in ICU patients with ventilator-associated pneumonia or ventilated hospital-acquired pneumonia. *Crit. Care Lond. Engl.* **2020**, *24*, 366. [CrossRef]
111. Maes, M.; Higginson, E.; Pereira-Dias, J.; Curran, M.D.; Parmar, S.; Khokhar, F.; Cuchet-Lourenço, D.; Lux, J.; Sharma-Hajela, S.; Ravenhill, B.; et al. Correction to: Ventilator-associated pneumonia in critically ill patients with COVID-19. *Crit. Care Lond. Engl.* **2021**, *25*, 130. [CrossRef]
112. Chang, D.W.; Dacosta, D.; Shapiro, M.F. Priority Levels in Medical Intensive Care at an Academic Public Hospital. *JAMA Intern. Med.* **2017**, *177*, 280–281. [CrossRef] [PubMed]
113. Hranjec, T.; Rosenberger, L.H.; Swenson, B.; Metzger, R.; Flohr, T.R.; Politano, A.D.; Riccio, L.M.; Popovsky, K.A.; Sawyer, R.G. Aggressive versus conservative initiation of antimicrobial treatment in critically ill surgical patients with suspected intensive-care-unit-acquired infection: A quasi-experimental, before and after observational cohort study. *Lancet Infect. Dis.* **2012**, *12*, 774–780. [CrossRef]

114. Falcone, M.; Russo, A.; Gentiloni Silverj, F.; Marzorati, D.; Bagarolo, R.; Monti, M.; Velleca, R.; D'Angelo, R.; Frustaglia, A.; Zuccarelli, G.C.; et al. Predictors of mortality in nursing-home residents with pneumonia: A multicentre study. *Clin. Microbiol. Infect.* **2018**, *24*, 72–77. [CrossRef] [PubMed]
115. Arzilli, G.; Scardina, G.; Casigliani, V.; Moi, M.; Lucenteforte, E.; Petri, D.; Rello, J.; Manissero, D.; Lopalco, P.L.; Tavoschi, L. Risk of infection in antimicrobial-resistant Gram-negative bacteria carriers: A systematic review. *Eur. J. Public Health* **2020**, *30*, ckaa165.319. [CrossRef]
116. Bonten, M.J.; Gaillard, C.A.; Johanson, W.G.; van Tiel, F.H.; Smeets, H.G.; van der Geest, S.; Stobberingh, E.E. Colonization in patients receiving and not receiving topical antimicrobial prophylaxis. *Am. J. Respir. Crit. Care Med.* **1994**, *150*, 1332–1340. [CrossRef] [PubMed]
117. Webb, B.J.; Dascomb, K.; Stenehjem, E.; Vikram, H.R.; Agrwal, N.; Sakata, K.; Williams, K.; Bockorny, B.; Bagavathy, K.; Mirza, S.; et al. Derivation and Multicenter Validation of the Drug Resistance in Pneumonia Clinical Prediction Score. *Antimicrob. Agents Chemother.* **2016**, *60*, 2652–2663. [CrossRef]
118. Restrepo, M.I.; Peterson, J.; Fernandez, J.F.; Qin, Z.; Fisher, A.C.; Nicholson, S.C. Comparison of the bacterial etiology of early-onset and late-onset ventilator-associated pneumonia in subjects enrolled in 2 large clinical studies. *Respir. Care* **2013**, *58*, 1220–1225. [CrossRef]

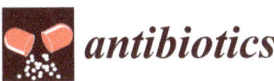

Review

Use of Antimicrobials for Bloodstream Infections in the Intensive Care Unit, a Clinically Oriented Review

Alexis Tabah [1,2,3,*], Jeffrey Lipman [3,4,5], François Barbier [6], Niccolò Buetti [7,8], Jean-François Timsit [7,9] and on behalf of the ESCMID Study Group for Infections in Critically Ill Patients—ESGCIP [†]

1. Intensive Care Unit, Redcliffe Hospital, Metro North Hospital and Health Services, Redcliffe, QLD 4020, Australia
2. School of Clinical Sciences, Queensland University of Technology, Brisbane, QLD 4000, Australia
3. Antimicrobial Optimisation Group, UQ Centre for Clinical Research, The University of Queensland, Brisbane, QLD 4029, Australia; j.lipman@uq.edu.au
4. Jamieson Trauma Institute and Intensive Care Services, Royal Brisbane and Women's Hospital, Metro North Hospital and Health Services, Brisbane, QLD 4029, Australia
5. Division of Anaesthesiology Critical Care Emergency and Pain Medicine, Nîmes University Hospital, University of Montpellier, 30029 Nîmes, France
6. Medical Intensive Care Unit, CHR Orléans, 45100 Orléans, France; barbierfrancois.chro@gmail.com
7. IAME, INSERM, Université de Paris, 75018 Paris, France; niccolo.buetti@hcuge.ch (N.B.); jean-francois.timsit@aphp.fr (J.-F.T.)
8. Infection Control Program and WHO Collaborating Centre on Patient Safety, Geneva University Hospitals and Faculty of Medicine, Rue Gabrielle-Perret-Gentil 4, 1205 Geneva, Switzerland
9. APHP Medical and Infectious Diseases Intensive Care Unit (MI), Bichat-Claude Bernard Hospital, 75018 Paris, France
* Correspondence: a.tabah@uq.edu.au; Tel.: +61-(0)-7-3883-7777
† ESCGIP study group listed in the acknowledgements.

Abstract: Bloodstream infections (BSIs) in critically ill patients are associated with significant mortality. For patients with septic shock, antibiotics should be administered within the hour. Probabilistic treatment should be targeted to the most likely pathogens, considering the source and risk factors for bacterial resistance including local epidemiology. Source control is a critical component of the management. Sending blood cultures (BCs) and other specimens before antibiotic administration, without delaying them, is key to microbiological diagnosis and subsequent opportunities for antimicrobial stewardship. Molecular rapid diagnostic testing may provide faster identification of pathogens and specific resistance patterns from the initial positive BC. Results allow for antibiotic optimisation, targeting the causative pathogen with escalation or de-escalation as required. Through this clinically oriented narrative review, we provide expert commentary for empirical and targeted antibiotic choice, including a review of the evidence and recommendations for the treatments of extended-spectrum β-lactamase-producing, AmpC-hyperproducing and carbapenem-resistant Enterobacterales; carbapenem-resistant *Acinetobacter baumannii*; and *Staphylococcus aureus*. In order to improve clinical outcomes, dosing recommendations and pharmacokinetics/pharmacodynamics specific to ICU patients must be followed, alongside therapeutic drug monitoring.

Keywords: bloodstream infection; bacteraemia; sepsis; septic shock; empirical; probabilistic antibiotics; source control; de-escalation; ICU; intensive care

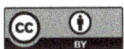

1. Introduction

A bloodstream infection (BSI) is defined as the microbial invasion of the blood stream. In clinical practice, this refers to a positive blood culture (BC) from a patient with clinical signs of infection [1]. Bloodstream infections can be categorised in a range of meaningful ways:

1. According to the origin of the infection, either community-acquired (CA-BSI), hospital-acquired (HA-BSI) or intensive care unit (ICU)–acquired (ICU-BSI).
2. Either secondary to a source of infection or primary, when there is no identified source [2].
3. Complicated or uncomplicated, which was recently defined as a having definite source (among urinary, catheter, intra-abdominal, pneumonia, skin or soft tissues), and effective source control, in a non-immunocompromised patient, and with clinical improvement after 72 h of antimicrobial therapy (at least defervescence and haemodynamic stability) [3].
4. By clinical severity, which is the absence or presence of organ failures and the need for organ supportive therapy in the ICU.

Critically ill patients are often debilitated and suffer from immune paresis caused by their initial reason for ICU admission [4]. Secondary infections are especially common in patients with higher severity of disease [5]. For ICU patients, BSIs are associated with significant mortality, ranging from 35% to more than 60% [6–8]. In a cohort study of 10,734 ICU patients with an ICU length of stay (LOS) of more than 3 days, 571 (5.3%) developed ICU-BSIs. In a multivariable COX model analysis, ICU-BSIs were independently associated with increased mortality [8].

This clinically oriented narrative review focusses on the antimicrobial management of BSIs, whose clinical severity requires ICU admission, or such infections that have been acquired in the ICU. We will review the importance of microbiology specimens, the timing and choice of the empirical antimicrobial therapy, the role of spectrum and dose optimisation, the importance for source control and, finally, strategies for stopping antimicrobials (Figure 1).

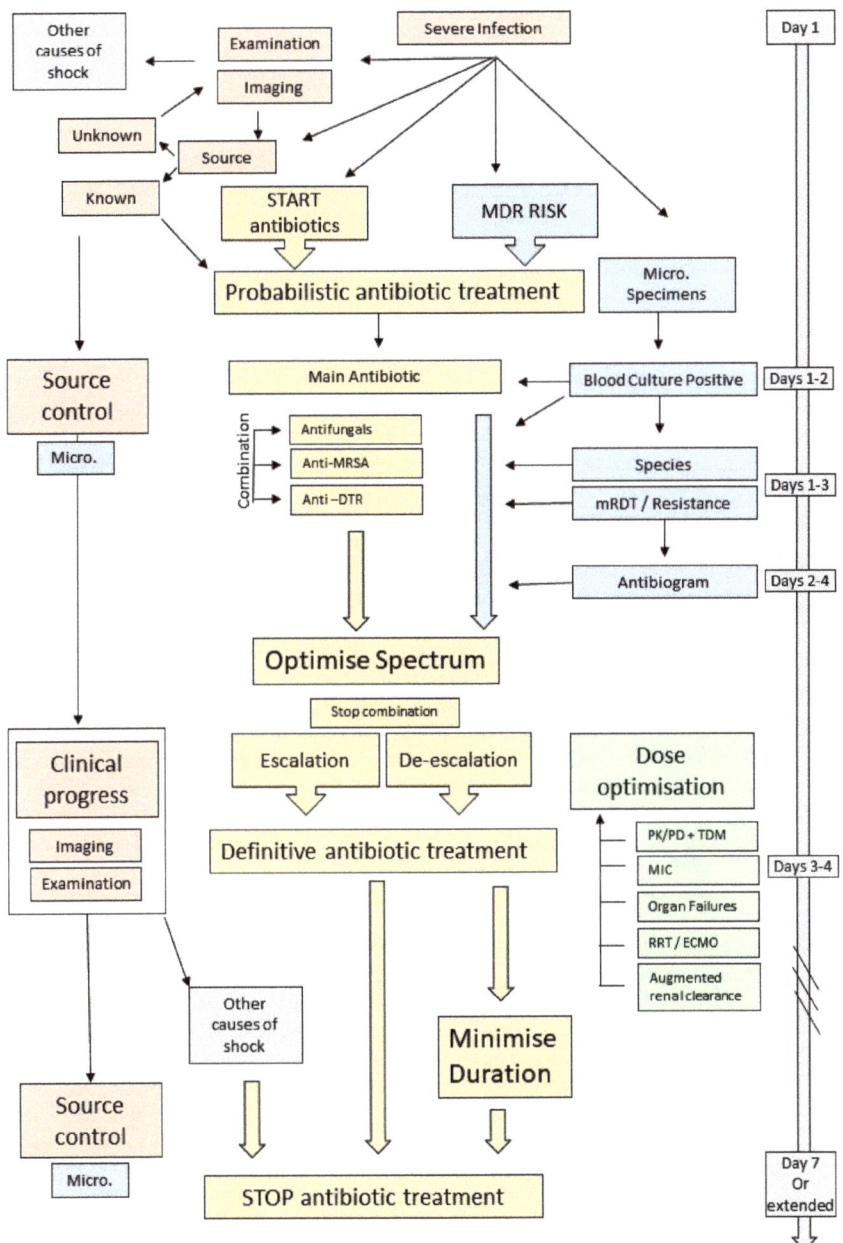

Figure 1. Management of an ICU patient with a blood stream infection. mRDT = molecular rapid diagnostic testing, Micro. = microbiology specimens, MDR = multidrug resistant, DTR = difficult-to-treat resistance, MRSA = methicillin-resistant *Staphylococcus aureus*.

2. Antimicrobial Therapy

2.1. Empirical Antimicrobial Therapy

2.1.1. The Importance of Getting It Right from the Start

For ICU patients with sepsis or septic shock, it is recommended to administer antimicrobials immediately, ideally within one hour of recognition [9]. This is supported by observational data. Kumar and colleagues described in 2006 a 12% increase in crude mortality for each hour of delay to administer antimicrobials from the onset of hypotension and septic shock [10]. The above-mentioned study by Adrie and colleagues shows a 30% increase in mortality when no adequate treatment is given in the first 24 h [8]. In the evaluation of a multifaceted intervention to decrease sepsis mortality in a group of 40 German hospitals, Bloos and colleagues report an increase in the risk of death of patients with sepsis or septic shock of 2% for each hour of delay of antimicrobial therapy and 1% for each hour of delay in source control [11]. However, not all research on time to antibiotics has been so positive [12]. Hranjec and colleagues investigated the issue with a before and after study in surgical ICU patients with sepsis but without shock [13]. They compared an aggressive approach where antibiotics were started as soon as sepsis was recognised to a conservative approach where they were started only if the infection was confirmed by positive microbiology. In the conservative period, immediate antibiotic therapy was recommended for patients with shock. The aggressive approach was associated with a lower time from fever and BC to start of treatment. The conservative approach was associated with more initially appropriate therapy, a shorter duration of antibiotics and lower mortality. This manuscript demonstrates the difficulty intensivists face daily in trying to differentiate infection from inflammation in the ICU patient population. It is conceivable that several patients were without infection and, therefore, did not require antibiotics. Delaying antibiotics to investigate the cause of "sepsis" may have multiple benefits for patients with low severity. It may improve outcomes through the diagnosis and management of non-infectious causes of inflammation and organ failures plus avoid harm from antibiotic overuse. Further, it will help in obtaining a diagnosis for a proportion of infections that would otherwise been labelled as "culture negative" or "from unknown source". Definitive clinical and microbiological diagnosis of an infection facilitates the provision of a targeted treatment and improves outcomes. While controversy remains and these data present all the biases inherent to observational studies, they highlight how important it is that patients with BSIs receive early appropriate antimicrobial therapy.

2.1.2. Broad-Spectrum Antibiotics and Combination Therapy?

The empirical regimen should be broad enough to maximise the likelihood of adequacy, especially in patients with septic shock. This may, however, lead to an unnecessary overuse of broad-spectrum antimicrobials and associated harms, including the promotion of antimicrobial resistance [14].

When the source is known, antibiotics should be targeted at the most common pathogens for the source as detailed in Table 1. Molecule choice takes into account risk factors for multidrug-resistant (MDR) or specific pathogens for the patient, according to their history and setting as shown in Table 2. For hospital-acquired infections, knowledge of colonisation from previous clinical or surveillance cultures is a valuable tool to optimise this choice [15,16].

Combination therapy can provide very broad empirical coverage for different classes of pathogens by adding anti-MRSA and antifungal agents or molecules targeted at MDR Gram-negative bacteria (GNB). These should be used with parsimony, in patients with significant risk factors, and only as part of the empirical regimen with a plan to subsequently de-escalate all drugs that are not required [17,18].

Table 1. Most common pathogen groups according to the presumed source of infection.

	Urinary	Respiratory	Intra-Abdominal	Intra Vascular Catheter
Community acquired	Enterobacterales *Enterococcus* sp. *P. aeruginosa* *	*Streptococcus pneumoniae* ++ *Legionella* sp. *** Enterobacterales *S. aureus* *P. aeruginosa* * *H. influenzae*	Enterobacterales *Enterococcus* sp. *Candida* sp. Anaerobes Polymicrobial	Coagulase neg. staphylococci *S. aureus* Enterobacterales
Hospital acquired	Enterobacterales *Candida* sp. *Enterococcus* sp. *P. aeruginosa* *Acinetobacter* sp.	Enterobacterales *S. aureus* *P. aeruginosa* *Acinetobacter* sp.	Enterobacterales *P. aeruginosa* *Enterococcus* sp. *Candida* sp. Anaerobes Polymicrobial	Enterobacterales *S. aureus* Coagulase neg. staphylococci *P. aeruginosa* *Acinetobacter* sp.

Describes the most common pathogens. Non-exhaustive list. ++ Largely predominant. * In patients with chronic respiratory disease and patients with long-term indwelling catheter for respiratory and urinary sources, respectively. *** *Legionella* sp. does not cause BSIs but should be included in severe community-acquired respiratory infections.

Table 2. Risk factors for multidrug-resistant bacteria.

Individual factors (history)	Recent hospitalisation (1 year) Exposure to antimicrobials (3–6 months) Severe co-morbidities (Charlson ≥ 4) Recent immunosuppression Chronic respiratory disease (COPD, cystic fibrosis) Recurrent urinary tract infections Urinary catheter
Individual factors (current)	Prior duration of hospital and ICU stay (continuous increase over time) High severity Known colonisation (surveillance cultures and previous infections)
Institution factors	Regional/institutional prevalence of MDR Overwhelmed health systems

COPD = chronic obstructive pulmonary disease, MDR = multidrug resistant, ICU = intensive care unit.

2.1.3. The Importance of Sending Blood Cultures before Starting Antimicrobials

The empirical antibiotic choice is made while differential diagnosis is still underway, including uncertainty on the pathogen. Microbiology results will be required to judge of the presence of an infection and to optimise antimicrobial therapy by targeting the causal pathogen(s) or to stop antibiotics if there is no infection.

Sending specimens before starting antimicrobials (without delaying the treatment) is key to avoiding false-negative results. Sheer and colleagues analysed the factors associated with BC positivity in a single centre cohort study of 599 patients with severe sepsis or septic shock who had at least two BC sets taken [19]. Patients with cultures sampled before antibiotics had a 50.6% positivity rate, almost double the 27.7% for those who had received antibiotics before. They showed that antibiotic therapy prior to BC sampling was an independent factor for BC negativity. In this cohort, 35 patients had cultures sampled both before and after antibiotics. The positivity rate was 57.1% (20/35) before antibiotics. After antibiotics, positivity decreased to 25.7% as 9 of those 20 patients still had positive cultures. This represents a loss of pathogen detection of 30.0% and highlights the importance of sending cultures prior to starting antibiotics.

When antibiotics are indicated, and the patient has septic shock, taking cultures must not delay the initiation of antimicrobials beyond a reasonable delay of 15 to 45 min [9]. Importantly, clinicians should not wait for culture results to start the treatment. When an

ICU patient develops new signs of sepsis, cultures should be sent from the likely source(s) of infection, from the blood and most often also from urine and sputum.

Sampling quality is very important. We recommend at least two sets of aerobic and anaerobic BCs, from two different sites, inoculating a sufficient amount of blood per bottle [2], usually, 8–10 mL per bottle. It is, however, good practice to check manufacturers' recommendations. Blood should be sampled peripherally following rigorous skin disinfection, and an aseptic non-touch technique for drawing the blood and inoculating the bottles is key to decreasing false-positive results from BC contamination with commensal micro-organisms [20].

2.1.4. The Advent of Molecular Rapid Diagnostic Testing

The rapidly expanding field of molecular rapid diagnostic testing (mRDT) provides a range of diagnostic tools for the faster identification of pathogens and specific resistance patterns from the initial positive BC [21]. A laboratory requires up to 1–2 days to identify the micro-organism from a positive BC and another 1–2 days to provide the antibiogram [22]. Accurate bacterial species identification is available in the matter of hours with techniques such as matrix-assisted laser desorption/ionisation–time of flight (MALDI-TOF) mass spectrometry [23]. Integrated solutions such as the Accelerate Pheno system automate both the identification and AST, providing accurate results in 90 min and 7 h, respectively. In a multicentre study, comparing with conventional BC processing, it accurately identified 14 common bacterial pathogens and 2 *Candida* sp. with sensitivities ranging from 94.6% to 100% [24]. The performance of AST results for methicillin-resistant *Staphylococcus aureus* (MRSA) and *Staphylococcus* sp. had an agreement of 97% with conventional processing. For GNB, the agreement on a panel of 15 antimicrobials was 94%, making this system suitable for prime clinical use [24].

Colorimetric assays are relatively inexpensive and extremely accurate benchtop solutions to detect extended-spectrum beta-lactamase-producing (ESBL-Es) or carbapenemase-producing Enterobacterales (CPEs) [21,25]. The newest kits such as the NitroSpeed-Carba NP can identify the presence and production of carbapenemase by GNB with a sensitivity of 100% and a specificity of 97%. It detects the type of carbapenemase with sensitivities ranging from 97% to 100%, even in cases with a very low level of carbapenemase activity [26]. These may allow for the urgent escalation of antibiotics, gaining several hours to days when compared with waiting for an antibiogram. When used within an antimicrobial stewardship (AMS) program, they may help to avoid the over prescription of the newer β-lactam–β-lactamase inhibitors (BL/BLIs) in the empirical regimen. Their use for ADE can (and should) be done, with caution as clinical evidence is only emerging [18].

2.2. What to Do with Culture Results

Patients with a suspected and then confirmed BSIs need to have microbiology results reviewed at least daily. The antibiotic treatment must be targeted to the pathogen in terms of molecule activity, with an adequate penetration at the source and sufficient dosing, as early as possible, and for the whole duration of the treatment, without exceeding the required duration. Effective communication with the microbiology laboratory is crucial. In our practice, we check for results during the morning and afternoon rounds, and the laboratory will call us almost immediately when they have a positive BC or any significant result. Antimicrobial stewardship programs and scheduled infectious diseases rounds help to ensure that no opportunities to optimise the treatment are missed.

The initial communication by the laboratory of a positive BC and Gram stain results may be the time when antibiotics are started or escalated. Identification of the pathogen comes a few hours to a day later and may include information on mechanisms of resistance depending on laboratory technique availability. Lastly, we will receive an antibiogram and final confirmation of the identified pathogen. At each step, we ensure the causative pathogen is covered by the administered treatment. With the final microbiology results, we make a definitive adjustment to the antibiotic regiment, including a decision on the duration of therapy.

Antimicrobial de-escalation (ADE) consists in either (i) replacing a broad-spectrum antimicrobial with an agent of a narrower clinical spectrum or a presumed lower ecological impact or (ii) stopping a component of an antimicrobial combination [18]. It is an important tool to reduce the exposure to broad-spectrum antibiotics and prevent the emergence of antimicrobial resistance. Antimicrobial de-escalation has demonstrated patient-level safety, with a meta-analysis suggesting improved outcomes in patients who received ADE [27]. Bloodstream infections are very specific as the causing pathogen is known with certainty, and this makes them perfect targets for ADE. Some sources, such as peritonitis or deep-seated abscesses may be polymicrobial, with sometimes the indication to maintain broader cover for some suspected—but not grown—pathogens. In nearly all other situations, we can safely select the molecules that provide the most adequate treatment for the pathogen causing the BSIs at the source, while having the lowest ecological impact. Importantly, outside specific extensively drug-resistant (XDR) pathogens, there is no benefit to continuing combination therapy for GNB infections [28].

2.2.1. Specific Pathogens

While ADE and narrow-spectrum antibiotics can be easily recommended for susceptible micro-organisms, globally increasing antimicrobial resistance (AMR) has significantly complicated antibiotic management as detailed in the examples below.

Extended-Spectrum β-Lactamase-Producing Enterobacterales

ESBL-producing Enterobacterales (ESBL-Es), and their surrogate, Enterobacterales resistant to third-generation cephalosporins should be treated with a carbapenem [29,30]. Carbapenem sparing in this context has been extensively investigated and was initially supported by observational studies [31]. The MERINO trial randomised 391 patients with a BSIs due to ceftriaxone-resistant *Escherichia coli* or *Klebsiella pneumoniae* to piperacillin–tazobactam or meropenem [32]. Mortality was 12.3% for piperacillin–tazobactam compared with 3.7% for meropenem, rejecting non-inferiority and not supporting the use of piperacillin–tazobactam in severe infections due to ESBL-Es. Alternatives for cases where a carbapenem cannot be used include fluoroquinolones and trimethoprim-sulphamethoxazole. Those are especially interesting for BSIs with a urinary source as they concentrate in the urine [30]. While ceftolozane–tazobactam and ceftazidime–avibactam (CAZ-AVI) are potential alternatives, their use should be restricted as reserve antibiotics for those pathogens that cannot be treated otherwise.

Inducible AmpC-Producing Enterobacterales

Enterobacterales including *Enterobacter cloacae*, *Klebsiella aerogenes* (ex. *Enterobacter aerogenes*) and *Citrobacter freundii* are the main pathogens of concern that carry a chromosomal inducible AmpC β-lactamase [33]. These are problematic because they initially show susceptibility to ceftriaxone. However, exposure to ceftriaxone and other β-lactams such as piperacillin–tazobactam or imipenem will induce a sufficient increase in the production of AmpC to cause resistance to ceftriaxone, leading to treatment failure [33,34]. These enzymes effectively hydrolyse ceftriaxone and ceftazidime. Tazobactam has weak efficacy against AmpC β-lactamases, and observational studies were equivocal [35]. The MERINO-2 pilot trial randomised patients with AmpC BSIs to piperacillin–tazobactam or meropenem. There was numerically higher mortality and clinical and microbiological failure with piperacillin–tazobactam but more relapses with meropenem. Pending further data, we should avoid using piperacillin–tazobactam in patients with severe infections due to pathogens with inducible AmpC [36,37]. Cefepime is a good treatment choice as it is a weak inducer, and it is relatively stable against AmpC β-lactamases. Caution is warranted in pathogens with a MIC ≥ 4 µg/mL for cefepime as they may harbour an ESBL, making them prone to treatment failure. All carbapenems are stable and recommended for the treatment of AmpC-hyperproducing Enterobacterales. New β-lactamase inhibitors (BLIs), such as avibactam, are very effective, but their use should be restricted to pathogens that do not have other treatment options [33]. For pathogens that are susceptible, fluoroquinolones and trimethoprim-sulphamethoxazole can be considered as alternatives [36].

Carbapenem-Resistant Enterobacterales

Carbapenem-resistant Enterobacterales (CREs) are defined by resistance to at least one carbapenem [38]. This can be either due to the production of a carbapenemase, such as *Klebsiella pneumoniae* carbapenemases (KPCs), oxacillinase (e.g., OXA-48), and metallo-β-lactamases (MBLs) (e.g., New Delhi metallo-β-lactamases), or a combination of other mechanisms, such as a mutation in porin genes that limit the entry of the antibiotic into the bacteria associated with upregulated production of other β-lactamases [39].

Recently, combinations of older β-lactams with a new BLI and a novel cephalosporin have been marketed specifically for the management of CREs. Avibactam, in CAZ-AVI is targeted to the inhibition of KPCs and OXA-48 carbapenemases. It is inactive against MBLs. Ceftazidime–avibactam was shown to be effective in a cohort study of 137 patients with infections caused by a CRE. There was an inverse probability of treatment weighting (IPTW)–adjusted probability of a better outcome of 64% with CAZ-AVI when compared with colistin [40]. While no randomised controlled trial (RCT) is available to date, these results are concordant with other studies comparing CAZ-AVI with other antibiotics [41,42].

Meropenem–vaborbactam is targeted at KPCs but is inactive against OXA-48 and MBLs. It was investigated in a 77-patient phase-3 RCT against the best available treatment (BAT) [43]. Forty-four patients had confirmed CRE infections. In this subpopulation, meropenem-vaborbactam was associated with improved cure rates (59.4% vs. 26.7%, $p = 0.002$) and a numerically but not statistically lower mortality (15.6% vs. 33.3%, $p = 0.2$).

There is less evidence for cefiderocol, a siderophore cephalosporin active in vitro against all CPEs including MBLs. The CREDIBLE-CR RCT included 118 patients with a CR-GNB at baseline (46% *A. baumannii*, 33% *K. pneumoniae* and 19% *P. aeruginosa*) compared cefiderocol and BAT for CR-GNB [44]. Mortality was higher in the cefiderocol arm (24.8% vs. 18.4%). A subgroup analysis showed that higher mortality was found in patients with carbapenem-resistant *Acinetobacter baumannii* (CRAB) but not in those with CREs [30]. When comparing cefiderocol with BAT, clinical cure was 66% vs. 45% in the CRE subgroup and 75% vs. 29% in the MBL subgroup. Aztreonam–avibactam is a very promising combination with potent activity against multiple carbapenemases including MBLs [45]. It is unfortunately not yet available for broad clinical use. Some MBLs that are resistant to cefiderocol, CAZ-AVI and other BL/BLIs remain susceptible in vitro to the combination of ceftazidime–avibactam–aztreonam. This treatment was independently associated with lower 30-day morality in an observational study of 102 patients with MBL-producing CRE BSIs and, with cefiderocol, may be, one of the only available treatment options for MBL producers [46,47].

Given the specific activity of each of those antimicrobials, effective AMS and use of phenotypic tests to determine the presence of each resistance mechanism are important to manage CRE BSIs in the ICU.

For CRE strains that are susceptible to BL/BLIs, there is no indication to add a second antibiotic as part of combination therapy, and if one was started, we suggest ADE [30]. A recent propensity-matched cohort study of 577 patients with KPC-producing *K. pneumoniae* (KPC-Kp) treated with CAZ-AVI combination therapy did not show benefit versus CAZ-AVI monotherapy [41]. This contrasts with studies published before the advent of the new generation of BL/BLIs. The INCREMENT cohort showed in the high-mortality risk strata of patients with CRE-BSIs an independent association between combination therapy and a lower risk of death [48]. When antibiotics such as polymyxin and tigecycline are used as pivotal antibiotics, combination therapy remains advised [30,48].

Carbapenem-Resistant *Acinetobacter baumannii*

Carbapenem-resistant *Acinetobacter baumannii*, and other *Acinetobacter* sp. resistant to carbapenems have very limited treatment options and subsequently high risks of treatment failure and mortality [49]. This is due to the common co-existence of multiple mechanisms conferring combined resistance to most or all antibiotic classes [36,49]. Further, the efficacy of novel BL/BLI combinations is disappointing. Vaborbactam does not restore the activity of meropenem against CRAB. Relebactam does not improve the activity of imipenem. Noting that CAZ-AVI is not indicated for CRAB, we refer to a study of 71 U.S. hospitals in 2012–13 finding that up to 73.6% of CRAB from ICU isolates were resistant to CAZ-AVI [50].

This pathogen remains one of the few indications in which it may be indicated to continue combination therapy for the duration of the treatment or at least until clinical improvement [36]. Combinations should include in vitro active drugs, where available. Given the paucity of treatment options, multiple combinations have been tested. A multi-centre RCT compared colistin alone or combined with meropenem (both administered at high doses) and found no difference in terms of clinical failure or 28-day mortality [51], not supporting the addition of meropenem to colistin for CRAB. Sulbactam has specific intrinsic antibiotic activity against *Acinetobacter* sp. For susceptible isolates, ampicillin–sulbactam is the preferred choice as the pivotal antibiotic of a combination regimen [52]. These strains are, however, becoming rare, and polymyxins are often one of the few available options. Polymyxin B is recommended for systemic infections because of better pharmacokinetic (PK) characteristics and less nephrotoxicity than colistin methane sulphonate (CMS), which is preferred for urinary sources [36]. Dosing recommendations from the latest guidelines should be followed given their narrow therapeutic index [53]. Tigecycline, if used, should be part of a combination as its clinical efficacy remains debated and its PK profile is unfavourable, especially in the blood and lung tissues [49]. High dosing schemes (200 mg loading followed by 100 mg 12 h) must be employed with caution, and fibrinogen levels must be followed due to time-dependent associated risk of coagulopathy, and dose-dependent gastro-intestinal side effects [54,55]. The adjunction of sulbactam as part of combination therapy for severe infections with strains that are non-susceptible to ampicillin–sulbactam might be considered due to its capacity to saturate altered penicillin-binding protein targets [56].

Staphylococcus aureus and MRSA

Staphylococcus aureus has a propensity for causing HA-BSIs as a complication of medical and surgical procedures or intra-vascular catheters. It often leads to complicated infections, seeding into abscesses, osteoarticular infections and endocarditis, thus, often requiring an extended duration of antibiotics. *S. aureus* can be susceptible to methicillin and many other β-lactam antibiotics (MSSA) or resistant to almost the whole class for MRSA. Newer cephalosporins such as ceftaroline and ceftobiprole have specific anti-MRSA activity. The therapeutic standard for MSSA is a narrow-spectrum anti-staphylococcal β-lactam such as flucloxacillin, oxacillin or a first-generation cephalosporin such as cephazolin [57]. Monotherapy with vancomycin is inferior to β-lactams [58]. In high-prevalence settings, probabilistic treatment should include optimal cover for both MSSA and MRSA. This can be achieved with a combination of flucloxacillin and vancomycin, ceftaroline or daptomycin. There must be a plan for ADE and only the targeted molecule should be retained once the antibiogram is available.

Vancomycin is the first-line antibiotic for MRSA BSIs [59]. Daptomycin is proposed as a first-line alternative to vancomycin by the Infectious Diseases Society of America (IDSA) guidelines [60]. Linezolid is not recommended as it failed to show non-inferiority to vancomycin in an RCT of MRSA catheter-related BSIs (CR-BSIs) [61]. It may be an option for oral step-down when extended treatments are indicated [62]. Daptomycin was associated with significantly lower rates of clinical failure and 30-day mortality in a propensity-matched cohort of 262 MRSA BSIs [63]. Further, it causes less AKI than vancomycin [64]. However, daptomycin is inactivated by pulmonary surfactant, limiting its indications. The emergence of resistance to daptomycin during treatment may lead to failure and warrants caution. Combination of daptomycin plus ceftaroline as rescue therapy for refractory MRSA BSIs has been reported [65]. Adjunctive rifampicin has long been advocated in MRSA infections to reduce the risk of treatment failure and recurrences but was recently shown to be of no benefit in a large multicentre RCT [66].

There is a strong relationship between the duration of bacteraemia and subsequent risk of death [67]. *Staphylococcus aureus* requires extended treatment durations as discussed below. Persisting BSIs may be secondary to endocarditis, and all *S. aureus* BSIs should have a cardiac echocardiography. Transoesophageal echocardiography can only be avoided in cases with specific protective factors [68].

3. Do Not Forget Source Control

Source control is equally essential with antibiotics in the treatment of BSIs. Surgical or percutaneous management of any abscess, deep-space infection or infected material such as intra-vascular catheters is a matter of urgency. In the EUROBACT International Cohort Study of ICU patients with HA-BSIs, not achieving source control was an independent predictor of day-28 mortality [6]. In a large multicentre observational study of *S. aureus* BSIs, delayed source control was associated with persistent BSIs [57]. In a cohort study of patients with peritonitis and septic shock, delay to surgical source control was an independent predictor of mortality [58]. In unstable patients, the multidisciplinary discussion with the surgical team revolves around timing and choice of the intervention. Damage-control surgery is often indicated. The essential parts of the operation are urgently performed, and a reoperation is planned after clinical stabilisation, 24–48 h later, for a second look and, where possible, anatomical reconstruction [59]. We must emphasise the need to send specimens from the foci of infection at each intervention.

4. Optimisation and Dosing Strategies

Sufficient antibiotic concentrations at the site of infection are required for optimal clinical outcomes. The initial and/or loading dose should be given in full, not adjusting for renal impairment [60]. Sepsis alters the PK properties of hydrophilic molecules (β-lactams, glycopeptides and aminoglycosides). They have an increased volume of distribution (Vd) leading to a lower-than-expected maximum serum concentration during a dosing interval (Cmax) [61]. Additionally, augmented renal clearance (ARC), the increase in renal blood flow that often arises in septic shock, leads to the augmented elimination of renally excreted antibiotics. This causes a lower-than-expected trough serum concentration (Cmin). Conversely, renal or hepatic dysfunction may alter the metabolism and elimination of antibiotics, leading to increased concentrations and potential toxicity. Renal replacement therapy (RRT) and extracorporeal membrane oxygenation (ECMO) will also affect the PK of antibiotics, often in unpredictable ways, and require additional monitoring [62].

Further, different PD targets need to be taken in account to ensure maximum bacterial killing and decrease the emergence of resistance. As shown in Figure 2, some antibiotics are concentration dependent (aminoglycosides) and require a high peak concentration obtained with a single daily loading dose. β-Lactams are both concentration and time dependent, requiring sufficient time with a free unbound drug minimum concentration (fCmin) above the MIC for targeted bacteria (fCmin/MIC) [63]. Others such as fluoroquinolones and vancomycin are both time and concentration dependent, and adjustment is based on the ratio of the area under the concentration–time curve from 0 to 24 h to minimum inhibitory concentration (AUC0–24/MIC) [64]. Based on those PK/PD considerations and a meta-analysis of three RCTs suggesting improved short-term mortality [65], it is now suggested to use a prolonged infusion for β-lactams following an initial bolus dose [9]. Further, initial dosing should follow recommendations tailored for critically ill patients (when they are available) rather than following package inserts (Table 3).

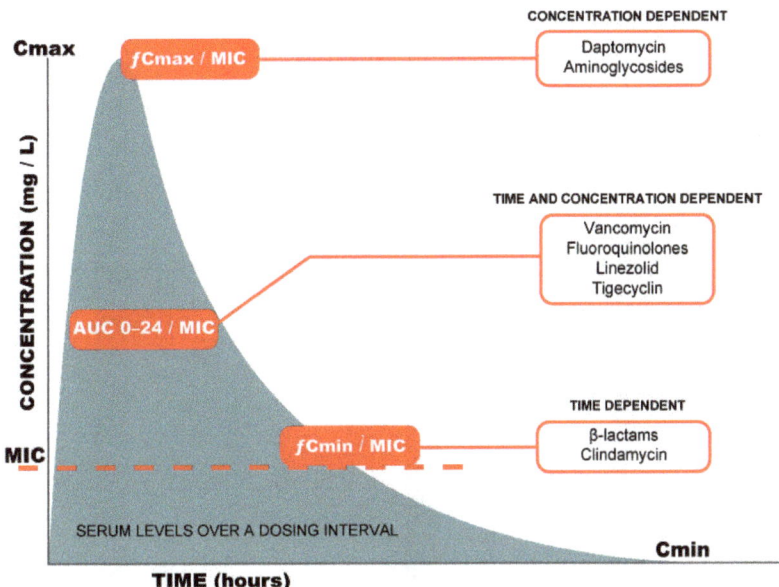

Figure 2. Pharmacokinetic targets for main antibiotic classes. Cmax = maximum serum concentration during a dosing interval, Cmin = trough (minimum) serum concentration over a dosing interval, MIC = minimum inhibitory concentration of the pathogen for the considered antibiotic, fCmax/MIC = ratio of free peak plasma concentration to MIC, fAUC/MIC = ratio of free unbound drug concentration area under the curve to MIC, fT > MIC = free unbound drug concentration time above the MIC.

Drug concentrations are usually measured for two reasons, to prevent (or explain) toxicity and to measure for efficacy. Aminoglycosides and glycopeptides have significant side effects at higher concentrations, and hence, measurement facilities are commonly available. More recently, efficacy targets have been set for these antibiotics. Beta-lactams have a high therapeutic ratio with some, but limited, toxicity. Recently, measurements of these compounds have become more relevant in view of underdosing, i.e., therapeutic drug monitoring (TDM) used for the efficacy of these agents [66]. Whilst beta-lactam concentration targets were obtained initially from animal data, there is still debate on what target beta-lactam levels should be used for clinical efficacy [64].

Table 3. Targets and dosing strategies for most commonly used antibiotics.

Antimicrobial	Specific Targets	Dosing Strategies	Caution
Beta-lactam antibiotics			
Ampicillin–sulbactam	CRAB	9 g q8h (CI/EI)	High dosing increases risk of neurotoxicity
Ampicillin or amoxicillin	Narrow-spectrum targeted therapy	2 g q6h (EI)	
Amoxicillin–clavulanic acid	Narrow-spectrum targeted therapy CA-peritonitis	2 g/200 mg q6h (EI)	
Piperacillin–tazobactam	Broad-spectrum antipseudomonal probabilistic for HAI	4.5 g q6h EI/CI preferred, loading dose req.	Biliary excretion Resistance promotion
Antistaphylococcal molecules			
Flucloxacillin	MSSA	2 g q4–6h (EI/CI)	
Cefazolin	MSSA	2 g q8h	
Ceftaroline	MRSA/VISA/VRSE	600 mg q8h	Neutropenia especially in longer treatments
Ceftobiprole	MRSA, MRSE, non-MDR GNB	500 mg q8h (2h EI)	Q4–6 h depending on degree of ARC Dose adjust in renal impairment
Vancomycin	MRSA/MRSE/ *E. faecium*	LD 30 mg/kg followed by 30 mg/kg (CI) or 15 mg/kg q12h(EI)	TDM required
Daptomycin	MRSA/MRSE/VRE	8–10 mg/kg q24h	
Linezolid	MRSA/MRSE/VRE	600 mg q12h	
Cephalosporins			
Ceftriaxone	CAP Susceptible Enterobacterales	1 g q12h EI	
Cefotaxime	CAP Susceptible Enterobacterales	1 g q6h EI CI suggested	
Ceftazidime	*Pseudomonas* sp., *Acinetobacter* sp.	2 g q8h ((EI/CI)	
Cefepime	AmpC-Es	2 g q8h EI	MIC ≥ 4 risk of ESBL-Es and treatment failure Most neurotoxic β-lactam, especially in overdose
Cefiderocol	CREs (KPCs, OXA48, MBLs), DTR-PA	2 g q8h EI (3 h)	Poor efficacy for CRAB
Carbapenems			

Table 3. Cont.

Antimicrobial	Specific Targets	Dosing Strategies	Caution
Imipenem-cilastatin	Broad spectrum Probabilistic for HAI Targeted ESBL-Es	1 g q6-8h (II)	
Meropenem	*Pseudomonas* sp., *Acinetobacter* sp.	1–2 g q8h (II, EI, CI)	Poor efficacy against *Enterococcus* sp.
Ertapenem	ESBLE-Es	1–2 g/24 h (II)	
New combinations *			
Ceftazidime–avibactam	CREs (KPCs, OXA-48)	2 g/500 mg q8h (II/EI)	
Aztreonam (+CAZ-AVI)	MBL-CREs, DTR-PA, *Stenotrophomonas maltophilia*	2 g q8h	Infuse aztreonam at same time with CAZ-AVI
Ceftolozane–tazobactam	DTR-PA	2 g/1 g q8h (II)	
Aztreonam–avibactam	MBL-CREs	2 g/500 mg q8h (II)	
Meropenem–vaborbactam	KPC-CREs, DTR-PA	2 g/2 g q8h IV (II/EI)	
Imipenem–relebactam	KPC-CREs, DTR-PA	500 mg/250 mg q6h (II)	
Aminoglycosides	Combination to extend spectrum when at risk for MDR. ESBL-Es, AmpC-Es, CREs, CRAB, DTR-PA.		Nephrotoxicity Ototoxicity TDM required
Amikacin		Once-Daily dose 25–30 mg/kg (/24h)	
Gentamicin		7–8 mg/kg (/24h)	
Polymyxins	CREs (KPCs, OXA48, MBLs) CRAB, DTR-PA Resistant to new/targeted antibiotics		Last-line antimicrobials Nephrotoxicity Use TDM if available
Polymyxin B	Systemic infections	Loading dose 2–2.5 mg/kg (20,000–25,000 IU/kg) 12-hourly injections of 1.25–1.5 mg/kg (12,500–15,000 IU/kg TBW)	Not renally adjusted Very few data on DTR BSIs
Colistin (CMS)	Urinary source	Loading dose of 300 mg CBA (9 MUI) then 12–24 h later: 300–360 mg CBA/day (9–10 MUI/day) divided in 2 injections	Renally adjusted More nephrotoxicity than polymyxin B
Other classes			

Table 3. *Cont.*

Antimicrobial	Specific Targets	Dosing Strategies	Caution
Ciprofloxacin	ESBL-Es, AmpC-Es, MDR-PA, *Stenotrophomonas maltophilia*	400 mg q8–12h (II/EI)	
Fosfomycin	CREs (KPCs, OXA48, MBLs) CRAB, DTR-PA		Salvage therapy if susceptible Combination if possible
Tigecycline	CREs (KPCs, OXA48, MBLs) CRAB	100 mg LD then 50 mg q12h OR 200 mg (LD) then 100 mg q12h	Caution with coagulopathy if high dose Use as part of combination
Eravacycline	CREs (KPCs, OXA48, MBLs), CRAB	1 mg/kg q12h (II)	
Cotrimoxazole (TMP/SMX)	ESBL-Es, AmpC-Es, *Stenotrophomonas maltophilia*	1.2–1.6 g SMX q8h (II)	

BSI = blood stream infection, HAI = hospital-acquired infection, CA = community acquired, CAP = community-acquired pneumonia, MDR = multidrug resistant, DTR = difficult-to-treat resistance, MSSA = methicillin-susceptible *Staphylococcus aureus*, MRSA = methicillin-resistant *Staphylococcus aureus*, VISA = vancomycin-intermediate *Staphylococcus aureus*, VRSA = vancomycin-resistant *Staphylococcus aureus*, VRE = vancomycin-resistant *Enterococcus*, PA = *Pseudomonas aeruginosa*, ESBL-Es = ESBL-producing Enterobacterales, CREs = carbapenem-resistant Enterobacterales, CRAB = carbapenem-resistant *Acinetobacter baumannii*, ARC = augmented renal clearance, TDM = therapeutic drug monitoring, LD = loading dose II = intermittent infusion, EI = extended infusion (3 to 4 h), CI = continuous infusion. All EI and CI require a LD, TBW = total body weight, * new refers to recently available BL/BLI combinations targeting specific resistance mechanisms.

5. When and How to Stop Therapy

Minimising the duration of exposure to antimicrobials is important to optimise patient outcomes. A recent umbrella review established how each additional day of therapy is associated with measurable harm [67]. This includes a 4% daily increase in the odds of an adverse drug reaction (OR 1.04, 95% CI 1.02–1.07) and a 3% increase in the odds of antimicrobial resistance (OR 1.03, 95% CI 0.98–1.07).

Since 2019, three multicentre RCTs with concordant results have established that a 7-day treatment was not inferior to a 10- or 14-day treatment for patients with an uncomplicated GNB BSIs [68–70]. We highlight that all patients included in all three RCTs were immunocompetent, afebrile after 3 days of therapy and without uncontrolled infectious sources or prosthetic devices. For ICU patients with BSIs, the duration of therapy should be individualised based on clinical response. A rapid decrease of biomarkers such as PCT or CRP might be interesting to reduce the duration of therapy [68,71,72]. For uncomplicated GNB BSIs, it is not necessary to send repeat BC to ensure bacterial clearance [3]. Otherwise, at least one set of BCs sent at day 2–4 is required. For *S. aureus*, multiple negative BCs may be required to ensure BSIs clearance [73].

Persisting bacteraemia is defined as 2 days or more with positive BC despite active antibiotics [74]. For those cases, after ensuring the pathogen is not resistant to the administered antibiotic, we need to repeat clinical examination and investigations (e.g., CT scanner) looking for a source that had been missed such as a deep-seated abscess. A cardiac echography may be necessary to exclude endocarditis. A review/removal of all suspect intravascular lines and material is likely indicated at this stage. In cases with initially incomplete source control, we suggest increasing the duration of antibiotics by 5–7 days from the time at which all the sources and septic metastasis were treated and microbiological clearance and clinical improvement were obtained. Some sources require longer antibiotic treatments, such as empyema (4–6 weeks), brain abscesses (6–8 weeks), joint infections including seeding from the BSIs (4–8 weeks) or prosthetic valve endocarditis (4–8 weeks) [2,75].

For some pathogens, extended durations of treatment are warranted. Uncomplicated *S. aureus* BSIs require 2 weeks of antibiotics [76]. Cases with incomplete or ineffective source control or with persisting bacteraemia require 4 and sometimes up to 8 weeks of antibiotics or longer, especially when infected devices or material cannot be removed [2]. For uncomplicated candidaemia, current guidelines recommend 14 days of treatment after the first negative BC [77]. Little data are available for XDR pathogens that have very limited treatment options or that are treated with antibiotics that have lesser activity [72]. For those, it is reasonable to focus on optimal source control and continue treatment for several days after microbiological clearance and clinical improvement.

Severely immunosuppressed patients deserve specific attention. In a cohort study of allogeneic–haematopoietic cell transplant (HCT) recipients with *P. aeruginosa* BSIs or and/or pneumonia, treatment durations of less than 14 days were associated with more recurrent infections [78]. This may not apply to other types of immunosuppression. A cohort study of 249 uncomplicated *P. aeruginosa* BSIs in which 65% of the patients were severely immunosuppressed (3% AIDS, 13% HCT, 21% recent chemotherapy, 16% neutropenia on day 1, 11% other immunosuppressive therapy) did not show any difference in outcomes with shorter compared to longer treatment durations (9 vs. 16 days) [79].

Conversely, for CR-BSIs caused by coagulase-negative staphylococci, a very short treatment of 3 days (or even antibiotic withdrawal) after catheter removal may be sufficient [80,81], highlighting the importance of individualising the treatment duration.

We emphasise that fever and persisting haemodynamic instability after treatment of a BSIs may be also due to an infection at another site or to a non-infectious cause. For all patients who do not show rapid improvement or for those with relapsing sepsis, it is crucial to include those diagnoses in a thorough differential before deciding to continue or escalate antibiotics.

6. Conclusions

Blood stream infections in critically ill patients are associated with significant morbidity and mortality. Early adequate antimicrobial therapy, sufficient dosing following ICU specific PK/PD principles and source control are key to improving prognosis. Aggressive ADE and shorter treatments should be used to decrease antibiotic-associated harms.

Author Contributions: A.T.: conceptualisation, writing—original draft. J.L., N.B., F.B. and J.-F.T.: writing—review and editing. All authors have read and agreed to the published version of the manuscript.

Funding: This research received no external funding.

Institutional Review Board Statement: Not applicable.

Informed Consent Statement: Not applicable.

Acknowledgments: ESCMID Study Group for Infections in Critically Ill Patients—ESGCIP: Alexis Tabah, Niccolò Buetti, Jean-François Timsit, Daniele Roberto Giacobbe, George Dimopoulos, Patricia Muñoz García.

Conflicts of Interest: A.T. has nothing to disclose. J.L. has received lecture fees and honoraria from MSD. N.B. received a fellowship grant (grant number: P4P4PM_194449) from the Swiss National Science Foundation. F.B. reported consulting and lecture fees, conference invitation from MSD and lecture fees from bioMérieux. J.-F.T. reported advisory board participation for Merck, Gilead, Becton Dickinson, Pfizer, Medimune, Paratek; lectures for Merck, bioMérieux, Shionogi, Pfizer and research grants to his department from Merck, Pfizer and Thermo Fisher.

References

1. Laupland, K.B.; Leal, J.R. Defining microbial invasion of the bloodstream: A structured review. *Infect. Dis.* **2020**, *52*, 391–395. [CrossRef] [PubMed]
2. Timsit, J.F.; Ruppe, E.; Barbier, F.; Tabah, A.; Bassetti, M. Bloodstream infections in critically ill patients: An expert statement. *Intensive Care Med.* **2020**, *46*, 266–284. [CrossRef] [PubMed]
3. Heil, E.L.; Bork, J.T.; Abbo, L.M.; Barlam, T.F.; Cosgrove, S.E.; Davis, A.; Ha, D.R.; Jenkins, T.C.; Kaye, K.S.; Lewis, J.S., 2nd; et al. Optimizing the Management of Uncomplicated Gram-Negative Bloodstream Infections: Consensus Guidance Using a Modified Delphi Process. *Open Forum Infect. Dis.* **2021**, *8*, ofab434. [CrossRef] [PubMed]
4. Angus, D.C.; Opal, S. Immunosuppression and Secondary Infection in Sepsis: Part, Not All, of the Story. *JAMA* **2016**, *315*, 1457–1459. [CrossRef] [PubMed]
5. Van Vught, L.A.; Klein Klouwenberg, P.M.; Spitoni, C.; Scicluna, B.P.; Wiewel, M.A.; Horn, J.; Schultz, M.J.; Nurnberg, P.; Bonten, M.J.; Cremer, O.L.; et al. Incidence, Risk Factors, and Attributable Mortality of Secondary Infections in the Intensive Care Unit After Admission for Sepsis. *JAMA* **2016**, *315*, 1469–1479. [CrossRef]
6. Tabah, A.; Koulenti, D.; Laupland, K.; Misset, B.; Valles, J.; Bruzzi de Carvalho, F.; Paiva, J.A.; Cakar, N.; Ma, X.; Eggimann, P.; et al. Characteristics and determinants of outcome of hospital-acquired bloodstream infections in intensive care units: The EUROBACT International Cohort Study. *Intensive Care Med.* **2012**, *38*, 1930–1945. [CrossRef]
7. Garrouste-Orgeas, M.; Timsit, J.F.; Tafflet, M.; Misset, B.; Zahar, J.R.; Soufir, L.; Lazard, T.; Jamali, S.; Mourvillier, B.; Cohen, Y.; et al. Excess risk of death from intensive care unit-acquired nosocomial bloodstream infections: A reappraisal. *Clin. Infect. Dis.* **2006**, *42*, 1118–1126. [CrossRef] [PubMed]
8. Adrie, C.; Garrouste-Orgeas, M.; Ibn Essaied, W.; Schwebel, C.; Darmon, M.; Mourvillier, B.; Ruckly, S.; Dumenil, A.S.; Kallel, H.; Argaud, L.; et al. Attributable mortality of ICU-acquired bloodstream infections: Impact of the source, causative micro-organism, resistance profile and antimicrobial therapy. *J. Infect.* **2017**, *74*, 131–141. [CrossRef]
9. Evans, L.; Rhodes, A.; Alhazzani, W.; Antonelli, M.; Coopersmith, C.M.; French, C.; Machado, F.R.; McIntyre, L.; Ostermann, M.; Prescott, H.C.; et al. Surviving sepsis campaign: International guidelines for management of sepsis and septic shock 2021. *Intensive Care Med.* **2021**, *47*, 1181–1247. [CrossRef]
10. Kumar, A.; Roberts, D.; Wood, K.E.; Light, B.; Parrillo, J.E.; Sharma, S.; Suppes, R.; Feinstein, D.; Zanotti, S.; Taiberg, L.; et al. Duration of hypotension before initiation of effective antimicrobial therapy is the critical determinant of survival in human septic shock. *Crit. Care Med.* **2006**, *34*, 1589–1596. [CrossRef]
11. Bloos, F.; Ruddel, H.; Thomas-Ruddel, D.; Schwarzkopf, D.; Pausch, C.; Harbarth, S.; Schreiber, T.; Grundling, M.; Marshall, J.; Simon, P.; et al. Effect of a multifaceted educational intervention for anti-infectious measures on sepsis mortality: A cluster randomized trial. *Intensive Care Med.* **2017**, *43*, 1602–1612. [CrossRef] [PubMed]
12. Singer, M. Antibiotics for Sepsis: Does Each Hour Really Count, or Is It Incestuous Amplification? *Am. J. Respir. Crit. Care Med.* **2017**, *196*, 800–802. [CrossRef] [PubMed]

13. Hranjec, T.; Rosenberger, L.H.; Swenson, B.; Metzger, R.; Flohr, T.R.; Politano, A.D.; Riccio, L.M.; Popovsky, K.A.; Sawyer, R.G. Aggressive versus conservative initiation of antimicrobial treatment in critically ill surgical patients with suspected intensive-care-unit-acquired infection: A quasi-experimental, before and after observational cohort study. *Lancet Infect. Dis.* **2012**, *12*, 774–780. [CrossRef]
14. Arulkumaran, N.; Routledge, M.; Schlebusch, S.; Lipman, J.; Conway Morris, A. Antimicrobial-associated harm in critical care: A narrative review. *Intensive Care Med.* **2020**, *46*, 225–235. [CrossRef]
15. MacFadden, D.R.; Coburn, B.; Shah, N.; Robicsek, A.; Savage, R.; Elligsen, M.; Daneman, N. Utility of prior cultures in predicting antibiotic resistance of bloodstream infections due to Gram-negative pathogens: A multicentre observational cohort study. *Clin. Microbiol. Infect.* **2018**, *24*, 493–499. [CrossRef]
16. Depuydt, P.; Benoit, D.; Vogelaers, D.; Decruyenaere, J.; Vandijck, D.; Claeys, G.; Verschraegen, G.; Blot, S. Systematic surveillance cultures as a tool to predict involvement of multidrug antibiotic resistant bacteria in ventilator-associated pneumonia. *Intensive Care Med.* **2008**, *34*, 675–682. [CrossRef]
17. Alhazzani, W.; Moller, M.H.; Arabi, Y.M.; Loeb, M.; Gong, M.N.; Fan, E.; Oczkowski, S.; Levy, M.M.; Derde, L.; Dzierba, A.; et al. Surviving Sepsis Campaign: Guidelines on the management of critically ill adults with Coronavirus Disease 2019 (COVID-19). *Intensive Care Med.* **2020**, *46*, 854–887. [CrossRef]
18. Tabah, A.; Bassetti, M.; Kollef, M.H.; Zahar, J.R.; Paiva, J.A.; Timsit, J.F.; Roberts, J.A.; Schouten, J.; Giamarellou, H.; Rello, J.; et al. Antimicrobial de-escalation in critically ill patients: A position statement from a task force of the European Society of Intensive Care Medicine (ESICM) and European Society of Clinical Microbiology and Infectious Diseases (ESCMID) Critically Ill Patients Study Group (ESGCIP). *Intensive Care Med.* **2020**, *46*, 245–265. [CrossRef]
19. Scheer, C.S.; Fuchs, C.; Grundling, M.; Vollmer, M.; Bast, J.; Bohnert, J.A.; Zimmermann, K.; Hahnenkamp, K.; Rehberg, S.; Kuhn, S.O. Impact of antibiotic administration on blood culture positivity at the beginning of sepsis: A prospective clinical cohort study. *Clin. Microbiol. Infect.* **2019**, *25*, 326–331. [CrossRef]
20. Dargere, S.; Cormier, H.; Verdon, R. Contaminants in blood cultures: Importance, implications, interpretation and prevention. *Clin. Microbiol. Infect.* **2018**, *24*, 964–969. [CrossRef]
21. Noster, J.; Thelen, P.; Hamprecht, A. Detection of Multidrug-Resistant *Enterobacterales*-From ESBLs to Carbapenemases. *Antibiotics* **2021**, *10*, 1140. [CrossRef] [PubMed]
22. Tabah, A.; Buetti, N.; Barbier, F.; Timsit, J.F. Current opinion in management of septic shock due to Gram-negative bacteria. *Curr. Opin. Infect. Dis.* **2021**, *34*, 718–727. [CrossRef] [PubMed]
23. Giacobbe, D.R.; Giani, T.; Bassetti, M.; Marchese, A.; Viscoli, C.; Rossolini, G.M. Rapid microbiological tests for bloodstream infections due to multidrug resistant Gram-negative bacteria: Therapeutic implications. *Clin. Microbiol. Infect.* **2020**, *26*, 713–722. [CrossRef] [PubMed]
24. Pancholi, P.; Carroll, K.C.; Buchan, B.W.; Chan, R.C.; Dhiman, N.; Ford, B.; Granato, P.A.; Harrington, A.T.; Hernandez, D.R.; Humphries, R.M.; et al. Multicenter Evaluation of the Accelerate PhenoTest BC Kit for Rapid Identification and Phenotypic Antimicrobial Susceptibility Testing Using Morphokinetic Cellular Analysis. *J. Clin. Microbiol.* **2018**, *56*, e01317–e01329. [CrossRef]
25. Meier, M.; Hamprecht, A. Systematic Comparison of Four Methods for Detection of Carbapenemase-Producing Enterobacterales Directly from Blood Cultures. *J. Clin. Microbiol.* **2019**, *57*, e00709–e00719. [CrossRef]
26. Nordmann, P.; Sadek, M.; Demord, A.; Poirel, L. NitroSpeed-Carba NP Test for Rapid Detection and Differentiation between Different Classes of Carbapenemases in Enterobacterales. *J. Clin. Microbiol.* **2020**, *58*, e00920–e00932. [CrossRef]
27. Tabah, A.; Cotta, M.O.; Garnacho-Montero, J.; Schouten, J.; Roberts, J.A.; Lipman, J.; Tacey, M.; Timsit, J.F.; Leone, M.; Zahar, J.R.; et al. A Systematic Review of the Definitions, Determinants, and Clinical Outcomes of Antimicrobial De-escalation in the Intensive Care Unit. *Clin. Infect. Dis.* **2016**, *62*, 1009–1017. [CrossRef]
28. Sjovall, F.; Perner, A.; Hylander Moller, M. Empirical mono- versus combination antibiotic therapy in adult intensive care patients with severe sepsis–A systematic review with meta-analysis and trial sequential analysis. *J. Infect.* **2017**, *74*, 331–344. [CrossRef]
29. Tamma, P.D.; Aitken, S.L.; Bonomo, R.A.; Mathers, A.J.; van Duin, D.; Clancy, C.J. Infectious Diseases Society of America Guidance on the Treatment of Extended-Spectrum beta-lactamase Producing Enterobacterales (ESBL-E), Carbapenem-Resistant Enterobacterales (CRE), and *Pseudomonas aeruginosa* with Difficult-to-Treat Resistance (DTR-*P. aeruginosa*). *Clin. Infect. Dis.* **2021**, *72*, 1109–1116. [CrossRef]
30. Paul, M.; Carrara, E.; Retamar, P.; Tangden, T.; Bitterman, R.; Bonomo, R.A.; de Waele, J.; Daikos, G.L.; Akova, M.; Harbarth, S.; et al. European Society of clinical microbiology and infectious diseases (ESCMID) guidelines for the treatment of infections caused by Multidrug-resistant Gram-negative bacilli (endorsed by ESICM -European Society of intensive care Medicine). *Clin. Microbiol. Infect.* **2021**. [CrossRef]
31. Pilmis, B.; Jullien, V.; Tabah, A.; Zahar, J.R.; Brun-Buisson, C. Piperacillin-tazobactam as alternative to carbapenems for ICU patients. *Ann. Intensive Care* **2017**, *7*, 113. [CrossRef] [PubMed]
32. Harris, P.N.A.; Tambyah, P.A.; Lye, D.C.; Mo, Y.; Lee, T.H.; Yilmaz, M.; Alenazi, T.H.; Arabi, Y.; Falcone, M.; Bassetti, M.; et al. Effect of Piperacillin-Tazobactam vs Meropenem on 30-Day Mortality for Patients with *E. coli* or *Klebsiella pneumoniae* Bloodstream Infection and Ceftriaxone Resistance: A Randomized Clinical Trial. *JAMA* **2018**, *320*, 984–994. [CrossRef] [PubMed]
33. Tamma, P.D.; Doi, Y.; Bonomo, R.A.; Johnson, J.K.; Simner, P.J.; Antibacterial Resistance Leadership Group. A Primer on AmpC beta-Lactamases: Necessary Knowledge for an Increasingly Multidrug-resistant World. *Clin. Infect. Dis.* **2019**, *69*, 1446–1455. [CrossRef] [PubMed]

34. Fung-Tomc, J.C.; Gradelski, E.; Huczko, E.; Dougherty, T.J.; Kessler, R.E.; Bonner, D.P. Differences in the resistant variants of Enterobacter cloacae selected by extended-spectrum cephalosporins. *Antimicrob. Agents Chemother.* **1996**, *40*, 1289–1293. [CrossRef]
35. Cheng, L.; Nelson, B.C.; Mehta, M.; Seval, N.; Park, S.; Giddins, M.J.; Shi, Q.; Whittier, S.; Gomez-Simmonds, A.; Uhlemann, A.C. Piperacillin-Tazobactam versus Other Antibacterial Agents for Treatment of Bloodstream Infections Due to AmpC beta-Lactamase-Producing Enterobacteriaceae. *Antimicrob. Agents Chemother.* **2017**, *61*, e00276-17. [CrossRef]
36. Tamma, P.D.; Aitken, S.L.; Bonomo, R.A.; Mathers, A.J.; van Duin, D.; Clancy, C.J. Infectious Diseases Society of America Guidance on the Treatment of AmpC beta-lactamase-Producing Enterobacterales, Carbapenem-Resistant *Acinetobacter baumannii*, and *Stenotrophomonas maltophilia* Infections. *Clin. Infect. Dis.* **2021**, ciab1013. [CrossRef]
37. Stewart, A.G.; Paterson, D.L.; Young, B.; Lye, D.C.; Davis, J.S.; Schneider, K.; Yilmaz, M.; Dinleyici, R.; Runnegar, N.; Henderson, A.; et al. Meropenem Versus Piperacillin-Tazobactam for Definitive Treatment of Bloodstream Infections Caused by AmpC beta-Lactamase-Producing *Enterobacter* spp., *Citrobacter freundii*, *Morganella morganii*, *Providencia* spp., or *Serratia marcescens*: A Pilot Multicenter Randomized Controlled Trial (MERINO-2). *Open Forum Infect. Dis.* **2021**, *8*, ofab387. [CrossRef]
38. Center for Disease Control and Prevention. Carbapenem-Resistant Enterobacterales (CRE): CRE Technical Information. Available online: https://www.cdc.gov/hai/organisms/cre/technical-info.html#Definition (accessed on 22 December 2021).
39. Van Duin, D.; Arias, C.A.; Komarow, L.; Chen, L.; Hanson, B.M.; Weston, G.; Cober, E.; Garner, O.B.; Jacob, J.T.; Satlin, M.J.; et al. Molecular and clinical epidemiology of carbapenem-resistant Enterobacterales in the USA (CRACKLE-2): A prospective cohort study. *Lancet Infect. Dis.* **2020**, *20*, 731–741. [CrossRef]
40. Van Duin, D.; Lok, J.J.; Earley, M.; Cober, E.; Richter, S.S.; Perez, F.; Salata, R.A.; Kalayjian, R.C.; Watkins, R.R.; Doi, Y.; et al. Colistin Versus Ceftazidime-Avibactam in the Treatment of Infections Due to Carbapenem-Resistant Enterobacteriaceae. *Clin. Infect. Dis.* **2018**, *66*, 163–171. [CrossRef]
41. Tumbarello, M.; Raffaelli, F.; Giannella, M.; Mantengoli, E.; Mularoni, A.; Venditti, M.; De Rosa, F.G.; Sarmati, L.; Bassetti, M.; Brindicci, G.; et al. Ceftazidime-Avibactam Use for *Klebsiella pneumoniae* Carbapenemase-Producing *K. pneumoniae* Infections: A Retrospective Observational Multicenter Study. *Clin. Infect. Dis.* **2021**, *73*, 1664–1676. [CrossRef]
42. Shields, R.K.; Nguyen, M.H.; Chen, L.; Press, E.G.; Potoski, B.A.; Marini, R.V.; Doi, Y.; Kreiswirth, B.N.; Clancy, C.J. Ceftazidime-avibactam is superior to other treatment regimens against carbapenem-resistant *Klebsiella pneumoniae* bacteremia. *Antimicrob. Agents Chemother.* **2017**, *61*, e00817–e00883. [CrossRef] [PubMed]
43. Wunderink, R.G.; Giamarellos-Bourboulis, E.J.; Rahav, G.; Mathers, A.J.; Bassetti, M.; Vazquez, J.; Cornely, O.A.; Solomkin, J.; Bhowmick, T.; Bishara, J.; et al. Effect and Safety of Meropenem-Vaborbactam versus Best-Available Therapy in Patients with Carbapenem-Resistant Enterobacteriaceae Infections: The TANGO II Randomized Clinical Trial. *Infect. Dis. Ther.* **2018**, *7*, 439–455. [CrossRef] [PubMed]
44. Bassetti, M.; Echols, R.; Matsunaga, Y.; Ariyasu, M.; Doi, Y.; Ferrer, R.; Lodise, T.P.; Naas, T.; Niki, Y.; Paterson, D.L.; et al. Efficacy and safety of cefiderocol or best available therapy for the treatment of serious infections caused by carbapenem-resistant Gram-negative bacteria (CREDIBLE-CR): A randomised, open-label, multicentre, pathogen-focused, descriptive, phase 3 trial. *Lancet Infect. Dis.* **2021**, *21*, 226–240. [CrossRef]
45. Shields, R.K.; Doi, Y. Aztreonam Combination Therapy: An Answer to Metallo-beta-Lactamase-Producing Gram-Negative Bacteria? *Clin. Infect. Dis.* **2020**, *71*, 1099–1101. [CrossRef] [PubMed]
46. Falcone, M.; Daikos, G.L.; Tiseo, G.; Bassoulis, D.; Giordano, C.; Galfo, V.; Leonildi, A.; Tagliaferri, E.; Barnini, S.; Sani, S.; et al. Efficacy of Ceftazidime-avibactam Plus Aztreonam in Patients with Bloodstream Infections Caused by Metallo-β-lactamase-Producing Enterobacterales. *Clin. Infect. Dis.* **2021**, *72*, 1871–1878. [CrossRef]
47. Timsit, J.-F.; Wicky, P.-H.; de Montmollin, E. Treatment of Severe Infections Due to Metallo-Betalactamases Enterobacterales in Critically Ill Patients. *Antibiotics* **2022**, *11*, 144. [CrossRef]
48. Gutierrez-Gutierrez, B.; Salamanca, E.; de Cueto, M.; Hsueh, P.R.; Viale, P.; Pano-Pardo, J.R.; Venditti, M.; Tumbarello, M.; Daikos, G.; Canton, R.; et al. Effect of appropriate combination therapy on mortality of patients with bloodstream infections due to carbapenemase-producing Enterobacteriaceae (INCREMENT): A retrospective cohort study. *Lancet Infect. Dis.* **2017**, *17*, 726–734. [CrossRef]
49. Piperaki, E.T.; Tzouvelekis, L.S.; Miriagou, V.; Daikos, G.L. Carbapenem-resistant *Acinetobacter baumannii*: In pursuit of an effective treatment. *Clin. Microbiol. Infect.* **2019**, *25*, 951–957. [CrossRef]
50. Sader, H.S.; Castanheira, M.; Flamm, R.K.; Mendes, R.E.; Farrell, D.J.; Jones, R.N. Ceftazidime/avibactam tested against Gram-negative bacteria from intensive care unit (ICU) and non-ICU patients, including those with ventilator-associated pneumonia. *Int. J. Antimicrob. Agents* **2015**, *46*, 53–59. [CrossRef]
51. Paul, M.; Daikos, G.L.; Durante-Mangoni, E.; Yahav, D.; Carmeli, Y.; Benattar, Y.D.; Skiada, A.; Andini, R.; Eliakim-Raz, N.; Nutman, A.; et al. Colistin alone versus colistin plus meropenem for treatment of severe infections caused by carbapenem-resistant Gram-negative bacteria: An open-label, randomised controlled trial. *Lancet Infect. Dis.* **2018**, *18*, 391–400. [CrossRef]
52. Oliveira, M.S.; Prado, G.V.; Costa, S.F.; Grinbaum, R.S.; Levin, A.S. Ampicillin/sulbactam compared with polymyxins for the treatment of infections caused by carbapenem-resistant *Acinetobacter* spp. *J. Antimicrob. Chemother.* **2008**, *61*, 1369–1375. [CrossRef] [PubMed]

53. Tsuji, B.T.; Pogue, J.M.; Zavascki, A.P.; Paul, M.; Daikos, G.L.; Forrest, A.; Giacobbe, D.R.; Viscoli, C.; Giamarellou, H.; Karaiskos, I.; et al. International Consensus Guidelines for the Optimal Use of the Polymyxins: Endorsed by the American College of Clinical Pharmacy (ACCP), European Society of Clinical Microbiology and Infectious Diseases (ESCMID), Infectious Diseases Society of America (IDSA), International Society for Anti-infective Pharmacology (ISAP), Society of Critical Care Medicine (SCCM), and Society of Infectious Diseases Pharmacists (SIDP). *Pharmacotherapy* **2019**, *39*, 10–39. [CrossRef] [PubMed]
54. Routsi, C.; Kokkoris, S.; Douka, E.; Ekonomidou, F.; Karaiskos, I.; Giamarellou, H. High-dose tigecycline-associated alterations in coagulation parameters in critically ill patients with severe infections. *Int. J. Antimicrob. Agents* **2015**, *45*, 90–93. [CrossRef] [PubMed]
55. Muralidharan, G.; Micalizzi, M.; Speth, J.; Raible, D.; Troy, S. Pharmacokinetics of tigecycline after single and multiple doses in healthy subjects. *Antimicrob. Agents Chemother.* **2005**, *49*, 220–229. [CrossRef] [PubMed]
56. Lenhard, J.R.; Smith, N.M.; Bulman, Z.P.; Tao, X.; Thamlikitkul, V.; Shin, B.S.; Nation, R.L.; Li, J.; Bulitta, J.B.; Tsuji, B.T. High-Dose Ampicillin-Sulbactam Combinations Combat Polymyxin-Resistant *Acinetobacter baumannii* in a Hollow-Fiber Infection Model. *Antimicrob. Agents Chemother.* **2017**, *61*, e01268-16. [CrossRef] [PubMed]
57. Minejima, E.; Mai, N.; Bui, N.; Mert, M.; Mack, W.J.; She, R.C.; Nieberg, P.; Spellberg, B.; Wong-Beringer, A. Defining the Breakpoint Duration of *Staphylococcus aureus* Bacteremia Predictive of Poor Outcomes. *Clin. Infect. Dis.* **2020**, *70*, 566–573. [CrossRef] [PubMed]
58. Azuhata, T.; Kinoshita, K.; Kawano, D.; Komatsu, T.; Sakurai, A.; Chiba, Y.; Tanjho, K. Time from admission to initiation of surgery for source control is a critical determinant of survival in patients with gastrointestinal perforation with associated septic shock. *Crit. Care* **2014**, *18*, R87. [CrossRef]
59. Sartelli, M.; Catena, F.; Abu-Zidan, F.M.; Ansaloni, L.; Biffl, W.L.; Boermeester, M.A.; Ceresoli, M.; Chiara, O.; Coccolini, F.; De Waele, J.; et al. Management of intra-abdominal infections: Recommendations by the WSES 2016 consensus conference. *World J. Emerg. Surg.* **2017**, *12*, 22. [CrossRef]
60. Timsit, J.F.; Bassetti, M.; Cremer, O.; Daikos, G.; de Waele, J.; Kallil, A.; Kipnis, E.; Kollef, M.; Laupland, K.; Paiva, J.A.; et al. Rationalizing antimicrobial therapy in the ICU: A narrative review. *Intensive Care Med.* **2019**, *45*, 172–189. [CrossRef]
61. Roberts, J.A.; Paul, S.K.; Akova, M.; Bassetti, M.; De Waele, J.J.; Dimopoulos, G.; Kaukonen, K.M.; Koulenti, D.; Martin, C.; Montravers, P.; et al. DALI: Defining antibiotic levels in intensive care unit patients: Are current beta-lactam antibiotic doses sufficient for critically ill patients? *Clin. Infect. Dis.* **2014**, *58*, 1072–1083. [CrossRef]
62. Matusik, E.; Boidin, C.; Friggeri, A.; Richard, J.C.; Bitker, L.; Roberts, J.A.; Goutelle, S. Therapeutic Drug Monitoring of Antibiotic Drugs in Patients Receiving Continuous Renal Replacement Therapy or Intermittent Hemodialysis: A Critical Review. *Ther. Drug Monit.* **2022**, *44*, 86–102. [CrossRef] [PubMed]
63. Wong, G.; Taccone, F.; Villois, P.; Scheetz, M.H.; Rhodes, N.J.; Briscoe, S.; McWhinney, B.; Nunez-Nunez, M.; Ungerer, J.; Lipman, J.; et al. β-Lactam pharmacodynamics in Gram-negative bloodstream infections in the critically ill. *J. Antimicrob. Chemother.* **2020**, *75*, 429–433. [CrossRef] [PubMed]
64. Roberts, J.A.; Abdul-Aziz, M.H.; Lipman, J.; Mouton, J.W.; Vinks, A.A.; Felton, T.W.; Hope, W.W.; Farkas, A.; Neely, M.N.; Schentag, J.J.; et al. Individualised antibiotic dosing for patients who are critically ill: Challenges and potential solutions. *Lancet Infect. Dis.* **2014**, *14*, 498–509. [CrossRef]
65. Roberts, J.A.; Abdul-Aziz, M.H.; Davis, J.S.; Dulhunty, J.M.; Cotta, M.O.; Myburgh, J.; Bellomo, R.; Lipman, J. Continuous versus Intermittent beta-Lactam Infusion in Severe Sepsis. A Meta-analysis of Individual Patient Data from Randomized Trials. *Am. J. Respir. Crit. Care Med.* **2016**, *194*, 681–691. [CrossRef] [PubMed]
66. Huttner, A.; Harbarth, S.; Hope, W.W.; Lipman, J.; Roberts, J.A. Therapeutic drug monitoring of the beta-lactam antibiotics: What is the evidence and which patients should we be using it for? *J. Antimicrob. Chemother.* **2015**, *70*, 3178–3183. [CrossRef] [PubMed]
67. Curran, J.; Lo, J.; Leung, V.; Brown, K.; Schwartz, K.L.; Daneman, N.; Garber, G.; Wu, J.H.C.; Langford, B.J. Estimating daily antibiotic harms: An umbrella review with individual study meta-analysis. *Clin. Microbiol. Infect.* **2021**. [CrossRef]
68. von Dach, E.; Albrich, W.C.; Brunel, A.S.; Prendki, V.; Cuvelier, C.; Flury, D.; Gayet-Ageron, A.; Huttner, B.; Kohler, P.; Lemmenmeier, E.; et al. Effect of C-Reactive Protein-Guided Antibiotic Treatment Duration, 7-Day Treatment, or 14-Day Treatment on 30-Day Clinical Failure Rate in Patients with Uncomplicated Gram-Negative Bacteremia: A Randomized Clinical Trial. *JAMA* **2020**, *323*, 2160–2169. [CrossRef]
69. Yahav, D.; Franceschini, E.; Koppel, F.; Turjeman, A.; Babich, T.; Bitterman, R.; Neuberger, A.; Ghanem-Zoubi, N.; Santoro, A.; Eliakim-Raz, N.; et al. Seven Versus 14 Days of Antibiotic Therapy for Uncomplicated Gram-negative Bacteremia: A Noninferiority Randomized Controlled Trial. *Clin. Infect. Dis.* **2019**, *69*, 1091–1098. [CrossRef]
70. Molina, J.; Montero-Mateos, E.; Praena-Segovia, J.; Leon-Jimenez, E.; Natera, C.; Lopez-Cortes, L.E.; Valiente, L.; Rosso-Fernandez, C.M.; Herrero, M.; Aller-Garcia, A.I.; et al. Seven-versus 14-day course of antibiotics for the treatment of bloodstream infections by Enterobacterales: A randomized, controlled trial. *Clin. Microbiol. Infect.* **2021**. [CrossRef]
71. Meier, M.A.; Branche, A.; Neeser, O.L.; Wirz, Y.; Haubitz, S.; Bouadma, L.; Wolff, M.; Luyt, C.E.; Chastre, J.; Tubach, F.; et al. Procalcitonin-guided Antibiotic Treatment in Patients with Positive Blood Cultures: A Patient-level Meta-analysis of Randomized Trials. *Clin. Infect. Dis.* **2019**, *69*, 388–396. [CrossRef]
72. Le Fevre, L.; Timsit, J.F. Duration of antimicrobial therapy for Gram-negative infections. *Curr. Opin. Infect. Dis.* **2020**, *33*, 511–516. [CrossRef] [PubMed]

73. Fiala, J.; Palraj, B.R.; Sohail, M.R.; Lahr, B.; Baddour, L.M. Is a single set of negative blood cultures sufficient to ensure clearance of bloodstream infection in patients with *Staphylococcus aureus* bacteremia? The skip phenomenon. *Infection* 2019, *47*, 1047–1053. [CrossRef] [PubMed]
74. Kuehl, R.; Morata, L.; Boeing, C.; Subirana, I.; Seifert, H.; Rieg, S.; Kern, W.V.; Kim, H.B.; Kim, E.S.; Liao, C.-H.; et al. Defining persistent *Staphylococcus aureus* bacteraemia: Secondary analysis of a prospective cohort study. *Lancet Infect. Dis.* 2020, *20*, 1409–1417. [CrossRef]
75. Brouwer, M.C.; Tunkel, A.R.; McKhann, G.M., 2nd; van de Beek, D. Brain abscess. *N. Engl. J. Med.* 2014, *371*, 447–456. [CrossRef]
76. Liu, C.; Bayer, A.; Cosgrove, S.E.; Daum, R.S.; Fridkin, S.K.; Gorwitz, R.J.; Kaplan, S.L.; Karchmer, A.W.; Levine, D.P.; Murray, B.E. Clinical practice guidelines by the Infectious Diseases Society of America for the treatment of methicillin-resistant *Staphylococcus aureus* infections in adults and children. *Clin. Infect. Dis.* 2011, *52*, e18–e55. [CrossRef] [PubMed]
77. Martin-Loeches, I.; Antonelli, M.; Cuenca-Estrella, M.; Dimopoulos, G.; Einav, S.; De Waele, J.J.; Garnacho-Montero, J.; Kanj, S.S.; Machado, F.R.; Montravers, P.; et al. ESICM/ESCMID task force on practical management of invasive candidiasis in critically ill patients. *Intensive Care Med.* 2019, *45*, 789–805. [CrossRef]
78. Olearo, F.; Kronig, I.; Masouridi-Levrat, S.; Chalandon, Y.; Khanna, N.; Passweg, J.; Medinger, M.; Mueller, N.J.; Schanz, U.; Van Delden, C.; et al. Optimal Treatment Duration of *Pseudomonas aeruginosa* Infections in Allogeneic Hematopoietic Cell Transplant Recipients. *Open Forum Infect. Dis.* 2020, *7*, ofaa246. [CrossRef]
79. Fabre, V.; Amoah, J.; Cosgrove, S.E.; Tamma, P.D. Antibiotic Therapy for *Pseudomonas aeruginosa* Bloodstream Infections: How Long Is Long Enough? *Clin. Infect. Dis.* 2019, *69*, 2011–2014. [CrossRef]
80. Muff, S.; Tabah, A.; Que, Y.A.; Timsit, J.F.; Mermel, L.; Harbarth, S.; Buetti, N. Short-Course Versus Long-Course Systemic Antibiotic Treatment for Uncomplicated Intravascular Catheter-Related Bloodstream Infections due to Gram-Negative Bacteria, Enterococci or Coagulase-Negative Staphylococci: A Systematic Review. *Infect. Dis. Ther.* 2021, *10*, 1591–1605. [CrossRef]
81. Hebeisen, U.P.; Atkinson, A.; Marschall, J.; Buetti, N. Catheter-related bloodstream infections with coagulase-negative staphylococci: Are antibiotics necessary if the catheter is removed? *Antimicrob. Resist. Infect. Control.* 2019, *8*, 21. [CrossRef]

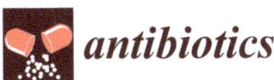

Review

Antibiotics and ECMO in the Adult Population—Persistent Challenges and Practical Guides

Francisco Gomez [1], Jesyree Veita [2] and Krzysztof Laudanski [3,4,5,*]

1. Department of Neurology, University of Missouri, Columbia, MO 65021, USA; fegyr7@umsystem.edu
2. Society for Healthcare Innovation, Philadelphia, PA 19146, USA; jassy.veita@shci.org
3. Department of Anesthesiology and Critical Care, University of Pennsylvania, Philadelphia, PA 19146, USA
4. Leonard Davis Institute for HealthCare Economics, University of Pennsylvania, Philadelphia, PA 19146, USA
5. Department of Neurology, University of Pennsylvania, Philadelphia, PA 19146, USA
* Correspondence: klaudanski@gmail.com; Tel.: +1-215-6628200

Abstract: Extracorporeal membrane oxygenation (ECMO) is an emerging treatment modality associated with a high frequency of antibiotic use. However, several covariables emerge during ECMO implementation, potentially jeopardizing the success of antimicrobial therapy. These variables include but are not limited to: the increased volume of distribution, altered clearance, and adsorption into circuit components, in addition to complex interactions of antibiotics in critical care illness. Furthermore, ECMO complicates the assessment of antibiotic effectiveness as fever, or other signs may not be easily detected, the immunogenicity of the circuit affects procalcitonin levels and other inflammatory markers while disrupting the immune system. We provided a review of pharmacokinetics and pharmacodynamics during ECMO, emphasizing practical application and review of patient-, illness-, and ECMO hardware-related factors.

Keywords: extracorporeal membrane oxygenation; ECMO; antibiotics; pharmacodynamics; pharmacokinetics; critical illness

Citation: Gomez, F.; Veita, J.; Laudanski, K. Antibiotics and ECMO in the Adult Population—Persistent Challenges and Practical Guides. *Antibiotics* 2022, 11, 338. https://doi.org/10.3390/antibiotics11030338

Academic Editors: Elizabeth Paramythiotou, Christina Routsi and Antoine Andremont

Received: 27 January 2022
Accepted: 26 February 2022
Published: 4 March 2022

Publisher's Note: MDPI stays neutral with regard to jurisdictional claims in published maps and institutional affiliations.

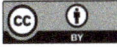

Copyright: © 2022 by the authors. Licensee MDPI, Basel, Switzerland. This article is an open access article distributed under the terms and conditions of the Creative Commons Attribution (CC BY) license (https://creativecommons.org/licenses/by/4.0/).

1. Introduction

Extracorporeal membrane oxygenation (ECMO) has been increasingly employed in critical care, showing a reduction in 90-day mortality in ARDS vs. conventional care in mixed metanalysis [1]. However, other randomized control trials have failed to show benefits for ECMO deployment [2–4]. The interest in this emerging technology and widespread use seems to be slightly out of synchrony with the amount of supporting evidence [4–6]. In general, ECMO has found applications in several conditions characterized by unsustainable pathophysiology refractory to traditional therapies, including failures of pulmonary gas exchange or cardiac ability to maintain circulation [6–9].

The primary advantage of ECMO is to provide ventilatory or hemodynamic support in severely critically ill patients as a bridge to recovery in otherwise irrecoverable patients. The presumption is that stress related to ECMO implementation is less deleterious than mechanical ventilation or classical circulatory system support via implanted devices or medical therapy [6,10]. In that respect, ECMO provides "a bridge" to recovery by allowing sufficient time to surmount otherwise unsurvivable injury. A less common indication is to provide support during cardiopulmonary resuscitation or to preserve the viability of organs in donors [11,12].

A common indication for ECMO is acute respiratory distress syndrome (ARDS), most commonly from infectious etiopathogenesis [5,7,8]. In addition, sepsis is considered the indication for ECMO deployment in some cases [10,13]. Alternatively, patients undergoing ECMO may develop infectious complications that are byproducts of implementations [6,7,14].

The risk is relatively elevated considering the presence of invasive cannulation and emergence of immunosuppression secondary to critical care illness and considering the introduction of mechanical support devices [15–17].

ECMO introduces several variables into antibiotic pharmacokinetics and pharmacodynamics, which must be considered to maximize therapeutic benefit and minimize risks. Moreover, the effect of ECMO on said parameters may be further complicated by patient characteristics and concomitant illnesses or organ failure [18–21]. Therefore, adequate selection, management, and dosing of antibiotics and chemotherapeutics are challenging. Conversely, our review will clearly demonstrate that most of the data suggest that underdosing of antibiotics may lead to suboptimal outcomes. Alternatively, bactericidal antibiotics may attain a level typical for bacteriostatic levels rendering the adequate immune system critical for therapeutic success.

The need for understanding how to optimize antibiotics effectiveness in ECMO-related situations is critical as the implementation and indications of the ECMO continues to progress, while the emergence of ECMO-derivative techniques such as a CO_2-removal device, Impella, intra-aortic balloon counterpulsation, and cytokine scavengers add other variables to understanding distribution, activity and metabolism of antibiotics in these situations [6,7,22–25]. Given the increasing utilization of ECMO in the setting of systemic infection, an understanding of the interactions between said therapies and antibiotics is paramount to successful patient care.

2. The ECMO Ins and Outs

ECMO is a relatively young modality that evolved from cardiopulmonary bypass [23]. In essence, ECMO can be considered as a protracted bypass and therapeutic takeover of pulmonary or cardiac function by mechanical devices. Driven by therapeutic goals, cannula configuration is applied to support the heart, lungs, or both. Venovenous VV-ECMO places both inflow and outflow cannulas in the venous system, allowing for gas exchange support in the absence of severe cardiac function impairment [23,26,27]. The ECMO circuit is integrated serially into the patient's circulation in this configuration. Conversely, venoarterial ECMO (VA-ECMO) places the intake cannula in the venous system while the outflow is placed into an arterial vessel. This configuration supports lung and cardiac functions [14,23,27]. The circuit is placed in parallel to the heart, allowing for differential support of the cardiac function.

Cannulas provide an access port to the patient's vascular system. They are single lumen and dual lumen [27,28]. To prevent kinking, they are made of metal coils embedded in protective shielding. Dual lumen cannulas need a precise placement but allow for higher mobility.

The ECMO system comprises several items in the circuit, with a pump and a membrane allowing for gas exchange as main components, connected via relatively high bore tubing [29] (Figure 1). The tubing is made of polyvinylchloride (PVC) with several coatings. Significant effort is taken to reduce a circuit-induced hypercoagulable state and immunogenicity via heparin or alternative coatings [30–32]. Transparency of the plastic tubing allows for visual inspection. Tubing pliability may lead to kinking and flow interruption, especially at 37 °C. A reinforced wire may be woven into the plastic to increase mechanical strength and to prevent kinking. The length of the tubing is dependent on circuit configuration, including additional elements (bridge, cytokine absorption devices, continuous renal replacement therapy bypass, access ports, and others) [33–35]. The length of the tubing is a compromise between ergonomics and patient mobility versus the overall need to minimize length [36]. The length of the tubing has several consequences. Apart from hemodynamics (i.e., shear stress, resistance to flow), tubing length determines the surface area coated by the biofilm, while length and diameter (3/8 inch) determine the fluid volume needed for priming as well as radiant heat loss.

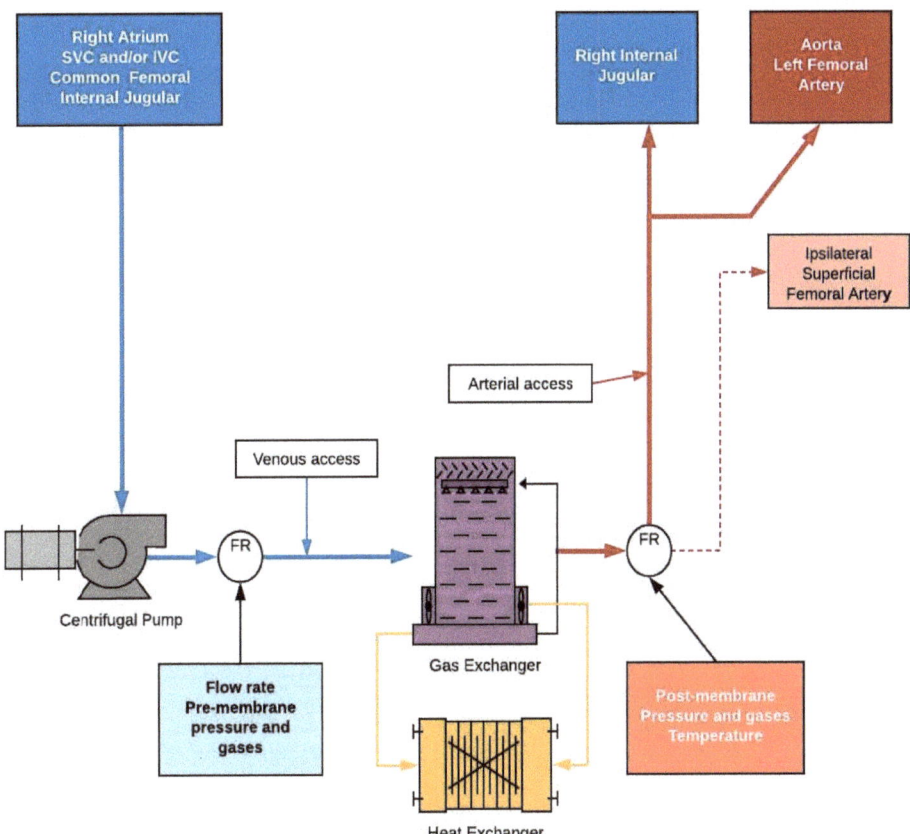

Figure 1. Sample VV ECMO circuit and possible cannulation sites.

The pump allows for high throughput, from the high bore intake cannula, through the oxygenator into the return cannula. There are two main types of pumps: roller and centrifugal [29]. The latter confers the advantage of minimized shear stress exerted upon erythrocytes [37,38]. The pump suctions venous blood from the patient, and a bladder may be introduced in front of the pump to prevent excessive negative pressure and venous collapse. The said pump produces the driving pressure necessary for blood to advance through the circuit and oxygenator while supporting perfusion pressure on the patient side. The pump design contributes to susceptibility of the circuity to kinking as the centrifugal pumps incur effluence with rising resistance, wherein the mechanical energy is lost as heat. In contrast, a roller pump, commonly found in CPB, will significantly increase pressure in a kinked circuit, leading to rupture. Safe pressure within the circuit is usually 300 mmHg, wherein 600 mmHg incurs the risk of rupture.

The membrane oxygenator's function is to provide a large surface area allowing for efficient gas exchange [39]. The effectiveness of the exchanger is measured as the amount of 75% saturated blood that can be further oxygenated to 95%. A gaseous mixture (usually oxygen and nitrogen) is injected into a gas exchanger. Carbon dioxide can be added for specific indications. The gas mixture is pumped through capillary tubing infused with blood, which flows counter to the gas [39]. Carbon dioxide exchange is quite efficient, while oxygen transfer is more limited due to the gases' respective water solubility. The same principles govern this phenomenon as the gas exchange in the lungs. The reduction in the size of the oxygenators due to technological advances has resulted in fewer chances for blood pooling and thrombus formation.

Finally, a heat exchanger allows for precise and dynamic thermoregulation, and several in-line monitors and couplings allow for drug administration or system sampling [14,29]. There is also an increasing interest in providing additional support by introducing Impella, intra-aortic balloon counterpulsation, and bioabsorption devices, with significant implications for drug distribution [40].

In general, the evolution of the ECMO circuitry is reflected in a decreased form factor and lower immunogenicity of the hardware [41]. The former element has resulted in declining needs for volume fluid priming with direct effects on drug volume of distribution, including antibiotics. More compact form factors and lower immunogenicity limit the biofilm formation and drug absorption in the circuit. The design difference between leading manufacturers is usually related to user interface and design peculiarities with unclear, potentially negligible pharmacokinetics and pharmacodynamics.

Infection and ECMO

Infection is the main driver for ECMO initiation, with meta-analysis of the CESAR and EOLIA trials finding ARDS to be the main indication for initiation of said therapy, with >60% being precipitated by pneumonia [1,6–8,13,23]. The risks factors for developing infection include more severally sick patients, ongoing immunosuppressive treatment targeting autoimmune diseases, prolonged cannulation, and VA ECMO [8,14]. In addition, critically ill patients develop a state of immunosuppression or anergy contributing to the infection's risk [15,17]. At the same time, antibiotic effectiveness relies on the bactericidal effect instead of bacteriostatic or past-antibiotics effect in most critical care situations.

Given the implantation of multiple invasive devices, ECMO itself confers risk for development of infections, including bloodstream infection at risk linearly related to the duration of therapy [14]. The prevalence of nosocomial infections in ECMO patients may range from 10–12% in registry data to 9–65% in single-center studies. Development of said infectious complications has been shown to increase morbidity and mortality, the latter by up to 38–63% [42]. In recent data, the most common sites of infection were respiratory at 56%, followed by bloodstream at 29%, and other sites, including urinary tract or soft tissues at 14% [43]. In more recent data, *Candida* sp. may have superseded other organisms [44]. Coagulase-negative staphylococci (15.9%), pseudomonas (10.5%), staphylococcus (9.4%), and *Enterococcus* (4%) are common pathogens [45]. Each hospital should have its profile for organism development.

Currently, there is no recommendation for routine infection prophylaxis in ECMO patients [29], although some centers conduct routine blood cultures for surveillance [14]. Compounding the issue of cannula-related infection, cannulas cannot be easily, or in some cases feasibly, replaced [29]. Thus, appropriate care for cannulas and insertion sites is paramount to prevent iatrogenic infections.

3. Antibiotics Therapy Principles

Antibiotic mechanisms of action can be classically divided into bacteriostatic, which inhibit bacterial replication while relying on the host's immune system to clear the infection, and bactericidal, which lyse bacteria. These effects are highly dependent on free drug plasma concentrations and hence not only antibiotic selection. Dosing is also paramount to effective therapy. As bacteriostatic antibiotics rely on host mechanisms, immunosuppression or existence of a nidus or niche allowing unimpeded bacterial replication results in resumption of bacterial growth once the bacteriostatic compound reaches subtherapeutic levels. Thus, the application of said antibiotics in critical care is somewhat limited. However, many bactericidal antibiotics exercise bacteriostatic effects below their bactericidal concentration. Considering that ECMO and routine dosing of antibiotics depresses the concentration of antibiotics to bacteriostatic levels, thus maintaining the adequate function of the immune system, may be the next step in assessing the effectiveness of the antibiotic.

3.1. Pharmacokinetics and Pharmacodynamics of Antibiotics

Antibiotic efficacy depends on several factors [46]. Most importantly, the concentration and the duration of exposure to antibiotics are critical. Pharmacodynamic properties of antibiotics will determine whether the majority of their bactericidal effects are concentration dependent, e.g., fluoroquinolones; time-dependent, e.g., beta-lactams; or a combination thereof, as the area under the curve dependent, such as glycopeptides [46,47].

The concentration of antibiotics is determined by the dose and the medium volume where the antibiotics are being diluted. Thus, the volume of distribution (Vd) is critical for determining antibiotic concentration [48]. The amount of the free drug is also determined by binding to circulating proteins or other molecules. The drug is then metabolized via several pathways involving liver, kidney, and other peripheral tissues [46]. Clearance (CL) is the fluid volume cleared from drug over a unit of time [46]. Most drugs undergo first-order kinetics, wherein a constant fraction of the drug is metabolized if the mechanism is not saturated. This is one of the critical determinants of the steady-state concentration of the drug [48,49].

Antibiotic concentrations can exert several actions depending on specific drug properties. The minimal bacteriostatic concentration (MBsC) relates to the minimum concentration that will inhibit bacterial replication in vitro and is utilized as a surrogate determinant of a specific antibiotic's potency. Furthermore, bacteriostatic concentrations need to be sustained over time, as replication is impeded only under therapeutic concentrations. Consequently, antibiotic dosing must be frequent enough to prevent levels from dropping below MBC to maintain effectiveness. Conversely, increasing antibiotic concentrations diminishes returns despite bacteriostatic antibiotics exhibiting bactericidal activity at higher concentrations. However, the concentrations necessary for this effect to occur for these types of antibiotics are not feasible in this clinical setting. However, what is critical is the immune system's performance to eradicate the bacteria. Bacteriostatic antibiotics retard bacteria growth, but eliminating the pathogens relies on immune system function.

The bactericidal effect refers to the direct killing of the pathogen. However, this effect depends on several factors. Minimal bactericidal concentration (MBC) is the level at which bacterial lysis begins to occur and is the determinant of a specific drug's potency against the pathogen. As drug levels vary, a fall in concentration results in a predominant inhibitory, or bacteriostatic, action of the antibiotics, finally reaching a minimal inhibitory concentration (MIC) [46] (Figure 2). At this point, the bactericidal drug becomes bacteriostatic, and host defenses are necessary for the clearance of the microorganisms.

Below MIC, drug actions do not necessarily cease. Several other antibacterial effects emerge, and the minimal concentration at which this effect occurs is called minimal antibacterial concentration (MAC). The post-antibiotic effect (PAE) refers to suppression of bacterial growth after a short pulse dose and has been previously described with several antibiotics and different bacterial strains [50–52] (Figure 2). Although MAC may guide antibiotic dosing, post-antibiotics effects are relatively short lived. In linezolid and ampicillin, the inhibition lasted between 1–3 h, depending on the type of bacteria treated [53,54]. For quinolones, the said effect may persist for up to 6 h [54]. Mechanisms are myriad and include inflicting sublethal damage, the persistence of antibiotics in periplasmic space, or efflux inhibition [55–57]. Post antibiotic leukocyte enhancement refers to increased bacterial susceptibility to immune system phagocytic activity [58]. Both bacteriostatic and bactericidal antibiotics can exercise this effect, but not all antibiotics can induce these effects [59–63]. The effect can be quite long for some aminoglycosides (tobramycin), allowing for one dose every 24 h [62]. Finally, MAC can trigger a reduction in pathogen virulence by modulating the immune response, altering chemotaxis adhesion, and decreasing pathogenic factor release [64–67]. These effects are sometimes grouped as post-antibiotics leukocyte enhancement (PALE) (Figure 2). The clinical effects of this phenomenon are unclear, as suppression of the immune system may occur concomitantly [68].

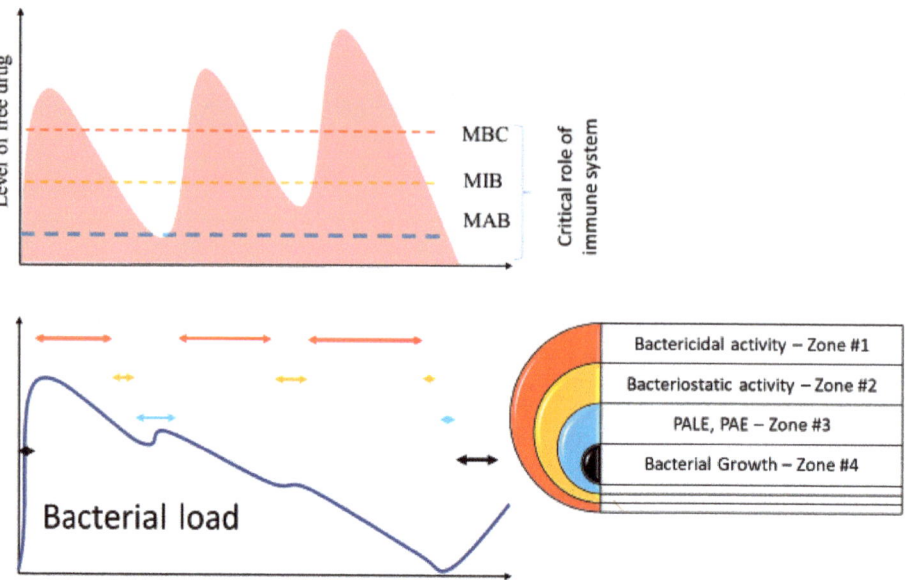

Figure 2. The level of the antibiotics are gradually increasing over the time to cross the MAB, MIB and MBC threshold, but only above MBC thresholds can the antibiotics eradicate infection instead of augmenting the immune system function.

3.2. Limitations of Current Approaches to Monitoring Antibiotic Dosing

However, one must realize that antibiotic potency is measured in vitro under artificial conditions. The killing or bacteriostatic activity assessment is performed at pH of 7.2, in a protein-free, aerobic medium. Antibiotic activity is measured against 10^5 of CFU during overnight exposure. These conditions diverge from physiological conditions in vivo. Notably, a plasma pH of 7.2 would signify severe acidosis and be considered an emergency. Catabolic processes during inflammation affect the circulating protein concentrations, while constant alterations in pH affect the electrostatic charge. Proteins abound in plasma, interacting with antibiotics in several ways, are highly variable in level and type, resulting from the ICU illness. Said factors are critical in dictating the amount of free antibiotic molecules that are critical for the antibacterial action as well as its potency.

The testing condition diverges substantially from the clinical reality of antibiotic dosing. A single dose of antibiotics is exceedingly rare in critical care situations. The bacterial load may be several-fold higher, and penicillin bactericidal properties are particularly sensitive to bacterial load. Most importantly, the in vitro test measures bacteria in the exponential growth phase, which is not necessarily the host's phase. Measurement of antibiotic success is a change in physical properties of the growth medium, which may not be the best measurements of drug action or concentration translatable to the bedside.

Conversely, measurements of antibiotics in serum in relation to antimicrobial activity may also be subjected to several biases. Poor penetration into bacterial nidus or sanctuary sites may necessitate increased dosages to achieve therapeutic concentrations within the target area. The ECMO circuit itself may offer a sanctuary for a pathogen to grow [69]. Furthermore, cellular antibiotic concentrations achieved are several-fold higher in some cases than those in plasma [70,71]. Certain biological compounds may inactivate other antibiotics. Measurements of sensitivity of bacteria rely on growth inhibition, but the concentration of antibiotics may change greatly depending on the fluid or compartment [70,72].

4. Critical Care Illness-Induced Changes in Antibiotics Levels

Several factors specific to ECMO further complicate the understanding of pharmacokinetics and pharmacodynamics of antibiotics in this setting. Some are related to critical care illness, while others are specific to the ECMO circuit itself.

Fluid resuscitation affects the volume of distribution, especially in the case of septic shock, where a large amount of fluid needs to be given to defend perfusion pressure despite venodilation and increase in vascular capacitance [73,74]. Endothelial activation secondary to an extracorporeal support circuit may promote capillary leakage increasing Vd [75]. Adding circuit volume and frequently pre-loading the patient to preserve the preload leads to a further increase in the volume of distribution (Vd) [36]. Liver and kidney failure can influence drug metabolism and excretion, and their function is highly dependent on ECMO performance, especially in VA ECMO [76]. Liver clearance is affected by blood stasis, which is highly dependent on the performance of the right ventricle [77]. Said performance may be affected by the emergence of cor pulmonale due to hypoxia, one of the primary reasons of ECMO implementation [6–8]. Fluid resuscitation can further exacerbate venous liver congestion [77,78]. The significant increase in fluid balance results in excessive mortality in ECMO [74]. Several factors mentioned above likely play a role. Secondarily sick patients may suffer from hypoalbuminemia, unpredictably affecting the level of free antibiotics [79]. Furthermore, the composition of the protein and the charge may be significantly different as seen in the nominal condition.

5. Antibiotics in ECMO

The interaction of the antibiotics during ECMO is complex and most likely results in a suboptimal level of the antibiotics (Figure 3). In addition, concomitant immunosuppressive conditions further hamper the ability of the patients to recover fully.

5.1. Pharmacokinetics

Notably, since ECMO is an emergent treatment, large, randomized trials or even case series testing for pharmacodynamic or pharmacokinetic alterations concerning antibiotic microbial effectiveness in this population are lacking. Most of the data reported arise from observational trials.

Patients on ECMO may exhibit various and wide-ranging alterations in pharmacokinetics, some attributable to said treatment and others related to the critical illness itself [75,80]. Altered parameters noted ex vivo have included decreased half-lives and clearance and increased Vd. Some of these effects may be attributable to circuit sequestration [75,81]. For example, it has been well described that patients on ECMO may require higher doses of sedatives and analgesics, a phenomenon that carries over to several antibiotics. In addition, numerous studies in animals, neonates, and adults have shown significant variability and unpredictability in antibiotic pharmacodynamics during ECMO therapy [80–83].

Antibiotic strategies not accounting for these changes carry an increased chance of treatment failure, both instances of underdosing and supratherapeutic levels causing side effects, which have been reported [43]. In addition, suboptimal antibiotic dosing becomes dire in these patients due to the progression of the primary process, while selective pressure for the development of antibiotic resistance renders antibiotics less useful on the population level [82].

5.2. ECMO Specific Patient-Related Factors Affecting Antibiotics Distribution

The critical illness itself may incur fluid status dysregulation, thus an increase in the volume of distribution [80]. It has been noted previously that large variations in pharmacokinetics in critically ill patients occur between and even within the same patient [75]. Renal or hepatic impairment may decrease drug clearance and decrease pulmonary blood flow [44,82]. Setups producing no pulsatile flow may stimulate the renin–angiotensin–aldosterone axis, increasing fluid retention [44]. Additionally, lack of pulsatile flow decreases the glomerular filtration rate [81]. These patients' conditions are dynamic and fluctuate rapidly.

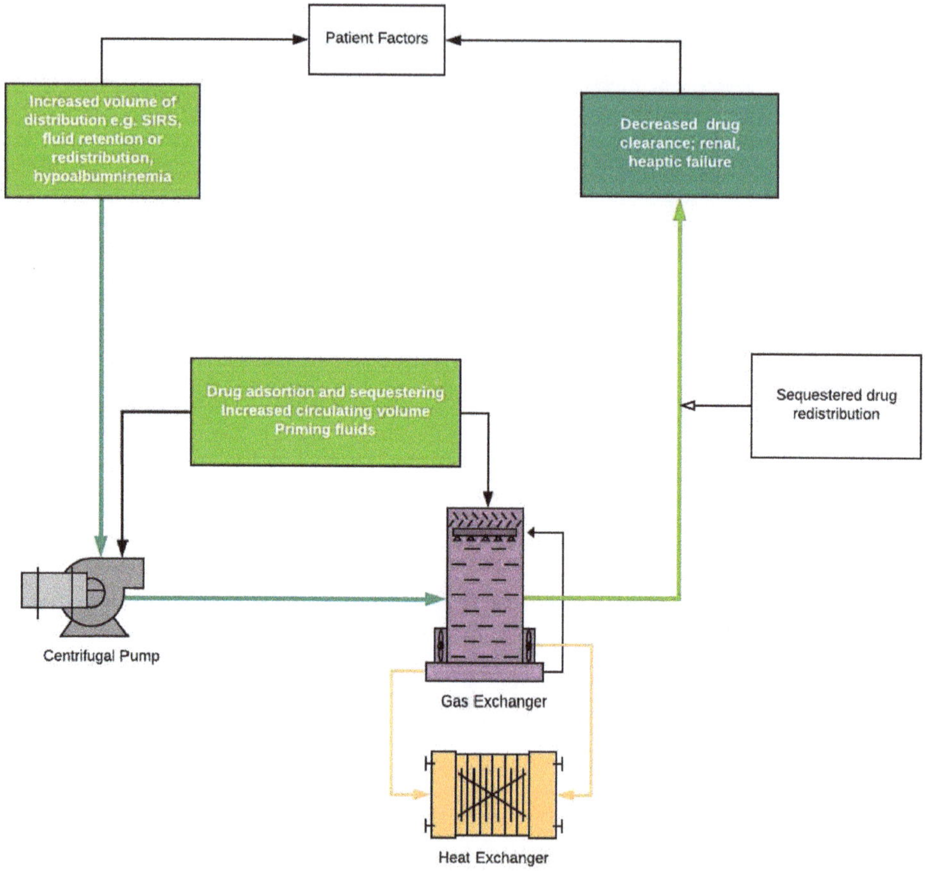

Figure 3. ECMO-specific factor affecting drug distribution.

5.3. Performance of the Immune System

Activation of the immune system may be altered in a way that is difficult to characterize at the current state of knowledge. This may significantly affect antibiotics' MIC and MAB levels. In addition, some of the medications administered during ECMO may have additional antibacterial effects. For example, non-inflammatory nonsteroidal drugs alter the activity of Gram(+) bacteria and may enhance the antibiotic's effect and modulate immune system activity [84–86]. In addition, proton pump inhibitors have additional antimicrobial activities, which are difficult to assess in terms of clinical efficiency [87].

5.4. ECMO Specific Hardware-Related Factors Affecting Antibiotics Distribution
5.4.1. Circuit-Related Factors

Various circuit parameters may alter pharmacokinetics (Figure 3). These phenomena depend on drug properties, circuit type, roller, and biofilm formation [3,4]. The ECMO circuit comprises a large surface area that may sequester drugs, with circuit coatings and components themselves allowing for the adsorption of antimicrobials, thus reducing bioavailability [18]. This effect may be more pronounced in lipophilic drugs, although this effect may wane as binding sites saturate. This may also result in the circuit acting as a reservoir with subsequent redistribution into plasma [82,88]. Lipophilic drugs tend to be most readily sequestered in the circuit [80,82]. Meropenem is heavily sequestered (80%), most likely affecting its anti-bacterial potency [89–91]. Similar sequestration is seen for cefazolin, ampicillin, gentamycin, voriconazole, and vancomycin, but most of the studies were performed in vitro [89,91–94]. However, in the case of cefazolin, the in vivo study failed to demonstrate a lower level of drug [95]. Oxygenator seems to be particularly absorbent for some antibiotics, which is related to high surface area of the device and properties of membranes [96–98]. Silicone-constructed membranes have exhibited more drug residues than those composed of hollow fibers [44]. Other ECMO-dependent factors include priming fluid selection, which may incur less pronounced effects in adults than in neonates [44,75]. However, the effect of biofilm formation on the ability of the membrane to sequester antibiotics cannot be ascertained. These factors may be further complicated by concomitant cytokine absorption techniques or co-existing renal replacement therapies [22,34,99–101].

5.4.2. Drug-Related Factors

Various properties of specific antibiotics directly influence ECMO effects on their pharmacodynamics. These include whether the antibiotic itself is lipophilic or hydrophilic, the tendency for protein binding, and the site of metabolic breakdown (Table 1) [82,102,103]. Furthermore, target MIC may vary by an agent or pathogen sensitivity.

Table 1. Selected antibiotics are divided into hydrophilic and lipophilic.

Hydrophilic	Lipophilic
Aminoglycosides	Fluoroquinolones *
β-lactams	Clindamycin
Glycopeptides	Tigecycline
Linezolid	Caspofungin
Colistin	Voriconazole

* Note that despite fluoroquinolones being described as lipophilic, the circuit loss rate for ciprofloxacin has been described as negligible. Thus, lipophilicity is not the only predictive factor for circuit sequestration [47,82].

6. Selected Antibiotics

Vancomycin is a hydrophilic glycopeptide antibiotic with bactericidal properties and low protein binding [43,47]. As clearance of this antibiotic is closely related to that of creatinine, it is usually dosed [47]. A wide variability for vancomycin Vd in ECMO patients has been noted previously [81]. An in vitro study suggested sequestration of vancomycin [94]. Analysis of retrospective data suggested no significant difference in drug concentration, Vd or clearance in ECMO vs. non-ECMO patients [104]. Vancomycin pharmacodynamics are largely unaffected by ECMO in several studies [103,105,106]. These results are not universal, as Park et al. demonstrated decreased levels in ECMO patients despite similar elimination rates, as seen in prior studies [106,107]. Wu et al. showed the opposite result in the affected clearance rate but showed unchanged pharmacokinetics parameters [108]. Differences in age or hardware use may account for these extremely heterogeneous conclusions. Current recommendations are: loading dose of 25–30 mg/kg followed by 15–20 mg/kg q8–12h dosage, as guided by therapeutic monitoring [43]. Another proposed regimen specifically for methicillin-resistant staphylococcus aureus recommended 400 mg q8h for MIC ≤ 0.5 μg/mL, or 600 mg q8h if the MIC was ≤ 1 μg/mL [103].

Amikacin is a hydrophilic aminoglycoside with bactericidal and post-antibiotic inhibition effects [47], with a low degree of protein binding [43]. While it has been posited the effects of ECMO on amikacin pharmacodynamics may be minimal, critically ill patients exhibit an increased volume of distribution. Studies involving gentamicin, another aminoglycoside, have noted a slight increase to a 1.5-fold increase in Vd for this population [81]. This said phenomenon exhibits a linear relationship in disease severity. One prospective observational study compared nine ECMO patients vs. 30 undergoing RRT vs. 50 with preserved renal function, wherein pre- and post-dosing amikacin concentrations were measured within 96 h. An increased volume of distribution and decreased clearance was observed in the ECMO group [109]. A similar study included 46 ECMO patients and controls and measured peak levels at 30 min after dosing and at 24 h, finding no significant differences in either measurement between said groups. An amikacin loading dose of 45–30 mg/kg is recommended [29,43], and given the narrow therapeutic window for aminoglycosides, routine therapeutic monitoring and further dosing are recommended as guided by achieved levels [43]. Given its narrow therapeutic window, the latter is paramount [47].

Meropenem is a carbapenem antibiotic, with effects similar to that of beta-lactams, exhibiting both bactericidal and post-antibiotic inhibitory effects [47,60]. Protein binding is low [47]. Several studies have demonstrated significant sequestration of the drug by circuit in vitro [110]. While increases in both volumes of distribution and clearance are likely, several trials failed to show a significant difference in pharmacodynamics in ECMO patients [47,75,80]. One study comparing 26 ECMO patients with 51 matched controls, wherein peak meropenem concentrations were drawn at 2 h after infusion and immediately prior to a subsequent dose, found no differences in distribution volume, half-life, or clearance [73]. Another study comparing 11 ECMO patients to historical controls sampled meropenem at 15, 30, 45, 60, 120, 360 and 480 min, finding a slight decrease in clearance and increase in volume of distribution [110]. Recommended dosing in this population involves a 1 g load followed by 1 g q8h [43], or 2 g q8h [110]. Higher doses of meropenem may be employed, and a regimen totaling 6g/d showed to be slightly superior in achieving MIC to standard dosing. Continuous infusion of 3–6/g has been recommended in patients with increased clearance or resistant organisms [110]. Notably, 6.1% of patients did not achieve target MIC compared to 0% of those receiving a higher-dose regimen [80]. High dosage may be considered in patients necessitating higher MICs [111]. Notably, in one study involving patients undergoing renal replacement therapy, MIC levels < 1 were associated with increased mortality [112].

Imipenem, also within the carbapenem classification, has also been studied. One study including 247 ECMO patients found lower plasma levels and higher dosing recommendable [111]. Others trialed 0.5 g every 6 h in 10 ECMO vs. 18 non-ECMO patients, sampling after the fourth dose and finding an increased distribution volume yet decreased clearance, which also recommended increased dosing [112]. Overall, increased dosing may be required, up to 4 g/day in reported cases [43,103], with prolonged infusion of 1 g over 4 h q6h as a recommendable strategy [112].

Cefazolin was reported as being sequestered in the ECMO circuit, although the physical properties of the circuit were critical [3,109]. Up to 84% of the cefazolin in vitro studies could be sequestered [3]. In the case series of ECMO patients, cefazolin clearance was significantly higher. The level of unbound cefazolin was higher and was most likely compensated by high Pk variability and changes in the volume of distribution [93]. In another case report, cefazolin pharmacokinetics was not changed [95]. These two studies may be reconciled, as Booke et al. demonstrated high interindividual variability in cefazolin kinetics [93]. In summary, adjusting cefazolin does not need to be performed in ECMO patients.

Ceftazidime demonstrated to be unaffected in serum dynamics in 30 ECMO patients compared to 75 non-ECMO ICU patients (from a mean age of ECMO 47.7 vs. 61.2 for non-ECMO in a prospective study). Consequently, adult dosing recommendations are to use a loading dose of 2 g intravenously and to adjust the dosing based on GFR (more than 30 = 6 g/24 h; less than 30 = 4 g/24 h) [80].

For teicoplanin, 89% of the drug can be sequestered, according to an in vitro study of the primed circuit [110]. Two in vivo studies agreed that the drug's loading has to be increased to 12 mg/kg to achieve therapeutic concentrations [113,114].

Ciprofloxacin belongs to the fluoroquinolone family. These drugs are lipophilic bactericidal, exhibiting a volume of distribution mostly unaffected by critical illness [47] and low protein binding [43]. The half-life of fluoroquinolones may be decreased in critical illness, necessitating more frequent dosage [47]. Although lipophilic, ciprofloxacin has exhibited minimal circuit sequestration in studies [82]. A recommended loading dose of ciprofloxacin is 800 mg followed by 400–600 mg q8h [43].

Piperacillin should be used with caution in ECMO patients, wherein they tend not to achieve the desired therapeutic targets in these patients. One single-center study showcased this phenomenon, wherein piperacillin–tazobactam-treated patients were less likely to achieve a prespecified ×4 MIC (48% vs. 13% in non-ECMO patients) [75]. A loading dose of 4.5 g is recommended, followed by 4.5 g q6h or doses as per clearance [43].

Linezolid patients receiving linezolid may also show a tendency to not achieve desired plasma levels (35% vs. 15%) [80]. Nevertheless, if selected, a linezolid loading dose of 600 mg followed by 1800 mg/d continuous infusion is recommended [111].

Caspofungin falls under the echinocandin classification as a lipophilic antifungal. However, reports regarding circuit sequestration are conflicting. For example, circuit loss secondary to sequestration may be as high as 43%, while others have deemed this drug as unaffected by ECMO [44,82]. One prospective observational study in post-transplant patients compared 12 ECMO patients to seven matched controls. Sampling was performed after the second and third caspofungin dose, finding no significant pharmacokinetics [114]. Hence, the usual dosing of 70 mg loading with subsequent 50 mg/d dosing may be sufficient [111]. Prior studies have noted a Vd for caspofungin within normal parameters in these patients [81].

Micafungin, another echinocandin, exhibited similar results, with sequestration gauged around 45–99% [110]. However, in one observational study on 12 ECMO patients, micafungin sampling at 1, 3, 5, 8, 18 and 24 h after infusion yielded no differences in clearance or distribution volume [115]. No consensus on dosing recommendations for micafungin were available at the time of writing [111].

Voriconazole is a triazole antifungal commonly employed in *Aspergillus* sp. infection. While it was previously assumed that high circuit losses could be expected due to the drug being highly lipophilic, one large retrospective study found no significant pharmacokinetic changes during ECMO. The in vitro study showed significant absorption by circuit [94,110]. Some demonstrated sequestration with up to 71% circuit losses, with later saturation and redistribution reported [82]. The median dose was 9.2 mg/kg; however, higher dosing might be necessary, given that a total of 56% of patients in this study did not reach target levels compared to 39% of the control group [102].

In addition, a member of the triazole family, fluconazole, has exhibited minimal sequestration. However, data sufficient for dosing recommendations remain lacking [111].

7. Interaction of Antibiotics with Other Treatments

Standard precautions regarding drug interactions apply, as patients on ECMO are bound to receive diverse agents during their course. More importantly, nearly 50% of all ECMO patients may necessitate renal replacement therapy (RRT) during their illness, further confounding antibiotic dosing [80,83]. The renal replacement circuit may be spliced into that of the ECMO, foregoing the need for further cannulation, although various access strategies have been employed [83]. Similar to ECMO, RRT mediates pharmacodynamic changes that must be accounted for when dosing strategies are selected. These alterations may be secondary to both drug properties or may be inherent to the RRT circuit itself.

Further compounding this issue in patients receiving concurrent ECMO and RRT, commonly utilized formulae employed for dosing calculations such as EGFR and Cockcroft-Gault may lose accuracy in this setting [19]. In addition, subtherapeutic levels may be observed in up to 25% of patients undergoing RRT alone [112]. This further highlights the exquisite need for therapeutic drug monitoring as necessary for management.

Various drug properties, including molecular size, protein binding, distribution volume, and metabolism, affect dialysis-mediated removal. In general, highly protein-bound drugs possess large molecular weight or volume of distribution, and/or non-renally cleared medications are least likely to be impacted by RRT [19]. Both the schedule or duration of RRT and effects exerted by the RRT circuit itself, including the use of high flow filters, may affect RRT-mediated clearance [19]. A rising estimated total renal clearance (eTRCL) correlated with lower trough concentrations for all antibiotics in one recent study [112].

While there is a paucity of data regarding pharmacodynamics in patients receiving concurrent ECMO and RRT, it is safe to suggest that the importance of therapeutic monitoring is further enhanced in these patients. A sieving coefficient can be determined for a drug if both plasma and ultrafiltrate concentrations are known (ultrafiltrate/plasma) [83]. This could be a potential avenue for further determining the interplay between ECMO, RRT, and antibiotic levels in the future.

Impala and other devices are not present in the data pertinent to the concomitant application of ECMO and cytokine absorption technique.

8. Effectiveness of Antibiotic Therapy in ECMO Patients

Several reports demonstrated that ECMO did not interfere with successful treatment of bacterial infections. However, given that these are mostly case reports, there is a lack of randomized controlled studies comparing success rates between patients treated with a similar regimen of antibiotics on ECMO vs. patients treated with mechanical ventilation. The CEASAR study was the only one designed in a way that demonstrated the superiority of transferring the patient to the specialized center vs. regional care [4]. There was no significant difference between the mechanical ventilation arm and ECMO once patients were transported to the reference center. Another study demonstrated a lack of mortality as well [115]. Although this study was followed by metanalysis incorporating large case reports, CEASAR may suggest that antibiotic therapy may be equally effective while the patient is on ECMO [1]. This is somewhat puzzling considering the large body of evidence suggesting sequestration of the antibiotic's changes in Vd and Pk among many antibiotics. However, in at least one study, free antibiotics were significantly higher, offsetting the lower overall levels [93]. Another hypothesis is that bactericidal antibiotics are high enough to provide a bacteriostatic level while the immune system can clear the pathogen.

The definite answer may be difficult to study as comparing study design in the CEASAR format may be unfeasible due to the ethical constraint. However, it is also interesting that since the study's conclusion, no similar study design was followed, while ECMO proponents relied on case reports.

9. Conclusions

Antibiotic therapy success may be difficult to achieve in the ECMO patient. The emergence of critical care illness creates a difficult condition at the baseline. The variability introduced by the circuit further complicates clinical decision making. Although we suggest utilizing good stewardship in antibiotic dosing combined with drug level monitoring, one must realize that these methods are likely to be insufficient to predict the appropriate regimen in the ECMO situation (Figure 4). Utilizing the software targeting the drug therapy may not be helpful, as several variables seem to compensate for each other, in cases of cefazolin at least [93]. The monitoring of the clinical response may be optimal yet difficult, considering that ECMO may blunt some responses (fever) while unpredictably affecting others (procalcitonin levels).

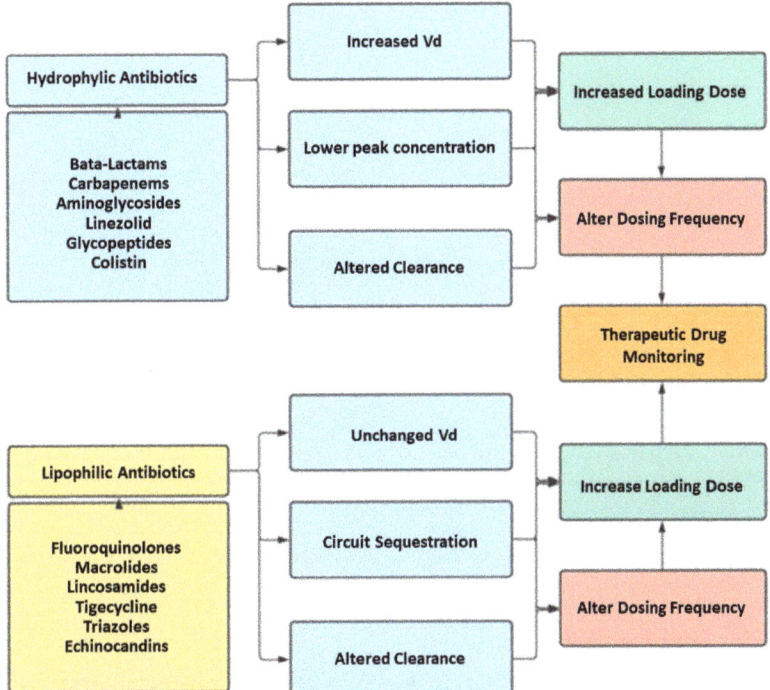

Figure 4. General recommendations regarding antibiotics as classified by hydrophilicity or lipophilicity [47,81,82,102].

Author Contributions: Conceptualization, K.L.; formal analysis, K.L. and F.G.; resources, K.L.; data curation, K.L. and F.G.; writing—original draft preparation, K.L., F.G. and J.V.; writing—review and editing, J.V.; visualization, K.L.; supervision. All authors have read and agreed to the published version of the manuscript.

Funding: This research received no external funding.

Data Availability Statement: Not applicable.

Acknowledgments: The authors would like to thank Justin Wain for his able assistance.

Conflicts of Interest: The authors declare no conflict of interest.

References

1. Combes, A.; Peek, G.J.; Hajage, D.; Hardy, P.; Abrams, D.; Schmidt, M.; Dechartres, A.; Elbourne, D. ECMO for severe ARDS: Systematic review and individual patient data meta-analysis. *Intensive Care Med.* **2020**, *46*, 2048–2057. [CrossRef] [PubMed]
2. Dagan, O.; Klein, J.; Gruenwald, C.; Bohn, D.; Barker, G.; Koren, G. Preliminary studies of the effects of extracorporeal membrane oxygenator on the disposition of common pediatric drugs. *Ther. Drug Monit.* **1993**, *15*, 263–266. [CrossRef]
3. Wildschut, E.D.; Ahsman, M.J.; Allegaert, K.; Mathot, R.A.; Tibboel, D. Determinants of drug absorption in different ECMO circuits. *Intensive Care Med.* **2010**, *36*, 2109–2116. [CrossRef] [PubMed]
4. Zapol, W.M.; Snider, M.T.; Hill, J.D.; Fallat, R.J.; Bartlett, R.H.; Edmunds, L.H.; Morris, A.H.; Peirce, E.C.; Thomas, A.N.; Proctor, H.J. Extracorporeal membrane oxygenation in severe acute respiratory failure: A randomized prospective study. *JAMA* **1979**, *242*, 2193–2196. [CrossRef] [PubMed]
5. Tramm, R.; Ilic, D.; Davies, A.R.; Pellegrino, V.A.; Romero, L.; Hodgson, C. Extracorporeal membrane oxygenation for critically ill adults. *Cochrane Database Syst. Rev.* **2015**, *1*, Cd010381. [CrossRef] [PubMed]
6. Boeken, U.; Assmann, A.; Beckmann, A.; Schmid, C.; Werdan, K.; Michels, G.; Miera, O.; Schmidt, F.; Klotz, S.; Starck, C.; et al. Extracorporeal Circulation (ECLS/ECMO) for Cardio-circulatory Failure—Summary of the S3 Guideline. *Thorac. Cardiovasc. Surg.* **2021**, *69*, 483–489. [CrossRef] [PubMed]

7. Bercker, S.; Petroff, D.; Polze, N.; Karagianidis, C.; Bein, T.; Laudi, S.; Stehr, S.N.; Voelker, M.T. ECMO use in Germany: An analysis of 29,929 ECMO runs. *PLoS ONE* **2021**, *16*, e0260324. [CrossRef]
8. Raffa, G.; Kowalewski, M.; Meani, P.; Pilato, M.; Lorusso, R. Oc39 meta-analysis of peripheral or central ECMO in postcardiotomy and non-postcardiotomy shock. *J. Cardiovasc. Med.* **2018**, *19*, e27. [CrossRef]
9. Kim, J.H.; Pieri, M.; Landoni, G.; Scandroglio, A.M.; Calabrò, M.G.; Fominskiy, E.; Lembo, R.; Heo, M.H.; Zangrillo, A. Venovenous ECMO treatment, outcomes, and complications in adults according to large case series: A systematic review. *Int. J. Artif. Organs* **2020**, *44*, 481–488. [CrossRef]
10. Butt, W.; MacLaren, G. Extracorporeal membrane oxygenation and sepsis. *Crit. Care Resusc.* **2007**, *9*, 76–80.
11. Abrams, D.; MacLaren, G.; Lorusso, R.; Price, S.; Yannopoulos, D.; Vercaemst, L.; Bělohlávek, J.; Taccone, F.S.; Aissaoui, N.; Shekar, K.; et al. Extracorporeal cardiopulmonary resuscitation in adults: Evidence and implications. *Intensive Care Med.* **2022**, *48*, 1–15. [CrossRef] [PubMed]
12. Gardiner, D.; Charlesworth, M.; Rubino, A.; Madden, S. The rise of organ donation after circulatory death: A narrative review. *Anaesthesia* **2020**, *75*, 1215–1222. [CrossRef] [PubMed]
13. Gopalakrishnan, R.; Vashisht, R. Sepsis and ECMO. *Indian J. Thorac. Cardiovasc. Surg.* **2021**, *37* (Suppl. 2), 267. [CrossRef]
14. Chaves, R.C.F.; Rabello Filho, R.; Timenetsky, K.T.; Moreira, F.T.; Vilanova, L.; Bravim, B.A.; Serpa Neto, A.; Correa, T.D. Extracorporeal membrane oxygenation: A literature review. *Rev. Bras Ter. Intensiva.* **2019**, *31*, 410–424. [CrossRef] [PubMed]
15. Hall, M.W.; Greathouse, K.C.; Thakkar, R.K.; Sribnick, E.A.; Muszynski, J.A. Immunoparalysis in pediatric critical care. *Pediatric Clin.* **2017**, *64*, 1089–1102. [CrossRef] [PubMed]
16. Grigoryev, E.; Matveeva, V.; Ivkin, A.; Khanova, M. Induced Immunosuppression in Critical Care. In *Immunosuppression*; IntechOpen: London, UK, 2020.
17. Al-Omari, A.; Aljamaan, F.; Alhazzani, W.; Salih, S.; Arabi, Y. Cytomegalovirus infection in immunocompetent critically ill adults: Literature review. *Ann. Intensive Care* **2016**, *6*, 110. [CrossRef] [PubMed]
18. Cota, J.M.; FakhriRavari, A.; Rowan, M.P.; Chung, K.K.; Murray, C.K.; Akers, K.S. Intravenous Antibiotic and Antifungal Agent Pharmacokinetic-Pharmacodynamic Dosing in Adults with Severe Burn Injury. *Clin. Ther.* **2016**, *38*, 2016–2031. [CrossRef]
19. Hoff, B.M.; Maker, J.H.; Dager, W.E.; Heintz, B.H. Antibiotic Dosing for Critically Ill Adult Patients Receiving Intermittent Hemodialysis, Prolonged Intermittent Renal Replacement Therapy, and Continuous Renal Replacement Therapy: An Update. *Ann. Pharm.* **2020**, *54*, 43–55. [CrossRef]
20. Meng, L.; Mui, E.; Holubar, M.K.; Deresinski, S.C. Comprehensive Guidance for Antibiotic Dosing in Obese Adults. *Pharmacotherapy* **2017**, *37*, 1415–1431. [CrossRef]
21. Pea, F. Pharmacokinetics and drug metabolism of antibiotics in the elderly. *Expert Opin. Drug Metab. Toxicol.* **2018**, *14*, 1087–1100. [CrossRef]
22. Akil, A.; Ziegeler, S.; Reichelt, J.; Rehers, S.; Abdalla, O.; Semik, M.; Fischer, S. Combined Use of CytoSorb and ECMO in Patients with Severe Pneumogenic Sepsis. *Thorac. Cardiovasc. Surg.* **2021**, *69*, 246–251. [CrossRef] [PubMed]
23. Kavita, M.; Ramanathan, K.R. Extracorporeal Lung Assist Devices. In *Thoracic Surgery: Cervical, Thoracic and Abdominal Approaches*; Nistor, C.E., Tsui, S., Kırali, K., Ciuche, A., Aresu, G., Kocher, G.J., Eds.; Springer International Publishing: Cham, Switzerland, 2020; pp. 995–1010.
24. Barge-Caballero, G.; Castel-Lavilla, M.A.; Almenar-Bonet, L.; Garrido-Bravo, I.P.; Delgado, J.F.; Rangel-Sousa, D.; González-Costello, J.; Segovia-Cubero, J.; Farrero-Torres, M.; Lambert-Rodríguez, J.L. Venoarterial extracorporeal membrane oxygenation with or without simultaneous intra-aortic balloon pump support as a direct bridge to heart transplantation: Results from a nationwide Spanish registry. *Interact. Cardiovasc. Thorac. Surg.* **2019**, *29*, 670–677. [CrossRef] [PubMed]
25. Fiorelli, F.; Panoulas, V. Impella as unloading strategy during VA-ECMO: Systematic review and meta-analysis. *Rev. Cardiovasc. Med.* **2021**, *22*, 1503–1511. [CrossRef] [PubMed]
26. Delnoij, T.S.; Driessen, R.; Sharma, A.S.; Bouman, E.A.; Strauch, U.; Roekaerts, P.M. Venovenous Extracorporeal Membrane Oxygenation in Intractable Pulmonary Insufficiency: Practical Issues and Future Directions. *Biomed Res. Int.* **2016**, *2016*, 9367464. [CrossRef]
27. Lindholm, J.A. Cannulation for veno-venous extracorporeal membrane oxygenation. *J. Thorac. Dis.* **2018**, *10* (Suppl. 5), S606. [CrossRef]
28. Pooboni, S.K.; Gulla, K.M. Vascular access in ECMO. *Indian J. Thorac. Cardiovasc. Surg.* **2021**, *37*, 221–231. [CrossRef]
29. Extracorporeal Life Support Organization. *ELSO Guidelines for Cardiopulmonary Extracorporeal Life Support*; ELSO: Ann Arbor, MI, USA, 2017.
30. Mangoush, O.; Purkayastha, S.; Haj-Yahia, S.; Kinross, J.; Hayward, M.; Bartolozzi, F.; Darzi, A.; Athanasiou, T. Heparin-bonded circuits versus nonheparin-bonded circuits: An evaluation of their effect on clinical outcomes. *Eur. J. Cardiothorac. Surg.* **2007**, *31*, 1058–1069. [CrossRef]
31. He, T.; He, J.; Wang, Z.; Cui, Z. Modification strategies to improve the membrane hemocompatibility in extracorporeal membrane oxygenator (ECMO). *Adv. Compos. Hybrid. Mater.* **2021**, *4*, 847–864. [CrossRef]
32. Zhang, M.; Pauls, J.P.; Bartnikowski, N.; Haymet, A.B.; Chan, C.H.H.; Suen, J.Y.; Schneider, B.; Ki, K.K.; Whittaker, A.K.; Dargusch, M.S.; et al. Anti-thrombogenic Surface Coatings for Extracorporeal Membrane Oxygenation: A Narrative Review. *ACS Biomater. Sci. Eng.* **2021**, *7*, 4402–4419. [CrossRef]
33. Van Dyk, M. The use of CRRT in ECMO patients. *Egypt. J. Crit. Care Med.* **2018**, *6*, 95–100. [CrossRef]

34. Selewski, D.T.; Wille, K.M. Seminars in dialysis. In *Continuous Renal Replacement Therapy in Patients Treated with Extracorporeal Membrane Oxygenation*; Wiley Online Library: Hoboken, NJ, USA, 2021.
35. Lüsebrink, E.; Stremmel, C.; Stark, K.; Joskowiak, D.; Czermak, T.; Born, F.; Kupka, D.; Scherer, C.; Orban, M.; Petzold, T. Update on weaning from veno-arterial extracorporeal membrane oxygenation. *J. Clin. Med.* **2020**, *9*, 992. [CrossRef]
36. Connelly, J.; Blinman, T. Seminars in perinatology. In *Special Equipment Considerations for Neonatal ECMO*; Elsevier: Amsterdam, The Netherlands, 2018; pp. 89–95.
37. Palanzo, D.A.; Baer, L.D.; El-Banayosy, A.; Wang, S.; Undar, A.; Pae, W.E. Choosing a pump for extracorporeal membrane oxygenation in the USA. *Artif. Organs* **2014**, *38*, 1–4. [CrossRef] [PubMed]
38. Wang, S.; Moroi, M.K.; Kunselman, A.R.; Myers, J.L.; Ündar, A. Evaluation of centrifugal blood pumps in term of hemodynamic performance using simulated neonatal and pediatric ECMO circuits. *Artif. Organs* **2020**, *44*, 16–27. [CrossRef] [PubMed]
39. Wrisinger, W.C.; Thompson, S.L. Basics of Extracorporeal Membrane Oxygenation. *Surg. Clin.* **2022**, *102*, 23–35. [CrossRef] [PubMed]
40. Affas, Z.R.; Touza, G.G.; Affas, S. A Meta-Analysis Comparing Venoarterial (VA) Extracorporeal Membrane Oxygenation (ECMO) to Impella for Acute Right Ventricle Failure. *Cureus* **2021**, *13*, e19622. [CrossRef] [PubMed]
41. Betit, P. Technical Advances in the Field of ECMO. *Respir. Care* **2018**, *63*, 1162–1173. [CrossRef]
42. Biffi, S.; Di Bella, S.; Scaravilli, V.; Peri, A.M.; Grasselli, G.; Alagna, L.; Pesenti, A.; Gori, A. Infections during extracorporeal membrane oxygenation: Epidemiology, risk factors, pathogenesis and prevention. *Int. J. Antimicrob. Agents* **2017**, *50*, 9–16. [CrossRef]
43. Abdul-Aziz, M.H.; Roberts, J.A. Antibiotic dosing during extracorporeal membrane oxygenation: Does the system matter? *Curr. Opin. Anaesthesiol.* **2020**, *33*, 71–82. [CrossRef]
44. Hahn, J.; Choi, J.H.; Chang, M.J. Pharmacokinetic changes of antibiotic, antiviral, antituberculosis and antifungal agents during extracorporeal membrane oxygenation in critically ill adult patients. *J. Clin. Pharm. Ther.* **2017**, *42*, 661–671. [CrossRef]
45. Bizzarro, M.J.; Conrad, S.A.; Kaufman, D.A.; Rycus, P.; Extracorporeal Life Support Organization Task Force on Infections, E.M.O. Infections acquired during extracorporeal membrane oxygenation in neonates, children, and adults. *Pediatr. Crit. Care Med.* **2011**, *12*, 277–281. [CrossRef]
46. Levy, S.B.; Chávez, A.D.; Rosenberg, A.S. Antimicrobial Therapy. In *Mount Sinai Expert Guides: Critical Care*; Wiley Online Library: Hoboken, NJ, USA, 2020; pp. 429–448.
47. Roberts, J.A.; Lipman, J. Pharmacokinetic issues for antibiotics in the critically ill patient. *Crit. Care Med.* **2009**, *37*, 840–851, quiz 859. [CrossRef] [PubMed]
48. Mansoor, A.; Mahabadi, N. *Volume of Distribution*; StatPearls: Bethesda, MD, USA, 2021.
49. Smith, D.A.; Beaumont, K.; Maurer, T.S.; Di, L. Clearance in Drug Design: Miniperspective. *J. Med. Chem.* **2018**, *62*, 2245–2255. [CrossRef] [PubMed]
50. Bundtzen, R.W.; Gerber, A.U.; Cohn, D.L.; Craig, W.A. Postantibiotic suppression of bacterial growth. *Rev. Infect. Dis.* **1981**, *3*, 28–37. [CrossRef]
51. Bigger, J. Treatment of staphylococcal infections with penicillin by intermittent sterilisation. *Lancet* **1944**, *244*, 497–500. [CrossRef]
52. Eagle, H. The Recovery of Bacteria from the Toxic Effects of Penicillin. *J. Clin. Invest.* **1949**, *28*, 832–836. [CrossRef] [PubMed]
53. Munckhof, W.J.; Giles, C.; Turnidge, J.D. Post-antibiotic growth suppression of linezolid against Gram-positive bacteria. *J. Antimicrob. Chemother.* **2001**, *47*, 879–883. [CrossRef] [PubMed]
54. Proma, F.H.; Shourav, M.K.; Choi, J. Post-Antibiotic Effect of Ampicillin and Levofloxacin to Escherichia coli and Staphylococcus aureus Based on Microscopic Imaging Analysis. *Antibiotics* **2020**, *9*, 458. [CrossRef]
55. Srimani, J.K.; Huang, S.; Lopatkin, A.J.; You, L. Drug detoxification dynamics explain the postantibiotic effect. *Mol. Syst. Biol.* **2017**, *13*, 948. [CrossRef]
56. Li, R.C.; Lee, S.W.; Kong, C.H. Correlation between bactericidal activity and postantibiotic effect for five antibiotics with different mechanisms of action. *J. Antimicrob. Chemother.* **1997**, *40*, 39–45. [CrossRef]
57. Wen, X.; Langevin, A.M.; Dunlop, M.J. Antibiotic export by efflux pumps affects growth of neighboring bacteria. *Sci. Rep.* **2018**, *8*, 15120. [CrossRef]
58. McDonald, P.J.; Wetherall, B.L.; Pruul, H. Postantibiotic leukocyte enhancement: Increased susceptibility of bacteria pretreated with antibiotics to activity of leukocytes. *Rev. Infect. Dis.* **1981**, *3*, 38–44. [CrossRef] [PubMed]
59. Ramadan, M.A.; Tawfik, A.F.; Shibl, A.M.; Gemmell, C.G. Post-antibiotic effect of azithromycin and erythromycin on streptococcal susceptibility to phagocytosis. *J. Med. Microbiol.* **1995**, *42*, 362–366. [CrossRef]
60. Novelli, A.; Fallani, S.; Cassetta, M.I.; Conti, S.; Mazzei, T. Postantibiotic leukocyte enhancement of meropenem against gram-positive and gram-negative strains. *Antimicrob. Agents Chemother.* **2000**, *44*, 3174–3176. [CrossRef] [PubMed]
61. Horgen, L.; Jerome, A.; Rastogi, N. Pulsed-exposure and postantibiotic leukocyte enhancement effects of amikacin, clarithromycin, clofazimine, and rifampin against intracellular Mycobacterium avium. *Antimicrob. Agents Chemother.* **1998**, *42*, 3006–3008. [CrossRef] [PubMed]
62. Novelli, A.; Mazzei, T.; Fallani, S.; Cassetta, M.I.; Conti, S. In vitro postantibiotic effect and postantibiotic leukocyte enhancement of tobramycin. *J. Chemother.* **1995**, *7*, 355–362. [CrossRef]
63. Pérez Fernández, P.; Herrera, I.; Martínez, P.; Gómez-Lus, M.L.; Prieto, J. Enhancement of the susceptibility of Staphylococcus aureus to phagocytosis after treatment with fosfomycin compared with other antimicrobial agents. *Chemotherapy* **1995**, *41*, 45–49. [CrossRef]

64. Bernardo, K.; Pakulat, N.; Fleer, S.; Schnaith, A.; Utermöhlen, O.; Krut, O.; Müller, S.; Krönke, M. Subinhibitory concentrations of linezolid reduce Staphylococcus aureus virulence factor expression. *Antimicrob. Agents Chemother.* **2004**, *48*, 546–555. [CrossRef]
65. Atshan, S.S.; Hamat, R.A.; Coolen, M.J.L.; Dykes, G.; Sekawi, Z.; Mullins, B.J.; Than, L.T.L.; Abduljaleel, S.A.; Kicic, A. The Role of Subinhibitory Concentrations of Daptomycin and Tigecycline in Modulating Virulence in Staphylococcus aureus. *Antibiotics* **2021**, *10*, 39. [CrossRef]
66. Chen, J.; Zhou, H.; Huang, J.; Zhang, R.; Rao, X. Virulence alterations in staphylococcus aureus upon treatment with the sub-inhibitory concentrations of antibiotics. *J. Adv. Res.* **2021**, *31*, 165–175. [CrossRef]
67. Mahmoudi, H.; Alikhani, M.Y.; Imani Fooladi, A.A. Synergistic antimicrobial activity of melittin with clindamycin on the expression of encoding exfoliative toxin in Staphylococcus aureus. *Toxicon* **2020**, *183*, 11–19. [CrossRef]
68. Evans, S.J.; Roberts, A.E.L.; Morris, A.C.; Simpson, A.J.; Harris, L.G.; Mack, D.; Jenkins, R.E.; Wilkinson, T.S. Contrasting effects of linezolid on healthy and dysfunctional human neutrophils: Reducing C5a-induced injury. *Sci. Rep.* **2020**, *10*, 16377. [CrossRef] [PubMed]
69. Schilcher, G.; Eisner, F.; Hackl, G.; Eller, P.; Valentin, T.; Zollner-Schwetz, I.; Krause, R.; Brcic, L. Candida infection of membrane oxygenator during ECMO therapy. *J. Infect.* **2019**, *78*, 75–86. [CrossRef] [PubMed]
70. Kobuchi, S.; Kabata, T.; Maeda, K.; Ito, Y.; Sakaeda, T. Pharmacokinetics of macrolide antibiotics and transport into the interstitial fluid: Comparison among erythromycin, clarithromycin, and azithromycin. *Antibiotics* **2020**, *9*, 199. [CrossRef]
71. Fernandes, P.; Pereira, D.; Watkins, P.B.; Bertrand, D. Differentiating the Pharmacodynamics and Toxicology of Macrolide and Ketolide Antibiotics. *J. Med. Chem.* **2020**, *63*, 6462–6473. [CrossRef] [PubMed]
72. Li, X. Long Journey on Daptomycin. *Synlett* **2022**, *33*, 27–33. [CrossRef]
73. Charlton, M.; Thompson, J. Pharmacokinetics in sepsis. *BJA Educ.* **2019**, *19*, 7. [CrossRef] [PubMed]
74. Fong, K.M.; Au, S.Y.; Ng, G.W.Y.; Leung, A.K.H. Positive fluid balance and mortality in adult patients treated with extracorporeal membrane oxygenation: A retrospective study. *J. Intensive Care Soc.* **2020**, *21*, 210–220. [CrossRef]
75. Donadello, K.; Antonucci, E.; Cristallini, S.; Roberts, J.A.; Beumier, M.; Scolletta, S.; Jacobs, F.; Rondelet, B.; de Backer, D.; Vincent, J.L.; et al. beta-Lactam pharmacokinetics during extracorporeal membrane oxygenation therapy: A case-control study. *Int. J. Antimicrob. Agents* **2015**, *45*, 278–282. [CrossRef]
76. Elena Puerto, E.; Guido Tavazzi, G.; Alessia Gambaro, A.; Chiara Cirillo, C.; Alessandro Pecoraro, A.; Roberto Martin-Asenjo, R.; Juan Delgado, J.; Hector Bueno, H.; Susanna Price, S. Interaction between veno-arterial extracorporeal membrane oxygenation and the right ventricle. *Eur. Heart J. Acute Cardiovasc. Care* **2021**, *10* (Suppl. 1), zuab020-173. [CrossRef]
77. Coleman, R.D.; Chartan, C.A.; Mourani, P.M. Intensive care management of right ventricular failure and pulmonary hypertension crises. *Pediatric Pulmonol.* **2021**, *56*, 636–648. [CrossRef]
78. Zoratti, C.; Moretti, R.; Rebuzzi, L.; Albergati, I.V.; Di Somma, A.; Decorti, G.; Di Bella, S.; Crocè, L.S.; Giuffrè, M. Antibiotics and Liver Cirrhosis: What the Physicians Need to Know. *Antibiotics* **2022**, *11*, 31. [CrossRef] [PubMed]
79. Ulldemolins, M.; Roberts, J.A.; Lipman, J.; Rello, J. Antibiotic dosing in multiple organ dysfunction syndrome. *Chest* **2011**, *139*, 1210–1220. [CrossRef] [PubMed]
80. Kuhn, D.; Metz, C.; Seiler, F.; Wehrfritz, H.; Roth, S.; Alqudrah, M.; Becker, A.; Bracht, H.; Wagenpfeil, S.; Hoffmann, M.; et al. Antibiotic therapeutic drug monitoring in intensive care patients treated with different modalities of extracorporeal membrane oxygenation (ECMO) and renal replacement therapy: A prospective, observational single-center study. *Crit. Care* **2020**, *24*, 664. [CrossRef]
81. Shekar, K.; Fraser, J.F.; Smith, M.T.; Roberts, J.A. Pharmacokinetic changes in patients receiving extracorporeal membrane oxygenation. *J. Crit. Care* **2012**, *27*, 741.e9–741.e18. [CrossRef] [PubMed]
82. Cheng, V.; Abdul-Aziz, M.H.; Roberts, J.A.; Shekar, K. Optimising drug dosing in patients receiving extracorporeal membrane oxygenation. *J. Thorac. Dis.* **2018**, *10* (Suppl. 5), S629–S641. [CrossRef]
83. Worku, B.; Khin, S.; Gaudino, M.; Gambardella, I.; Iannacone, E.; Ebrahimi, H.; Savy, S.; Voevidko, L.; Oribabor, C.; Hadjiangelis, N.; et al. Renal replacement therapy in patients on extracorporeal membrane oxygenation support: Who and how. *Int. J. Artif. Organs* **2021**, *44*, 531–538. [CrossRef] [PubMed]
84. Ozturk, I.; Erac, Y.; Ballar Kirmizibayrak, P.; Ermertcan, S. Nonsteroidal antiinflammatory drugs alter antibiotic susceptibility and expression of virulence-related genes and protein A of Staphylococcus aureus. *Turk. J. Med. Sci.* **2021**, *51*, 835–847. [CrossRef]
85. Riordan, J.T.; Dupre, J.M.; Cantore-Matyi, S.A.; Kumar-Singh, A.; Song, Y.; Zaman, S.; Horan, S.; Helal, N.S.; Nagarajan, V.; Elasri, M.O.; et al. Alterations in the transcriptome and antibiotic susceptibility of Staphylococcus aureus grown in the presence of diclofenac. *Ann. Clin. Microbiol. Antimicrob.* **2011**, *10*, 30. [CrossRef]
86. Chan, E.W.L.; Yee, Z.Y.; Raja, I.; Yap, J.K.Y. Synergistic effect of non-steroidal anti-inflammatory drugs (NSAIDs) on antibacterial activity of cefuroxime and chloramphenicol against methicillin-resistant Staphylococcus aureus. *J. Glob. Antimicrob. Resist.* **2017**, *10*, 70–74. [CrossRef]
87. da Rosa, T.F.; Foletto, V.S.; Serafin, M.B.; Bottega, A.; Horner, R. Anti-infective properties of proton pump inhibitors: Perspectives. *Int. Microbiol.* **2022**, *25*, 217–222. [CrossRef]
88. Bertholee, D.; ter Horst, P.G.; Hijmering, M.L.; Spanjersberg, A.J.; Hospes, W.; Wilffert, B. Blood concentrations of cefuroxime in cardiopulmonary bypass surgery. *Int. J. Clin. Pharm.* **2013**, *35*, 798–804. [CrossRef] [PubMed]
89. Denooz, R.; Charlier, C. Simultaneous determination of five beta-lactam antibiotics (cefepim, ceftazidim, cefuroxim, meropenem and piperacillin) in human plasma by high-performance liquid chromatography with ultraviolet detection. *J. Chromatogr. B Analyt. Technol. Biomed Life Sci.* **2008**, *864*, 161–167. [CrossRef] [PubMed]

90. Shekar, K.; Fraser, J.F.; Taccone, F.S.; Welch, S.; Wallis, S.C.; Mullany, D.V.; Lipman, J.; Roberts, J.A. The combined effects of extracorporeal membrane oxygenation and renal replacement therapy on meropenem pharmacokinetics: A matched cohort study. *Crit. Care* **2014**, *18*, 565. [CrossRef] [PubMed]
91. Cies, J.J.; Nikolos, P.; Moore, W.S.; Giliam, N.; Low, T.; Marino, D.; Deacon, J.; Enache, A.; Chopra, A. Oxygenator impact on meropenem/vaborbactam in extracorporeal membrane oxygenation circuits. *Perfusion* **2021**, 02676591211018985. [CrossRef] [PubMed]
92. Moffett, B.S.; Morris, J.; Galati, M.; Munoz, F.M.; Arikan, A.A. Population Pharmacokinetic Analysis of Gentamicin in Pediatric Extracorporeal Membrane Oxygenation. *Ther. Drug Monit.* **2018**, *40*, 581–588. [CrossRef]
93. Booke, H.; Frey, O.R.; Röhr, A.C.; Chiriac, U.; Zacharowski, K.; Holubec, T.; Adam, E.H. Excessive unbound cefazolin concentrations in critically ill patients receiving veno-arterial extracorporeal membrane oxygenation (vaECMO): An observational study. *Sci. Rep.* **2021**, *11*, 16981. [CrossRef]
94. Raffaeli, G.; Cavallaro, G.; Allegaert, K.; Koch, B.C.; Mosca, F.; Tibboel, D.; Wildschut, E.D. Sequestration of voriconazole and vancomycin into contemporary extracorporeal membrane oxygenation circuits: An in vitro study. *Front. Pediatrics* **2020**, *8*, 468. [CrossRef]
95. Dhanani, J.A.; Lipman, J.; Pincus, J.; Townsend, S.; Livermore, A.; Wallis, S.C.; Abdul-Aziz, M.H.; Roberts, J.A. Pharmacokinetics of Total and Unbound Cefazolin during Veno-Arterial Extracorporeal Membrane Oxygenation: A Case Report. *Chemotherapy* **2019**, *64*, 115–118. [CrossRef]
96. Cies, J.J.; Moore, W.S.; Giliam, N.; Low, T.; Enache, A.; Chopra, A. Oxygenator Impact on Ceftolozane and Tazobactam in Extracorporeal Membrane Oxygenation Circuits. *Pediatric Crit. Care Med.* **2020**, *21*, 276–282. [CrossRef]
97. Cies, J.J.; Moore, W.S.I.; Giliam, N.; Low, T.; Enache, A.; Chopra, A. Oxygenator Impact on Ceftaroline in Extracorporeal Membrane Oxygenation Circuits. *Pediatric Crit. Care Med.* **2018**, *19*, 1077–1082. [CrossRef]
98. Cies, J.; Moore, W.; Marino, D.; Deacon, J.; Enache, A.; Chopra, A. 1005: Oxygenator impact on peramivir in extracorporeal membrane oxygenation circuits. *Crit. Care Med.* **2022**, *50*, 499. [CrossRef]
99. Ruiz-Rodríguez, J.C.; Molnar, Z.; Deliargyris, E.N.; Ferrer, R. The Use of CytoSorb Therapy in Critically Ill COVID-19 Patients: Review of the Rationale and Current Clinical Experiences. *Crit. Care Res. Pract.* **2021**, *2021*, 7769516. [CrossRef] [PubMed]
100. Gacitua, I.; Frias, A.; Sanhueza, M.E.; Bustamante, S.; Cornejo, R.; Salas, A.; Guajardo, X.; Torres, K.; Figueroa Canales, E.; Tobar, E.; et al. Extracorporeal CO_2 removal and renal replacement therapy in acute severe respiratory failure in COVID-19 pneumonia: Case report. *Semin. Dial.* **2021**, *34*, 257–262. [CrossRef] [PubMed]
101. Cau, A.; Cheng, M.P.; Lee, T.; Levin, A.; Lee, T.C.; Vinh, D.C.; Lamontagne, F.; Singer, J.; Walley, K.R.; Murthy, S.; et al. Acute Kidney Injury and Renal Replacement Therapy in COVID-19 Versus Other Respiratory Viruses: A Systematic Review and Meta-Analysis. *Can. J. Kidney Health Dis.* **2021**, *8*, 20543581211052185. [CrossRef] [PubMed]
102. Van Daele, R.; Bekkers, B.; Lindfors, M.; Broman, L.M.; Schauwvlieghe, A.; Rijnders, B.; Hunfeld, N.G.M.; Juffermans, N.P.; Taccone, F.S.; Coimbra Sousa, C.A.; et al. A Large Retrospective Assessment of Voriconazole Exposure in Patients Treated with Extracorporeal Membrane Oxygenation. *Microorganisms* **2021**, *9*, 1543. [CrossRef] [PubMed]
103. Liu, D.; Chen, W.; Wang, Q.; Li, M.; Zhang, Z.; Cui, G.; Li, P.; Zhang, X.; Ma, Y.; Zhan, Q.; et al. Influence of venovenous extracorporeal membrane oxygenation on pharmacokinetics of vancomycin in lung transplant recipients. *J. Clin. Pharm. Ther.* **2020**, *45*, 1066–1075. [CrossRef] [PubMed]
104. Donadello, K.; Roberts, J.A.; Cristallini, S.; Beumier, M.; Shekar, K.; Jacobs, F.; Belhaj, A.; Vincent, J.L.; de Backer, D.; Taccone, F.S. Vancomycin population pharmacokinetics during extracorporeal membrane oxygenation therapy: A matched cohort study. *Crit. Care* **2014**, *18*, 632. [CrossRef] [PubMed]
105. Jung, Y.; Lee, D.H.; Kim, H.S. Prospective Cohort Study of Population Pharmacokinetics and Pharmacodynamic Target Attainment of Vancomycin in Adults on Extracorporeal Membrane Oxygenation. *Antimicrob. Agents Chemother.* **2021**, *65*, e02408-20. [CrossRef]
106. Mulla, H.; Pooboni, S. Population pharmacokinetics of vancomycin in patients receiving extracorporeal membrane oxygenation. *Br. J. Clin. Pharmacol.* **2005**, *60*, 265–275. [CrossRef]
107. Park, S.J.; Yang, J.H.; Park, H.J.; In, Y.W.; Lee, Y.M.; Cho, Y.H.; Chung, C.R.; Park, C.-M.; Jeon, K.; Suh, G.Y. Trough Concentrations of Vancomycin in Patients Undergoing Extracorporeal Membrane Oxygenation. *PLoS ONE* **2015**, *10*, e0141016. [CrossRef]
108. Wu, C.-C.; Shen, L.-J.; Hsu, L.-F.; Ko, W.-J.; Wu, F.-L.L. Pharmacokinetics of vancomycin in adults receiving extracorporeal membrane oxygenation. *J. Formos. Med. Assoc.* **2016**, *115*, 560–570. [CrossRef] [PubMed]
109. Mehta, N.M.; Halwick, D.R.; Dodson, B.L.; Thompson, J.E.; Arnold, J.H. Potential drug sequestration during extracorporeal membrane oxygenation: Results from an ex vivo experiment. *Intensive Care Med.* **2007**, *33*, 1018–1024. [CrossRef] [PubMed]
110. Zhang, Y.; Hu, H.; Zhang, Q.; Ou, Q.; Zhou, H.; Sha, T.; Zeng, Z.; Wu, J.; Lu, J.; Chen, Z. Effects of ex vivo Extracorporeal Membrane Oxygenation Circuits on Sequestration of Antimicrobial Agents. *Front. Med.* **2021**, *8*, 748769. [CrossRef] [PubMed]
111. Duceppe, M.A.; Kanji, S.; Do, A.T.; Ruo, N.; Cavayas, Y.A.; Albert, M.; Robert-Halabi, M.; Zavalkoff, S.; Dupont, P.; Samoukovic, G.; et al. Pharmacokinetics of Commonly Used Antimicrobials in Critically Ill Adults During Extracorporeal Membrane Oxygenation: A Systematic Review. *Drugs* **2021**, *81*, 1307–1329. [CrossRef]
112. Roberts, J.A.; Joynt, G.M.; Lee, A.; Choi, G.; Bellomo, R.; Kanji, S.; Mudaliar, M.Y.; Peake, S.L.; Stephens, D.; Taccone, F.S.; et al. The Effect of Renal Replacement Therapy and Antibiotic Dose on Antibiotic Concentrations in Critically Ill Patients: Data From the Multinational Sampling Antibiotics in Renal Replacement Therapy Study. *Clin. Infect. Dis.* **2021**, *72*, 1369–1378. [CrossRef]

113. Kroh, U.F.; Holl, T.; Feussner, K.D. Pharmacokinetics and dosage adjustment of antibiotics during continuous extracorporeal lung assistance and hemofiltration. *Artif. Organs* **1992**, *16*, 457–460. [CrossRef]
114. Wi, J.; Noh, H.; Min, K.L.; Yang, S.; Jin, B.H.; Hahn, J.; Bae, S.K.; Kim, J.; Park, M.S.; Choi, D.; et al. Population Pharmacokinetics and Dose Optimization of Teicoplanin during Venoarterial Extracorporeal Membrane Oxygenation. *Antimicrob. Agents Chemother.* **2017**, *61*, e01015-17. [CrossRef]
115. Combes, A.; Hajage, D.; Capellier, G.; Demoule, A.; Lavoué, S.; Guervilly, C.; Da Silva, D.; Zafrani, L.; Tirot, P.; Veber, B.; et al. Extracorporeal Membrane Oxygenation for Severe Acute Respiratory Distress Syndrome. *N. Engl. J. Med.* **2018**, *378*, 1965–1975. [CrossRef]

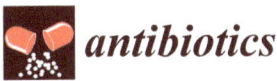

Review

Probiotics in the Intensive Care Unit

Alex R. Schuurman [1,†], Robert F. J. Kullberg [1,†] and Willem Joost Wiersinga [1,2,*]

[1] Center for Experimental and Molecular Medicine (CEMM), Amsterdam University Medical Centers, University of Amsterdam, 1105 AZ Amsterdam, The Netherlands; a.r.schuurman@amsterdamumc.nl (A.R.S.); r.f.j.kullberg@amsterdamumc.nl (R.F.J.K.)
[2] Division of Infectious Diseases, Department of Medicine, Amsterdam University Medical Centers, University of Amsterdam, 1105 AZ Amsterdam, The Netherlands
[*] Correspondence: w.j.wiersinga@amsterdamumc.nl
[†] These authors contributed equally to this work.

Abstract: The understanding of the gut microbiome in health and disease has shown tremendous progress in the last decade. Shaped and balanced throughout life, the gut microbiome is intricately related to the local and systemic immune system and a multitude of mechanisms through which the gut microbiome contributes to the host's defense against pathogens have been revealed. Similarly, a plethora of negative consequences, such as superinfections and an increased rate of hospital re-admissions, have been identified when the gut microbiome is disturbed by disease or by the iatrogenic effects of antibiotic treatment and other interventions. In this review, we describe the role that probiotics may play in the intensive care unit (ICU). We discuss what is known about the gut microbiome of the critically ill, and the concept of probiotic intervention to positively modulate the gut microbiome. We summarize the evidence derived from randomized clinical trials in this context, with a focus on the prevention of ventilator-associated pneumonia. Finally, we consider what lessons we can learn in terms of the current challenges, efficacy and safety of probiotics in the ICU and what we may expect from the future. Throughout the review, we highlight studies that have provided conceptual advances to the field or have revealed a specific mechanism; this narrative review is not intended as a comprehensive summary of the literature.

Keywords: microbiome; probiotics; intensive care unit; dysbiosis; ventilator-associated pneumonia

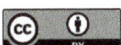

1. Introduction

The gut microbiome harbors complex communities of bacteria which together fulfill a wide range of functions within the human body. A balanced gut microbiome enhances the host defense against infection by finetuning the local and systemic immune system [1,2], repressing enteric pathogens [3,4], and supporting epithelial barrier integrity [5]. Conversely, perturbation of the microbiome (called 'dysbiosis') appears to have detrimental effects on the host and is associated with a wide range of diseases [6]. This is of particular relevance in the intensive care unit (ICU) where patients with life-threatening conditions (such as respiratory failure, sepsis, myocardial infarction, cardiovascular procedures, intracranial hemorrhage and cerebral infarction) are treated [7].

The microbiome of such critically ill patients is continually assaulted by the disease itself and by iatrogenic effects of clinical intervention [2,8]. As a result, the gut microbiome of virtually all patients admitted to the ICU is severely disrupted [8–10]. These disruptions have associated with a multitude of negative consequences such as ventilator-associated pneumonia (VAP) and increased re-infection and re-admission rates [10–12]. The field of probiotics—the administration of selected, live bacteria that are of potential benefit to the host (see Section 1.1)—strives to address dysbiosis-related problems by reinforcing or reconstituting the gut microbiome, both in preventative and therapeutic approaches. In this review, we will first explore the causes and putative consequences of dysbiosis in

ICU patients. Next, we summarize the experimental data, mainly comprising studies in mice, that support the rationale for probiotic administration in the critically ill. We proceed by discussing the current clinical evidence for probiotic intervention in the ICU, with a focus on the prevention of VAP in adults. Herein, we combine meta-analyses and a recent landmark clinical trial to evaluate the efficacy and safety of probiotics in the ICU. We close with a reflection on current opportunities and pitfalls in the field, and an outlook on the potential future positioning of probiotics in the ICU.

1.1. A Brief Overview of Modalities Used in the ICU to Modulate the Gut Microbiome

Several (partly experimental) strategies are used in the ICU to modulate the microbiome in order to prevent or treat infections. Examples are the use of pre/synbiotics, probiotics, fecal microbiota transplantation (FMT) and antibiotic prophylaxis. Briefly, probiotics are selected "live microorganisms that, when administered in adequate amounts, confer a health benefit on the host" [13]. Prebiotics are nutrients—often oligosaccharides—that can selectively feed certain bacterial colonies, while a combination of probiotics and prebiotics is called synbiotics. FMT comprises the transfer of a stool sample, autologous or from a donor, to a recipient in order to (re)introduce healthy bacterial flora. Probiotics can be administered in various ways, such as in a soluble powder or in pill form, which can contain billions of bacteria per dose. Often, such probiotics include bacterial strains from the *Lactobacillus* and *Bifidobacterium* species—sometimes genetically modified to have less virulent factors.

2. Gut Microbiota in Critically Ill Patients

2.1. Causes of Gut Microbiota Disruptions

Critically ill patients have a severely disturbed microbiome, characterized by a loss of diversity, depletion of commensal bacteria (e.g., *Ruminococcus*, *Pseudobutyrivibrio*, *Blautia*, *Faecalibacterium*) and domination by pathogens (e.g., *Enterococcus*, *Staphylococcus*, *Enterobacteriaceae*) [2,8,9]. These disruptions extend to kingdoms beyond bacteria (e.g., bacteriophages, eukaryotic viruses, fungi and protozoa) and enable the overgrowth of viruses and opportunistic yeasts [14]. A multitude of endogenous and iatrogenic factors contribute to these extensive alterations in the microbiota composition of ICU patients, including gastrointestinal dysmotility, shifts in intraluminal pH values, increased production of catecholamines, treatment with antibiotics, proton pump inhibitors, opioids and (par)enteral feeding [2,8]. In addition, infection of the gastrointestinal tract by pathogenic bacteria or viruses could drive microbiome alterations. Recently, several studies showed that SARS-CoV-2 can infect human enterocytes and that gut microbiota are disrupted during COVID-19 [15,16].

The exact effect of any of these disruptive factors on the composition of the gut microbiota varies highly per individual [17]. For example, Rashidi et al. analyzed 260 stool samples of patients with acute leukemia receiving multiple antibiotics and demonstrated that pre-treatment microbiota composition (specifically the earlier described health-promoting bacteria such as *Roseburia*, *Blautia* and *Eggerthella*) was the most important determinant of antibiotic-induced microbiota alterations. Even under intense antibiotic pressure, gut microbiota maintained a highly personalized composition [18]. Besides the iatrogenic changes and disruptive effects of critical illness itself, demographic variables also influence the microbiome during critical illness. In a cohort of 155 critically ill patients in the ICU, age and sex were associated with the differential abundance of a large number of bacterial taxa, while less associations were found between bacterial taxa and the length of ICU stay or disease severity (quantified by SOFA score) [19]. This is in line with a large study that analyzed three cohorts of healthy adults across different continents, describing relatively low microbial diversity in males and elderly people [20].

Thus, although microbiome disruptions are common in the ICU and general patterns are observed, the range of factors contributing to these alterations in ICU patients results in highly individual patterns of intestinal microbiota [9].

2.2. Potential Negative Consequences of Gut Microbiota Disruptions

Dysbiosis of the gut microbiome, and specifically overgrowth by pathobionts (commensal microbes with pathogenic potential), has been associated with adverse clinical outcomes. For example, in eight patients that underwent allogeneic hematopoietic cell transplant, intestinal domination by Proteobacteria or Candida resulted in translocation and subsequent invasive bacterial and fungal infections [21]. In a larger study that followed 708 recipients of allogeneic hematopoietic cell transplant, it was found that overrepresentation of Gram-negative bacteria was strongly associated with the development of bloodstream infections [22]. A study in 301 critically ill patients found that Enteroccocus domination (>30% relative abundance) of the gut microbiome was associated with a 19% increased probability of death, significant after correction for disease severity [23].

In addition, gut microbiome perturbations potentially have negative long-term health consequences and could be of clinical relevance following a hospitalization and ICU stay. Large observational studies described associations between presumed disrupted microbiota (based on antibiotic exposure or diseases associated with dysbiosis) and subsequent increased risks of sepsis [24,25]. One observational study from the US used data from over 12 million hospitalized patients and found a doubled risk of severe sepsis in the 90 days following hospitalization in patients exposed to ≥ 4 antibiotic classes or ≥ 14 days of antibiotic therapy, compared to those without antibiotic exposure [24]. Exposure to high-risk antibiotics (e.g., third- or fourth-generation cephalosporin or fluoroquinolones) was associated with a 1.65-fold greater risk of severe sepsis in the 90 days following discharge [24]. Although the aforementioned studies suggest a link between intestinal microbiota disruptions and critical illness in humans, whether this links implies a causal relation and—most importantly—a modifiable one remains undetermined.

2.3. Mechanisms Underlying the Beneficial Role of Probiotics in Critical Illness

Probiotics are hypothesized to reconstitute the disrupted intestinal microbiome and may provide health benefits through two main mechanisms. First, probiotics would inhibit pathogen growth or replace pathogenic bacteria with non-pathogenic bacteria (the probiotic) and create a more favorable microbial environment in the stomach and gut. Thus, oropharyngeal colonization by pathogenic bacteria could be prevented, thereby diminishing the risk of pneumonia caused by micro-aspiration. Moreover, transloca-tion of intestinal bacteria to the blood and distant organs might be avoided by replac-ing pathogenic gut bacteria [26]. Second, a re-established microbiome could provide health benefits by influencing immune responses outside the gut [13,27].

However, as the mechanisms underlying the role of gut microbiota perturbation in critical illness are not yet fully understood, the exact mechanisms of action of most probiotics are not yet known either. Animal models revealed some potential mechanisms through which gut microbiota disruptions result in reduced colonization resistance against pathogens and immune derangements. As an example, in health, commensal bacteria prevent the expansion of pathogens through a competition for nutrients, enhancement of immunoglobulin A production, and by stimulating the release of antimicrobial peptides such as regenerating islet-derived protein IIIγ (REGIIIγ) from epithelial cells [28,29]. In addition, commensal-derived short-chain fatty acids (SCFAs) serve as the main nutrient of gut enterocytes, which maintain intestinal barrier function, thereby protecting against systemic dissemination of pathogenic bacteria. During critical illness, the decrease of commensal bacteria leads to a loss of colonization resistance and increased gut permeability, resulting in an overgrowth of harmful microbes and subsequent translocation to blood and distant organs, specifically the lungs and brain [30,31]. Thus, probiotic supplementation might re-establish the disrupted intestinal microbiome and provide colonization resistance against pathogens.

The beneficial effects of a reconstituted microbiome extend beyond the intestine, through the production of immunomodulatory metabolites. Gut derived SCFAs can, for instance, affect the immunological environment in the lung and increase the bactericidal activity of alveolar macrophages [32]. Another microbial metabolite, D-lactate, translocates from the gut to the liver through the portal vein and promotes pathogen clearance by Kupffer cells (the resident macrophages of the liver) [33]. In addition, murine studies suggested the involvement of gut microbiota in complications of critical illness such as acute kidney injury induced by ischemia-reperfusion, acute respiratory distress syndrome (ARDS) and liver injury [30,34,35]. Together, probiotics are hypothesized to prevent the detrimental consequences of gut dysbiosis and support a healthy enteric and systemic immune response [13].

However, whether commonly used probiotics actually approximate these functions of commensal microbiota, and whether these mechanisms are of equal importance in humans—where the microbiome is much more complex, and circumstances are not standardized—remains somewhat speculative. In a randomized controlled trial aiming to translate such preclinical evidence to healthy humans, gut microbiota disruption with broad-spectrum antibiotics had no effect on the surrogate markers of sepsis (e.g., vital signs and systemic cytokine responses) upon intravenous lipopolysaccharide injection [36]. Similarly, existing interindividual differences in gut microbiota composition were not associated with variation in cytokine responses (TNF-α, IL-6, IL-8 and IL-10) during the same model of experimental endotoxemia [37]. This underscores the notion that the gut microbiota is just one of the many factors that regulate the systemic immune response, and also highlights the difficulty of translating findings from animals to humans.

3. Microbiome Modulation in the ICU

3.1. Preclinical Data on the Efficacy of Probiotics

Preclinical findings, specifically mouse models of severe infection, have further built the rationale for probiotic approaches in the ICU. For example, administration of *Lactobacillus* and *Bifidobacterium* blunted the pro-inflammatory response, decreased lung injury and improved survival in a mouse model of sepsis induced by cecal ligation and puncture [38,39]. In comparable sepsis models, mice pretreated with *L. rhamnosus* GG showed improved survival compared to controls [40]. In more comprehensive follow-up studies, the same research group showed that pretreatment with *L. rhamnosus* GG limited sepsis-induced dysbiosis, improved read-outs of the intestinal barrier function, decreased inflammatory cytokine levels, and prevented changes in some fecal metabolites, such as lysophosphatidylcholine and eicosatetraenoic acid lipids of which the (patho)physiological relevance remain uncertain [41,42]. In neonatal mice, administration of *L. murinus* protected against gut overgrowth of the pathobiont *Klebsiella pneumoniae*, thereby preventing subsequent systemic translocation and late-onset sepsis. Interestingly, only selected lactobacilli, namely, *L. murinus*, were effective probiotics, while the commonly used commercial strains, *L. rhamnosus* GG and *L. plantarum*, did not protect against dysbiosis [43]. Together, experimental data in murine models of sepsis showed beneficial effects of (specific strains of) probiotic intervention in modulating the gut microbiome, although the exact mechanisms largely remain to be elucidated.

3.2. Prevention of Ventilator-Associated Pneumonia

The negative outcomes associated with dysbiosis in the ICU, together with the beneficial effects of probiotics in murine studies, have provided the rationale for probiotic intervention to prevent secondary infections in the critically ill. Specifically, in recent years most attention has be paid to the use of probiotics for the prevention of VAP.

VAP is defined by the American Thoracic Society as hospital-acquired pneumonia in patients that have been on mechanical ventilation for at least 48 h [44]. VAP is reported to affect 10–25% of all mechanically ventilated patients, with the incidence ranging from 2 to 15 cases per 1000 ventilator-days [45]. The pathogenesis of VAP is complex and multi-facetted, involving an interplay between (endogenous) bacteria, the detrimental physiological effects of intubation, and decreased immunological resilience during critical illness [46]. The endotracheal tube facilitates the entry of pathogenic bacteria—

either translocated from the digestive tract or via inhalation—to the lower respiratory tract through micro-aspiration, biofilm formation and impaired mucociliary clearance. A dysregulated immune response during critical illness and mechanical ventilation further contributes to the development of VAP, including a role being played by the decreased phagocytic activity of macrophages [47], impaired type I interferon signaling [48], and neutrophil dysfunction [49]. Overall, the translocation of bacteria from the digestive tract to the lungs might be a core mechanism in VAP [50], and altering the composition of the gut microbiome through probiotics aims at combatting this mechanism.

Over the last decades, a multitude of trials have been performed in this rapidly expanding field. A recent meta-analysis pooled the results of nine randomized controlled trials, together reporting on 1127 patients (564 receiving probiotics and 563 receiving placebo), all investigating probiotic intervention in the ICU, with the primary aim of reducing the incidence of VAP [51]. The studies included used myriad probiotics, including *Lactobacillus*, *Bifidobacterium* and *Streptococcus* spp., and two specific probiotic formulas (containing *Bacillus* and *Enterococcus* spp., or *Pediococcus* and *Lactobacillus* spp.).

An overall positive effect of probiotic intervention was found with a lower incidence of VAP (odds ratio 0.70, confidence interval 0.56–0.88), shorter duration of mechanical ventilation (mean difference of 3.75 days), shorter ICU stay (mean difference of 4.20 days) and lower in-hospital mortality (odds ratio 0.73, confidence interval 0.54–0.98). The total length of hospital stay was unaffected. This systematic review assessed several forms of bias and performed subgroup analyses, which did not reveal apparent publication bias, nor significant differences between trials with a high vs. low risk of bias, or between trials undertaken in a trauma vs. mixed population of patients. The studies included in the meta-analysis did show heterogeneity in terms of the definition of VAP and in the intervention, as some studies employed a single-strain probiotic (such as *L. rhamnosus*), while others used multiple probiotics (e.g., a combination of three *Lactobacillus* species and *B. bifidum*), or a synbiotic product (e.g., 'Synbiotic 2000Forte' which contains *Pediococcus* and *Lactobacillus* spp. along with inulin, betaglucan, pectin, and resistant starch as the prebiotic). Notably, the route, timing, and length of intervention was also variable. The conclusion of this meta-analysis—that VAP incidence was lower in the probiotic group—is in line with several earlier systematic reviews [52–56]. Together, almost all systematic reviews conclude that any result must be interpreted with caution. The heterogeneity in cohort characteristics, type of probiotic intervention and study design warranted a large, multi-center randomized controlled trial [51–56]. Recently, such a trial has been published.

In the randomized, placebo-controlled PROSPECT trial in 44 hospitals across three countries, Johnstone et al. investigated whether probiotic administration could lower the incidence of VAP [57]. The study included 2653 patients in the ICU—expected to be on mechanical ventilation for at least 72 h—split evenly between 1×10^{10} colony forming units of *L. rhamnosus GG* or placebo twice daily, for a period of sixty days or until discharge. The results were clear: the probiotic intervention did not lower the incidence of VAP (21.9% in the probiotic group, 21.3% in the placebo group). Furthermore, no differences were found when they used alternative definitions for pneumonia. The discrepancy between these findings and results from previous studies and meta-analyses, often including *L. rhamnosus* as a probiotic intervention too, is remarkable. This may be a product of the inter-study heterogeneity in terms of design and patient population, or differences between the probiotic formulae. The importance of this heterogeneity is highlighted by a recent, smaller study with a different design and in this placebo-controlled trial, 112 multi-trauma patients—expected to be on mechanical ventilation for at least 10 days—were randomized between either a probiotic formula (consisting of *L. acidophilus*, *L. plantarum*, *B. lactis* and *Saccharomyces boulardii*) or placebo twice daily for two days [58]. The incidence of VAP (11.9% vs. 28.3%, respectively) and sepsis (6.8% vs. 24.5%, respectively) was significantly lower in the probiotic group, while the length of hospital and ICU stay were also reduced. Notably, the study stopped prematurely and included less than half of the intended number of patients. Although this limitation may preclude robust conclusions, the contrast between the findings of these studies is stark and may in part be explained by a different patient population and the use of a multi-strain probiotic formula. Overall, the current level of evidence tempers the initial enthusiasm on the use of probiotic therapy for the prevention of VAP, and more work is needed to identify which probiotic intervention may be beneficial for specific patient groups.

3.3. Other Indications in the ICU

While the prevention of VAP has been the main focus in probiotic research, several other outcome measures have also been investigated including diarrhea, other infections, length of hospital stay and mortality. A recent placebo-controlled randomized controlled trial in 218 Australian ICU patients by Litton et al. assessed the effect of early daily *Lactobacillus plantarum* 299v supplementation [59]. The primary outcome was days alive and out of hospital to day 60, a composite endpoint of death, hospital length of stay and hospital re-admissions. Early and sustained administration of *L. plantarum* 299v did not improve the primary outcome measure (49.5 (IQR 37–53) in the probiotic group and 49 (IQR 43.8–53) in the placebo group, $p = 0.55$) [59]. Several subgroup analyses, including the evaluation of antibiotic treatment, the presence of sepsis and type of ICU admission, did not reveal significant differences either. This is in line with the recent findings by Johnstone et al. that found no differences in ICU and hospital length of stay, or mortality [57]. Moreover, while a meta-analysis of 14 trials reporting on a total of 1233 critically ill patients found a reduction in infections following probiotic treatment (risk ratio 0.80, confidence interval 0.68–0.95) [55], the incidence of infections was not different between groups in the two recent trials (by Johnstone et al. and Litton et al.) [57,59]. The incidence of any infection was 31.4% in both the placebo and the probiotic group (hazard ratio 0.97, confidence interval 0.84–1.11) [57], and nosocomial infections occurred in 7.3% and 4.6 of the probiotic and placebo group patients, respectively (odds ratio 1.62, confidence interval 0.51–5.10) [59]. Together, as we noted for VAP, the results of recent high-quality trials appear to deviate from the conclusions of meta-analyses.

Given the often detrimental effects of antibiotics on the gut microbiome and their wide use in ICU patients, multiple trials have investigated whether probiotics could mitigate the negative consequences of antibiotic perturbation such as antibiotic-associated diarrhea and *Clostridium difficile* infection. A meta-analysis of nine trials and 1259 ICU patients did not demonstrate a treatment benefit of probiotics on diarrhea (risk ratio 0.97, confidence interval 0.82–1.15) [55]. Likewise, in the aforementioned trial by Johnstone et al. there were no differences in the incidence of antibiotic-associated diarrhea (hazard ratio 1.02, confidence interval 0.93–1.15) or *C. difficile* infection (odds ratio 1.15, confidence interval 0.69–1.93) [57]; however, in meta-analyses including both out- and in-patients, rather than focusing solely on ICU patients, probiotics reduced the risk of *C. difficile* infection and antibiotic-associated diarrhea [60,61]. Among 13 trials enrolling 2454 participants with a high baseline risk of *C. difficile* associated disease (>5%), probiotics reduced the risk of *C. difficile* associated disease by 70%, but no significant effect of probiotics was found in trials with a lower baseline risk ($\leq$5%) [60]. Due to the lack of conclusive high-quality evidence, probiotics are currently not included in treatment guidelines for *C. difficile* infections [62,63].

Since the start of the COVID-19 pandemic, multiple randomized-controlled trials assessing the potential role of probiotic treatment in COVID-19 have been registered [64]. Of those, only one investigates the effect of probiotics (*Streptococcus salivarius* K12 combined with *L. brevis*) in ICU patients with COVID-19 (clinicaltrials.gov: NCT05175833). Thus far, no results of this trial are available and the role of probiotics in critically ill COVID-19 patients remains unclear.

Overall, current evidence does not unambiguously support the use of probiotics for the prevention or treatment of antibiotic-associated diarrhea and *C. difficile* infection in ICU patients. The identification of subgroups that could potentially benefit from probiotics is an important future challenge.

4. Current Challenges

4.1. Safety

In addition to the unclear efficacy, the implementation of probiotic treatment in the ICU has been hampered by safety concerns. These concerns stem in part from the frequently debated and re-analyzed results of the PROPATRIA study [65–67], a double-blind, placebo-controlled trial in which patients with predicted severe acute pancreatitis received either enteral probiotics (a combination of *three Lactobacillus* spp., two *Bifidobacterium* spp. and one *Lactococcus* spp.) or placebo. The probiotic treatment resulted in higher mortality (16%, 24 of 152 patients) compared to the placebo (6%, 9 of 144 patients), which was presumably—albeit still a subject of debate—caused by intestinal ischemia and translocation of gut bacteria to the bloodstream, resulting in multiorgan failure.

Although probiotic supplementation has earlier been associated with higher risks of sepsis and fungemia in critically ill patients [68], it was only recently shown that probiotics supplementation in pediatric ICU patients could result in the systemic translocation of probiotic bacteria. Epidemiological data of 22,174 ICU patients showed that patients receiving *Lactobacillus rhamnosus* GG were at increased risk of Lactobacillus bacteremia (6 out of 522 patients, compared to 0 out of 21,652). Whole-genome-based phylogeny analysis confirmed that *Lactobacilli* isolated from the blood of patients treated with probiotics were phylogenetically inseparable from the probiotic product [69]. Similarly, in the aforementioned trial by Johnstone et al. that investigated 2653 ICU patients, the incidence of adverse events (including the sequencing-confirmed presence of *Lactobacillus rhamnosus* GG in previously sterile sites) was significantly higher in the probiotic group (1.1% versus 0.1% in the placebo group) [57].

Together, these studies raise valid questions regarding the potential harm of probiotic supplementation in the critically ill, and a thorough examination of adverse effects is warranted. Of note, it was recently reported that out of 53 studies investigating probiotic, prebiotic or synbiotic intervention in hospitalized and/or critically ill patients, only 7 reported the number of serious adverse events per group [70].

4.2. Other Pitfalls in the Field

Despite the many links between microbiome disruption and adverse outcomes in the ICU, and the apparent beneficial effect of probiotics on mortality and inflammation in numerous animal models of severe infection, probiotic treatment has not unequivocally proven to be of clear clinical benefit in critically ill patients. Therefore, what challenges need to be addressed, in order for probiotics to reach their full clinical potential in the ICU (Table 1)?

Table 1. Current challenges for probiotics in the ICU.

Efficacy	While the majority of meta-analyses find a positive effect, the negative results of the recent PROSPECT trial cast doubt on the efficacy of probiotics for preventing ventilator-associated pneumonia [57].
Safety	Overall lack of safety reporting, coupled with recent reports of probiotic bacteremia, together warrant increased attention for monitoring potential harm.
Mechanisms	Causal links between probiotic intervention and improved outcome in experimental models remain largely elusive.
Microbiome Effects	Microbiome diversity and composition are often not among the (secondary) outcome measurements in clinical trials, which cloud our understanding of the (long-term) effects of probiotics on gut microbiota.
Heterogeneity	Gut microbiota, and the negative effect of antibiotics thereon, show inter-individual differences which may call for more personalized therapy.

First, practical issues such as dosage, treatment duration, timing and the effects of concurrent administration with antibiotics—potentially directly eliminating the administered bacteria—need to be considered and ideally standardized to improve the interpretation and comparability of RCTs. Next, microorganisms that are used as a probiotic should be adequately characterized in terms of their genome and functional repertoire, as strain level differences influence their health-promoting functions [43]. A recent study revealed enormous genetic and functional inter- and intra-species diversity within a single commensal gut family. Through whole-genome sequencing and gene annotation in 20 human donors, the authors found remarkable differences within the Lachnospiraceae family, which are likely to influence butyrate production of a specific strain and thereby its contribution to colonization resistance and the host's mucosal immune response [71]. These findings indicate that proper genomic and metabolic analyses of microbes is essential to identify the strain-specific qualities that could be harnessed in effective new probiotics.

Furthermore, although an altered microbiome could be assumed to be a prerequisite for any beneficial effects of probiotics, the actual effect of probiotic supplementation on gut communities is very often not reported in human trials [72]. A systematic review found no effect of probiotics on the fecal microbiota composition of healthy adults in six out of seven randomized controlled trials [73]. Recently, two key studies described the effect of probiotics on the gut microbiome in much more detail. Zmora et al. described the impact of probiotics on the human gut mucosa-associated microbiome [74]. By characterizing the microbiome in mucosal stool samples before and during the administration of a placebo or an 11-strain probiotic preparation (existing of *Lactobacillus*, *Bifidobacterium*, *Lactococcus* and *Streptococcus* spp.), they found a transient and highly individualized effect of probiotics on the mucosal communities and the gut transcriptome—approximately half of the participants showed significantly higher abundances of probiotics in their gut mucosa, while others were not colonized by probiotics. This person-specific susceptibility to gut colonization by probiotics was associated with baseline host transcriptional and microbiome characteristics and could explain the high interpersonal variability in probiotic effects. Of significance, Suez et al. showed that a four-week administration of the same multi-strain probiotic formula after broad-spectrum antibiotic exposure resulted in a delayed microbiome reconstitution when compared to watchful waiting and autologous FMT [75]. Intestinal, mucosal and stool samples indicated that the probiotics inhibited the repopulation of the indigenous communities, both in terms of microbial diversity and transcriptional profile. These findings shed light on the longitudinal effects of probiotic intervention and indicate that temporarily boosting the gut microbiome with probiotics may result in a stunted recovery of the microbiome in the long-term. This previously underestimated trade-off is seldom taken into account in current studies and warrants an extended monitoring of the microbiome and outcome of patients treated with probiotics.

Finally, what constitutes a "healthy microbiome"—or similarly, dysbiosis [76]—remains ill-defined [77]. While a core human microbiome may exist, it is known that each individual carries a personalized microbial signature that evolves throughout life. The heterogeneous consequences of ICU treatment on gut microbiota composition and the person-specific gut mucosal colonization resistance against probiotics [8,70], highlight the need for personalized approaches to reconstitute the disrupted microbiome rather than a standardized, single-strain probiotic intervention in the highly diverse ICU population. In other words, one size will probably not fit all.

5. Future Perspectives

It is notable that although indirect evidence for the importance of the gut microbiome is abundant (associations with clinical outcome, in vitro work and mouse models), proven mechanistic links between gut microbiome changes and the (patho)physiology of critically ill humans remain absent. Nevertheless, many randomized-controlled trials have been performed over the last decade. The fact that probiotics are classified as food supplements, and not as medication, could perhaps partly explain this early transition to human intervention trials. A focus on the mechanistic, causal effects of specific features of the human microbiome is advised to be the basis for future interventional trials (Figure 1) [78].

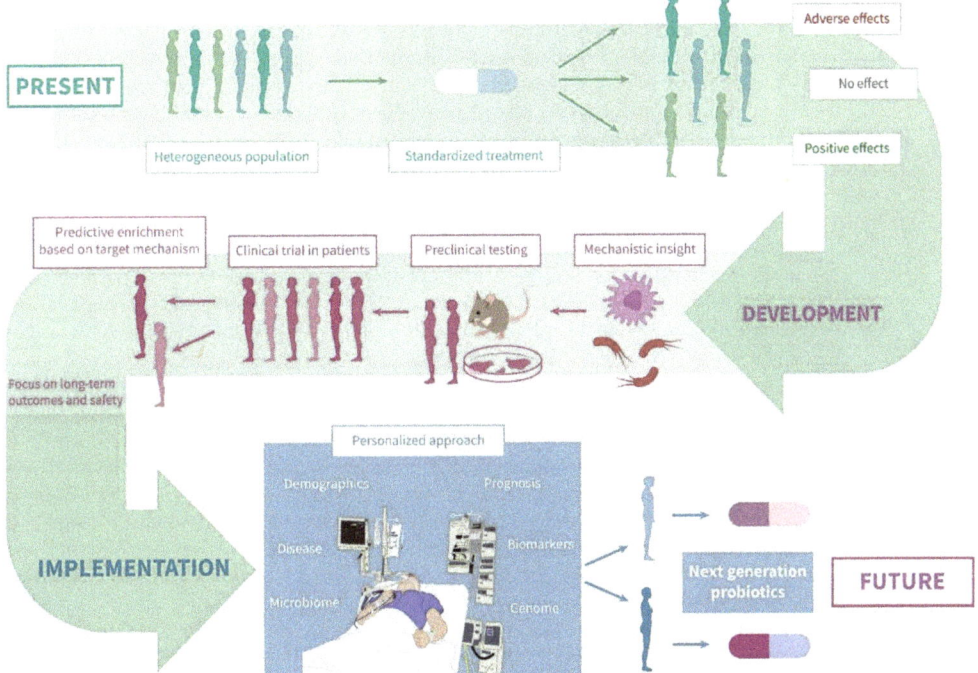

Figure 1. Current and future role of probiotics in the ICU. Current practice involves a standardized intervention in the highly diverse ICU population, with inconsistent clinical effects. A focus on a mechanistic understanding, combined with rigorous preclinical testing—including in healthy volunteers—can lay the groundwork for new probiotics with well-documented biological effects. The clinical efficacy of these next-generation probiotics should be tested in clinical trials with a focus on long-term outcomes and safety. Herein, dividing patients into specific subgroups (predictive enrichment) based on the target mechanism can increase the chance of finding positive effects. Eventually, the use of patient-specific data may allow clinicians to tailor probiotic treatment in the ICU to individual patients.

In recent years, several preclinical studies have described novel live microorganisms that have not been used to promote health to date. These non-standard probiotics—also known as next-generation probiotics [79]—often comprise gut commensals rather than the currently used *Lactobacillus* or *Bifidobacterium* species and might affect the gut microbiome and protect against infections. For example, murine studies demonstrated that a combination of four gut commensals (*Bacteroides sartorii*, *Parabacteroides distasonis*, *Clostridium boltea* and *Blautia producta*) restored colonization resistance against vancomycin-resistant Enterococci through cooperativity between these commensals [80]. In addition, *Clostridium scindens* (another gut commensal) could reduce enteric colonization by *C. difficile* through synthesizing *C. difficile*-inhibiting metabolites from bile salts [81].

Studies could also focus more on the prevention of microbiota disruption by antibiotics, aside from reconstituting the microbiome after iatrogenic dysbiosis. In this context, a recent investigation screened potential antidotes that may specifically mitigate the collateral damage of antibiotics on commensals [82]. By analyzing a library of 1197 pharmaceuticals, it was reported that an anticoagulant drug (dicumarol), an uricosuric agent (benzbromarone) and two non-steroidal anti-inflammatory drugs (tolfenamic acid and diflunisal) could protect *Bacteroides* species from the negative effects of erythromycin and doxycycline. Importantly, it was shown in human-stool-derived communities and gnotobiotic mice (i.e. animals containing only known microorganisms) that these antidotes did not affect antibiotic efficacy against the pathogens for which erythromycin and doxycycline were prescribed [82]. Further development of these next-generation probiotics and antidotes could result in new therapeutics that limit antibiotic-induced damage to the microbiome, enhance colonization resistance and reduce (antibiotic-resistant) infections [28]. Ideally, future trials assessing such interventions should comprehensively measure the effects on the microbiota composition over an extended period of time.

6. Conclusions

Altogether, we can conclude that the field of microbiota research has comprehensively shown that the gut microbiome is severely disrupted in critically ill patients in the ICU. The resulting dysbiosis has been associated with worse clinical outcomes, re-infections and re-admissions, but causal relationships remain elusive. Similarly, there are strong indications from experimental data that probiotic intervention may improve outcomes in models of severe infection, but the underlying mechanisms are still unclear. Substantial heterogeneity between randomized controlled trials, concerns about safety and a recent high-quality trial with negative results with regards to VAP prevention reflect that a beneficial role for probiotics in the ICU remains uncertain. Future experimental and clinical studies focused on mechanistic evidence, are needed to determine how the full potential of the microbiome in terms of its diagnostic and therapeutic value can be unlocked in the ICU setting. While we may have to go back to the drawing board and rethink our approach, microbiome modulation in intensive care remains a promising clinical tool to improve long-term outcomes.

Author Contributions: Conceptualization, A.R.S., R.F.J.K. and W.J.W.; writing—original draft preparation, A.R.S. and R.F.J.K.; writing—review and editing, A.R.S., R.F.J.K. and W.J.W.; visualization, A.R.S. and R.F.J.K.; supervision, W.J.W.; project administration, W.J.W.; funding acquisition, W.J.W. All authors have read and agreed to the published version of the manuscript.

Funding: This research was funded by the Top Consortia for Knowledge and Innovations and Top Sector Life Sciences & Health (TKI-LSH), and the Netherlands Organization for Scientific Research (Nederlandse Organisatie voor Wetenschappelijk Onderzoek) under VIDI grant 91716475 to W.J.W.

Conflicts of Interest: The authors declare no conflict of interest. The funders had no role in the writing of this review, or in the decision to publish.

References

1. Chung, H.; Pamp, S.J.; Hill, J.A.; Surana, N.K.; Edelman, S.M.; Troy, E.B.; Reading, N.C.; Villablanca, E.J.; Wang, S.; Mora, J.R. Gut immune maturation depends on colonization with a host-specific microbiota. *Cell* **2012**, *149*, 1578–1593. [CrossRef]
2. Haak, B.W.; Wiersinga, W.J. The role of the gut microbiota in sepsis. *Lancet Gastroenterol. Hepatol.* **2017**, *2*, 135–143. [CrossRef]
3. Kim, S.; Covington, A.; Pamer, E.G. The intestinal microbiota: Antibiotics, colonization resistance, and enteric pathogens. *Immunol. Rev.* **2017**, *279*, 90–105. [CrossRef]
4. Byndloss, M.X.; Olsan, E.E.; Rivera-Chávez, F.; Tiffany, C.R.; Cevallos, S.A.; Lokken, K.L.; Torres, T.P.; Byndloss, A.J.; Faber, F.; Gao, Y. Microbiota-activated PPAR-γ signaling inhibits dysbiotic Enterobacteriaceae expansion. *Science* **2017**, *357*, 570–575. [CrossRef]
5. Odenwald, M.A.; Turner, J.R. The intestinal epithelial barrier: A therapeutic target? *Nat. Rev. Gastroenterol. Hepatol.* **2017**, *14*, 9–21. [CrossRef] [PubMed]
6. Lynch, S.V.; Pedersen, O. The human intestinal microbiome in health and disease. *N. Engl. J. Med.* **2016**, *15*, 2369–2379. [CrossRef]
7. Wunsch, H.; Angus, D.C.; Harrison, D.A.; Linde-Zwirble, W.T.; Rowan, K.M. Comparison of medical admissions to intensive care units in the United States and United Kingdom. *Am. J. Respir. Crit. Care Med.* **2011**, *183*, 1666–1673. [CrossRef] [PubMed]
8. Dickson, R.P. The microbiome and critical illness. *Lancet Respir. Med.* **2016**, *4*, 59–72. [CrossRef]
9. Lankelma, J.M.; van Vught, L.A.; Belzer, C.; Schultz, M.J.; van der Poll, T.; de Vos, W.M.; Wiersinga, W.J. Critically ill patients demonstrate large interpersonal variation in intestinal microbiota dysregulation: A pilot study. *Intensive Care Med.* **2017**, *43*, 59–68. [CrossRef] [PubMed]

10. McDonald, D.; Ackermann, G.; Khailova, L.; Baird, C.; Heyland, D.; Kozar, R.; Lemieux, M.; Derenski, K.; King, J.; Vis-Kampen, C. Extreme Dysbiosis of the Microbiome in Critical Illness. *Msphere* **2016**, *1*, e00199-16. [CrossRef] [PubMed]
11. Wolff, N.S.; Hugenholtz, F.; Wiersinga, W.J. The emerging role of the microbiota in the ICU. *Crit. Care* **2018**, *22*, 78. [CrossRef]
12. Adelman, M.W.; Woodworth, M.H.; Langelier, C.; Busch, L.M.; Kempker, J.A.; Kraft, C.S.; Martin, G.S. The gut microbiome's role in the development, maintenance, and outcomes of sepsis. *Crit. Care* **2020**, *24*, 278. [CrossRef]
13. Hill, C.; Guarner, F.; Reid, G.; Gibson, G.R.; Merenstein, D.J.; Pot, B.; Morelli, L.; Canani, R.B.; Flint, H.J.; Salminen, S.; et al. Expert consensus document. The International Scientific Association for Probiotics and Prebiotics consensus statement on the scope and appropriate use of the term probiotic. *Nat. Rev. Gastroenterol. Hepatol.* **2014**, *11*, 506–514. [CrossRef] [PubMed]
14. Haak, B.W.; Argelaguet, R.; Kinsella, C.M.; Kullberg, R.F.J.; Lankelma, J.M.; Deijs, M.; Klein, M.; Jebbink, M.F.; Hugenholtz, F.; Kostidis, S.; et al. Integrative Transkingdom Analysis of the Gut Microbiome in Antibiotic Perturbation and Critical Illness. *Msystems* **2021**, *6*, e01148-20. [CrossRef] [PubMed]
15. Lamers, M.M.; Beumer, J.; van der Vaart, J.; Knoops, K.; Puschhof, J.; Breugem, T.I.; Ravelli, R.; Paul van Schayck, J.; Mykytyn, A.Z.; Duimel, H.Q.; et al. SARS-CoV-2 productively infects human gut enterocytes. *Science* **2020**, *369*, 50–54. [CrossRef] [PubMed]
16. Zuo, T.; Zhang, F.; Lui, G.; Yeoh, Y.K.; Li, A.; Zhan, H.; Wan, Y.; Chung, A.; Cheung, C.P.; Chen, N.; et al. Alterations in Gut Microbiota of Patients with COVID-19 during Time of Hospitalization. *Gastroenterology* **2020**, *159*, 944–955.e8. [CrossRef]
17. Dethlefsen, L.; Relman, D.A. Incomplete recovery and individualized responses of the human distal gut microbiota to repeated antibiotic perturbation. *Proc. Natl. Acad. Sci. USA* **2011**, *108* (Suppl. 1), 4554–4561. [CrossRef]
18. Rashidi, A.; Ebadi, M.; Rehman, T.U.; Elhusseini, H.; Nalluri, H.; Kaiser, T.; Holtan, S.G.; Khoruts, A.; Weisdorf, D.J.; Staley, C. Gut microbiota response to antibiotics is personalized and depends on baseline microbiota. *Microbiome* **2021**, *9*, 211. [CrossRef]
19. Agudelo-Ochoa, G.M.; Valdés-Duque, B.E.; Giraldo-Giraldo, N.A.; Jaillier-Ramírez, A.M.; Giraldo-Villa, A.; Acevedo-Castaño, I.; Yepes-Molina, M.A.; Barbosa-Barbosa, J.; Benítez-Paéz, A. Gut microbiota profiles in critically ill patients potential biomarkers and risk variables for sepsis. *Gut Microbes* **2020**, *12*, 1707610. [CrossRef]
20. De la Cuesta-Zuluaga, J.; Kelley, S.T.; Chen, Y.; Escobar, J.S.; Mueller, N.T.; Ley, R.E.; McDonald, D.; Huang, S.; Swafford, A.D.; Knight, R.; et al. Age- and Sex-Dependent Patterns of Gut Microbial Diversity in Human Adults. *Msystems* **2019**, *4*, e00261-19. [CrossRef]
21. Zhai, B.; Ola, M.; Rolling, T.; Tosini, N.L.; Joshowitz, S.; Littmann, E.R.; Amoretti, L.A.; Fontana, E.; Wright, R.J.; Miranda, E.; et al. High-resolution mycobiota analysis reveals dynamic intestinal translocation preceding invasive candidiasis. *Nat. Med.* **2020**, *26*, 59–64. [CrossRef]
22. Stoma, I.; Littmann, E.R.; Peled, J.U.; Giralt, S.; van den Brink, M.R.M.; Pamer, E.G.; Taur, Y. Compositional flux within the intestinal microbiota and risk for bloodstream infection with gram-negative bacteria. *Clin. Infect. Dis.* **2020**, *73*, e4627–e4635. [CrossRef] [PubMed]
23. Freedberg, D.E.; Zhou, M.J.; Cohen, M.E.; Annavajhala, M.K.; Khan, S.; Moscoso, D.I.; Brooks, C.; Whittier, S.; Chong, D.H.; Uhlemann, A.C.; et al. Pathogen colonization of the gastrointestinal microbiome at intensive care unit admission and risk for subsequent death or infection. *Intensive Care Med.* **2018**, *44*, 1203–1211. [CrossRef] [PubMed]
24. Baggs, J.; Jernigan, J.A.; Laufer Halpin, A.; Epstein, L.; Hatfield, K.M.; McDonald, L.C. Risk of Subsequent Sepsis within 90 Days After a Hospital Stay by Type of Antibiotic Exposure. *Clin. Infect. Dis.* **2018**, *66*, 1004–1012. [CrossRef] [PubMed]
25. Prescott, H.C.; Dickson, R.P.; Rogers, M.A.M.; Langa, K.M.; Iwashyna, T.J. Hospitalization Type and Subsequent Severe Sepsis. *Am. J. Respir. Crit. Care Med.* **2015**, *192*, 581–588. [CrossRef] [PubMed]
26. van Ruissen, M.C.E.; Bos, L.D.; Dickson, R.P.; Dondorp, A.M.; Schultsz, C.; Schultz, M.J. Manipulation of the microbiome in critical illness-probiotics as a preventive measure against ventilator-associated pneumonia. *Intensive Care Med. Exp.* **2019**, *7* (Suppl. 1), 37. [CrossRef]
27. Shimizu, K.; Ojima, M.; Ogura, H. Gut Microbiota and Probiotics/Synbiotics for Modulation of Immunity in Critically Ill Patients. *Nutrients* **2021**, *13*, 2439. [CrossRef]
28. Pamer, E.G. Resurrecting the intestinal microbiota to combat antibiotic-resistant pathogens. *Science* **2016**, *352*, 535–538. [CrossRef] [PubMed]
29. Kamada, N.; Seo, S.U.; Chen, G.Y.; Núñez, G. Role of the gut microbiota in immunity and inflammatory disease. *Nat. Rev. Immunol.* **2013**, *13*, 321–335. [CrossRef] [PubMed]
30. Dickson, R.P.; Singer, B.H.; Newstead, M.W.; Falkowski, N.R.; Erb-Downward, J.R.; Standiford, T.J.; Huffnagle, G.B. Enrichment of the lung microbiome with gut bacteria in sepsis and the acute respiratory distress syndrome. *Nat. Microbiol.* **2016**, *1*, 16113. [CrossRef] [PubMed]
31. Singer, B.H.; Dickson, R.P.; Denstaedt, S.J.; Newstead, M.W.; Kim, K.; Falkowski, N.R.; Erb-Downward, J.R.; Schmidt, T.M.; Huffnagle, G.B.; Standiford, T.J. Bacterial Dissemination to the Brain in Sepsis. *Am. J. Respir. Crit. Care Med.* **2018**, *197*, 747–756. [CrossRef]
32. Sencio, V.; Barthelemy, A.; Tavares, L.P.; Machado, M.G.; Soulard, D.; Cuinat, C.; Queiroz-Junior, C.M.; Noordine, M.L.; Salomé-Desnoulez, S.; Deryuter, L.; et al. Gut Dysbiosis during Influenza Contributes to Pulmonary Pneumococcal Superinfection through Altered Short-Chain Fatty Acid Production. *Cell Rep.* **2020**, *30*, 2934–2947.e6. [CrossRef] [PubMed]
33. McDonald, B.; Zucoloto, A.Z.; Yu, I.L.; Burkhard, R.; Brown, K.; Geuking, M.B.; McCoy, K.D. Programing of an Intravascular Immune Firewall by the Gut Microbiota Protects against Pathogen Dissemination during Infection. *Cell Host Microbe* **2020**, *28*, 660–668.e4. [CrossRef]

34. Andrade-Oliveira, V.; Amano, M.T.; Correa-Costa, M.; Castoldi, A.; Felizardo, R.J.; de Almeida, D.C.; Bassi, E.J.; Moraes-Vieira, P.M.; Hiyane, M.I.; Rodas, A.C.; et al. Gut Bacteria Products Prevent AKI Induced by Ischemia-Reperfusion. *J. Am. Soc. Nephrol.* **2015**, *26*, 1877–1888. [CrossRef]
35. Gong, S.; Yan, Z.; Liu, Z.; Niu, M.; Fang, H.; Li, N.; Huang, C.; Li, L.; Chen, G.; Luo, H.; et al. Intestinal Microbiota Mediates the Susceptibility to Polymicrobial Sepsis-Induced Liver Injury by Granisetron Generation in Mice. *Hepatology* **2019**, *69*, 1751–1767. [CrossRef]
36. Lankelma, J.M.; Cranendonk, D.R.; Belzer, C.; de Vos, A.F.; de Vos, W.M.; van der Poll, T.; Wiersinga, W.J. Antibiotic-induced gut microbiota disruption during human endotoxemia: A randomised controlled study. *Gut* **2017**, *66*, 1623–1630. [CrossRef]
37. Habes, Q.L.; Konstanti, P.; Kiers, H.D.; Koch, R.M.; Stolk, R.F.; Belzer, C.; Kox, M.; Pickkers, P. No interplay between gut microbiota composition and the lipopolysaccharide-induced innate immune response in humans in vivo. *Clin. Transl. Immunol.* **2021**, *10*, e1278. [CrossRef] [PubMed]
38. Khailova, L.; Frank, D.N.; Dominguez, J.A.; Wischmeyer, P.E. Probiotic administration reduces mortality and improves intestinal epithelial homeostasis in experimental sepsis. *Anesthesiology* **2013**, *119*, 166–177. [CrossRef] [PubMed]
39. Khailova, L.; Petrie, B.; Baird, C.H.; Dominguez Rieg, J.A.; Wischmeyer, P.E. Lactobacillus rhamnosus GG and Bifidobacterium longum attenuate lung injury and inflammatory response in experimental sepsis. *PLoS ONE* **2014**, *9*, e97861. [CrossRef] [PubMed]
40. Chen, L.; Xu, K.; Gui, Q.; Chen, Y.; Chen, D.; Yang, Y. Probiotic pre-administration reduces mortality in a mouse model of cecal ligation and puncture-induced sepsis. *Exp. Ther. Med.* **2016**, *12*, 1836–1842. [CrossRef]
41. Chen, L.; Li, H.; Li, J.; Chen, Y.; Yang, Y. Lactobacillus rhamnosus GG treatment improves intestinal permeability and modulates microbiota dysbiosis in an experimental model of sepsis. *Int. J. Mol. Med.* **2019**, *43*, 1139–1148. [CrossRef] [PubMed]
42. Chen, L.; Li, H.; Li, J.; Chen, Y.; Yang, Y. Probiotic Lactobacillus rhamnosus GG reduces mortality of septic mice by modulating gut microbiota composition and metabolic profiles. *Nutrition* **2020**, *78*, 110863. [CrossRef] [PubMed]
43. Singer, J.R.; Blosser, E.G.; Zindl, C.L.; Silberger, D.J.; Conlan, S.; Laufer, V.A.; DiToro, D.; Deming, C.; Kumar, R.; Morrow, C.; et al. Preventing dysbiosis of the neonatal mouse intestinal microbiome protects against late-onset sepsis. *Nat. Med.* **2019**, *25*, 1772–1782. [CrossRef]
44. Kalil, A.C.; Metersky, M.L.; Klompas, M.; Muscedere, J.; Sweeney, D.A.; Palmer, L.B.; Napolitano, L.M.; O'Grady, N.P.; Bartlett, J.G.; Carratalà, J.; et al. Management of Adults With Hospital-acquired and Ventilator-associated Pneumonia: 2016 Clinical Practice Guidelines by the Infectious Diseases Society of America and the American Thoracic Society. *Clin. Infect. Dis.* **2016**, *63*, e61–e111. [CrossRef] [PubMed]
45. Torres, A.; Cilloniz, C.; Niederman, M.S.; Menéndez, R.; Chalmers, J.D.; Wunderink, R.G.; van der Poll, T. Pneumonia. *Nat. Rev. Dis. Prim.* **2021**, *7*, 25. [CrossRef]
46. Kalanuria, A.A.; Zai, W.; Mirski, M. Ventilator-associated pneumonia in the ICU. *Crit. Care* **2014**, *18*, 208. [CrossRef]
47. Bielen, K.; Jongers, B.; Boddaert, J.; Lammens, C.; Jorens, P.G.; Malhotra-Kumar, S.; Goossens, H.; Kumar-Singh, S. Mechanical Ventilation Induces Interleukin 4 Secretion in Lungs and Reduces the Phagocytic Capacity of Lung Macrophages. *J. Infect. Dis.* **2018**, *217*, 1645–1655. [CrossRef] [PubMed]
48. van Vught, L.A.; Scicluna, B.P.; Wiewel, M.A.; Hoogendijk, A.J.; Klein Klouwenberg, P.M.; Franitza, M.; Toliat, M.R.; Nürnberg, P.; Cremer, O.L.; Horn, J.; et al. Comparative Analysis of the Host Response to Community-acquired and Hospital-acquired Pneumonia in Critically Ill Patients. *Am. J. Respir. Crit. Care Med.* **2016**, *194*, 1366–1374. [CrossRef] [PubMed]
49. Conway Morris, A.; Anderson, N.; Brittan, M.; Wilkinson, T.S.; McAuley, D.F.; Antonelli, J.; McCulloch, C.; Barr, L.C.; Dhaliwal, K.; Jones, R.O. Combined dysfunctions of immune cells predict nosocomial infection in critically ill patients. *Br. J. Anaesth.* **2013**, *111*, 778–787. [CrossRef] [PubMed]
50. Soussan, R.; Schimpf, C.; Pilmis, B.; Degroote, T.; Tran, M.; Bruel, C.; Philippart, F.; RESIST Study Group. Ventilator-associated pneumonia: The central role of transcolonization. *J. Crit. Care* **2019**, *50*, 155–161. [CrossRef] [PubMed]
51. Batra, P.; Soni, K.D.; Mathur, P. Efficacy of probiotics in the prevention of VAP in critically ill ICU patients: An updated systematic review and meta-analysis of randomized control trials. *J. Intensive Care* **2020**, *8*, 81. [CrossRef]
52. Bo, L.; Li, J.; Tao, T.; Bai, Y.; Ye, X.; Hotchkiss, R.S.; Kollef, M.H.; Crooks, N.H.; Deng, X. Probiotics for preventing ventilator-associated pneumonia. *Cochrane Database Syst. Rev.* **2014**, *10*, CD009066. [CrossRef]
53. Weng, H.; Li, J.G.; Mao, Z.; Feng, Y.; Wang, C.Y.; Ren, X.Q.; Zeng, X.T. Probiotics for Preventing Ventilator-Associated Pneumonia in Mechanically Ventilated Patients: A Meta-Analysis with Trial Sequential Analysis. *Front. Pharmacol.* **2017**, *8*, 717. [PubMed]
54. Liu, K.X.; Zhu, Y.G.; Zhang, J.; Tao, L.L.; Lee, J.W.; Wang, X.D.; Qu, J.M. Probiotics' effects on the incidence of nosocomial pneumonia in critically ill patients: A systematic review and meta-analysis. *Crit. Care* **2012**, *16*, R109. [CrossRef] [PubMed]
55. Manzanares, W.; Lemieux, M.; Langlois, P.L.; Wischmeyer, P.E. Probiotic and synbiotic therapy in critical illness: A systematic review and meta-analysis. *Crit. Care* **2016**, *20*, 262. [CrossRef] [PubMed]
56. Su, M.; Jia, Y.; Li, Y.; Zhou, D.; Jia, J. Probiotics for the Prevention of Ventilator-Associated Pneumonia: A Meta-Analysis of Randomized Controlled Trials. *Respir. Care* **2020**, *65*, 673–685. [CrossRef] [PubMed]
57. Johnstone, J.; Meade, M.; Lauzier, F.; Marshall, J.; Duan, E.; Dionne, J.; Arabi, Y.M.; Heels-Ansdell, D.; Thabane, L.; Lamarche, D.; et al. Effect of Probiotics on Incident Ventilator-Associated Pneumonia in Critically Ill Patients: A Randomized Clinical Trial. *JAMA* **2021**, *326*, 1024–1033. [CrossRef] [PubMed]

58. Tsilika, M.; Thoma, G.; Aidoni, Z.; Tsaousi, G.; Fotiadis, K.; Stavrou, G.; Malliou, P.; Chorti, A.; Massa, H.; Antypa, E.; et al. A four-probiotic preparation for ventilator-associated pneumonia in multi-trauma patients: Results of a randomized clinical trial. *Int. J. Antimicrob. Agents* **2021**, *59*, 106471. [CrossRef] [PubMed]
59. Litton, E.; Anstey, M.; Broadhurst, D.; Chapman, A.; Currie, A.; Ferrier, J.; Gummer, J.; Higgins, A.; Lim, J.; Manning, L.; et al. Early and sustained Lactobacillus plantarum probiotic therapy in critical illness: The randomised, placebo-controlled, restoration of gut microflora in critical illness trial (ROCIT). *Intensive Care Med.* **2021**, *47*, 307–315. [CrossRef]
60. Hempel, S.; Newberry, S.J.; Maher, A.R.; Wang, Z.; Miles, J.N.; Shanman, R.; Johnsen, B.; Shekelle, P.G. Probiotics for the prevention and treatment of antibiotic-associated diarrhea: A systematic review and meta-analysis. *JAMA* **2012**, *307*, 1959–1969.
61. Goldenberg, J.Z.; Yap, C.; Lytvyn, L.; Lo, C.K.; Beardsley, J.; Mertz, D.; Johnston, B.C. Probiotics for the prevention of Clostridium difficile-associated diarrhea in adults and children. *Cochrane Database Syst. Rev.* **2017**, *12*, CD006095. [CrossRef]
62. McDonald, L.C.; Gerding, D.N.; Johnson, S.; Bakken, J.S.; Carroll, K.C.; Coffin, S.E.; Dubberke, E.R.; Garey, K.W.; Gould, C.V.; Kelly, C. Clinical Practice Guidelines for Clostridium difficile Infection in Adults and Children: 2017 Update by the Infectious Diseases Society of America (IDSA) and Society for Healthcare Epidemiology of America (SHEA). *Clin. Infect. Dis.* **2018**, *66*, e1–e48. [CrossRef] [PubMed]
63. van Prehn, J.; Reigadas, E.; Vogelzang, E.H.; Bouza, E.; Hristea, A.; Guery, B.; Krutova, M.; Norén, T.; Allerberger, F.; Coia, J.; et al. European Society of Clinical Microbiology and Infectious Diseases: 2021 update on the treatment guidance document for Clostridioides difficile infection in adults. *Clin. Microbiol. Infect.* **2021**, *27* (Suppl. 2), S1–S21. [CrossRef] [PubMed]
64. Din, A.U.; Mazhar, M.; Waseem, M.; Ahmad, W.; Bibi, A.; Hassan, A.; Ali, N.; Gang, W.; Qian, G.; Ullah, R.; et al. SARS-CoV-2 microbiome dysbiosis linked disorders and possible probiotics role. *Biomed. Pharmacother.* **2021**, *133*, 110947. [CrossRef] [PubMed]
65. Besselink, M.G.; van Santvoort, H.C.; Buskens, E.; Boermeester, M.A.; van Goor, H.; Timmerman, H.M.; Nieuwenhuijs, V.B.; Bollen, T.L.; van Ramshorst, B.; Witteman, B.J.; et al. Probiotic prophylaxis in predicted severe acute pancreatitis: A randomised, double-blind, placebo-controlled trial. *Lancet* **2008**, *371*, 651–659. [CrossRef]
66. Bongaerts, G.P.; Severijnen, R.S. A reassessment of the PROPATRIA study and its implications for probiotic therapy. *Nat. Biotechnol.* **2016**, *34*, 55–63. [CrossRef] [PubMed]
67. The Editors of the Lancet. Expression of concern—Probiotic prophylaxis in predicted severe acute pancreatitis: A randomised, double-blind, placebo-controlled trial. *Lancet* **2010**, *375*, 875–876. [CrossRef]
68. Didari, T.; Solki, S.; Mozaffari, S.; Nikfar, S.; Abdollahi, M. A systematic review of the safety of probiotics. *Expert Opin. Drug Saf.* **2014**, *13*, 227–239. [CrossRef]
69. Yelin, I.; Flett, K.B.; Merakou, C.; Mehrotra, P.; Stam, J.; Snesrud, E.; Hinkle, M.; Lesho, E.; McGann, P.; McAdam, A.J.; et al. Genomic and epidemiological evidence of bacterial transmission from probiotic capsule to blood in ICU patients. *Nat. Med.* **2019**, *25*, 1728–1732. [CrossRef]
70. Bafeta, A.; Koh, M.; Riveros, C.; Ravaud, P. Harms reporting in randomized controlled trials of interventions aimed at modifying microbiota: A systematic review. *Ann. Intern. Med.* **2018**, *169*, 240–247. [CrossRef]
71. Sorbara, M.T.; Littmann, E.R.; Fontana, E.; Moody, T.U.; Kohout, C.E.; Gjonbalaj, M.; Eaton, V.; Seok, R.; Leiner, I.M.; Pamer, E.G. Functional and Genomic Variation between Human-Derived Isolates of Lachnospiraceae Reveals Inter- and Intra-Species Diversity. *Cell Host Microbe.* **2020**, *28*, 134–146.e4. [CrossRef]
72. Morrow, L.E.; Wishmeyer, P. Blurred Lines: Dysbiosis and Probiotics in the ICU. *Chest* **2017**, *151*, 492–499. [CrossRef]
73. Kristensen, N.B.; Bryrup, T.; Allin, K.H.; Nielsen, T.; Hansen, T.H.; Pedersen, O. Alterations in fecal microbiota composition by probiotic supplementation in healthy adults: A systematic review of randomized controlled trials. *Genome med.* **2016**, *8*, 52. [CrossRef]
74. Zmora, N.; Zilberman-Schapira, G.; Suez, J.; Mor, U.; Dori-Bachash, M.; Bashiardes, S.; Kotler, E.; Zur, M.; Regev-Lehavi, D.; Brik, R.B.; et al. Personalized Gut Mucosal Colonization Resistance to Empiric Probiotics Is Associated with Unique Host and Microbiome Features. *Cell* **2018**, *174*, 1388–1405.e21. [CrossRef] [PubMed]
75. Suez, J.; Zmora, N.; Zilberman-Schapira, G.; Mor, U.; Dori-Bachash, M.; Bashiardes, S.; Zur, M.; Regev-Lehavi, D.; Ben-Zeev Brik, R.; Federici, S.; et al. Post-Antibiotic Gut Mucosal Microbiome Reconstitution Is Impaired by Probiotics and Improved by Autologous FMT. *Cell* **2017**, *174*, 1406–1423.e16. [CrossRef] [PubMed]
76. Hooks, K.B.; O'Malley, M.A. Dysbiosis and Its Discontents. *MBio* **2017**, *8*, e01492-17. [CrossRef] [PubMed]
77. McBurney, M.I.; Davis, C.; Fraser, C.M.; Schneeman, B.O.; Huttenhower, C.; Verbeke, K.; Walter, J.; Latulippe, M.E. Establishing What Constitutes a Healthy Human Gut Microbiome: State of the Science, Regulatory Considerations, and Future Directions. *J. Nutr.* **2019**, *149*, 1882–1895. [CrossRef]
78. Fischbach, M.A. Microbiome: Focus on Causation and Mechanism. *Cell* **2018**, *174*, 785–790. [CrossRef]
79. O'Toole, P.W.; Marchesi, J.R.; Hill, C. Next-generation probiotics: The spectrum from probiotics to live biotherapeutics. *Nat. Microbiol.* **2017**, *2*, 17057. [CrossRef]
80. Caballero, S.; Kim, S.; Carter, R.A.; Leiner, I.M.; Sušac, B.; Miller, L.; Kim, G.J.; Ling, L.; Pamer, E.G. Cooperating Commensals Restore Colonization Resistance to Vancomycin-Resistant Enterococcus faecium. *Cell Host Microbe.* **2017**, *21*, 592–602.e4. [CrossRef]

81. Buffie, C.G.; Bucci, V.; Stein, R.R.; McKenney, P.T.; Ling, L.; Gobourne, A.; No, D.; Liu, H.; Kinnebrew, M.; Viale, A.; et al. Precision microbiome reconstitution restores bile acid mediated resistance to *Clostridium difficile*. *Nature* **2015**, *517*, 205–208. [CrossRef] [PubMed]
82. Maier, L.; Goemans, C.V.; Wirbel, J.; Kuhn, M.; Eberl, C.; Pruteanu, M.; Müller, P.; Garcia-Santamarina, S.; Cacace, E.; Zhang, B.; et al. Unravelling the collateral damage of antibiotics on gut bacteria. *Nature* **2021**, *599*, 120–124. [CrossRef] [PubMed]

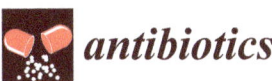

Article

Size Matters: The Influence of Patient Size on Antibiotics Exposure Profiles in Critically Ill Patients on Continuous Renal Replacement Therapy

Soo-Min Jang [1,*], Alex R. Shaw [2] and Bruce A. Mueller [3]

1. Department of Pharmacy Practice, Loma Linda University School of Pharmacy, Loma Linda, CA 92350, USA
2. Medical Strategist, Ironwood Pharmaceuticals, Boston, MA 02110, USA; arshaw89@gmail.com
3. Department of Clinical Pharmacy, University of Michigan College of Pharmacy, Ann Arbor, MI 48109, USA; muellerb@med.umich.edu
* Correspondence: smjang@llu.edu

Abstract: (1) Purpose of this study: To determine whether patient weight influences the probability of target attainment (PTA) over 72 h of initial therapy with beta-lactam (cefepime, ceftazidime, piperacillin/tazobactam) and carbapenem (imipenem, ertapenem, meropenem) antibiotics in the critical care setting. This is the first paper to address the question of whether patient size affects antibiotic PTA in the ICU. (2) Methods: We performed a post hoc analysis of Monte Carlo simulations conducted in virtual critically ill patients receiving antibiotics and continuous renal replacement therapy. The PTA was calculated for each antibiotic on the following pharmacodynamic (PD) targets: (a) were above the target organism's minimum inhibitory concentration ($\geq$%fT$\geq$1×MIC), (b) were above four times the MIC ($\geq$%fT$\geq$4×MIC), and (c) were always above the MIC ($\geq$100%fT$\geq$MIC) for the first 72 h of antibiotic therapy. The PTA was analyzed in patient weight quartiles [Q1 (lightest)-Q4 (heaviest)]. Optimal doses were defined as the lowest dose achieving $\geq$90% PTA. (3) Results: The PTA for fT$\geq$1×MIC led to similarly high rates regardless of weight quartiles. Yet, patient weight influenced the PTA for higher PD targets (100%fT$\geq$MIC and fT$\geq$4×MIC) with commonly used beta-lactams and carbapenems. Reaching the optimal PTA was more difficult with a PD target of 100%fT$\geq$MIC compared to fT$\geq$4×MIC. (4) Conclusions: The Monte Carlo simulations showed patients in lower weight quartiles tended to achieve higher antibiotic pharmacodynamic target attainment compared to heavier patients.

Keywords: renal replacement therapy; Monte Carlo simulation; antibiotics; pharmacokinetics; pharmacodynamics

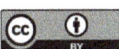

1. Introduction

Continuous renal replacement therapy (CRRT) is the preferred renal replacement therapy (RRT) over intermittent hemodialysis in patients with acute kidney injury (AKI) due to hemodynamic instability [1]. The multicenter study Veterans Affairs/National Institutes of Health Acute Renal Failure Trial Network Study (ATN trial) showed that there was no difference in clinical outcomes when patients received less-intensive or intensive effluent rates for CRRT [2]. Since the antibiotic doses were used in both intensity arms, some suggested that patients with intensive CRRT may have had lower overall antibiotic exposures due to a higher drug removal rate [3,4]. Our previous study showed there were no significant differences in the probability of target attainment (PTA) between less-intensive (20–25 mL/kg/h) vs. intensive (35–45 mL/kg/h) effluent rate arms [5].

The combination of AKI and aggressive fluid resuscitation for sepsis leads to a considerable amount of fluid weight gain, increasing the volume of distribution (Vd) in drugs [6]. Increased Vd leads to a lower plasma concentration, requiring higher doses of a drug. This is noteworthy because altered Vd in AKI patients receiving CRRT can cause high interindividual and interoccasion variability in antibiotic serum concentrations [7]. For example, interindividual variability was noted with piperacillin and tazobactam trough levels by ≥123-fold and ≥192-fold, respectively, in critically ill patients [8]. Moreover, the majority of clinical studies that derived dosing recommendations do not include larger patients (>100 kg), and obesity is a well-known risk factor of antibiotic therapy failure [9,10].

Antimicrobial activity is impacted by multiple factors, including drug dose regimen, potency of the drug against a specific organism, and pharmacokinetic (PK) parameters. For beta-lactam agents, in vitro and clinical studies suggest that maintaining free serum concentrations at least four times as high as the organism's minimum inhibitory concentration (MIC) (fT≥4×MIC) optimizes bactericidal activity and clinical response in critically ill patients compared to less stringent pharmacodynamic targets [11–13]. Moreover, clinical outcomes were superior when the PD target maintained free drug concentrations above the 1×MIC (fT≥1×MIC) level for 100% of the dosing interval in critically ill patients [14]. The objective of this post-hoc study was to determine PTA over the first 72 h of commonly prescribed doses of beta-lactams (cefepime, ceftazidime, and piperacillin/tazobactam) and carbapenems (imipenem, meropenem) in different patient weight quartiles using Monte Carlo simulation (MCS) techniques.

2. Results

The PTA rates in overall (for all 10,000 virtual patients) and in different weight quartiles [Q1 (lightest) to Q4 (heaviest)] for cefepime, ceftazidime, piperacillin, and tazobactam are reported in Table 1. Table 2 lists the PTA for overall virtual patients and different weight quartiles for the meropenem, imipenem, and ertapenem dosing regimens. Three different pharmacodynamic targets were assessed, from the least stringent %fT≥1×MIC to the most stringent target of 100%fT≥MIC.

Table 1. Probability of target attainment comparison among weight quartiles for key beta-lactams used in the ATN trial: Cefepime, ceftazidime, piperacillin, and tazobactam.

	ATN Less Intensive				ATN Intensive		
Weight Quartile	1×MIC	4×MIC	100% fT>1×MIC	Weight Quartile	1×MIC	4×MIC	100% fT>1×MIC
Cefepime 1 g every 12 h							
Overall	100%	7.8%	10.8%	Overall	99.9%	2.3%	8.4%
Q1 (40–70 kg)	100%	18.2%	31%	Q1 (40–70 kg)	99.8%	6.5%	24.4%
Q2 (70–82 kg)	100%	8.6%	9.6%	Q2 (70–82 kg)	100%	2.2%	7.7%
Q3 (82–95 kg)	100%	3.7%	2.3%	Q3 (82–96 kg)	100%	0.6%	1.3%
Q4 (95–177 kg)	100%	0.6%	0.4%	Q4 (96–204 kg)	100%	0.0%	0.1%
Cefepime 1 g every 8 h							
Overall	100%	57.4%	15.5%	Overall	100%	33%	15.6%
Q1 (40–70 kg)	100%	79.6%	43.7%	Q1 (40–70 kg)	100%	59.7%	44.9%
Q2 (70–82 kg)	100%	68.6%	14.2%	Q2 (70–82 kg)	100%	39.8%	13.5%
Q3 (82–95 kg)	100%	54.5%	4%	Q3 (82–96 kg)	100%	24.4%	3.8%
Q4 (95–189 kg)	100%	27.1%	0.2%	Q4 (96–213 kg)	100%	8.2%	0.4%
Cefepime 2 g every 12 h							
Overall	100%	86.5%	56.3%	Overall	100%	77.2%	55.2%
Q1 (40–70 kg)	100%	94.04%	90.3%	Q1 (40–70 kg)	100%	88.7%	88.1%
Q2 (70–82 kg)	100%	93.9%	71%	Q2 (70–82 kg)	100%	86.9%	70.6%
Q3 (82–95 kg)	100%	89.04%	46.4%	Q3 (82–96 kg)	100%	79.2%	44.9%
Q4 (95–180 kg)	100%	69.04%	17.3%	Q4 (96–183 kg)	100%	53.9%	17.0%

Table 1. Cont.

	ATN Less Intensive				ATN Intensive		
Weight Quartile	1×MIC	4×MIC	100% fT>1×MIC	Weight Quartile	1×MIC	4×MIC	100% fT>1×MIC
Cefepime 2 g every 8 h							
Overall	100%	100%	57%	Overall	100%	99%	56.9%
Q1 (40–70 kg)	100%	100%	92.4%	Q1 (40–70 kg)	100%	99.7%	92.4%
Q2 (70–82 kg)	100%	100%	72.6%	Q2 (70–82 kg)	100%	100.0%	71.4%
Q3 (82–96 kg)	100%	100%	45.6%	Q3 (82–96 kg)	100%	99.8%	46.2%
Q4 (96–185 kg)	100%	98.9%	17.3%	Q4 (96–217 kg)	100%	96.3%	17.5%
Ceftazidime 1 g every 12 h							
Overall	100%	31.3%	31.2%	Overall	100%	16.9%	24.7%
Q1 (40–70 kg)	100%	54.5%	51.8%	Q1 (40–70 kg)	100%	37.6%	46.3%
Q2 (70–82 kg)	100%	37%	34.8%	Q2 (70–82 kg)	100%	18.3%	29.3%
Q3 (82–95 kg)	100%	23.8%	25.7%	Q3 (82–96 kg)	100%	8.8%	16.5%
Q4 (95–200 kg)	100%	9.7%	12.5%	Q4 (96–204 kg)	99.9%	2.9%	6.8%
Ceftazidime 2 g every 12 h							
Overall	100%	95.7%	81.1%	Overall	100%	88%	78.3%
Q1 (40–70 kg)	100%	97.9%	93.2%	Q1 (40–70 kg)	100%	88.1%	78.5%
Q2 (70–82 kg)	100%	97.4%	86.7%	Q2 (70–82 kg)	100%	87.7%	78.4%
Q3 (82–95 kg)	100%	96.7%	81.0%	Q3 (82–96 kg)	100%	88%	78.2%
Q4 (95–183 kg)	100%	90.9%	63.5%	Q4 (96–193 kg)	100%	88.2%	78.3%
Piperacillin 3 g every 12 h							
Overall	93.4%	30.7%	23.8%	Overall	91.9%	24.4%	20.5%
Q1 (41–71 kg)	91%	38%	35.2%	Q1 (40–70 kg)	90.1%	33.0%	32.6%
Q2 (71–82 kg)	93.3%	33%	27.6%	Q2 (70–82 kg)	91.4%	25.8%	23.3%
Q3 (82–96 kg)	94.5%	28.9%	20.4%	Q3 (82–96 kg)	92.2%	22.9%	16.2%
Q4 (96–191 kg)	94.6%	22.9%	11.9%	Q4 (96–204 kg)	93.8%	16.1%	9.7%
Piperacillin 4 g every 12 h							
Overall	96.3%	50%	42.8%	Overall	95.4%	44.6%	38.4%
Q1 (40–70 kg)	94.7%	49%	55.7%	Q1 (40–70 kg)	93.8%	53.0%	51.2%
Q2 (70–82 kg)	95.3%	48.8%	46.8%	Q2 (70–82 kg)	94.8%	48.3%	43.6%
Q3 (82–95 kg)	97.3%	51.7%	40.8%	Q3 (82–96 kg)	96.2%	43.0%	34.6%
Q4 (95–184 kg)	97.8%	50.4%	28%	Q4 (96–213 kg)	96.6%	34.0%	24.0%
Piperacillin 3 g every 8 h							
Overall	99%	61%	33.5%	Overall	98.8%	56.6%	33.1%
Q1 (40–71 kg)	98.7%	66.1%	50.9%	Q1 (40–70 kg)	97.4%	62.0%	50.1%
Q2 (71–82 kg)	98.8%	63.5%	37.2%	Q2 (70–82 kg)	99.2%	60.2%	37.5%
Q3 (82–95 kg)	99%	59.8%	29%	Q3 (82–96 kg)	99.3%	56.6%	28.6%
Q4 (95–191 kg)	99.4%	54.4%	17%	Q4 (96–183 kg)	99.4%	47.3%	16.0%

Table 1. Cont.

	ATN Less Intensive				ATN Intensive		
Weight Quartile	1×MIC	4×MIC	100% fT>1×MIC	Weight Quartile	1×MIC	4×MIC	100% fT>1×MIC
Piperacillin 4 g every 8 h							
Overall	99.5%	77.9%	54.6%	Overall	99.3%	75.1%	52.9%
Q1 (40–70 kg)	99%	81%	72%	Q1 (40–70 kg)	98.5%	77.6%	69.4%
Q2 (70–82 kg)	99.5%	78.2%	59.2%	Q2 (70–82 kg)	99.3%	76.9%	59.2%
Q3 (82–96 kg)	99.5%	77.2%	49.2%	Q3 (82–96 kg)	99.6%	74.8%	49.0%
Q4 (96–206 kg)	99.8%	75.2%	37.9%	Q4 (96–217 kg)	99.7%	71.1%	33.7%
Piperacillin 3 g every 6 h							
Overall	99.9%	80%	39.2%	Overall	99.8%	77.1%	37.9%
Q1 (40–70 kg)	99.8%	83.6%	60%	Q1 (40–70 kg)	99.6%	80.4%	58.4%
Q2 (70–82 kg)	99.8%	81.6%	43.6%	Q2 (70–82 kg)	99.9%	77.9%	42.7%
Q3 (82–96 kg)	99.9%	79.4%	32.8%	Q3 (82–96 kg)	99.7%	78.4%	31.8%
Q4 (96–217 kg)	100%	75.5%	20.2%	Q4 (96–217 kg)	100%	71.5%	18.6%
Piperacillin 4 g every 6 h							
Overall	99.9%	89.9%	60%	Overall	99.9%	88.5%	57.6%
Q1 (40–71 kg)	99.8%	89.9%	77.9%	Q1 (40–70 kg)	99.8%	90.7%	76.2%
Q2 (71–82 kg)	100%	89.5%	66.2%	Q2 (70–82 kg)	99.8%	89.0%	63.4%
Q3 (82–95 kg)	99.9%	90.4%	56%	Q3 (82–96 kg)	99.9%	87.8%	54.5%
Q4 (95–184 kg)	100%	89.8%	39.8%	Q4 (96–217 kg)	100%	86.4%	36.0%
Tazobactam 375 mg every 12 h							
Overall	76.8%	10%	3.6%	Overall	73%	5.4%	2.3%
Q1 (40–71 kg)	79.4%	17.5%	7.2%	Q1 (40–70 kg)	76.5%	10.4%	4.6%
Q2 (71–82 kg)	78.2%	10.6%	3.6%	Q2 (70–82 kg)	76.1%	5.5%	2.4%
Q3 (82–95 kg)	76.4%	7.4%	2.3%	Q3 (82–96 kg)	72.9%	3.9%	1.6%
Q4 (95–199 kg)	73%	4.4%	1.2%	Q4 (96–202 kg)	66.2%	1.8%	0.7%
Tazobactam 500 mg every 12 h							
Overall	84.7%	21.8%	8.5%	Overall	82.9%	14.8%	7%
Q1 (40–71 kg)	85.4%	30.5%	13.8%	Q1 (40–70 kg)	84.5%	23.7%	13.1%
Q2 (71–82 kg)	84.2%	23.6%	9.6%	Q2 (70–82 kg)	84.5%	16.5%	7.7%
Q3 (82–96 kg)	85.7%	19.6%	6.6%	Q3 (82–96 kg)	81.4%	12.5%	5.0%
Q4 (96–187 kg)	83.6%	13.4%	4.1%	Q4 (96–204 kg)	80.6%	6.7%	2.2%
Tazobactam 375 mg every 8 h							
Overall	89.1%	27.9%	4.7%	Overall	87.8%	20.9%	4.6%
Q1 (40–71 kg)	89.5%	36.1%	8.8%	Q1 (40–70 kg)	88.6%	30.3%	9.2%
Q2 (71–82 kg)	89.4%	31.8%	4.9%	Q2 (70–82 kg)	87.6%	25.0%	5.5%
Q3 (82–95 kg)	88.9%	25.1%	3.2%	Q3 (82–96 kg)	88.1%	17.2%	2.4%
Q4 (95–222 kg)	88.5%	18.7%	1.9%	Q4 (96–184 kg)	86.6%	11.2%	1.3%

Table 1. Cont.

	ATN Less Intensive				ATN Intensive		
Weight Quartile	1×MIC	4×MIC	100% fT>1×MIC	Weight Quartile	1×MIC	4×MIC	100% fT>1×MIC
Tazobactam 375 mg every 6 h							
Overall	93.4%	44.8%	6.6%	Overall	93.6%	38.8%	6.2%
Q1 (40–70 kg)	93.8%	53.8%	11.5%	Q1 (40–70 kg)	94.2%	50.5%	12.0%
Q2 (70–82 kg)	92.8%	47.5%	6.7%	Q2 (70–82 kg)	93.6%	42.1%	6.8%
Q3 (82–95 kg)	94%	43%	5.2%	Q3 (82–96 kg)	94.1%	37.1%	4.0%
Q4 (95–225 kg)	93%	35.1%	2.9%	Q4 (96–185 kg)	92.4%	25.3%	1.9%
Tazobactam 500 mg every 8 h							
Overall	93.2%	45.5%	11.7%	Overall	92.3%	38%	10.3%
Q1 (40–70 kg)	93%	56.2%	19.3%	Q1 (40–70 kg)	92.5%	48.5%	17.8%
Q2 (70–82 kg)	93.7%	48.6%	13.6%	Q2 (70–82 kg)	92.9%	42.6%	10.5%
Q3 (82–96 kg)	92.3%	43.2%	8.8%	Q3 (82–96 kg)	92.1%	35.5%	8.4%
Q4 (96–181 kg)	93.4%	34.2%	5%	Q4 (96–181 kg)	91.6%	25.5%	4.6%
Tazobactam 500 mg every 6 h							
Overall	96.1%	61.3%	13.3%	Overall	95.8%	55.3%	12.3%
Q1 (40–71 kg)	96%	68.9%	22.6%	Q1 (40–70 kg)	95.8%	64.8%	20.1%
Q2 (71–82 kg)	96%	63.8%	14.8%	Q2 (70–82 kg)	96.2%	60.5%	13.5%
Q3 (82–96 kg)	96.2%	59.4%	9.6%	Q3 (82–96 kg)	96.0%	53.3%	10.1%
Q4 (96–182 kg)	96.4%	53%	6.4%	Q4 (96–209 kg)	94.9%	42.6%	5.6%

Shaded to represent probability of target attainment ≥90% (green), 60 < 90% (orange), and <60% (red).

Table 2. Probability of target attainment comparison among weight quartiles for key carbapenems used in the ATN trial: ertapenem, imipenem, and meropenem.

	ATN Less Intensive				ATN Intensive		
Wt. Quartile	1×MIC	4×MIC	100% fT≥1×MIC	Wt. Quartile	1×MIC	4×MIC	100% fT≥1×MIC
Ertapenem 1 g every 24 h (MIC 1)							
Overall	100%	100%	99.72%	Overall	100%	99.98%	99.17%
Q1 (40–70 kg)	100%	100%	99%	Q1 (40–70 kg)	100%	100%	97.5%
Q2 (70–82 kg)	100%	100%	99.9%	Q2 (70–82 kg)	100%	100%	99.6%
Q3 (82–96 kg)	100%	100%	100%	Q3 (82–96 kg)	100%	100%	99.7%
Q4 (96–204 kg)	99.9%	99.9%	100%	Q4 (96–212 kg)	99.9%	99.8%	99.8%
Ertapenem 1 g every 24 h (MIC 2)							
Overall	100%	98.2%	93.7%	Overall	98.2%	87.32%	87.73%
Q1 (40–70 kg)	100%	99.7%	91.2%	Q1 (40–70 kg)	100%	98.6%	82%
Q2 (70–82 kg)	100%	99.6%	97.6%	Q2 (70–82 kg)	100%	96%	91.8%
Q3 (82–96 kg)	100%	98.8%	97.8%	Q3 (82–96 kg)	100%	89.8%	93.4%
Q4 (96–213 kg)	99.9%	94.6%	87.2%	Q4 (96–212 kg)	99.9%	64.7%	83.7%
Imipenem 500 mg every 12 h							
Overall	98%	3.3%	5.8%	Overall	97.3%	1.8%	3.6%
Q1 (40–70 kg)	95%	3.8%	3.2%	Q1 (40–70 kg)	92.2%	2.7%	2.2%
Q2 (70–82 kg)	98%	3.8%	5.5%	Q2 (70–82 kg)	98.1%	2.0%	3.9%
Q3 (82–95 kg)	99.2%	3.5%	7.9%	Q3 (82–96 kg)	99.2%	1.4%	3.9%
Q4 (95–199 kg)	99.9%	2.1%	6.4%	Q4 (96–201 kg)	99.6%	1.1%	4.4%
Imipenem 500 mg every 8 h							
Overall	100%	40%	39.9%	Overall	100%	32.8%	33.4%
Q1 (40–71 kg)	100%	44%	36.2%	Q1 (40–70 kg)	100%	36.2%	29.2%
Q2 (71–82 kg)	100%	43.7%	46.8%	Q2 (70–82 kg)	100%	36.2%	38.2%
Q3 (82–95 kg)	100%	39.2%	46.2%	Q3 (82–96 kg)	100%	33.9%	38.9%
Q4 (95–196 kg)	100%	33.2%	30.4%	Q4 (96–212 kg)	100%	24.6%	27.2%

Table 2. Cont.

	ATN Less Intensive				ATN Intensive		
Wt. Quartile	1×MIC	4×MIC	100% fT≥1×MIC	Wt. Quartile	1×MIC	4×MIC	100% fT≥1×MIC
Imipenem 500 mg every 6 h							
Overall	100%	78.3%	61.6%	Overall	97.3%	74.6%	60%
Q1 (40–71 kg)	100%	80.5%	71.3%	Q1 (40–70 kg)	100%	77.5%	68.1%
Q2 (71–82 kg)	100%	80%	71.7%	Q2 (70–82 kg)	100%	77.4%	70.6%
Q3 (82–95 kg)	100%	78%	61.8%	Q3 (82–96 kg)	100%	75%	60.7%
Q4 (95–191 kg)	100%	74.8%	41.8%	Q4 (96–187 kg)	100%	68.5%	40.9%
Imipenem 1 g every 8 h							
Overall	100%	98%	87%	Overall	100%	97.3%	82.3%
Q1 (40–71 kg)	100%	96.8%	71.4%	Q1 (40–70 kg)	100%	96.6%	65.6%
Q2 (71–82 kg)	100%	98.4%	87%	Q2 (70–82 kg)	100%	96.8%	81.0%
Q3 (82–96 kg)	100%	98.8%	93.5%	Q3 (82–96 kg)	100%	98.1%	88.9%
Q4 (96–193 kg)	100%	98.2%	96%	Q4 (96–202 kg)	100%	97.8%	93.8%
Meropenem 500 mg every 12 h							
Overall	97.6%	63.3%	45.7%	Overall	97.4%	58.1%	45.7%
Q1 (40–71 kg)	96.1%	66.4%	58.4%	Q1 (40–70 kg)	95.8%	65.1%	54.6%
Q2 (71–82 kg)	97.6%	65.8%	52.4%	Q2 (70–82 kg)	96.8%	60.0%	47.9%
Q3 (82–96 kg)	97.9%	63.8%	43.4%	Q3 (82–96 kg)	98.1%	57.8%	40.9%
Q4 (96–173 kg)	98.8%	57.2%	28.6%	Q4 (96–217 kg)	98.9%	49.6%	24.5%
Meropenem 500 mg every 8 h							
Overall	99.8%	84.8%	57.9%	Overall	99.7%	82.6%	55.8%
Q1 (40–71 kg)	99.5%	87.2%	77.6%	Q1 (40–70 kg)	99.2%	85.6%	74.1%
Q2 (71–82 kg)	99.8%	85.08%	64.9%	Q2 (70–82 kg)	99.8%	83.6%	63.8%
Q3 (82–96 kg)	100%	84.9%	55.1%	Q3 (82–96 kg)	99.7%	82.2%	52.8%
Q4 (96–189 kg)	99.8%	81.8%	33.9%	Q4 (96–206 kg)	99.9%	78.8%	32.5%
Meropenem 1 g every 12 h							
Overall	99.4%	90.6%	82%	Overall	99.2%	89.8%	79.5%
Q1 (40–70 kg)	98.6%	88.6%	77.6%	Q1 (40–70 kg)	98%	87.5%	74.2%
Q2 (70–82 kg)	99.3%	90.7%	84.4%	Q2 (70–82 kg)	99%	90%	81%
Q3 (82–95 kg)	99.8%	91.8%	85.8%	Q3 (82–96 kg)	100%	90.6%	82.8%
Q4 (95–183 kg)	99.9%	91.1%	80%	Q4 (96–206 kg)	100%	90.8%	79.8%
Meropenem 1 g every 8 h							
Overall	100%	98.1%	92.2%	Overall	99.9%	97.6%	90.8%
Q1 (40–70 kg)	99.9%	97.3%	91.5%	Q1 (40–70 kg)	99.8%	97%	90.3%
Q2 (70–82 kg)	100%	98%	94.2%	Q2 (70–82 kg)	100%	100%	93.8%
Q3 (82–95 kg)	100%	98.9%	94.8%	Q3 (82–96 kg)	100%	97.9%	93%
Q4 (95–195 kg)	100%	98.2%	88.3%	Q4 (96–202 kg)	100%	97.9%	86.2%
Meropenem 2 g every 12 h							
Overall	99.8%	98.1%	91.4%	Overall	99.7%	97.4%	89.5%
Q1 (40–71 kg)	99.6%	97.1%	86.5%	Q1 (40–70 kg)	99.4%	95.8%	83.2%
Q2 (71–82 kg)	99.8%	97.9%	89.7%	Q2 (70–82 kg)	99.6%	97.5%	89.4%
Q3 (82–95 kg)	99.8%	98.3%	93.3%	Q3 (82–96 kg)	99.8%	97.8%	91.6%
Q4 (95–199 kg)	100%	99%	96%	Q4 (96–206 kg)	100%	98.6%	93.7%

Shaded to represent probability of target attainment: ≥90% (green), 60 ≤ 89% (orange), and <60% (red).

As reported in Table 1 (cefepime, ceftazidime, piperacillin/tazobactam), the PTA against *P. aeruginosa* consistently decreases as the weight quartile increases. The PTA in less-intensive CRRT effluent rate arms was higher than the PTA in intensive CRRT effluent rate arms for all drugs. Nevertheless, these differences were usually small within any weight quartile for any drug. Table 2 illustrates similar findings for carbapenem antibiotics. With a few exceptions, the carbapenem PTA decreased as the weight quartiles increased. The intensity of the CRRT effluent rate also influenced the PTA such that lower PTA rates were observed in the intensive CRRT than in the analogous lower CRRT intensity groups. Again, the differences observed with CRRT intensity were not large. Two drug dosing regimens (imipenem 1 g every 8 h and meropenem 2 g every 12 h) showed a different trend, namely that their PTAs increased as the weight quartile increased.

3. Discussion

This is the first MCS to examine the influence of subject weights on antibiotic PTA in patients receiving CRRT. Our hypothesis for the present study was that antibiotic exposures will be significantly lower (resulting in a lower PTA) in heavier virtual critically ill patients (obesity and/or fluid overloaded) receiving CRRT when the same daily antibiotic dose is used. Our results showed virtual patients who were in Q1 (the lightest quartile) had a higher PTA for its PD target; the PTA gradually decreased as the weight quartile increased [the heaviest (Q4) had the lowest PTA] for all drugs in this study (cefepime, ceftazidime, piperacillin, tazobactam, ertapenem, imipenem, and meropenem) with few exceptions.

The lowest modeled cefepime dosing regimen (1 g every 12 h) met acceptable PTA rates at the least stringent (%fT$\geq$1$\times$MIC) target but poor PTA achievement in both the less-intensive and intensive CRRT groups for the more stringent PD targets (fT$\geq$4$\times$MIC and 100%fT$\geq$MIC). For cefepime, the PTA significantly decreased as the weight quartiles (heavier patients) increased. For example, the overall PTA for 100%fT$\geq$MIC with cefepime 2 g every 12 h in the less-intensive group was 56.3%. Yet, in the first quartile (weight: 40–70 kg) and the last quartile (weight: 95–180 kg) in the less-intensive group achieved PTA values of 90.3% and 17.3%, respectively. Ceftazidime followed a similarly lower PTA with a higher weight trend. Ceftazidime 2 g every 12 h, in the less-intensive group for the PD target of 100%fT$\geq$1$\times$MIC, yielded an overall PTA of 81.1%. However, it exhibited large differences between weight quartiles: 93.2% (in Q1: 40–70 kg) and 63.5% (in Q4: 95–187 kg). Weights influenced piperacillin/tazobactam, as the PTA decreased as the weight quartile increased. For instance, the overall PTA was 60%, but Q1 (40–71 kg) and Q4 (95–184 kg) were 77.9% and 39.8%, respectively, for the PD target of 100%fT$\geq$MIC with piperacillin 4 g every 6 h.

In our study, a few carbapenem dosing regimens demonstrated interesting results, for example, ertapenem 1 g every 24 h with the PD target of 100%fT$\geq$MIC. Subjects in the intensive CRRT arm in Q1 (the lightest) exhibited the lowest PTA compared to larger virtual patients. The PTAs were: Q1 82%, Q2 91.8%, Q3 93.4%, and Q4 83.7%. One potential explanation is that Q1 subjects had the smallest Vd, which may have led to a higher relative drug clearance by intensive CRRT. Imipenem also showed unusual results within the 1 g every 8 h dosing regimen model. The PTA increased as the weight quartiles increased for the PD target of 100%fT$\geq$MIC: PTA Q1 66%; Q2 81%; Q3 89%, and Q4 94% in the intensive CRRT group. With further PK analysis with this cohort, the mean Vd for Q1 was 0.33 L/kg (20.39 L) and in Q4 was 0.37 L/kg (40.36 L). Moreover, the mean nonrenal clearance (CL_{NR}) for Q1 subjects was 98.5 mL/min when CL_{NR} for Q4 subjects was 97.9 mL/min. This phenomenon (increased PTA with higher weight) may be explained by a combination of smaller Vd leading to more drug removal by CRRT and higher CL_{NR} in the Q1 cohort. The other standard dosing regimens for carbapenem results were consistent with our hypothesis (lower PTA with higher weight quartiles).

This study is consistent with Hites et al. [15], who evaluated beta-lactam standard dosing regimens in critically ill patients (both obese and nonobese patients). They found the standard dosing regimens resulted in subtherapeutic plasma concentrations in 32% of their patients and supratherapeutic plasma concentrations in 25% overall. It was evident for meropenem that more obese patients had subtherapeutic antibiotic concentrations compared to nonobese patients (35% vs. 0%, p = 0.02) [15]. The authors did not find statistical differences between obese and nonobese patients for cefepime and piperacillin/tazobactam. Lastly, patients receiving CRRT were more likely to result in supratherapeutic levels than patients who were not receiving CRRT (44.1% vs. 8.8%; p = 0.002) in this study. Moreover, obese patients receiving CRRT were more likely to have supratherapeutic levels compared to nonobese patients receiving CRRT.

Taccone et al. [16] shared a case report that illustrated that obese patients require a much higher antibiotic dosing regimen compared to nonobese patients. This case report was regarding a patient who had a body mass index (BMI) of 35 who presented with septic shock due to extensively drug-resistant *P. aeruginosa*. The PD target was 40%T$\geq$4$\times$MIC, and the standard meropenem dosing regimen did not reach the PD target. The patient required meropenem of 12 g/d (3 g every 6 h with 3 h extended infusion), which resulted in meropenem resolution without any adverse events and no abnormal electroencephalogram.

Cheatham et al. [17] evaluated pharmacokinetics and pharmacodynamics with meropenem use in morbidly obese patients. Nine patients were included with a total body weight of 152.3 ± 31.0 kg (ideal body weight: 60.3 ± 10.6 kg) and a BMI of 54.7 ± 8.6 kg/m^2. The authors found appropriate meropenem dosing regimens for morbidly obese patients were 1 g every 8 h, 2 g every 8 h, 500 mg every 6 h, and 1 g every 6 h when the PD target was 40%fT≥1×MIC (2 mg/mL). For a more stringent PD target (40%fT≥4×MIC), 2 g every 8 h and 1 g every 6 h were necessary for this special population. Even though this study did not include critically ill patients receiving CRRT, it highlights that morbidly obese patients require a higher meropenem dose.

This study has several limitations, including not having BMI information since the study was based on MCS (virtual patients). The PK parameters were derived in different patient populations other than the American patients (ATN trial). However, our objective was not to determine the PTA for patients with obesity but rather determine if there were any differences among weight quartiles. Moreover, our data may not be applicable in non-ICU patients who are underweight (weight: <40 kg) because our minimum weight was set as 40 kg, and pharmacokinetic data were derived from critically ill patients. Lastly, we have not further analyzed any toxicity profiles nor outcome data. These PTA tables will provide better guidance to clinicians who have different antimicrobial PD benchmarks (fT≥1×MIC vs. 100%fT≥1×MIC vs. fT≥4×MIC) for their critically ill patients undergoing CRRT.

4. Materials and Methods

This study was a post-hoc analysis of a previously published paper determining the influence of CRRT's intensity (less intensive vs. intensive) on antibiotic exposure profiles [5]. Institutional review board approval was not required since pharmacokinetic and demographic data were applied to computer-generated "virtual" patients.

4.1. Pharmacokinetic Model and Simulations

The initial study [5] utilized one-compartment, first-order, and multiple-dose pharmacokinetic models to simulate antibiotic plasma concentration–time profiles based on demographic and CRRT dose information from the ATN trials [2,18]. Pertinent pharmacokinetic data in critically ill patients (Vd, unbound fraction, and nonrenal clearance (CL_{NR})) were collected from primary literature sources and incorporated in the MCS (Table 3). Beta-lactams (cefepime, ceftazidime, and piperacillin/tazobactam) and carbapenems (imipenem, ertapenem, and meropenem) were chosen for analysis because they were commonly used during the time of the ATN trial. The commonly recommended antibiotic dosing regimens for CRRT were simulated for 72 h in MCS. Drug concentration–time profiles were generated in a log-Gaussian distribution with preset limits using the mean and SD of the pharmacokinetic parameters outlined in Table 3 by the MCS (Crystal Ball, Oracle©, Santa Clara, CA, USA). The mean and SD of subject weight and delivered effluent rates from each study were used for that study's MCS. Detailed descriptions of the PK model and MCS are included in the previous report [5].

4.2. Pharmacodynamic Targets

We used the Clinical and Laboratory Standards Institute (CLSI) susceptibility breakpoints against *P. aeruginosa* which are: 2 mg/L for meropenem and imipenem, 8 mg/L for cefepime and ceftazidime, and 16 mg/L for piperacillin (4 mg/L for tazobactam threshold). The susceptibility breakpoint for ertapenem against *S. pneumoniae* is 1 mg/L [35]. The PD targets were: ≥40%fT≥1×MIC of 2 mg/L for meropenem and imipenem (4×MIC = 8 mg/L), ≥40%fT≥1×MIC of 1 mg/L for ertapenem (4×MIC = 4 mg/L), ≥50%fT≥1×MIC of 16 mg/L for piperacillin (4×MIC = 64 mg/L), ≥50% fT>4 mg/L for tazobactam, and ≥60% fT≥1×MIC of 8 mg/L for cefepime and ceftazidime (4×MIC = 32 mg/L) over the first 72 h of antibiotic therapy [36,37]. Delattre and colleagues have recommended the use of %fT≥4×MIC as the benchmark for beta-lactams [36]. In order to implement in vitro, animal, and clinical data regarding optimal beta-lactam PD targets, we tested %fT≥MIC targets (1×MIC and 4×MIC) and 100%fT≥MIC in the present analysis.

Table 3. Adapted pharmacokinetic parameters used in Monte Carlo simulations [5].

Drug [Ref]	Cefepime [18–23]	Ceftazidime [24–29]	Ertapenem [5,30]	Imipenem [5,30]	Meropenem [5,30]	Piperacillin [23,31–34]	Tazobactam [23,33]
Vd (L/kg)	0.48 ± 0.24 (0.16–1.11)	0.34 ± 0.20 (0.13–1.1)	0.19 ± 0.07 (0.13–0.34)	0.34 ± 0.1 (0.21–0.63)	0.41 ± 0.18 (0.08–1.07)	0.40 ± 0.21 (0–1.11)	0.50 ± 0.37 (0–2.13)
Free Fraction	0.79 ± 0.09 (0.72–0.85)	0.86 ± 0.05 (0.75–0.94)	0.25 ± 0.45 (0–1)	0.8 ± 0.16 (0–1)	0.79 ± 0.09 (0–1)	0.76 ± 0.2 (0–1)	0.74 ± 0.27 (0–1)
NR CL (mL/min)	24.33 ± 11.25 (13–44)	15.9 ± 9.9 (8–37.7)	11 ± 3 (10–19)	100.5 ± 28 (53–160)	54.9 ± 49 (0–251)	48.5 ± 37 (0–187)	40.4 ± 70 (0–381)
Sieving coefficient	0.67 ± 0.13 (0–1)	0.85 ± 0.05 (0–1)	0.2 ± 0.06 (0–1)	0.57 ± 0.1 (0–1)	0.63 ± 0.13 (0–1)	0.6 ± 0.28 (0–1)	0.8 ± 0.36 (0–1)
r^2 weight and Vd	0.4197	0.0237	0.3318	0.17	0.1435	0.0567	0.0049
r^2 weight and NR CL	0.038	0.1254	0.1156	0.013	0.0072	0.036	0.0098
Weight ± SD (kg)	Less intensive: 84.1 ± 18.9; Intensive: 84.1 ± 19.6						
CRRT % delivered	Less intensive: 0.95 ± 0.35 (0–1); Intensive: 0.89 ± 0.39 (0–1)						
Q_{eff} (mL/kg/h)	Less intensive: 22 ± 6.1 (0–47.5) vs. Intensive: 35.8 ± 6.4 (0–47.5)						
Q_{rep} (L/h)	Less intensive: 0.83 ± 0.25 (0.33–1.33); Intensive: 0.89 ± 0.39 (0–1)						

All values are mean ± standard deviation (minimum–maximum limits). Abbreviations: CL = clearance; NR = nonrenal; r^2 = correlation; Vd = volume of distribution; Q_{eff} = effluent flow rate; Q_{rep} = replacement fluid rate.

4.3. Optimal Dosing Regimen

Drug dosing regimen was considered optimal if it reached a PTA of 90%, which is a standard threshold in simulation studies [5,23,30,38]. This means the virtual patients will achieve 90% of predetermined pharmacodynamic targets with simulated dosing regimens. Antibiotic toxicity profiles were not analyzed in this experiment, as the threshold for toxicity is poorly characterized [37,38].

4.4. Weight Quartile Analysis

The weight for 10,000 virtual subjects was limited to a minimum of 40 kg with no maximum limit set. The 10,000 virtual patients were organized by body weight, and their PTA analyses were divided into four quartiles. The lightest group was "Q1" (the 2500 virtual patients with the lowest weight) through the heaviest group called "Q4" (the 2500 virtual patients with the highest weight). Since there were 10,000 virtual subjects for each drug and dosing regimen and each was modeled separately, the weights within each quartile differ slightly between regimens.

5. Conclusions

Our post-hoc analysis shows that the patient's weight influences antibiotic drugs' pharmacodynamic target attainment related to antimicrobial efficacy. One-size-fits-all dosing should not be applied to large critically ill patients who might be obese, fluid overloaded, or both. This analysis does not include toxicity analysis but rather includes the PTA for 10,000 virtual patients to achieve different pharmacodynamic targets. Thus, we are not recommending any specific drug dosing regimen.

Author Contributions: B.A.M. and S.-M.J. designed experiments, derived the models, and analyzed the data. S.-M.J. and A.R.S. assisted with data collection. S.-M.J. analyzed samples for data analysis. B.A.M. and S.-M.J. wrote the manuscript. All authors have read and agreed to the published version of the manuscript.

Funding: This research did not receive any specific grant from funding agencies in the public, commercial, or not-for-profit sectors.

Institutional Review Board Statement: This study protocol did not require institutional review board approval.

Data Availability Statement: Data are available and stored at the University of Michigan College of Pharmacy.

Conflicts of Interest: Bruce Mueller has grants from Merck and NxStage. He is a consultant for Wolters Kluwer.

References

1. Eyler, R.F.; Mueller, B.A.; Medscape. Antibiotic dosing in critically ill patients with acute kidney injury. *Nat. Rev. Nephrol.* **2011**, *7*, 226–235. [CrossRef]
2. Palevsky, P.M.; Zhang, J.H.; O'Connor, T.Z.; Chertow, G.M.; Crowley, S.T.; Choudhury, D.; Finkel, K.; Kellum, J.A.; Paganini, E.; Schein, R.M.; et al. Intensity of renal support in critically ill patients with acute kidney injury. *N. Engl. J. Med.* **2008**, *359*, 7–20. [CrossRef]
3. Kielstein, J.T.; David, S. Pro: Renal replacement trauma or Paracelsus 2.0. *Nephrol. Dial Transpl.* **2013**, *28*, 2728–2731. [CrossRef]
4. Lewis, S.J.; Mueller, B.A. Antibiotic dosing in critically ill patients receiving CRRT: Underdosing is overprevalent. *Semin. Dial* **2014**, *27*, 441–445. [CrossRef] [PubMed]
5. Jang, S.M.; Pai, M.P.; Shaw, A.R.; Mueller, B.A. Antibiotic Exposure Profiles in Trials Comparing Intensity of Continuous Renal Replacement Therapy. *Crit. Care Med.* **2019**, *47*, e863–e871. [CrossRef] [PubMed]
6. Jang, S.M.; Lewis, S.J.; Mueller, B.A. Harmonizing antibiotic regimens with renal replacement therapy. *Expert Rev. Anti Infect. Ther.* **2020**, *18*, 887–895. [CrossRef]
7. Roberts, D.M.; Liu, X.; Roberts, J.A.; Nair, P.; Cole, L.; Roberts, M.S.; Lipman, J.; Bellomo, R.; Investigators, R.R.T.S. A multicenter study on the effect of continuous hemodiafiltration intensity on antibiotic pharmacokinetics. *Crit. Care* **2015**, *19*, 84. [CrossRef] [PubMed]
8. Zander, J.; Dobbeler, G.; Nagel, D.; Scharf, C.; Huseyn-Zada, M.; Jung, J.; Frey, L.; Vogeser, M.; Zoller, M. Variability of piperacillin concentrations in relation to tazobactam concentrations in critically ill patients. *Int. J. Antimicrob. Agents* **2016**, *48*, 435–439. [CrossRef]
9. Longo, C.; Bartlett, G.; Macgibbon, B.; Mayo, N.; Rosenberg, E.; Nadeau, L.; Daskalopoulou, S.S. The effect of obesity on antibiotic treatment failure: A historical cohort study. *Pharmacoepidemiol. Drug Saf.* **2013**, *22*, 970–976. [CrossRef]
10. Al-Dorzi, H.M.; Al Harbi, S.A.; Arabi, Y.M. Antibiotic therapy of pneumonia in the obese patient: Dosing and delivery. *Curr. Opin. Infect. Dis.* **2014**, *27*, 165–173. [CrossRef]
11. Craig, W.A.; Ebert, S.C. Killing and regrowth of bacteria in vitro: A review. *Scand. J. Infect. Dis. Suppl.* **1990**, *74*, 63–70. [PubMed]
12. Vitrat, V.; Hautefeuille, S.; Janssen, C.; Bougon, D.; Sirodot, M.; Pagani, L. Optimizing antimicrobial therapy in critically ill patients. *Infect. Drug Resist.* **2014**, *7*, 261–271. [CrossRef]
13. Vogelman, B.; Craig, W.A. Kinetics of antimicrobial activity. *J. Pediatr.* **1986**, *108*, 835–840. [CrossRef]
14. Abdul-Aziz, M.H.; Sulaiman, H.; Mat-Nor, M.B.; Rai, V.; Wong, K.K.; Hasan, M.S.; Abd Rahman, A.N.; Jamal, J.A.; Wallis, S.C.; Lipman, J.; et al. Beta-Lactam Infusion in Severe Sepsis (BLISS): A prospective, two-centre, open-labelled randomised controlled trial of continuous versus intermittent beta-lactam infusion in critically ill patients with severe sepsis. *Intensive Care Med.* **2016**, *42*, 1535–1545. [CrossRef] [PubMed]
15. Hites, M.; Taccone, F.S.; Wolff, F.; Cotton, F.; Beumier, M.; De Backer, D.; Roisin, S.; Lorent, S.; Surin, R.; Seyler, L.; et al. Case-control study of drug monitoring of beta-lactams in obese critically ill patients. *Antimicrob. Agents Chemother.* **2013**, *57*, 708–715. [CrossRef]
16. Taccone, F.S.; Cotton, F.; Roisin, S.; Vincent, J.L.; Jacobs, F. Optimal meropenem concentrations to treat multidrug-resistant Pseudomonas aeruginosa septic shock. *Antimicrob. Agents Chemother.* **2012**, *56*, 2129–2131. [CrossRef]
17. Cheatham, S.C.; Fleming, M.R.; Healy, D.P.; Chung, E.K.; Shea, K.M.; Humphrey, M.L.; Kays, M.B. Steady-state pharmacokinetics and pharmacodynamics of meropenem in morbidly obese patients hospitalized in an intensive care unit. *J. Clin. Pharmacol.* **2014**, *54*, 324–330. [CrossRef]
18. Barbhaiya, R.H.; Knupp, C.A.; Forgue, S.T.; Matzke, G.R.; Guay, D.R.; Pittman, K.A. Pharmacokinetics of cefepime in subjects with renal insufficiency. *Clin. Pharmacol. Ther.* **1990**, *48*, 268–276. [CrossRef]
19. Park, J.T.; Lee, H.; Kee, Y.K.; Park, S.; Oh, H.J.; Han, S.H.; Joo, K.W.; Lim, C.S.; Kim, Y.S.; Kang, S.W.; et al. High-Dose Versus Conventional-Dose Continuous Venovenous Hemodiafiltration and Patient and Kidney Survival and Cytokine Removal in Sepsis-Associated Acute Kidney Injury: A Randomized Controlled Trial. *Am. J. Kidney Dis.* **2016**, *68*, 599–608. [CrossRef]
20. Allaouchiche, B.; Breilh, D.; Jaumain, H.; Gaillard, B.; Renard, S.; Saux, M.C. Pharmacokinetics of cefepime during continuous venovenous hemodiafiltration. *Antimicrob. Agents Chemother.* **1997**, *41*, 2424–2427. [CrossRef]
21. Isla, A.; Gascon, A.R.; Maynar, J.; Arzuaga, A.; Toral, D.; Pedraz, J.L. Cefepime and continuous renal replacement therapy (CRRT): In vitro permeability of two CRRT membranes and pharmacokinetics in four critically ill patients. *Clin. Ther.* **2005**, *27*, 599–608. [CrossRef]
22. Cronqvist, J.; Nilsson-Ehle, I.; Oqvist, B.; Norrby, S.R. Pharmacokinetics of cefepime dihydrochloride arginine in subjects with renal impairment. *Antimicrob. Agents Chemother.* **1992**, *36*, 2676–2680. [CrossRef]
23. Jang, S.M.; Gharibian, K.N.; Lewis, S.J.; Fissell, W.H.; Tolwani, A.J.; Mueller, B.A. A Monte Carlo Simulation Approach for Beta-Lactam Dosing in Critically Ill Patients Receiving Prolonged Intermittent Renal Replacement Therapy. *J. Clin. Pharmacol.* **2018**, *58*, 1254–1265. [CrossRef] [PubMed]

24. Schmaldienst, S.; Traunmuller, F.; Burgmann, H.; Rosenkranz, A.R.; Thalhammer-Scherrer, R.; Horl, W.H.; Thalhammer, F. Multiple-dose pharmacokinetics of cefepime in long-term hemodialysis with high-flux membranes. *Eur. J. Clin. Pharmacol.* **2000**, *56*, 61–64. [CrossRef] [PubMed]
25. Kinowski, J.M.; de la Coussaye, J.E.; Bressolle, F.; Fabre, D.; Saissi, G.; Bouvet, O.; Galtier, M.; Eledjam, J.J. Multiple-dose pharmacokinetics of amikacin and ceftazidime in critically ill patients with septic multiple-organ failure during intermittent hemofiltration. *Antimicrob. Agents Chemother.* **1993**, *37*, 464–473. [CrossRef] [PubMed]
26. Vincent, H.H.; Vos, M.C.; Akcahuseyin, E.; Goessens, W.H.; van Duyl, W.A.; Schalekamp, M.A. Drug clearance by continuous haemodiafiltration. Analysis of sieving coefficients and mass transfer coefficients of diffusion. *Blood Purif.* **1993**, *11*, 99–107. [CrossRef] [PubMed]
27. Traunmuller, F.; Schenk, P.; Mittermeyer, C.; Thalhammer-Scherrer, R.; Ratheiser, K.; Thalhammer, F. Clearance of ceftazidime during continuous venovenous haemofiltration in critically ill patients. *J Antimicrob. Chemother.* **2002**, *49*, 129–134. [CrossRef] [PubMed]
28. Mariat, C.; Venet, C.; Jehl, F.; Mwewa, S.; Lazarevic, V.; Diconne, E.; Fonsale, N.; Carricajo, A.; Guyomarc'h, S.; Vermesch, R.; et al. Continuous infusion of ceftazidime in critically ill patients undergoing continuous venovenous haemodiafiltration: Pharmacokinetic evaluation and dose recommendation. *Crit. Care* **2006**, *10*, R26. [CrossRef]
29. Isla, A.; Gascon, A.R.; Maynar, J.; Arzuaga, A.; Sanchez-Izquierdo, J.A.; Pedraz, J.L. In vitro AN69 and polysulphone membrane permeability to ceftazidime and in vivo pharmacokinetics during continuous renal replacement therapies. *Chemotherapy* **2007**, *53*, 194–201. [CrossRef]
30. Zelenitsky, S.A.; Ariano, R.E.; Zhanel, G.G. Pharmacodynamics of empirical antibiotic monotherapies for an intensive care unit (ICU) population based on Canadian surveillance data. *J. Antimicrob. Chemother.* **2011**, *66*, 343–349. [CrossRef]
31. Joos, B.; Schmidli, M.; Keusch, G. Pharmacokinetics of antimicrobial agents in anuric patients during continuous venovenous haemofiltration. *Nephrol. Dial Transplant.* **1996**, *11*, 1582–1585. [CrossRef]
32. Gashti, C.N.; Salcedo, S.; Robinson, V.; Rodby, R.A. Accelerated venovenous hemofiltration: Early technical and clinical experience. *Am. J. Kidney Dis.* **2008**, *51*, 804–810. [CrossRef] [PubMed]
33. Mueller, S.C.; Majcher-Peszynska, J.; Hickstein, H.; Francke, A.; Pertschy, A.; Schulz, M.; Mundkowski, R.; Drewelow, B. Pharmacokinetics of piperacillin-tazobactam in anuric intensive care patients during continuous venovenous hemodialysis. *Antimicrob. Agents Chemother.* **2002**, *46*, 1557–1560. [CrossRef] [PubMed]
34. Arzuaga, A.; Maynar, J.; Gascon, A.R.; Isla, A.; Corral, E.; Fonseca, F.; Sanchez-Izquierdo, J.A.; Rello, J.; Canut, A.; Pedraz, J.L. Influence of renal function on the pharmacokinetics of piperacillin/tazobactam in intensive care unit patients during continuous venovenous hemofiltration. *J. Clin. Pharmacol.* **2005**, *45*, 168–176. [CrossRef]
35. Wayne, P.A. Clinical and Laboratory Standards Institute. Performance Standards for Antimicrobial Susceptibility Testing. *Inform. Suppl.* **2011**, *31*, 100–121.
36. Delattre, I.K.; Taccone, F.S.; Jacobs, F.; Hites, M.; Dugernier, T.; Spapen, H.; Laterre, P.F.; Wallemacq, P.E.; Van Bambeke, F.; Tulkens, P.M. Optimizing beta-lactams treatment in critically-ill patients using pharmacokinetics/pharmacodynamics targets: Are first conventional doses effective? *Expert Rev. Anti Infect. Ther.* **2017**, *15*, 677–688. [CrossRef]
37. Drusano, G.L. Antimicrobial pharmacodynamics: Critical interactions of 'bug and drug'. *Nat. Rev. Microbiol.* **2004**, *2*, 289–300. [CrossRef]
38. Lewis, S.J.; Kays, M.B.; Mueller, B.A. Use of Monte Carlo Simulations to Determine Optimal Carbapenem Dosing in Critically Ill Patients Receiving Prolonged Intermittent Renal Replacement Therapy. *J. Clin. Pharmacol.* **2016**, *56*, 1277–1287. [CrossRef]

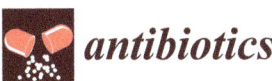

Systematic Review

Systematic Review of Antimicrobial Combination Options for Pandrug-Resistant *Acinetobacter baumannii*

Stamatis Karakonstantis *[ ], Petros Ioannou [ ], George Samonis and Diamantis P. Kofteridis

Department of Internal Medicine & Infectious Diseases, University Hospital of Heraklion, 71110 Heraklion, Crete, Greece; petros_io@hotmail.com (P.I.); samonis@med.uoc.gr (G.S.); kofterid@med.uoc.gr (D.P.K.)
* Correspondence: stamatiskarakonstantis@gmail.com

Abstract: Antimicrobial combinations are at the moment the only potential treatment option for pandrug-resistant *A. baumannii*. A systematic review was conducted in PubMed and Scopus for studies reporting the activity of antimicrobial combinations against *A. baumannii* resistant to all components of the combination. The clinical relevance of synergistic combinations was assessed based on concentrations achieving synergy and PK/PD models. Eighty-four studies were retrieved including 818 eligible isolates. A variety of combinations ($n = 141$ double, $n = 9$ triple) were tested, with a variety of methods. Polymyxin-based combinations were the most studied, either as double or triple combinations with cell-wall acting agents (including sulbactam, carbapenems, glycopeptides), rifamycins and fosfomycin. Non-polymyxin combinations were predominantly based on rifampicin, fosfomycin, sulbactam and avibactam. Several combinations were synergistic at clinically relevant concentrations, while triple combinations appeared more active than the double ones. However, no combination was consistently synergistic against all strains tested. Notably, several studies reported synergy but at concentrations unlikely to be clinically relevant, or the concentration that synergy was observed was unclear. Selecting the most appropriate combinations is likely strain-specific and should be guided by in vitro synergy evaluation. Furthermore, there is an urgent need for clinical studies on the efficacy and safety of such combinations.

Keywords: *Acinetobacter*; pandrug-resistant; antimicrobial combinations; synergy

1. Introduction

Pandrug-resistant (PDR) Gram-negative bacteria, resistant to all currently available antibiotics, including carbapenems, aminoglycosides, polymyxins and tigecycline, have been increasingly reported worldwide [1]. Especially problematic is the management of infections by PDR *A. baumannii* (PDRAB), since there are no monotherapy treatment options and associated mortality is very high [2]. Cefiderocol, where available, is a last resort option [3]. However, resistance to cefiderocol is already being reported and is likely to increase, considering the high prevalence of heteroresistance to this agent [4], as has occurred with polymyxins [5]. Therefore, pending approval of new antimicrobials, synergistic combinations are at the moment the only potential treatment option for PDRAB [6].

Combination antimicrobial therapy compared to monotherapy has not so far been proven in most studies to lead to better clinical outcomes of *A. baumannii* infections [7–11]. However, the available studies are predominantly based on combinations including at least one active antimicrobial and a potential benefit in PDRAB infections, with no monotherapy treatment options, should not be excluded [6,12,13]. Similar to clinical studies, prior systematic reviews that have assessed the in vitro synergy of various combinations (based on polymyxins [14–16], rifampin [14,16], meropenem [16,17] or tigecycline [16,18]) against *A. baumannii*, were predominantly based on studies testing combinations including at least one active antimicrobial. However, synergy testing may be most useful to identify

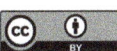

combinations for salvage therapy of infections by bacteria resistant to all monotherapy treatment options [19].

Therefore, the purpose of this systematic review is to identify synergistic combinations that may be used for treatment of infections caused by PDRAB, i.e., combinations based on antimicrobials to which *A. baumannii* is resistant. Furthermore, it was evaluated whether the identified combinations were synergistic at concentrations achievable in vivo, a major consideration when assessing the in vivo relevance of in vitro synergy [20], especially when referring to PDRAB. These data aim to aid microbiology laboratories and infectious disease clinicians to prioritize the potential combination options for evaluation for synergy against the local PDRAB strains.

2. Methods

2.1. Search Strategy

The following search was conducted in PubMed from inception to 20 April 2021: (*Acinetobacter* [ti] OR baumannii [ti] OR "*Acinetobacter*" [Mesh] OR "*Acinetobacter baumannii*" [Mesh]) AND (synerg* [ti] OR combin* [ti] OR "Drug Combinations" [Mesh] OR "Drug Synergism" [Mesh] OR "Drug Therapy, Combination" [Mesh]). The same search, without the MESH terms, was also conducted in Scopus.

2.2. Eligibility Criteria

Any study (including in vitro, animal models, and clinical studies) evaluating the activity of antimicrobial combinations against clinical *A. baumannii* isolates was eligible, provided that the *A. baumannii* isolates tested were resistant to all components of the antimicrobial combinations assessed. The following exclusion criteria were applied: (1) studies including only noneligible isolates (see below definition for eligibility), (2) studies including both eligible and noneligible isolates, but not possible to extract data for eligible isolates, (3) combinations of antimicrobials with adjuvant, nonantibiotic agents, or with investigational agents (not currently in use for the treatment of infections). (4) Clinical studies without any information on synergy. (5) Studies written in languages other than English (little impact [21,22], often at higher risk of bias [23], and data extraction can be inaccurate [23]). Deduplication and screening for eligibility of the retrieved articles was conducted by the first author using the Rayyan online platform [24].

2.3. Data Extraction

The following data were extracted from each eligible article: country where the study was conducted, number of participating hospitals, methods of synergy testing (readers are referred to relevant references for a more detailed overview of the different methods [19,20,25–27]), list of antimicrobials tested for synergy, number of eligible strains (as defined below), number of eligible strains against which each combination demonstrated synergy and antimicrobial concentrations achieving synergy. Data were extracted by the first author in duplicate.

2.4. Definition of Eligible Strains

A. baumannii isolates were eligible for this review if resistant to all components of the antimicrobial combinations tested. The following breakpoints were used to define resistance based on CLSI [28] or EUCAST [29] clinical breakpoints (whichever was higher): amikacin > 32 mg/L, ampicillin-sulbactam > 16/8 mg/L, cefepime > 16 mg/L, cefiderocol > 8 mg/L, ceftazidime > 16 mg/L, ciprofloxacin > 2 mg/L, colistin > 2 mg/L, gentamicin > 8 mg/L, imipenem > 4 mg/L, levofloxacin > 4 mg/L, meropenem > 8 mg/L, minocycline > 8 mg/L, piperacillin > 64 mg/L, piperacillin/tazobactam > 64/4 mg/L, polymyxin B > 2 mg/L, tobramycin > 8 mg/L, trimethoprim-sulfamethoxazole > 2/38 mg/L. For antibiotics without established breakpoints by either EUCAST or CLSI the following cut-offs were applied: azithromycin > 4 mg/L (based on CLSI breakpoints for *Staphylococci* [12,28]), aztreonam >16 mg/L (based on breakpoints for *P. aeruginosa* [28,29]), cefoperazone/sulbactam > 32/16 mg/L [30], ceftazidime/avibactam > 8/4 mg/dl (based on breakpoints for *P. aeruginosa* [28,29]), chloramphenicol > 16 mg/L (based on breakpoints for Enterobacterales [28]), fosfomycin > 32 mg/L (based on EUCAST breakpoints for Enterobacterales and *Staphylococcus* spp [29]), fusidic acid > 1 mg/L (based on EUCAST breakpoints for *Staphylococcus* spp [29]), moxifloxacin > 0.25 mg/L (based on EUCAST breakpoints for Enterobacterales [29]), plazomicin > 4 mg/L (FDA interpretive criteria for Enterobacteriaceae [31]), rifampicin > 2 mg/L (based on CLSI breakpoints for *Staphylococci* [28], although much lower cut-offs have been proposed for *A. baumannii* [32]), tigecycline > 2 mg/L [33], trimethoprim > 8 mg/L (based on CLSI breakpoints for Enterobacterales [28]), vancomycin > 20 mg/L (based on clinically achievable concentrations [34–36], noting that the CLSI breakpoints for coagulase-negative *Staphylococci* is > 16 mg/L [28]).

2.5. Evaluation of In Vivo Feasibility of the Identified Combinations

In vivo feasibility of each synergistic combination was assessed based on the following: (1) synergy present in vitro at concentrations equal to or lower than established breakpoints of resistance (as defined above) for all antimicrobials used in the combination, or (2) synergy demonstrated in dynamic drug concentration-time experiments (such as the hollow-fiber infection model, or animal infection models) simulating the pharmacokinetics of human treatment regimens, or (3) clinically-achievable synergy based on pharmacokinetic/pharmacodynamic (PK/PD) modelling and Monte Carlo simulations [37].

2.6. Data Synthesis and Analysis

A qualitative synthesis of the data was conducted. Meta-analysis of the data was not pursued (a post hoc decision), based on the following findings of the review; methodological heterogeneity in synergy testing methods and interpretation, small number of studies and eligible isolates per combination, clonal relatedness of *A. baumannii* isolates from single-center studies, potential differences between different *A. baumannii* strains (i.e., synergy against *A. baumannii* strains isolated from one institution does not necessarily predict synergy against different strains, with different mechanisms and level of resistance), potential for publication bias (studies with negative results are less likely to be published), selective performance of more cumbersome synergy testing methods (such as time-kill assay or animal models) only against strains for which synergy had been demonstrated by other methods (such as checkerboard), questionable clinical relevance of synergy in many studies (synergy present only at high antimicrobial concentrations, likely not relevant for in vivo use, or at unclear concentrations).

3. Results

3.1. Summary and Characteristics of Reviewed Studies

A flow chart of the review is depicted in Figure 1. Eighty-four relevant publications [12,35–117] were retrieved including 818 eligible *A. baumannii* isolates. The characteristics of the reviewed studies are summarized in the Supplementary Materials File S1 (Section 2). Most (73%) studies were published in the last 10 years, while about a third (35%) were published in the last 5 years (Appendix A, Table A1). Most studies were conducted in the European region (33%), America (29%) and the Western-Pacific region (24%) (Appendix A, Table A2). The number of eligible isolates per study was small in most studies, with most (79%) of them including ≤ 10 isolates (Supplementary Materials File S1 Section 2.4). Finally, most studies were single center (65%) and of the multicenter studies most (58%) were conducted in only two to five centers (Supplementary Materials File S1 Section 2.5), an important consideration as this reflects the clonal diversity of the *A. baumannii* isolates available for each study.

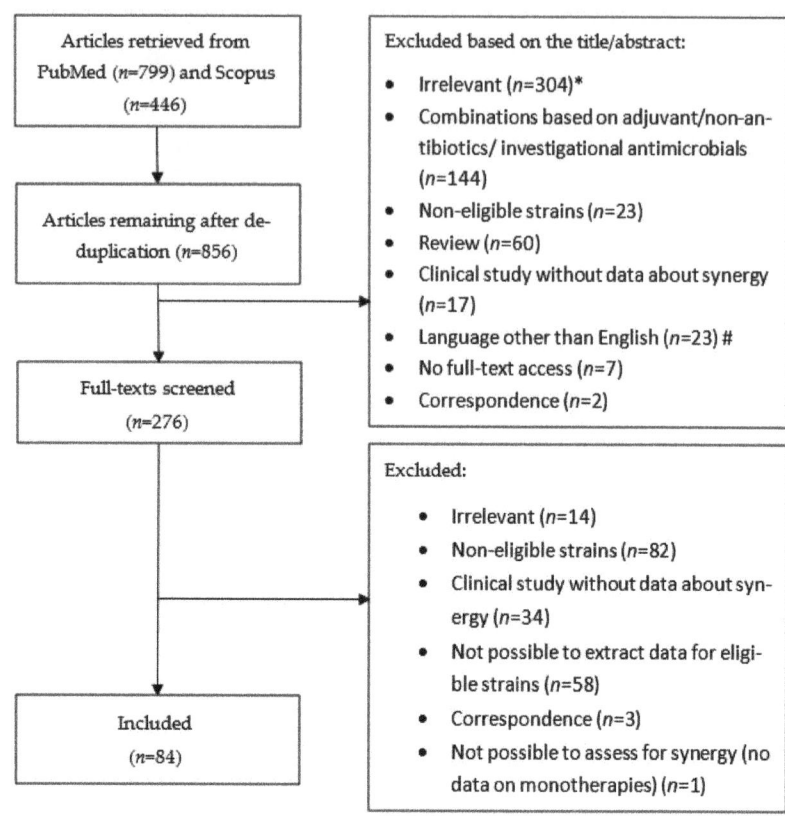

* See Supplementary materials File S1 (Section 5).

Chinese (*n*=9), Turkish (*n*=6), French (*n*=5), Korean (*n*=2), Japanese (*n*=1). The list of excluded non-English articles is available in the Supplementary materials File S1 (Section 6).

Figure 1. Flow chart of the review.

3.2. Overview of Methods for Assessment of Antimicrobial Combinations

A variety of methods were used for in vitro evaluation of antimicrobial combinations; disk diffusion methods (n = 4 studies, n = 18 eligible isolates), gradient strip methods (n = 11 studies, n = 229 eligible isolates), MIC determination by agar dilution (n = 2 studies, n = 42 eligible isolates), checkerboard assay (n = 44 studies, n = 599 eligible isolates), the multiple-combination bactericidal test (n = 1 study, n = 9 eligible isolates), time-kill assay (n = 51 studies, n = 259 eligible isolates), dynamic in vitro PK/PD models with antimicrobial concentrations simulating human treatment regimens (n = 6 studies, n = 10 isolates), and semi-mechanistic PK/PD modelling based on TKA data (n = 5 studies [37,54,102,107,118]). Finally, a few in vivo animal models (n = 11 studies, n = 18 isolates) eligible for review have been published [35,38,55,64,70,90,94,98,102,105,113]. No eligible clinical studies were retrieved.

3.3. Overview of Antimicrobial Combinations That have been Evaluated

Numerous different combinations (n = 141 double and n = 9 triple combinations) were evaluated predominantly based on polymyxins, rifamycins (predominantly rifampicin and recently rifabutin), sulbactam, fosfomycin and carbapenems. However, there were few available studies for most combinations with only 10 combinations having >3 studies available. Summarizing Tables of the number of studies and number of eligible isolates for

3.4. Overview of Polymyxin-Based Combinations

Polymyxin-based combinations were the most studied, with several studies demonstrating synergy against eligible *A. baumannii* isolates by combinations of polymyxins (either colistin or polymyxin-B) with cell-wall acting agents including: sulbactam (either alone or as ampicillin-sulbactam), beta-lactams (predominantly carbapenems, but also third generation cephalosporins, aztreonam, and ceftazidime/avibactam), glycopeptides (predominantly vancomycin, but also teicoplanin), and daptomycin. Furthermore, several studies have reported synergy between colistin and rifamycins against eligible strains (predominantly rifampicin and recently rifabutin). Isolated reports have also demonstrated synergy with trimethoprim/sulfamethoxazole, chloramphenicol, and fusidic acid.

The following triple polymyxin-based combinations have also been shown to be synergistic against selected eligible strains: polymyxin-B/meropenem/sulbactam [51,69], polymyxin-B/ meropenem/ampicillin/sulbactam [61,62], colistin/doripenem/sulbactam [82], polymyxin-B/ meropenem/fosfomycin [51,69] and polymyxin-B/doripenem/vancomycin [35]. Triple polymyxin- based combinations appear to be more active than double combinations and more likely to prevent regrowth during treatment [51,61,69,82], likely by preventing emergence of resistant subpopulations [61].

A variety of the above combinations (colistin/sulbactam, polymyxin-b/sulbactam, colistin/imipenem, colistin/meropenem, polymyxin-B/meropenem, colistin/doripenem, colistin/tigecycline, colistin/rifampicin, polymyxin-B/rifampicin, colistin/vancomycin, polymyxin-B/vancomycin, colistin/daptomycin, colistin/trimethoprim/sulfamethoxazole, colistin/chloramphenicol, colistin/fusidic acid, colistin/levofloxacin, polymyxin-B/ fosfomycin/meropenem, polymyxin-B/sulbactam/meropenem, polymyxin-B/ampicillin/ sulbactam/meropenem, colistin/sulbactam/doripenem, colistin/vancomycin/doripenem) have been shown to be synergistic at concentrations equal to or less than established breakpoints by a variety of methods, or in dynamic drug concentration-time experiments including animal models (Appendix A; Tables A3–A5, and Supplementary Materials File S1 Section 4). Nevertheless, the number of studies and eligible isolates per combination was small and most combinations were active at clinically relevant concentrations only against selected of the tested eligible strains (Appendix A; Tables A3–A5, and Supplementary Materials File S1 Sections 3–4).

3.5. Overview of Non-Polymyxin Based Combinations

Non-polymyxin-based combinations are predominantly based on combinations of the following antimicrobials (Supplementary Materials File S1 Section 3): sulbactam (either as sulbactam alone or in the form of ampicillin/sulbactam or cefoperazone/sulbactam), fosfomycin, rifampicin and carbapenems. However, a variety of other antimicrobials have been tried in combination regimens including aminoglycosides, tetracyclines (doxycycline, tigecycline, minocycline and eravacycline), fluoroquinolones, cephalosporins, aztreonam, trimethoprim/sulfamethoxazole, linezolid, teicoplanin and azithromycin.

The best data for non-polymyxin-based combinations come from four studies by Mohd Sazly Lim S et al. [37,44,45,118]. Fosfomycin/sulbactam (FOF/SUL), fosfomycin/meropenem (FOF/MEM), sulbactam/meropenem (SUL/MEM), fosfomycin/rifampin (FOF/RIF) and meropenem/rifampin (MEM/RIF) were evaluated for synergy against 50 eligible *A. baumannii* isolates characterized by high genetic diversity. The combinations were first evaluated by checkerboard assay [44]. Based on an FICI $\leq$ 0.5 the combinations were synergistic against 74% (FOF/SUL), 28% (FOF/MEM), 56% (SUL/MEM), 24% (FOF/RIF) and 20% (RIF/MEM) of eligible strains. Synergy was mostly detected at concentrations above established breakpoints of resistance. However, considering higher proposed breakpoints based on PK/PD models (32 mg/L for SUL [119,120] and 128 mg/L for FOF [45,121]) the combination FOF/SUL was active against 18 of 28 (64%) eligible isolates [37], the combination FOF/MEM was active against 9 of 33 (27%) eligible isolates [45], and the combination SUL/MEM was active against 9 of 46 (20%) eligible isolates [118]. FOF/SUL and SUL/MEM were further evaluated in TKA against selected isolates [37,44,118], but synergy was only reported at concentrations (128/128 mg/L for SUL/FOF and 64/32–128/64 for SUL/MEM) higher than established breakpoints.

Finally, Mohd Sazly Lim S et al. evaluated two of the above combinations with semi-mechanistic PK/PD modelling; FOF/SUL (simulated regimen: 8 g of fosfomycin given every 8 h as a 1 h infusion and 4 g of sulbactam given every 8 h as a 4 h infusion) [37] and SUL/MEM (simulated regimen: 2 gr of meropenem given every 8 h as a 3 h infusion, and 4 g of sulbactam given every 8 h as a 4 h infusion [118]). A high probability of target attainment was shown for FOF/SUL against the selected isolate (FOF MIC 2048, SUL MIC 128, combination MIC in checkerboard 32/16 mg/L); 81.6%, 76.4%, and 71.6% for stasis, 1-$\log_{10}$ kill and 2-$\log_{10}$ kill, respectively (compared to 23.3%, 19.8% and 15.5% for fosfomycin monotherapy, and 53.5%, 46.5%, and 32.5% for sulbactam monotherapy) [37]. In contrast, the probability of target attainment was at best moderate for SUL/MEM against the selected isolates (MEM MIC 128 mg/L, SUL MIC 256 mg/L, combination MICs 8/64 and 8/32 mg/L); 41%, 38% and 34% for stasis, 1-$\log_{10}$ kill and 2-$\log_{10}$ kill, respectively (compared to no killing with either of the monotherapies) [118].

Avibactam/sulbactam is another recently proposed promising combination. Rodriguez CH et al. [47] showed that avibactam at a fixed concentration of 4 mg/L reduced the MIC of sulbactam to ≤4 mg/L in all 35 non-metallo-β-lactamase (MBL)-producing sulbactam-resistant *A. baumannii* isolates in one study. The activity of sulbactam/avibactam (and to a lesser extent of sulbactam/relebactam) was also confirmed in a subsequent study [122]. The rationale of the combination is that avibactam may inhibit the β-lactamases that affect activity of sulbactam [47]. However, the combination is less effective against metallo-β-lactamase-producing isolates [47,122].

In contrast to non-MBL Enterobacterales [6], double carbapenem combinations are less likely to be clinically relevant for *A. baumannii* strains. Specifically, the combination meropenem/imipenem was synergistic against 6 of 21 eligible isolates according to checkerboard assay in one study, but synergy was only observed at concentration above established breakpoints of resistance (synergy was present at the following meropenem/imipenem concentrations: 16/4, 16/8, 32/16 and 32/32, 16/8 mg/L) and all isolates had relatively low MICs (mostly 32–64 mg/L) [46]. The combination imipenem/meropenem has also been shown to be effective in a murine intraperitoneal infection model (using two *A. baumannii* strains with meropenem-imipenem MICs 16–16 and 32–32 mg/L, respectively), but mortality and bacterial clearance were similar comparing meropenem monotherapy to combination therapy [38]. Additionally, the combination imipenem/ertapenem was not found to be synergistic in another study [73].

3.6. Evaluation of Clinical Relevance of Reported Synergy

Detailed data regarding the proportion of observed synergy for each combination (per study and method) and assessment of the clinical relevance are available in the Supplementary Materials File S1 (Section 4). In most cases, synergy was only reported at antimicrobial concentrations above the established breakpoints of resistance or the concentration at which synergy was observed was not reported. Specifically, of $n = 539$ cases of reported synergy in checkerboard assay, synergy was observed at concentrations ≤breakpoints in only 112 (21%) cases, synergy was reported at concentration >breakpoints in 194 (36%) cases, while in 233 (43%) cases the concentration at which synergy was present was unclear. Similarly, of $n = 185$ cases of reported synergy in TKA, synergy was observed at concentrations ≤breakpoints in only 65 (35%) cases, synergy was reported at concentration >breakpoints in 88 (48%) cases, while in 32 (17%) cases the concentration at which synergy was present was unclear.

Additionally, the clinical relevance of improved outcomes (survival, reduction of bacterial loads, sterilization of cultures) in animal models is unclear, despite simulation of human treatment regimens, considering the unexpectedly high efficacy of monotherapies in many cases [38,90,94,98,105,113], and potentially nonrelevant for humans mechanisms of action of antimicrobials [35]. Finally, dynamic in vitro PK/PD models [61,62,73,87,88,107] and semi-mechanistic PK/PD models were available for only a few combinations and selected isolates [37,54,102,107,118] but provided useful information about the killing activity of antimicrobial combinations at clinically relevant concentrations.

A summary of combinations that have been found synergistic at concentrations ≤established breakpoints of resistance are available in Table A3 of Appendix A. Studies using dynamic in vitro PK/PD models or animal models are summarized in Tables A4 and A5 of Appendix A.

3.7. Clinical Studies

Although several studies have assessed antimicrobial combination in *A. baumannii* infections (e.g., [7–11,123,124]) none was eligible for this review for the following reasons: (a) combinations were assessed in patients with noneligible isolates (i.e., isolates susceptible to at least one component of the combination) or the extraction of data for eligible isolates was not possible, and/or (b) lack of in vitro evaluation for the presence of synergy. The latter is important because, as demonstrated in this review, in vitro synergy observed against selected *A. baumannii* strains with a specific combination cannot be generalized to other *A. baumannii* strains. Furthermore, the very few available studies including patients with infections by PDRAB [1,6,124,125] have major limitations, including small study populations, retrospective designs, lack of a control group or direct comparison of different treatment regimens, and lack of correlation of in vitro susceptibility testing of the combinations with outcomes.

Notable among the available studies is a secondary analysis of the AIDA study (a randomized controlled trial comparing colistin monotherapy to colistin-meropenem combination in patients with carbapenem-resistant Gram-negative infections [9]) comparing monotherapy to combination therapy against colistin- and carbapenem-resistant *A. baumannii* infections [10]. Based on this study, the colistin-meropenem combination was paradoxically associated with higher mortality compared to monotherapy [10]. However, being an exploratory subgroup analysis, the study has several limitations and data on the presence (or absence) of synergy were not reported for the subgroup of patients with colistin- and carbapenem-resistant *A. baumannii* infections. Nevertheless, the study raises the hypothesis that blindly (in the absence of clinical data) using antimicrobial combinations could unexpectedly result in worse outcomes.

In contrast, favorable results have been reported in a few small series (with all the above-mentioned limitations) with selected combinations. For example, triple combination therapy with high-dose ampicillin/sulbactam, high-dose tigecycline and colistin in patients with ventilator-associated pneumonia by PDRAB resulted in clinical cure in 9 of 10 patients [125]. Similarly, in another series, all seven patients with ventilator-associated pneumonia or bacteremia by colistin-resistant *A. baumannii* were successfully treated with a triple combination including colistin, doripenem and ampicillin/sulbactam (although with one exception, all isolates had ampicillin/sulbactam MICs ≤ 16/8 mg/L, i.e., were not eligible for this review) [126]. Furthermore, the combination of colistin with rifampicin has been used successfully to treat post-neurosurgical meningitis after emergence of colistin resistance during treatment with colistin monotherapy [127,128]. However, eligibility of the included isolates in the latter studies could not be assessed due to lack of reporting of rifampicin MICs [127,128].

Therefore, clinical studies assessing antimicrobial combinations in infections by PDRAB are urgently needed. The selection of antimicrobial combinations for further clinical study should ideally be guided by in vitro susceptibility testing of the combinations against local *A. baumannii* strains, taking into account whether synergy is achievable at clinically relevant concentrations.

4. Discussion

4.1. Summary of Main Findings

The emergence of XDR/PDR *A. baumannii* [1], which is associated with high mortality [2] and limited treatment options [6], has resulted in an increasing number of publications evaluating the role of antimicrobial combination therapy. A vast number of potential combinations has been reported, although most combinations have been evaluated only against a limited number of eligible *A. baumannii* isolates. The most studied combinations are polymyxin-based combinations with cell-wall acting agents (including sulbactam, carbapenems and vancomycin), rifampicin and fosfomycin. Nevertheless, a variety of combinations have been reported to be synergistic at clinically achievable concentrations, at least against selected *A. baumannii* isolates. However, in most cases synergy was reported either at too high concentrations or at unclear concentrations.

4.2. Polymyxin-Based Combinations

Polymyxin-based combinations were originally proposed to prevent treatment failure due to the emergence of polymyxin-resistant *A. baumannii* during therapy [129], but may actually be most useful for PDRAB [5,125,127,128]. A proposed mechanism to explain the synergy between polymyxins and other antimicrobials is that polymyxins, even at subinhibitory concentrations, may increase the permeability of *A baumannii*'s cell wall to other antimicrobials, including antimicrobials that would otherwise be ineffective against Gram-negative pathogens (such as glycopeptides and lipopeptides) [12,34,56,88].

Polymyxins may be combined, either as double or as triple combinations, with a variety of antimicrobials, including carbapenems, sulbactam, fosfomycin, rifampicin, rifabutin (which has recently been shown to be much more potent than rifampicin [130] and may retain activity even against PDRAB [131]) and vancomycin. Synergy with many of these combinations was achievable at concentrations ≤established breakpoints of resistance and demonstratable in animal models and/or dynamic in vitro PK/PD studies simulating human treatment regimens.

However, synergy is not universal and not applicable to every *A. baumannii* strain. Clinically relevant synergy may be less likely for strains with very high MICs. For example, clinically-relevant synergy between polymyxins and carbapenems appears to be less likely for isolates with high carbapenem MIC (doripenem >64 mg/L [82], meropenem ≥64 mg/L [132]). Triple combinations may be more effective than double combinations, by lowering MICs of individual agents to even lower levels and preventing emergence of resistance during treatment [51,61,69,82].

4.3. Non-Polymyxin Combinations

A variety of non-polymyxin combinations have been reported, predominantly involving the following antimicrobials: carbapenems, fosfomycin, sulbactam and rifamycins. The combination fosfomycin/sulbactam and to a lesser extent meropenem/sulbactam are especially promising and most studied [37,44,118], but a variety of other combinations have been found synergistic against selected eligible *A. baumannii* isolates. Such combinations may be even more active as triple combinations with polymyxins [51,61,69,82]. Furthermore, among non-polymyxin combinations, the recently proposed avibactam/sulbactam combination (aiming to restore susceptibility to sulbactam by inhibition of non-MBL β-lactamases with avibactam) is particularly promising and warrants further study [47,122].

Tigecycline-based combinations are often used in clinical practice against PDRAB [124,133], probably because of MICs closer to the cut-off for susceptibility [12]. However, based on the limited available data, tigecycline-based (or other tetracyclines, including eravacycline and minocycline) combinations are seldomly synergistic against resistant *A. baumannii* strains at clinically achievable concentrations [12,53,63,71,77,89,96,103,104,117]. However, the lack of in vitro synergy does not preclude a role for tigecycline in the treatment of XDR/PDR *A. baumannii*, especially with higher dose regimens that are predicted to achieve PK/PD targets for isolates with MICs up to 4–8 mg/L [134].

4.4. Limitations of the Review and of the Available Evidence

Despite the abundance of in vitro studies evaluating a variety of antimicrobial combinations against XDR/PDR *A. baumannii*, in vivo data, PK/PD models and clinical data are still limited. Furthermore, there is no acceptable gold standard method (one that best predicts in vivo efficacy) for the in vitro evaluation of synergy, mainly due to the lack of studies correlating in vitro synergy to clinical outcomes [19], and the results of different methods are often conflicting [25,68].

Moreover, as demonstrated in this review, studies often fail to assess the clinical relevance of reported synergy, as evidenced by the evaluation for synergy at antimicrobial concentration unlikely to be clinically relevant or lack of reporting of concentrations at which synergy is present. For example, an FIC index ≤ 0.5 in checkerboard assay does not necessarily prove clinically relevant synergy if antimicrobials are synergistic at concentrations higher than those achievable in vivo at the site of the infection. Similarly, in time-kill assays antimicrobials should ideally be used in concentrations achievable at the site of infection [20], which is often not the case as demonstrated in this review.

However, although clinically-relevant synergy was defined as synergy achievable at concentrations $\leq$ breakpoints of resistance it should be acknowledged that potentially higher breakpoints have been estimated (based on PK/PD data and Monte Carlo simulations) for high-dose, prolonged-infusion regimens [6]. For example, a high probability of target attainment with such regimens has been reported up to the following maximum MICs: meropenem $\leq$128 mg/L [135], doripenem $\leq$8 mg/L [136], fosfomycin $\leq$128 mg/L [45,121], sulbactam $\leq$32 mg/L [119,120]. Furthermore, some studies have evaluated the feasibility of synergistic combinations based on maximum clinically achievable concentrations [44,59] but we believe this approach could result in overestimating the in vivo relevance of synergistic combinations. Finally, the clinical relevance of synergy in animal models, even when using dosing regimens simulating human pharmacokinetics, is unclear considering that in some studies high efficacy was seen even for monotherapies against resistant strains [38,113], while in some cases antimicrobials may have additional functions in animal models not relevant to humans [35].

Finally, another major limitation of this review is the limited clonal diversity of eligible *A. baumannii* isolates for most combinations evaluated, considering that most studies were single-center and that for most combinations only few eligible isolates were assessed. This, combined with the inconsistent activity of antimicrobial combinations highlight the need to confirm in vitro synergy against local *A. baumannii* strains before using any of these combinations in clinical practice.

4.5. Strengths of the Review

Despite the above limitations, this is an exhaustive review of antimicrobial combination options against PDRAB, aiming to aid clinicians, researchers and microbiology laboratories to prioritize the selection of the most promising combinations for further evaluation against PDRAB. Furthermore, a detailed assessment of the potential clinical relevance of each synergistic combination was conducted, based on the concentrations that synergy was observed and the availability of PK/PD or animal models.

5. Conclusions

Antimicrobial combinations may be the only treatment option against PDR *A. baumannii*. Numerous combinations have been evaluated and several appear to be active at clinically relevant concentrations, at least against selected eligible *A. baumannii* isolates. However, studies often do not report the concentrations at which synergy is observed or use antimicrobials at concentrations unlikely to be clinically relevant. This is an important limitation of the available literature and an important consideration for future studies evaluating antimicrobial combinations against PDRAB. Furthermore, no combination was consistently synergistic against all isolates evaluated. Therefore, selecting the most appropriate combination is likely strain-specific and should be guided by in vitro synergy evaluation. Combinations demonstrating activity at clinically relevant concentrations and/or supported by PK/PD data and animal models should be further evaluated in appropriately designed clinical studies, which are currently lacking.

Supplementary Materials: The following are available online at https://www.mdpi.com/article/10.3390/antibiotics10111344/s1, File S1: Table of Contents.

Author Contributions: Conceptualization, S.K., P.I. and D.P.K.; methodology, S.K.; literature search and data extraction, S.K.; data curation, S.K.; writing—original draft preparation, S.K.; writing—review and editing, P.I., G.S. and D.P.K.; supervision, D.P.K. and G.S. All authors have read and agreed to the published version of the manuscript.

Funding: This research received no external funding.

Data Availability Statement: The summary of characteristics and findings of each study included in this review is available in the Supplementary Materials File S1.

Conflicts of Interest: The authors declare no conflict of interest.

Appendix A

Table A1. Distribution of studies by year of publication.

Year of Publication	Number of Studies (%)
2017–2021	**29 (35%)**
2021	5 (6%)
2020	6 (7%)
2019	10 (12%)
2018	3 (4%)
2017	5 (6%)
2012–2016	**32 (38%)**
2016	10 (12%)
2015	6 (7%)
2014	7 (8%)
2013	6 (7%)
2012	3 (4%)
2007–2011	**15 (18%)**
2011	3 (4%)
2010	6 (7%)
2009	3 (4%)
2008	2 (2%)
2007	1 (1%)
2002–2006	**7 (8%)**
2005	2 (2%)
2004	4 (5%)
2003	1 (1%)
1995–2001	**1 (1%)**
1996	1 (1%)

Table A2. Distribution of studies by country and WHO regions.

WHO Regions	Number of Studies Per Region (%)
Americas	**24 (29%)**
Brazil	6 (7%)
USA	12 (14%)
Argentina	3 (4%)
Colombia	1 (1%)
Southeast Asia Region	**7 (8%)**
India	1 (1%)
Thailand	6 (7%)
European Region	**28 (33%)**
France	3 (4%)
Germany	1 (1%)
Greece	3 (4%)
Italy	3 (4%)
Spain	7 (8%)
Turkey	7 (8%)
Switzerland	1 (1%)
United Kingdom	1 (1%)
Eastern Mediterranean Region	**5 (6%)**
Iran	1 (1%)
Saudi Arabia	4 (5%)
United Arab Emirates	2 (2%)
Oman	2 (2%)
Kuwait	2 (2%)
Qatar	2 (2%)
Bahrain	3 (4%)
Western Pacific Region	**20 (24%)**
China	9 (11%)
South Korea	6 (7%)
Taiwan	3 (3%)

Table A3. Antimicrobial combinations shown to be synergistic in checkerboard (CHBD) and/or time-kill assay (TKA) at concentrations ≤ established breakpoints of resistance.

Antimicrobial Combinations	CHBD			CHBD: Concentration at which Synergy Was Present			TKA			TKA: Concentration at which Synergy Was Present		
	Studies n	Isolates n	Synergy n (% *)	≤Breakpoints n (% *)	>Breakpoints n (% *)	Unclear n (% *)	Studies n	Isolates n	Synergy n (% *)	≤Breakpoints n (% *)	>Breakpoints n (% *)	Unclear n (% *)
SUL-based												
SUL/CAZ	1	10	7 (70%)	1 (10%)	6 (60%)	0 (0%)						
SUL/CIP	1	10	8 (80%)	2 (20%)	6 (60%)	0 (0%)						
SUL/MEM	6	173	72 (42%)	2 (1%)	2 (1%)	68 (39%)	3	54	32 (59%)	0 (0%)	7 (22%)	25 (78%)
SUL/DOR							1	17	4 (24%)	4 (100%)	0 (0%)	0 (0%)
SUL/AVI							1	1	1 (100%)	1 (100%)	0 (0%)	0 (0%)
SUL/GEN	1	10	8 (80%)	2 (25%)	6 (75%)	0 (0%)						
SUL/CST							1	6	2 (33%)	2 (100%)	0 (0%)	0 (0%)
SUL/PMB	1	3	2 (67%)	2 (100%)	0 (0%)	0 (0%)						
SUL/FOF	2	56	41 (73%)	3 (7%)	37 (90%)	1 (2%)	2	10	7 (70%)	0 (0%)	7 (100%)	0 (0%)
SAM-based												
SAM/FEP	1	2	2 (100%)	1 (50%)	1 (50%)	0 (0%)						
SAM/LVX	1	7	7 (100%)	5 (71%)	2 (29%)	0 (0%)						
SAM/MEM	2	10	2 (20%)	2 (100%)	0 (0%)	0 (0%)	1	2	0 (0%)	0 (0%)	0 (0%)	0 (0%)
SAM/RIF	1	7	7 (100%)	4 (57%)	1 (14%)	2 (29%)						
IMP-based												
IMP/CFS	1	16	11 (69%)	9 (82%)	2 (18%)	0 (0%)						
IMP/CST	2	10	9 (90%)	2 (20%)	7 (70%)	0 (0%)	1	2	0 (0%)	0 (0%)	0 (0%)	0 (0%)
IMP/RIF	2	28	16 (57%)	11 (39%)	3 (11%)	2 (7%)	5	13	6 (46%)	0 (0%)	6 (46%)	0 (0%)
IMP/FOF	3	45	26 (58%)	9 (20%)	10 (22%)	7 (16%)	1	9	8 (89%)	0 (0%)	8 (89%)	0 (0%)
MEM-based												
MEM/SUL	6	173	72 (42%)	2 (1%)	2 (1%)	68 (39%)	3	54	32 (59%)	0 (0%)	7 (13%)	25 (46%)

Table A3. Cont.

Antimicrobial Combinations	CHBD			CHBD: Concentration at which Synergy Was Present				TKA		TKA: Concentration at which Synergy Was Present		
	Studies n	Isolates n	Synergy n (%*)	≤Breakpoints n (%*)	>Breakpoints n (%*)	Unclear n (%*)	Studies n	Isolates n	Synergy n (%*)	≤Breakpoints n (%*)	>Breakpoints n (%*)	Unclear n (%*)
MEM/SAM	2	10	2 (20%)	2 (20%)	0 (0%)	0 (0%)	1	2	0 (0%)	0 (0%)	0 (0%)	0 (0%)
MEM/AMK	4	47	16 (34%)	1 (2%)	2 (4%)	13 (28%)						
MEM/CST	6	29	21 (72%)	5 (17%)	11 (3%)	5 (17%)	3	4	4 (100%)	0 (0%)	4 (100%)	0 (0%)
MEM/PMB	1	3	3 (100%)	3 (100%)	0 (0%)	0 (0%)	1	2	0 (0%)	0 (0%)	0 (0%)	0 (0%)
MEM/FOF	4	79	15 (19%)	1 (1%)	14 (18%)	0 (0%)						
MEM/VAN	1	5	3 (60%)	1 (20%)	0 (0%)	2 (40%)						
DOR-based												
DOR/SUL							1	17	4 (24%)	4 (24%)	0 (0%)	0 (0%)
DOR/CST	3	6	2 (33%)	1 (17%)	1 (17%)	0 (0%)	5	33	23 (70%)	19 (58%)	4 (12%)	0 (0%)
DOR/TGC	1	3	3 (100%)	1 (33%)	0 (0%)	2 (67%)	1	45	5 (11%)	5 (11%)	0 (0%)	0 (0%)
DOR/RIF	1	1	0 (0%)	0 (0%)	0 (0%)	0 (0%)	1	5	2 (40%)	1 (20%)	1 (20%)	0 (0%)
CZA- or AVI-based												
AVI/SUL							1	1	1 (100%)	1 (100%)	0 (0%)	0 (0%)
CST-based												
CST/SUL	2	2	1 (50%)	1 (50%)	0 (0%)	0 (0%)	1	6	2 (33%)	2 (33%)	0 (0%)	0 (0%)
CST/LVX	2	10	9 (90%)	2 (20%)	7 (70%)	0 (0%)	2	2	1 (50%)	0 (0%)	1 (50%)	0 (0%)
CST/IMP	2	10	9 (90%)				1	2	0 (0%)	0 (0%)	0 (0%)	0 (0%)
CST/MEM	6	29	21 (72%)	5 (17%)	11 (38%)	5 (17%)	3	4	4 (100%)	0 (0%)	4 (100%)	0 (0%)
CST/DOR	3	6	2 (33%)	1 (17%)	1 (17%)	0 (0%)	5	33	23 (70%)	19 (58%)	4 (12%)	0 (0%)
CST/TGC	2	10	0 (0%)	0 (0%)	0 (0%)	0 (0%)	1	12	7 (100%)	7 (100%)	0 (0%)	0 (0%)
CST/RIF	5	40	31 (78%)	10 (25%)	10 (25%)	11 (28%)	3	7	7 (100%)	0 (0%)	6 (86%)	1 (14%)
CST/SXT	2	8	2 (25%)	1 (13%)	0 (0%)	1 (13%)	1	1	1 (100%)	0 (0%)	1 (100%)	0 (0%)
CST/CHL	1	2	2 (100%)	1 (50%)	1 (50%)	0 (0%)	1	2	2 (100%)	0 (0%)	2 (100%)	0 (0%)
CST/FA	2	6	6 (100%)	1 (17%)	2 (33%)	3 (50%)	2	4	3 (75%)	0 (0%)	3 (75%)	0 (0%)
CST/VAN	7	33	29 (88%)	2 (6%)	2 (6%)	25 (67%)	6	20	16 (80%)	13 (65%)	3 (15%)	0 (0%)
PMB-based												
PMB/SUL	1	3	2 (67%)	2 (67%)	0 (0%)	0 (0%)						
PMB/MEM	1	3	3 (100%)	3 (100%)	0 (0%)	0 (0%)	1	2	0 (0%)	0 (0%)	0 (0%)	0 (0%)

Table A3. *Cont.*

Antimicrobial Combinations	CHBD			CHBD: Concentration at which Synergy Was Present				TKA			TKA: Concentration at which Synergy Was Present		
	Studies n	Isolates n	Synergy n (%*)	≤Breakpoints n (%*)	>Breakpoints n (%*)	Unclear n (%*)		Studies n	Isolates n	Synergy n (%*)	≤Breakpoints n (%*)	>Breakpoints n (%*)	Unclear n (%*)
PMB/RIF	1	3	3 (100%)	1 (33%)	1 (33%)	1 (33%)		1	3	1 (33%)	1 (33%)	0 (0%)	0 (0%)
PMB/VAN	1	3	3 (100%)	3 (100%)	0 (0%)	0 (0%)		1	3	2 (67%)	0 (0%)	2 (67%)	0 (0%)
TGC-based													
TGC/DOR	1	3	3 (100%)	1 (33%)	0 (0%)	2 (67%)		1	45	5 (11%)	5 (11%)	0 (0%)	0 (0%)
TGC/AMK	1	14	2 (14%)	1 (7%)	1 (7%)	0 (0%)		1	1	1 (100%)	1 (100%)	0 (0%)	0 (0%)
TGC/CST	2	10	0 (0%)	0 (0%)	0 (0%)	0 (0%)		1	12	7 (58%)	7 (58%)	0 (0%)	0 (0%)
TGC/RIF	2	16	1 (6%)	0 (0%)	1 (6%)	0 (0%)		2	4	1 (25%)	1 (25%)	0 (0%)	0 (0%)
TGC/FOF	1	4	3 (75%)	1 (25%)	2 (50%)	0 (0%)		1	1	1 (100%)	0 (0%)	1 (100%)	0 (0%)
RIF-based													
RIF/SAM	1	7	7 (100%)	4 (57%)	1 (14%)	2 (29%)							
RIF/CFS	1	7	2 (29%)	1 (14%)	0 (0%)	1 (14%)							
RIF/IMP	2	28	16 (57%)	11 (39%)	3 (11%)	2 (7%)		5	13	6 (46%)	0 (0%)	6 (46%)	0 (0%)
RIF/DOR	1	1	0 (0%)	0 (0%)	0 (0%)	0 (0%)		1	5	2 (40%)	1 (20%)	1 (20%)	0 (0%)
RIF/CST	5	40	31 (78%)	10 (25%)	10 (25%)	11 (28%)		3	7	7 (100%)	0 (0%)	6 (85%)	1 (14%)
RIF/PMB	1	3	3 (100%)	1 (33%)	1 (33%)	1 (33%)		1	3	1 (33%)	1 (33%)	0 (0%)	0 (0%)
RIF/TGC	2	16	1 (100%)	0 (0%)	1 (100%)	0 (0%)		2	4	1 (25%)	1 (25%)	0 (0%)	0 (0%)
FOF-based													
FOF/SUL	2	56	41 (73%)	3 (5%)	37 (66%)	1 (2%)		2	10	7 (70%)	0 (0%)	7 (70%)	0 (0%)
FOF/IMP	3	45	26 (58%)	9 (20%)	10 (22%)	7 (16%)		1	9	8 (89%)	0 (0%)	8 (89%)	0 (0%)
FOF/MEM	4	79	15 (19%)	1 (1%)	14 (18%)	0 (0%)							
FOF/AMK	2	29	26 (90%)	11 (38%)	15 (52%)	0 (0%)							
FOF/GEN	2	13	12 (92%)	3 (32%)	9 (69%)	0 (0%)							
FOF/TGC	1	4	3 (75%)	1 (25%)	2 (50%)	0 (0%)		1	1	1 (100%)	0 (0%)	1 (100%)	0 (0%)

Table A3. Cont.

Antimicrobial Combinations	Studies n	CHBD Isolates n	Synergy n (% *)	CHBD: Concentration at which Synergy Was Present			Studies n	TKA Isolates n	Synergy n (% *)	TKA: Concentration at which Synergy Was Present		
				≤Breakpoints n (% *)	>Breakpoints n (% *)	Unclear n (% *)				≤Breakpoints n (% *)	>Breakpoints n (% *)	Unclear n (% *)
Triple combinations												
PMB/FOF/MEM	1	3	3 (100%)	3 (100%)	0 (0%)	0 (0%)						
PMB/SUL/MEM	1	3	3 (100%)	3 (100%)	0 (0%)	0 (0%)						
CST/DOR/SUL							1	6	6 (100%)	6 (100%)	0 (0%)	0 (0%)
CST/VAN/DOR							1	3	3 (100%)	3 (100%)	0 (0%)	0 (0%)

* Percentage over total number of isolates. Combinations only shown to be synergistic at concentrations > established breakpoints or at unclear concentrations are not included in this Table. A more complete (including all combinations) version of this Table as well as similar Tables for other methods are available in the Supplementary Materials File S1 Section 4. Abbreviations: AMK = amikacin, AVI = avibactam, ATM = aztreonam, AZM = azithromycin, CAZ = ceftazidime, CFS = cefoperazone/sulbactam, CHBD = checkerboard assay, CHL = chloramphenicol, CIP = ciprofloxacin, CST = colistin, CZA = ceftazidime/avibactam, DOR = doripenem, FA = fusidic acid, FEP = cefepime, FOF = fosfomycin, GEN = gentamicin, IMP = imipenem, LVX = levofloxacin, MEM = meropenem, PMB = polymyxin-B, RIF = rifampicin, SAM = ampicillin/sulbactam, SUL = sulbactam, SXT = trimethoprim/sulfamethoxazole, TEC = teicoplanin, TGC = tigecycline, TKA = time-kill assay, TMP = trimethoprim, VAN = vancomycin. In the single eligible study using multiple-combination bactericidal assay [12] (not shown in the Table) the following combinations were active at concentrations equal to breakpoints of resistance: SAM/RIF (synergistic against 1 of 8 eligible isolates), SAM/SXT (1/7), SAM/TEC (1/7), AMK/CAZ (1/6), AMK/SXT (1/8), AZM/CAZ (1/8), AZM/TEC (1/9), AZM/SXT (1/6), ATM/CAZ (1/9), ATM/TEC (1/9), CAZ/MEM (1/9), CAZ/RIF (1/9), CAZ/TGC (1/9), CAZ/SXT (1/7), CAZ/VAN (1/9), MEM/RIF (1/9), MEM/TEC (1/9), RIF/SXT (1/7), SXT/VAN (1/7), AMK/RIF (2/6), CAZ/TEC (2/9), CST/RIF (9/9), CST/TEC (9/9), CST/VAN (8/9), CST/MEM (8/9), CST/ATM (8/9), CST/CAZ (6/9), CST/SAM (5/8), CST/SXT (3/8), CST/AMK (4/6), CST/AZM (4/8).

Table A4. Studies using dynamic in vitro PK/PD models.

Study-Combinations	Method	Synergy % (n/N)	Comments
Lenhard, J.R., 2017 [61,62]			
PMB/MEM	HFIM	0 (0/1)	Doses simulating human regimens were used (PMB 3.33 mg/kg then 1.43 mg/kg every 12 h, MEM 2 gr every 8 h as 3 h infusions, SAM 8/4 g every 8 h as 3 h infusions).
PMB/SAM	HFIM	0 (0/1)	
MEM/SAM		0 (0/1)	
PMB/MEM/SAM		100 (1/1)	
Yuan, Z., 2010 [102] and Lim, T.P., 2008 [107]			
AMK/LVX	HFIM	0 (0/1)	Regrowth despite initial killing at 4 h.
AMK/FEP		0 (0/1)	Regrowth despite initial killing at 4 h.
Córdoba, J., 2015 [73]			
CST/IMP	Other dynamic in vitro PK/PD model	0 (0/1)	Simulation of human treatment regimens
CST/DAP		100 (1/1)	
IMP/ETP		0 (0/3)	
RIF/CFS		0 (0/7)	
Housman, S.T., 2013 [87]			Simulated regimens: SAM 9 g q8 h (3 h inf), DOR 2 gr q8 h (4 h inf), TGC 200 mg q12 h (0.5 h inf).
TGC/DOR	Other dynamic in vitro PK/PD model	0 (0/2)	
SAM/DOR		0 (0/3)	Increased killing with SAM/DOR vs. monotherapies against all 3 strains but with regrowth by 24 h.
SAM/TGC		0 (0/1)	
Lee, H.J., 2013 [88]			
CST/RIF	Other dynamic in vitro PK/PD model	100 (1/1)	Regimens mimicking human serum concentration after usual doses in critically-ill patients.

Abbreviations: AMK = amikacin, CFS = cefoperazone/sulbactam, CHBD = checkerboard assay, CST = colistin, CZA = ceftazidime/avibactam, DAP = daptomycin, DOR = doripenem, ETP = ertapenem, FEP = cefepime, FOF = fosfomycin, HFIM = hollow-fiber infection model, IMP = imipenem, LVX = levofloxacin, MEM = meropenem, n/N = number of isolates against which synergy was demonstrated/total number of eligible isolates, PK/PD = pharmacokinetic/pharmacodynamic, PMB = polymyxin-B, RIF = rifampicin, SAM = ampicillin/sulbactam, TGC = tigecycline.

Table A5. Studies using animal models.

Study-Combinations	Method	Synergy % (n/N)	Comments
Cebrero-Cangueiro, T., 2021 [38]			
MEM/IMP	Intraperitoneal infection mouse model	0 (0/2)	Decreased bacterial loads with combination vs. monotherapy, but similar mortality and bacterial clearance comparing meropenem monotherapy to combination therapy.
Poulakou, G., 2019 [55]			
CST/DAP	Intraperitoneal infection mouse model	100 (1/1)	The combination significantly improved survival and reduced bacterial loads in tissues compared to monotherapies.
Wei, W., 2017 [64]			
CST/LVX	*G. mellonella* model	0 (0/1)	Same survival comparing combination therapy to monotherapy
Yang, H., 2016 [70]			
CST/VAN	*G. mellonella* model	100 (1/1)	Survival rate in *G. mellonella* model higher with combination, but high survival even with monotherapies.
O'Hara, J.A., 2013 [35]			
CST/DOR	*G. mellonella* model	0 (0/3)	No synergy
CST/VAN		0 (0/3)	
DOR/VAN		100 (3/3)	The clinical relevance of the *G. mellonella* model is unclear because of mechanisms of action likely not relevant to humans; high survival even with DOR and VAN monotherapies, and high survival with DOR/VAN despite lack of in vitro synergy
CST/VAN/DOR		100 (3/3)	
Queenan, A.M., 2013 [90]			
DOR/CIP	intraperitoneal infection mouse model	0 (0/1)	No synergy
DOR/LVX		100 (1/1)	Improved survival in the mouse model (the isolate had relatively low MICs: DOR 16 mg/L and LVX 8 mg/L).
Pachón-Ibáñez, M.E., 2011 [94]			
RIF/IMP	Pneumonia mouse model	0 (0/2)	In the animal model survival with RIF/IMP (80 and 33%) and RIF/SUL (60 and 53%) did not differ significantly compared to RIF monotherapy (73 and 40%). Lung clearance and blood culture sterilization was higher against one of the two strains with RIF/SUL.
RIF/SUL		50 (1/2)	
Pachón-Ibáñez, M.E., 2010 [98]			
SUL/IMP	Pneumonia (mouse) and meningitis (rabbit) models	100 (1/1)	Higher survival and bacterial clearance in animal model compared to monotherapies.
RIF/IMP		0 (0/1)	Survival not improved comparing RIF monotherapy (71%) to combination therapy (60%), despite improved bacterial clearance.
RIF/SUL		0 (0/1)	Survival not improved comparing RIF monotherapy (71%) to combination therapy (47%), despite improved bacterial clearance.
Yuan, Z., 2010 [102]			
AMK/LVX	Pneumonia mouse model	0 (0/1)	Similar survival with AMK monotherapy.
AMK/FEP		1 (1/1)	Improved survival and reduction of tissue bacterial burden in the mouse model.
FEP/LVX		0 (0/1)	Similar survival with FEP monotherapy.
Song, Y.C., 2009 [105]			
IMP/RIF	Pneumonia mouse model	100 (3/3)	Synergistic ($\geq 2\Delta$log reduction in lung baterial loads compared to RIF monotherapy) against all 3 strains, but 100% survival with both monotherapy and combination.
RIF/AMK		0 (0/1)	Not better than monotherapy
IMP/AMK		0 (0/1)	Not better than monotherapy
Montero, A., 2004 [113]			
IMP/RIF	Pneumonia mouse model	50 (1/2)	Strain D: no differences compared to monotherapy in the mouse model. Strain E: significantly reduced lung bacterial counts, no significant reduction of bacteremia, similar survival (100% with the combination, 100% with RIF monotherapy).

Abbreviations: AMK = amikacin, CIP = ciprofloxacin, CST = colistin, DOR = doripenem, FEP = cefepime, IMP = imipenem, LVX = levofloxacin, MEM = meropenem, RIF = rifampicin, SUL = sulbactam, VAN = vancomycin.

References

1. Karakonstantis, S.; Kritsotakis, E.I.; Gikas, A. Pandrug-resistant Gram-negative bacteria: A systematic review of current epidemiology, prognosis and treatment options. *J. Antimicrob. Chemother.* **2019**, *75*, 271–282. [CrossRef] [PubMed]
2. Karakonstantis, S.; Gikas, A.; Astrinaki, E.; Kritsotakis, E.I. Excess mortality due to pandrug-resistant *Acinetobacter baumannii* infections in hospitalized patients. *J. Hosp. Infect.* **2020**, *106*, 447–453. [CrossRef] [PubMed]
3. McCreary, E.K.; Heil, E.L.; Tamma, P.D. New Perspectives on Antimicrobial Agents: Cefiderocol. *Antimicrob. Agents Chemother.* **2021**, *65*, e0217120. [CrossRef] [PubMed]
4. Choby, J.E.; Ozturk, T.; Satola, S.W.; Jacob, J.T.; Weiss, D.S. Widespread cefiderocol heteroresistance in carbapenem-resistant Gram-negative pathogens. *Lancet Infect. Dis.* **2021**, *21*, 597–598. [CrossRef]
5. Karakonstantis, S.; Saridakis, I. Colistin heteroresistance in *Acinetobacter* spp.: Systematic review and meta-analysis of the prevalence and discussion of the mechanisms and potential therapeutic implications. *Int. J. Antimicrob. Agents* **2020**, *56*, 106065. [CrossRef]
6. Karakonstantis, S.; Kritsotakis, E.I.; Gikas, A. Treatment options for K. pneumoniae, P. aeruginosa and *A. baumannii* co-resistant to carbapenems, aminoglycosides, polymyxins and tigecycline: An approach based on the mechanisms of resistance to carbapenems. *Infection* **2020**, *48*, 835–851. [CrossRef]
7. Wang, J.; Niu, H.; Wang, R.; Cai, Y. Safety and efficacy of colistin alone or in combination in adults with *Acinetobacter baumannii* infection: A systematic review and meta-analysis. *Int. J. Antimicrob. Agents* **2019**, *53*, 383–400. [CrossRef]
8. Salameh, M.; Daher, L.M.A.; Chartouny, M.; Hanna, P.A. Colistin monotherapy v/s colistin combination therapy for treatment of *Acinetobacter* infections, a systematic review. *J. Infect. Dev. Ctries.* **2018**, *12*, 23S. [CrossRef]
9. Paul, M.; Daikos, G.L.; Durante-Mangoni, E.; Yahav, D.; Carmeli, Y.; Benattar, Y.D.; Skiada, A.; Andini, R.; Eliakim-Raz, N.; Nutman, A.; et al. Colistin alone versus colistin plus meropenem for treatment of severe infections caused by carbapenem-resistant Gram-negative bacteria: An open-label, randomised controlled trial. *Lancet Infect. Dis.* **2018**, *18*, 391–400. [CrossRef]
10. Dickstein, Y.; Lellouche, J.; Amar, M.B.D.; Schwartz, D.; Nutman, A.; Daitch, V.; Yahav, D.; Leibovici, L.; Skiada, A.; Antoniadou, A.; et al. Treatment Outcomes of Colistin- and Carbapenem-resistant *Acinetobacter baumannii* Infections: An Exploratory Subgroup Analysis of a Randomized Clinical Trial. *Clin. Infect. Dis.* **2018**, *69*, 769–776. [CrossRef]
11. Poulikakos, P.; Tansarli, G.S.; Falagas, M.E. Combination antibiotic treatment versus monotherapy for multidrug-resistant, extensively drug-resistant, and pandrug-resistant *Acinetobacter* infections: A systematic review. *Eur. J. Clin. Microbiol. Infect. Dis.* **2014**, *33*, 1675–1685. [CrossRef]
12. Bae, S.; Kim, M.-C.; Park, S.-J.; Kim, H.S.; Sung, H.; Kim, S.-H.; Lee, S.-O.; Choi, S.-H.; Woo, J.H.; Kim, Y.S.; et al. In Vitro Synergistic Activity of Antimicrobial Agents in Combination against Clinical Isolates of Colistin-Resistant *Acinetobacter baumannii*. *Antimicrob. Agents Chemother.* **2016**, *60*, 6774–6779. [CrossRef]
13. Karakonstantis, S. Re: 'Colistin plus meropenem for carbapenem-resistant Gram-negative infections: In vitro synergism is not associated with better clinical outcomes' by Nutman et al. *Clin. Microbiol. Infect.* **2020**, *26*, 1274. [CrossRef]
14. Mohammadi, M.; Khayat, H.; Sayehmiri, K.; Soroush, S.; Sayehmiri, F.; Delfani, S.; Bogdanovic, L.; Taherikalani, M. Synergistic Effect of Colistin and Rifampin Against Multidrug Resistant *Acinetobacter baumannii*: A Systematic Review and Meta-Analysis. *Open Microbiol. J.* **2017**, *11*, 63–71. [CrossRef]
15. Ni, W.; Shao, X.; Di, X.; Cui, J.; Wang, R.; Liu, Y. In vitro synergy of polymyxins with other antibiotics for *Acinetobacter baumannii*: A systematic review and meta-analysis. *Int. J. Antimicrob. Agents* **2015**, *45*, 8–18. [CrossRef]
16. Scudeller, L.; Righi, E.; Chiamenti, M.; Bragantini, D.; Menchinelli, G.; Cattaneo, P.; Giske, C.G.; Lodise, T.; Sanguinetti, M.; Piddock, L.J.; et al. Systematic review and meta-analysis of in vitro efficacy of antibiotic combination therapy against carbapenem-resistant Gram-negative bacilli. *Int. J. Antimicrob. Agents* **2021**, *57*, 106344. [CrossRef]
17. Jiang, Z.; He, X.; Li, J. Synergy effect of meropenem-based combinations against *Acinetobacter baumannii*: A systematic review and meta-analysis. *Infect. Drug Resist.* **2018**, *11*, 1083–1095. [CrossRef]
18. Li, J.; Yang, X.; Chen, L.; Duan, X.; Jiang, Z. In Vitro Activity of Various Antibiotics in Combination with Tigecycline Against *Acinetobacter baumannii*: A Systematic Review and Meta-Analysis. *Microb. Drug Resist.* **2017**, *23*, 982–993. [CrossRef]
19. Brennan-Krohn, T.; Kirby, J.E. When One Drug Is Not Enough: Context, Methodology, and Future Prospects in Antibacterial Synergy Testing. *Clin. Lab. Med.* **2019**, *39*, 345–358. [CrossRef]
20. Pillai, S.K.; Moellering, R.C.; Eliopoulos, G.M. Antimicrobial combinations. In *Antibiotics in Laboratory Medicine*, 5th ed.; Lorian, V., Ed.; Lippincott Williams and Wilkins: Philadelphia, PA, USA, 2005.
21. Morrison, A.; Polisena, J.; Husereau, D.; Moulton, K.; Clark, M.; Fiander, M.; Mierzwinski-Urban, M.; Clifford, T.; Hutton, B.; Rabb, D. The effect of English-language restriction on systematic review-based meta-analyses: A systematic review of empirical studies. *Int. J. Technol. Assess. Health Care* **2012**, *28*, 138–144. [CrossRef]
22. Higgins, J.P.T.; Thomas, J.; Chandler, J.; Cumpston, M.; Li, T.; Page, M.J.; Welch, V.A.E. Cochrane Handbook for Systematic Reviews of Interventions Version 6.2 (updated February 2021). Available online: www.training.cochrane.org/handbook (accessed on 3 November 2021).
23. Balk, E.M.; Chung, M.; Chen, M.L.; Chang, L.K.W.; Trikalinos, T.A. Data extraction from machine-translated versus original language randomized trial reports: A comparative study. *Syst. Rev.* **2013**, *2*, 97. [CrossRef]
24. Ouzzani, M.; Hammady, H.; Fedorowicz, Z.; Elmagarmid, A. Rayyan—A web and mobile app for systematic reviews. *Syst. Rev.* **2016**, *5*, 1–10. [CrossRef]

25. Bonapace, C.R.; Bosso, J.A.; Friedrich, L.V.; White, R.L. Comparison of methods of interpretation of checkerboard synergy testing. *Diagn. Microbiol. Infect. Dis.* **2002**, *44*, 363–366. [CrossRef]
26. Brill, M.; Kristoffersson, A.; Zhao, C.; Nielsen, E.; Friberg, L. Semi-mechanistic pharmacokinetic–pharmacodynamic modelling of antibiotic drug combinations. *Clin. Microbiol. Infect.* **2018**, *24*, 697–706. [CrossRef]
27. Doern, C.D. When Does 2 Plus 2 Equal 5? A Review of Antimicrobial Synergy Testing. *J. Clin. Microbiol.* **2014**, *52*, 4124–4128. [CrossRef]
28. CLSI. *Performance Standards for Antimicrobial Susceptibility Testing*, 31st ed.; CLSI Supplement M100; Clinical Laboratory Standards Institute: Wayne, PA, USA, 2021.
29. The European Committee on Antimicrobial Susceptibility Testing. Breakpoint Tables for Interpretation of MICs and Zone Diameters. Version 11.0. Available online: http://www.eucast.org/ (accessed on 3 November 2021).
30. Sader, H.S.; Carvalhaes, C.; Streit, J.M.; Castanheira, M.; Flamm, R.K. Antimicrobial activity of cefoperazone-sulbactam tested against Gram-Negative organisms from Europe, Asia-Pacific, and Latin America. *Int. J. Infect. Dis.* **2020**, *91*, 32–37. [CrossRef]
31. FDA. Plazomicin Infection. FDA-Identified Interpretive Criteria. Available online: https://www.fda.gov/drugs/development-resources/plazomicin-injection (accessed on 23 June 2021).
32. Lepe, J.A.; García-Cabrera, E.; Gil-Navarro, M.V.; Aznar, J. Rifampin breakpoint for *Acinetobacter baumannii* based on pharmacokinetic-pharmacodynamic models with Monte Carlo simulation. *Rev. Esp. Quimioter. Publ. Soc. Esp. Quimioter.* **2012**, *25*, 134–138.
33. Food and Drug Administration (FDA). Tigecycline–Injection Products 2019. Available online: https://www.fda.gov/drugs/development-resources/tigecycline-injection-products (accessed on 26 June 2019).
34. Gordon, N.; Png, K.; Wareham, D.W. Potent Synergy and Sustained Bactericidal Activity of a Vancomycin-Colistin Combination versus Multidrug-Resistant Strains of *Acinetobacter baumannii*. *Antimicrob. Agents Chemother.* **2010**, *54*, 5316–5322. [CrossRef]
35. O'Hara, J.A.; Ambe, L.A.; Casella, L.G.; Townsend, B.M.; Pelletier, M.R.; Ernst, R.K.; Shanks, R.M.Q.; Doi, Y. Activities of Vancomycin-Containing Regimens against Colistin-Resistant *Acinetobacter baumannii* Clinical Strains. *Antimicrob. Agents Chemother.* **2013**, *57*, 2103–2108. [CrossRef]
36. Bowler, S.L.; Spychala, C.N.; McElheny, C.L.; Mettus, R.T.; Doi, Y. In Vitro Activity of Fusidic Acid-Containing Combinations against Carbapenem-Resistant *Acinetobacter baumannii* Clinical Strains. *Antimicrob. Agents Chemother.* **2016**, *60*, 5101. [CrossRef]
37. Lim, S.M.S.; Heffernan, A.J.; Roberts, J.A.; Sime, F.B. Semimechanistic Pharmacokinetic/Pharmacodynamic Modeling of Fosfomycin and Sulbactam Combination against Carbapenem-Resistant *Acinetobacter baumannii*. *Antimicrob. Agents Chemother.* **2021**, *65*, e02472-20. [CrossRef]
38. Cebrero-Cangueiro, T.; Nordmann, P.; Carretero-Ledesma, M.; Pachón, J.; Pachón-Ibáñez, M.E. Efficacy of dual carbapenem treatment in a murine sepsis model of infection due to carbapenemase-producing *Acinetobacter baumannii*. *J. Antimicrob. Chemother.* **2021**, *76*, 680–683. [CrossRef] [PubMed]
39. Cheng, J.; Yan, J.; Reyna, Z.; Slarve, M.; Lu, P.; Spellberg, B.; Luna, B. Synergistic Rifabutin and Colistin Reduce Emergence of Resistance When Treating *Acinetobacter baumannii*. *Antimicrob. Agents Chemother.* **2021**, *65*, e02204-20. [CrossRef] [PubMed]
40. Terbtothakun, P.; Voravuthikunchai, S.; Chusri, S. Evaluation of the Synergistic Antibacterial Effects of Fosfomycin in Combination with Selected Antibiotics against Carbapenem–Resistant *Acinetobacter baumannii*. *Pharmaceuticals* **2021**, *14*, 185. [CrossRef]
41. Armengol, E.; Asunción, T.; Viñas, M.; Sierra, J.M. When Combined with Colistin, an Otherwise Ineffective Rifampicin–Linezolid Combination Becomes Active in *Escherichia coli*, *Pseudomonas aeruginosa*, and *Acinetobacter baumannii*. *Microorganisms* **2020**, *8*, 86. [CrossRef]
42. Li, J.; Fu, Y.; Zhang, J.; Zhao, Y.; Fan, X.; Yu, L.; Wang, Y.; Zhang, X.; Li, C. The efficacy of colistin monotherapy versus combination therapy with other antimicrobials against carbapenem-resistant *Acinetobacter baumannii* ST2 isolates. *J. Chemother.* **2020**, *32*, 359–367. [CrossRef]
43. Limsrivanichakorn, S.; Ngamskulrungroj, P.; Leelaporn, A. Activity of Antimicrobial Combinations Against Extensively Drug-Resistant *Acinetobacter baumannii* as Determined by Checkerboard Method and E-test. *Siriraj Med. J.* **2020**, *72*, 214–218. [CrossRef]
44. Lim, S.M.S.; Naicker, S.; Ayfan, A.; Zowawi, H.; Roberts, J.; Sime, F. Non-polymyxin-based combinations as potential alternatives in treatment against carbapenem-resistant *Acinetobacter baumannii* infections. *Int. J. Antimicrob. Agents* **2020**, *56*, 106115. [CrossRef]
45. Lim, S.M.S.; Heffernan, A.J.; Roberts, J.A.; Sime, F.B. Pharmacodynamic Analysis of Meropenem and Fosfomycin Combination Against Carbapenem-Resistant *Acinetobacter baumannii* in Patients with Normal Renal Clearance: Can It Be a Treatment Option? *Microb. Drug Resist.* **2021**, *27*, 546–552. [CrossRef]
46. Nordmann, P.; Perler, J.; Kieffer, N.; Poirel, L. In-vitro evaluation of a dual carbapenem combination against carbapenemase-producing *Acinetobacter baumannii*. *J. Infect.* **2020**, *80*, 121–142. [CrossRef]
47. Rodriguez, C.H.; Brune, A.; Nastro, M.; Vay, C.; Famiglietti, A. In vitro synergistic activity of the sulbactam/avibactam combination against extensively drug-resistant *Acinetobacter baumannii*. *J. Med. Microbiol.* **2020**, *69*, 928–931. [CrossRef]
48. Gaudereto, J.J.; Neto, L.V.P.; Leite, G.C.; Martins, R.R.; Prado, G.V.B.D.; Rossi, F.; Guimarães, T.; Levin, A.S.; Costa, S.F. Synergistic Effect of Ceftazidime-Avibactam with Meropenem against Panresistant, Carbapenemase-Harboring *Acinetobacter baumannii* and *Serratia marcescens* Investigated Using Time-Kill and Disk Approximation Assays. *Antimicrob. Agents Chemother.* **2019**, *63*, e02367-18. [CrossRef]

49. Ghaith, D.; Hassan, R.; Dawoud, M.E.E.-D.; Eweis, M.; Metwally, R.; Zafer, M. Effect of rifampicin–colistin combination against XDR *Acinetobacter baumannii* harbouring blaOXA 23-like gene and showed reduced susceptibility to colistin at Cairo University Hospital, Cairo, Egypt. *Infect. Dis.* **2019**, *51*, 308–311. [CrossRef]
50. Kara, E.M.; Yılmaz, M.; Çelik, B. In vitro activities of ceftazidime/avibactam alone or in combination with antibiotics against multidrug-resistant *Acinetobacter baumannii* isolates. *J. Glob. Antimicrob. Resist.* **2019**, *17*, 137–141. [CrossRef]
51. Menegucci, T.C.; Fedrigo, N.H.; Lodi, F.G.; Albiero, J.; Nishiyama, S.A.B.; Mazucheli, J.; Carrara-Marroni, F.E.; Voelkner, N.M.F.; Gong, H.; Sy, S.; et al. Pharmacodynamic Effects of Sulbactam/Meropenem/Polymyxin-B Combination Against Extremely Drug Resistant *Acinetobacter baumannii* Using Checkerboard Information. *Microb. Drug Resist.* **2019**, *25*, 1266–1274. [CrossRef]
52. Oliva, A.; Garzoli, S.; De Angelis, M.; Marzuillo, C.; Vullo, V.; Mastroianni, C.M.; Ragno, R. In-Vitro Evaluation of Different Antimicrobial Combinations with and without Colistin Against Carbapenem-Resistant *Acinetobacter baumannii*. *Molecules* **2019**, *24*, 886. [CrossRef]
53. Ozger, H.S.; Cuhadar, T.; Yildiz, S.S.; Gulmez, Z.D.; Dizbay, M.; Tunccan, O.G.; Kalkanci, A.; Simsek, H.; Unaldi, O. In vitro activity of eravacycline in combination with colistin against carbapenem-resistant *A. baumannii* isolates. *J. Antibiot.* **2019**, *72*, 600–604. [CrossRef]
54. Phee, L.M.; Kloprogge, F.; Morris, R.; Barrett, J.; Wareham, D.W.; Standing, J.F. Pharmacokinetic-pharmacodynamic modelling to investigate in vitro synergy between colistin and fusidic acid against MDR *Acinetobacter baumannii*. *J. Antimicrob. Chemother.* **2019**, *74*, 961–969. [CrossRef]
55. Poulakou, G.; Renieris, G.; Sabrakos, L.; Zarkotou, O.; Themeli-Digalaki, K.; Perivolioti, E.; Kraniotaki, E.; Giamarellos-Bourboulis, E.J.; Zavras, N. Daptomycin as adjunctive treatment for experimental infection by *Acinetobacter baumannii* with resistance to colistin. *Int. J. Antimicrob. Agents* **2018**, *53*, 190–194. [CrossRef]
56. Shinohara, D.R.; Menegucci, T.C.; Fedrigo, N.H.; Migliorini, L.B.; Carrara-Marroni, F.E.; Anjos, M.; Cardoso, C.L.; Nishiyama, S.A.B.; Tognim, M.C.B. Synergistic activity of polymyxin B combined with vancomycin against carbapenem-resistant and polymyxin-resistant *Acinetobacter baumannii*: First in vitro study. *J. Med. Microbiol.* **2019**, *68*, 309–315. [CrossRef]
57. Wang, J.; Ning, Y.; Li, S.; Wang, Y.; Liang, J.; Jin, C.; Yan, H.; Huang, Y. Multidrug-resistant *Acinetobacter baumannii* strains with NDM-1: Molecular characterization and in vitro efficacy of meropenem-based combinations. *Exp. Ther. Med.* **2019**, *18*, 2924–2932. [CrossRef]
58. Chen, F.; Wang, L.; Wang, M.; Xie, Y.; Xia, X.; Li, X.; Liu, Y.; Cao, W.; Zhang, T.; Li, P.; et al. Genetic characterization and in vitro activity of antimicrobial combinations of multidrug-resistant *Acinetobacter baumannii* from a general hospital in China. *Oncol. Lett.* **2018**, *15*, 2305–2315. [CrossRef]
59. Singkham-In, U.; Chatsuwan, T. In vitro activities of carbapenems in combination with amikacin, colistin, or fosfomycin against carbapenem-resistant *Acinetobacter baumannii* clinical isolates. *Diagn. Microbiol. Infect. Dis.* **2018**, *91*, 169–174. [CrossRef]
60. Zhu, W.; Wang, Y.; Cao, W.; Cao, S.; Zhang, J. In vitro evaluation of antimicrobial combinations against imipenem-resistant *Acinetobacter baumannii* of different MICs. *J. Infect. Public Health* **2018**, *11*, 856–860. [CrossRef]
61. Lenhard, J.R.; Thamlikitkul, V.; Silveira, F.P.; Garonzik, S.M.; Tao, X.; Forrest, A.; Shin, B.S.; Kaye, K.S.; Bulitta, J.B.; Nation, R.L.; et al. Polymyxin-resistant, carbapenem-resistant *Acinetobacter baumannii* is eradicated by a triple combination of agents that lack individual activity. *J. Antimicrob. Chemother.* **2017**, *72*, 1415–1420. [CrossRef]
62. Lenhard, J.; Smith, N.M.; Bulman, Z.P.; Tao, X.; Thamlikitkul, V.; Shin, B.S.; Nation, R.L.; Li, J.; Bulitta, J.B.; Tsuji, B.T. High-Dose Ampicillin-Sulbactam Combinations Combat Polymyxin-Resistant *Acinetobacter baumannii* in a Hollow-Fiber Infection Model. *Antimicrob. Agents Chemother.* **2017**, *61*, e01268-16. [CrossRef]
63. Madadi-Goli, N.; Moniri, R.; Bagheri-Josheghani, S.; Dasteh-Goli, N. Sensitivity of levofloxacin in combination with ampicillin-sulbactam and tigecycline against multidrug-resistant *Acinetobacter baumannii*. *Iran. J. Microbiol.* **2017**, *9*, 19–25.
64. Wei, W.; Yang, H.; Hu, L.; Ye, Y.; Li, J. Activity of levofloxacin in combination with colistin against *Acinetobacter baumannii*: In vitro and in a Galleria mellonella model. *J. Microbiol. Immunol. Infect.* **2017**, *50*, 821–830. [CrossRef]
65. Wei, W.-J.; Yang, H.-F. Synergy against extensively drug-resistant *Acinetobacter baumannii* in vitro by two old antibiotics: Colistin and chloramphenicol. *Int. J. Antimicrob. Agents* **2017**, *49*, 321–326. [CrossRef]
66. Hong, D.J.; Kim, J.O.; Lee, H.; Yoon, E.-J.; Jeong, S.H.; Yong, D.; Lee, K. In vitro antimicrobial synergy of colistin with rifampicin and carbapenems against colistin-resistant *Acinetobacter baumannii* clinical isolates. *Diagn. Microbiol. Infect. Dis.* **2016**, *86*, 184–189. [CrossRef]
67. Laishram, S.; Anandan, S.; Devi, B.Y.; Elakkiya, M.; Priyanka, B.; Bhuvaneshwari, T.; Peter, J.V.; Subramani, K.; Balaji, V. Determination of synergy between sulbactam, meropenem and colistin in carbapenem-resistant *Klebsiella pneumoniae* and *Acinetobacter baumannii* isolates and correlation with the molecular mechanism of resistance. *J. Chemother.* **2016**, *28*, 297–303. [CrossRef] [PubMed]
68. Leite, G.C.; Oliveira, M.S.; Perdigão-Neto, L.V.; Rocha, C.K.D.; Guimarães, T.; Rizek, C.; Levin, A.; Costa, S.F. Antimicrobial Combinations against Pan-Resistant *Acinetobacter baumannii* Isolates with Different Resistance Mechanisms. *PLoS ONE* **2016**, *11*, e0151270. [CrossRef] [PubMed]
69. Menegucci, T.C.; Albiero, J.; Migliorini, L.B.; Alves, J.L.B.; Viana, G.F.; Mazucheli, J.; Carrara-Marroni, F.E.; Cardoso, C.L.; Tognim, M.C.B. Strategies for the treatment of polymyxin B-resistant *Acinetobacter baumannii* infections. *Int. J. Antimicrob. Agents* **2016**, *47*, 380–385. [CrossRef] [PubMed]

70. Yang, H.; Lv, N.; Hu, L.; Liu, Y.; Cheng, J.; Ye, Y.; Li, J. In vivoactivity of vancomycin combined with colistin against multidrug-resistant strains of *Acinetobacter baumannii* in aGalleriamellonellamodel. *Infect. Dis.* **2016**, *48*, 189–194. [CrossRef] [PubMed]
71. Yang, Y.-S.; Lee, Y.; Tseng, K.-C.; Huang, W.-C.; Chuang, M.-F.; Kuo, S.-C.; Lauderdale, T.-L.Y.; Chen, T.-L. In Vivo and In Vitro Efficacy of Minocycline-Based Combination Therapy for Minocycline-Resistant *Acinetobacter baumannii*. *Antimicrob. Agents Chemother.* **2016**, *60*, 4047–4054. [CrossRef] [PubMed]
72. Yavaş, S.; Yetkin, M.A.; Kayaaslan, B.; Baştuğ, A.; Aslaner, H.; But, A.; Kanyilmaz, D.; Sari, B.; Akinci, E.; Bodur, H. Investigating the in vitro synergistic activities of several antibiotic combinationsagainst carbapenem-resistant *Acinetobacter baumannii* isolates. *Turk. J. Med. Sci.* **2016**, *46*, 892–896. [CrossRef] [PubMed]
73. Córdoba, J.; Coronado-Álvarez, N.M.; Parra, D.; Parra-Ruiz, J. In Vitro Activities of Novel Antimicrobial Combinations against Extensively Drug-Resistant *Acinetobacter baumannii*. *Antimicrob. Agents Chemother.* **2015**, *59*, 7316–7319. [CrossRef] [PubMed]
74. García-Salguero, C.; Rodríguez-Avial, I.; Picazo, J.J.; Culebras, E. Can Plazomicin Alone or in Combination Be a Therapeutic Option against Carbapenem-Resistant *Acinetobacter baumannii*? *Antimicrob. Agents Chemother.* **2015**, *59*, 5959–5966. [CrossRef]
75. Marie, M.A.M.; Krishnappa, L.G.; Alzahrani, A.J.; Mubaraki, M.A.; Alyousef, A.A. A prospective evaluation of synergistic effect of sulbactam and tazobactam combination with meropenem or colistin against multidrug resistant *Acinetobacter baumannii*. *Bosn. J. Basic Med. Sci.* **2015**, *15*, 24–29. [CrossRef]
76. Phee, L.M.; Betts, J.; Bharathan, B.; Wareham, D.W. Colistin and Fusidic Acid, a Novel Potent Synergistic Combination for Treatment of Multidrug-Resistant *Acinetobacter baumannii* Infections. *Antimicrob. Agents Chemother.* **2015**, *59*, 4544–4550. [CrossRef]
77. Rodríguez, C.H.; Nastro, M.; Vay, C.; Famiglietti, A. In vitro activity of minocycline alone or in combination in multidrug-resistant *Acinetobacter baumannii* isolates. *J. Med. Microbiol.* **2015**, *64*, 1196–1200. [CrossRef]
78. Vourli, S.; Frantzeskaki, F.; Meletiadis, J.; Stournara, L.; Armaganidis, A.; Zerva, L.; Dimopoulos, G. Synergistic interactions between colistin and meropenem against extensively drug-resistant and pandrug-resistant *Acinetobacter baumannii* isolated from ICU patients. *Int. J. Antimicrob. Agents* **2015**, *45*, 670–671. [CrossRef]
79. Galani, I.; Orlandou, K.; Moraitou, H.; Petrikkos, G.; Souli, M. Colistin/daptomycin: An unconventional antimicrobial combination synergistic in vitro against multidrug-resistant *Acinetobacter baumannii*. *Int. J. Antimicrob. Agents* **2014**, *43*, 370–374. [CrossRef]
80. Majewski, P.; Wieczorek, P.; Ojdana, D.; Sacha, P.; Wieczorek, A.; Tryniszewska, E. In vitro activity of rifampicin alone and in combination with imipenem against multidrug-resistant *Acinetobacter baumannii* harboring theblaOXA-72resistance gene. *Scand. J. Infect. Dis.* **2014**, *46*, 260–264. [CrossRef]
81. Nastro, M.; Rodríguez, C.H.; Monge, R.; Zintgraff, J.; Neira, L.; Rebollo, M.; Vay, C.; Famiglietti, A. Activity of the colistin–rifampicin combination against colistin-resistant, carbapenemase-producing Gram-negative bacteria. *J. Chemother.* **2014**, *26*, 211–216. [CrossRef]
82. Oleksiuk, L.M.; Nguyen, M.H.; Press, E.G.; Updike, C.L.; O'Hara, J.A.; Doi, Y.; Clancy, C.J.; Shields, R.K. In VitroResponses of *Acinetobacter baumannii* to Two- and Three-Drug Combinations following Exposure to Colistin and Doripenem. *Antimicrob. Agents Chemother.* **2014**, *58*, 1195–1199. [CrossRef]
83. Percin, D.; Akyol, S.; Kalin, G. In vitro synergism of combinations of colistin with selected antibiotics against colistin-resistant *Acinetobacter baumannii*. *GMS Hyg. Infect. Control* **2014**, *9*, Doc14. [CrossRef]
84. Sun, Y.; Wang, L.; Li, J.; Zhao, C.; Zhao, J.; Liu, M.; Wang, S.; Lu, C.; Shang, G.; Jia, Y.; et al. Synergistic efficacy of meropenem and rifampicin in a murine model of sepsis caused by multidrug-resistant *Acinetobacter baumannii*. *Eur. J. Pharmacol.* **2014**, *729*, 116–122. [CrossRef]
85. Wang, Y.; Bao, W.; Guo, N.; Chen, H.; Cheng, W.; Jin, K.; Shen, F.; Xu, J.; Zhang, Q.; Wang, C.; et al. Antimicrobial activity of the imipenem/rifampicin combination against clinical isolates of *Acinetobacter baumannii* grown in planktonic and biofilm cultures. *World J. Microbiol. Biotechnol.* **2014**, *30*, 3015–3025. [CrossRef]
86. Cetin, E.S.; Tekeli, A.; Ozseven, A.G.; Us, E.; Aridogan, B.C. Determination of In Vitro Activities of Polymyxin B and Rifampin in Combination with Ampicillin/Sulbactam or Cefoperazone/Sulbactam against Multidrug-Resistant *Acinetobacter baumannii* by the E-test and Checkerboard Methods. *Jpn. J. Infect. Dis.* **2013**, *66*, 463–468. [CrossRef]
87. Housman, S.T.; Hagihara, M.; Nicolau, D.P.; Kuti, J.L. In vitro pharmacodynamics of human-simulated exposures of ampicillin/sulbactam, doripenem and tigecycline alone and in combination against multidrug-resistant *Acinetobacter baumannii*. *J. Antimicrob. Chemother.* **2013**, *68*, 2296–2304. [CrossRef] [PubMed]
88. Lee, H.J.; Bergen, P.J.; Bulitta, J.; Tsuji, B.; Forrest, A.; Nation, R.L.; Li, J. Synergistic Activity of Colistin and Rifampin Combination against Multidrug-Resistant *Acinetobacter baumannii* in anIn VitroPharmacokinetic/Pharmacodynamic Model. *Antimicrob. Agents Chemother.* **2013**, *57*, 3738–3745. [CrossRef] [PubMed]
89. Principe, L.; Capone, A.; Mazzarelli, A.; D'Arezzo, S.; Bordi, E.; Di Caro, A.; Petrosillo, N. In Vitro Activity of Doripenem in Combination with Various Antimicrobials Against Multidrug-Resistant *Acinetobacter baumannii*: Possible Options for the Treatment of Complicated Infection. *Microb. Drug Resist.* **2013**, *19*, 407–414. [CrossRef] [PubMed]
90. Queenan, A.M.; A Davies, T.; He, W.; Lynch, A.S. Assessment of the combination of doripenem plus a fluoroquinolone against non-susceptible *Acinetobacter baumannii* isolates from nosocomial pneumonia patients. *J. Chemother.* **2013**, *25*, 141–147. [CrossRef]
91. Deveci, A.; Coban, A.Y.; Acicbe, O.; Tanyel, E.; Yaman, G.; Durupinar, B. In vitro effects of sulbactam combinations with different antibiotic groups against clinical *Acinetobacter baumannii* isolates. *J. Chemother.* **2012**, *24*, 247–252. [CrossRef]

92. Peck, K.R.; Kim, M.J.; Choi, J.Y.; Kim, H.S.; Kang, C.-I.; Cho, Y.K.; Park, D.W.; Lee, H.J.; Lee, M.S.; Ko, K.S. In vitro time-kill studies of antimicrobial agents against blood isolates of imipenem-resistant *Acinetobacter baumannii*, including colistin- or tigecycline-resistant isolates. *J. Med. Microbiol.* **2012**, *61*, 353–360. [CrossRef]
93. Vidaillac, C.; Benichou, L.; Duval, R. In VitroSynergy of Colistin Combinations against Colistin-Resistant *Acinetobacter baumannii*, *Pseudomonas aeruginosa*, and *Klebsiella pneumoniae* Isolates. *Antimicrob. Agents Chemother.* **2012**, *56*, 4856–4861. [CrossRef]
94. Pachón-Ibáñez, M.E.; Docobo-Pérez, F.; Jiménez-Mejías, M.E.; Ibáñez-Martínez, J.; García-Curiel, A.; Pichardo, C.; Pachón, J. Efficacy of rifampin, in monotherapy and in combinations, in an experimental murine pneumonia model caused by panresistant *Acinetobacter baumannii* strains. *Eur. J. Clin. Microbiol. Infect. Dis.* **2011**, *30*, 895–901. [CrossRef]
95. Santimaleeworagun, W.; Wongpoowarak, P.; Chayakul, P.; Pattharachayakul, S.; Tansakul, P.; Garey, K.W. In vitro activity of colistin or sulbactam in combination with fosfomycin or imipenem against clinical isolates of carbapenem-resistant *Acinetobacter baumannii* producing OXA-23 carbapenemases. *Southeast Asian J. Trop. Med. Public Health* **2011**, *42*, 890–900.
96. Tan, T.Y.; Lim, T.P.; Lee, W.H.L.; Sasikala, S.; Hsu, L.Y.; Kwa, A.L.-H. In VitroAntibiotic Synergy in Extensively Drug-Resistant *Acinetobacter baumannii*: The Effect of Testing by Time-Kill, Checkerboard, and Etest Methods. *Antimicrob. Agents Chemother.* **2011**, *55*, 436–438. [CrossRef]
97. Kiratisin, P.; Apisarnthanarak, A.; Kaewdaeng, S. Synergistic activities between carbapenems and other antimicrobial agents against *Acinetobacter baumannii* including multidrug-resistant and extensively drug-resistant isolates. *Int. J. Antimicrob. Agents* **2010**, *36*, 243–246. [CrossRef]
98. Pachón-Ibáñez, M.E.; Docobo-Pérez, F.; López-Rojas, R.; Domínguez-Herrera, J.; Jiménez-Mejías, M.E.; García-Curiel, A.; Pichardo, C.; Jiménez, L.; Pachón, J. Efficacy of Rifampin and Its Combinations with Imipenem, Sulbactam, and Colistin in Experimental Models of Infection Caused by Imipenem-Resistant *Acinetobacter baumannii*. *Antimicrob. Agents Chemother.* **2010**, *54*, 1165–1172. [CrossRef]
99. Pankuch, G.A.; Seifert, H.; Appelbaum, P.C. Activity of doripenem with and without levofloxacin, amikacin, and colistin against *Pseudomonas aeruginosa* and *Acinetobacter baumannii*. *Diagn. Microbiol. Infect. Dis.* **2010**, *67*, 191–197. [CrossRef]
100. Rodriguez, C.H.; De Ambrosio, A.; Bajuk, M.; Spinozzi, M.; Nastro, M.; Bombicino, K.; Radice, M.; Gutkind, G.; Vay, C.; Famiglietti, A. In vitro antimicrobials activity against endemic *Acinetobacter baumannii* multiresistant clones. *J. Infect. Dev. Ctries.* **2010**, *4*, 164–167. [CrossRef]
101. Urban, C.; Mariano, N.; Rahal, J.J. In Vitro Double and Triple Bactericidal Activities of Doripenem, Polymyxin B, and Rifampin against Multidrug-Resistant *Acinetobacter baumannii*, *Pseudomonas aeruginosa*, *Klebsiella pneumoniae*, and *Escherichia coli*. *Antimicrob. Agents Chemother.* **2010**, *54*, 2732–2734. [CrossRef]
102. Yuan, Z.; Ledesma, K.R.; Singh, R.; Hou, J.; Prince, R.A.; Tam, V.H. Quantitative Assessment of Combination Antimicrobial Therapy against Multidrug-Resistant Bacteria in a Murine Pneumonia Model. *J. Infect. Dis.* **2010**, *201*, 889–897. [CrossRef]
103. Lim, T.-P.; Tan, T.-Y.; Lee, W.; Sasikala, S.; Tan, T.-T.; Hsu, L.-Y.; Kwa, A.L. In vitro activity of various combinations of antimicrobials against carbapenem-resistant *Acinetobacter* species in Singapore. *J. Antibiot.* **2009**, *62*, 675–679. [CrossRef]
104. Principe, L.; D'Arezzo, S.; Capone, A.; Petrosillo, N.; Visca, P. In vitro activity of tigecycline in combination with various antimicrobials against multidrug resistant *Acinetobacter baumannii*. *Ann. Clin. Microbiol. Antimicrob.* **2009**, *8*, 18. [CrossRef]
105. Song, J.Y.; Cheong, H.J.; Lee, J.; Sung, A.K.; Kim, W.J. Efficacy of monotherapy and combined antibiotic therapy for carbapenem-resistant *Acinetobacter baumannii* pneumonia in an immunosuppressed mouse model. *Int. J. Antimicrob. Agents* **2009**, *33*, 33–39. [CrossRef]
106. Lee, C.-H.; Tang, Y.-F.; Su, L.-H.; Chien, C.-C.; Liu, J.-W. Antimicrobial Effects of Varied Combinations of Meropenem, Sulbactam, and Colistin on a Multidrug-Resistant *Acinetobacter baumannii* Isolate That Caused Meningitis and Bacteremia. *Microb. Drug Resist.* **2008**, *14*, 233–237. [CrossRef]
107. Lim, T.-P.; Ledesma, K.R.; Chang, K.-T.; Hou, J.-G.; Kwa, A.L.; Nikolaou, M.; Quinn, J.P.; Prince, R.A.; Tam, V.H. Quantitative Assessment of Combination Antimicrobial Therapy against Multidrug-Resistant *Acinetobacter baumannii*. *Antimicrob. Agents Chemother.* **2008**, *52*, 2898–2904. [CrossRef]
108. Lee, N.-Y.; Wang, C.-L.; Chuang, Y.-C.; Yu, W.-L.; Lee, H.-C.; Chang, C.-M.; Wang, L.-R.; Ko, W.-C. Combination Carbapenem-Sulbactam Therapy for Critically Ill Patients with Multidrug-Resistant *Acinetobacter baumannii* Bacteremia: Four Case Reports and an In Vitro Combination Synergy Study. *Pharmacother. J. Hum. Pharmacol. Drug Ther.* **2007**, *27*, 1506–1511. [CrossRef]
109. Sader, H.S.; Rhomberg, P.; Jones, R.N. In Vitro Activity of β-Lactam Antimicrobial Agents in Combination with Aztreonam Tested Against Metallob-β-Lactamase-Producing *Pseudomonas aeruginosa* and *Acinetobacter baumannii*. *J. Chemother.* **2005**, *17*, 622–627. [CrossRef]
110. Sader, H.S.; Jones, R.N. Comprehensive in vitro evaluation of cefepime combined with aztreonam or ampicillin/sulbactam against multi-drug resistant *Pseudomonas aeruginosa* and *Acinetobacter* spp. *Int. J. Antimicrob. Agents* **2005**, *25*, 380–384. [CrossRef]
111. Choi, J.Y.; Park, Y.S.; Cho, C.H.; Shin, S.Y.; Song, Y.G.; Yong, D.; Lee, K.; Kim, J.M. Synergic in-vitro activity of imipenem and sulbactam against *Acinetobacter baumannii*. *Clin. Microbiol. Infect.* **2004**, *10*, 1098–1101. [CrossRef]
112. Jung, R.; Husain, M.; Choi, M.K.; Fish, D.N. Synergistic Activities of Moxifloxacin Combined with Piperacillin-Tazobactam or Cefepime against *Klebsiella pneumoniae*, *Enterobacter cloacae*, and *Acinetobacter baumannii* Clinical Isolates. *Antimicrob. Agents Chemother.* **2004**, *48*, 1055–1057. [CrossRef]

113. Montero, A.; Ariza, J.; Corbella, X.; Doménech, A.; Cabellos, C.; Ayats, J.; Tubau, F.; Borraz, C.; Gudiol, F. Antibiotic combinations for serious infections caused by carbapenem-resistant *Acinetobacter baumannii* in a mouse pneumonia model. *J. Antimicrob. Chemother.* **2004**, *54*, 1085–1091. [CrossRef]
114. Yoon, J.; Urban, C.; Terzian, C.; Mariano, N.; Rahal, J.J. In Vitro Double and Triple Synergistic Activities of Polymyxin B, Imipenem, and Rifampin against Multidrug-Resistant *Acinetobacter baumannii*. *Antimicrob. Agents Chemother.* **2004**, *48*, 753–757. [CrossRef]
115. Fernández-Cuenca, F.; Martínez, L.M.; Pascual, A.; Perea, E.J. In vitro Activity of Azithromycin in Combination with Amikacin, Ceftazidime, Ciprofloxacin or Imipenem against Clinical Isolates of *Acinetobacter baumannii*. *Chemotherapy* **2003**, *49*, 24–26. [CrossRef]
116. Roussel-Delvallez, M.; Wallet, F.; Delpierre, F.; Courcol, R. In Vitro Bactericidal Effect of a β-lactam + Aminoglycoside Combination Against Multiresistant *Pseudomonas aeruginosa* and *Acinetobacter baumannii*. *J. Chemother.* **1996**, *8*, 365–368. [CrossRef]
117. Park, G.C.; Choi, J.A.; Jang, S.J.; Jeong, S.H.; Kim, C.-M.; Choi, I.S.; Kang, S.H.; Park, G.; Moon, D.S. In Vitro Interactions of Antibiotic Combinations of Colistin, Tigecycline, and Doripenem Against Extensively Drug-Resistant and Multidrug-Resistant *Acinetobacter baumannii*. *Ann. Lab. Med.* **2016**, *36*, 124–130. [CrossRef] [PubMed]
118. Lim, S.M.S.; Heffernan, A.J.; Zowawi, H.M.; Roberts, J.A.; Sime, F.B. Semi-mechanistic PK/PD modelling of meropenem and sulbactam combination against carbapenem-resistant strains of *Acinetobacter baumannii*. *Eur. J. Clin. Microbiol. Infect. Dis.* **2021**, *40*, 1943–1952. [CrossRef]
119. Jaruratanasirikul, S.; Wongpoowarak, W.; Wattanavijitkul, T.; Sukarnjanaset, W.; Samaeng, M.; Nawakitrangsan, M.; Ingviya, N. Population Pharmacokinetics and Pharmacodynamics Modeling to Optimize Dosage Regimens of Sulbactam in Critically Ill Patients with Severe Sepsis Caused by *Acinetobacter baumannii*. *Antimicrob. Agents Chemother.* **2016**, *60*, 7236–7244. [CrossRef] [PubMed]
120. Jaruratanasirikul, S.; Nitchot, W.; Wongpoowarak, W.; Samaeng, M.; Nawakitrangsan, M. Population pharmacokinetics and Monte Carlo simulations of sulbactam to optimize dosage regimens in patients with ventilator-associated pneumonia caused by *Acinetobacter baumannii*. *Eur. J. Pharm. Sci.* **2019**, *136*, 104940. [CrossRef] [PubMed]
121. Asuphon, O.; Montakantikul, P.; Houngsaitong, J.; Kiratisin, P.; Sonthisombat, P. Optimizing intravenous fosfomycin dosing in combination with carbapenems for treatment of *Pseudomonas aeruginosa* infections in critically ill patients based on pharmacokinetic/pharmacodynamic (PK/PD) simulation. *Int. J. Infect. Dis.* **2016**, *50*, 23–29. [CrossRef] [PubMed]
122. Pasteran, F.; Cedano, J.; Baez, M.; Albornoz, E.; Rapoport, M.; Osteria, J.; Montaña, S.; Le, C.; Ra, G.; Bonomo, R.; et al. A New Twist: The Combination of Sulbactam/Avibactam Enhances Sulbactam Activity against Carbapenem-Resistant *Acinetobacter baumannii* (CRAB) Isolates. *Antibiotics* **2021**, *10*, 577. [CrossRef] [PubMed]
123. Savoldi, A.; Carrara, E.; Piddock, L.J.V.; Franceschi, F.; Ellis, S.; Chiamenti, M.; Bragantini, D.; Righi, E.; Tacconelli, E. The role of combination therapy in the treatment of severe infections caused by carbapenem resistant gram-negatives: A systematic review of clinical studies. *BMC Infect. Dis.* **2021**, *21*, 1–11. [CrossRef] [PubMed]
124. Kofteridis, D.P.; Andrianaki, A.M.; Maraki, S.; Mathioudaki, A.; Plataki, M.; Alexopoulou, C.; Ioannou, P.; Samonis, G.; Valachis, A. Treatment pattern, prognostic factors, and outcome in patients with infection due to pan-drug-resistant gram-negative bacteria. *Eur. J. Clin. Microbiol. Infect. Dis.* **2020**, *39*, 965–970. [CrossRef]
125. Assimakopoulos, S.F.; Karamouzos, V.; Lefkaditi, A.; Sklavou, C.; Kolonitsiou, F.; Christofidou, M.; Fligou, F.; Gogos, C.; Marangos, M. Triple combination therapy with high-dose ampicillin/sulbactam, high-dose tigecycline and colistin in the treatment of ventilator-associated pneumonia caused by pan-drug resistant *Acinetobacter baumannii*: A case series study. *Infez. Med.* **2019**, *27*, 11–16.
126. Qureshi, Z.A.; Hittle, L.E.; O'Hara, J.A.; Rivera, J.I.; Syed, A.; Shields, R.K.; Pasculle, A.W.; Ernst, R.; Doi, Y. Colistin-Resistant *Acinetobacter baumannii*: Beyond Carbapenem Resistance. *Clin. Infect. Dis.* **2015**, *60*, 1295–1303. [CrossRef]
127. Park, H.J.; Cho, J.H.; Kim, H.J.; Han, S.H.; Jeong, S.H.; Byun, M.K. Colistin monotherapy versus colistin/rifampicin combination therapy in pneumonia caused by colistin-resistant *Acinetobacter baumannii*: A randomised controlled trial. *J. Glob. Antimicrob. Resist.* **2019**, *17*, 66–71. [CrossRef]
128. Hernan, R.C.; Karina, B.; Gabriela, G.; Marcela, N.; Carlos, V.; Angela, F. Selection of colistin-resistant *Acinetobacter baumannii* isolates in postneurosurgical meningitis in an intensive care unit with high presence of heteroresistance to colistin. *Diagn. Microbiol. Infect. Dis.* **2009**, *65*, 188–191. [CrossRef]
129. Cai, Y.; Chai, D.; Wang, R.; Liang, B.; Bai, N. Colistin resistance of *Acinetobacter baumannii*: Clinical reports, mechanisms and antimicrobial strategies. *J. Antimicrob. Chemother.* **2012**, *67*, 1607–1615. [CrossRef]
130. Luna, B.; Trebosc, V.; Lee, B.; Bakowski, M.; Ulhaq, A.; Yan, J.; Lu, P.; Cheng, J.; Nielsen, T.; Lim, J.; et al. A nutrient-limited screen unmasks rifabutin hyperactivity for extensively drug-resistant *Acinetobacter baumannii*. *Nat. Microbiol.* **2020**, *5*, 1134–1143. [CrossRef]
131. Trebosc, V.; Schellhorn, B.; Schill, J.; Lucchini, V.; Bühler, J.; Bourotte, M.; Butcher, J.J.; Gitzinger, M.; Lociuro, S.; Kemmer, C.; et al. In vitro activity of rifabutin against 293 contemporary carbapenem-resistant *Acinetobacter baumannii* clinical isolates and characterization of rifabutin mode of action and resistance mechanisms. *J. Antimicrob. Chemother.* **2020**, *75*, 3552–3562. [CrossRef]
132. Fan, B.; Guan, J.; Wang, X.; Cong, Y. Activity of Colistin in Combination with Meropenem, Tigecycline, Fosfomycin, Fusidic Acid, Rifampin or Sulbactam against Extensively Drug-Resistant *Acinetobacter baumannii* in a Murine Thigh-Infection Model. *PLoS ONE* **2016**, *11*, e0157757. [CrossRef]
133. Elsayed, E.; Elarabi, M.A.; Sherif, D.A.; Elmorshedi, M.; El-Mashad, N. Extensive drug resistant *Acinetobacter baumannii*: A comparative study between non-colistin based combinations. *Int. J. Clin. Pharm.* **2020**, *42*, 80–88. [CrossRef]

134. Xie, J.; Roberts, J.A.; Alobaid, A.S.; Roger, C.; Wang, Y.; Yang, Q.; Sun, J.; Dong, H.; Wang, X.; Xing, J.; et al. Population Pharmacokinetics of Tigecycline in Critically Ill Patients with Severe Infections. *Antimicrob. Agents Chemother.* **2017**, *61*, e00345-17. [CrossRef]
135. Song, X.; Wu, Y.; Cao, L.; Yao, D.; Long, M. Is Meropenem as a Monotherapy Truly Incompetent for Meropenem-Nonsusceptible Bacterial Strains? A Pharmacokinetic/Pharmacodynamic Modeling With Monte Carlo Simulation. *Front. Microbiol.* **2019**, *10*, 2777. [CrossRef]
136. Van Wart, S.A.; Andes, D.; Ambrose, P.G.; Bhavnani, S.M. Pharmacokinetic–pharmacodynamic modeling to support doripenem dose regimen optimization for critically ill patients. *Diagn. Microbiol. Infect. Dis.* **2009**, *63*, 409–414. [CrossRef]

MDPI
St. Alban-Anlage 66
4052 Basel
Switzerland
Tel. +41 61 683 77 34
Fax +41 61 302 89 18
www.mdpi.com

Antibiotics Editorial Office
E-mail: antibiotics@mdpi.com
www.mdpi.com/journal/antibiotics

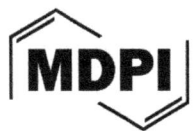

www.ingramcontent.com/pod-product-compliance
Lightning Source LLC
LaVergne TN
LVHW070452100526
838202LV00014B/1708